W9-ATN-721

Management of
Common Problems
in Obstetrics
and Gynecology

Management of Common Problems in Obstetrics and Gynecology

Edited by

DANIEL R. MISHELL, JR MD
The Lyle G. McNeile Professor and Chairman

and

PAUL F. BRENNER MD
Professor and Vice Chairman

Department of Obstetrics and Gynecology
University of Southern California
School of Medicine, Los Angeles, California

THIRD EDITION

BOSTON

Blackwell Scientific Publications

OXFORD LONDON EDINBURGH
MELBOURNE PARIS BERLIN VIENNA

© 1994 by
Blackwell Scientific Publications, Inc.
Editorial Offices:
238 Main Street, Cambridge
    Massachusetts 02142, USA
Osney Mead, Oxford OX2 0EL, England
25 John Street, London WC1N 2BL
    England
23 Ainslie Place, Edinburgh EH3 6AJ
    Scotland
54 University Street, Carlton
    Victoria 3053, Australia

Other Editorial Offices:
Librairie Arnette SA
1, rue de Lille
75007 Paris
France

Blackwell Wissenschafts-Verlag GmbH
Düsseldorfer Str. 38
D-10707 Berlin
Germany

Blackwell MZV
Feldgasse 13
A-1238 Wien
Austria

All rights reserved. No part of this book
may be reproduced in any form or by any
electronic or mechanical means, including
information storage and retrieval systems,
without permission in writing from the
publisher, except by a reviewer who may
quote brief passages in a review.

First published 1988
Second edition 1990
Third edition 1994

Set by Excel Typesetters Co., Hong Kong
Printed and bound in the United States of
America by Edwards Brothers, Ann Arbor,
Michigan

95 96 97 5 4 3 2

DISTRIBUTORS

USA
   Blackwell Scientific Publications, Inc.
   238 Main Street
   Cambridge, Massachusetts 02142
   (ORDERS: Tel: 800 759-6102
                    617 876-7000)

Canada
   Times Mirror Professional Publishing,
   Ltd
   130 Flaska Drive
   Markham, Ontario L6G 1B8
   (ORDERS: Tel: 800 268-4178
                    416 470-6739)

Australia
   Blackwell Scientific Publications Pty, Ltd
   54 University Street
   Carlton, Victoria 3053
   (ORDERS: Tel: 03 347-5552)

Outside North America and Australia
   Marston Book Services Ltd
   PO Box 87
   Oxford OX2 0DT
   (ORDERS: Tel: 0865 791155
                    Fax: 0865 791927
                    Telex: 837515)

Library of Congress
Cataloging-in-Publication Data

Management of common problems in
ob/gyn:
   edited by Daniel R. Mishell, Jr.,
   Paul F. Brenner. — 3rd ed.
         p.   cm.
   Includes bibliographical references
   and index.
   ISBN 0-86542-269-9
   1. Pregnancy—Complications.
   2. Generative organs, Female—Diseases.
   I. Mishell, Daniel R.
   II. Brenner, Paul F.
   [DNLM: 1. Genital Diseases, Female—
   therapy.
   2. Endocrine Diseases—therapy.
   3. Fetal Diseases—therapy.
   4. Pregnancy Complications—therapy.
   WP 140 M266 1994]
   RG571.M23   1994
   618—dc20

The editors wish to dedicate this volume to their mentor, colleague, and friend, Dr Val Davajan. Dr Davajan was the first Chief of the Division of Reproductive Endocrinology and Infertility in our Department. He was the consummate teacher and clinician. He combined wisdom, wit, and common sense to make learning enjoyable. For the anxiety-ridden, desperate infertility couple he was the beacon of integrity and practicality.

Contents

Part 3: Gynecology

Contributors

RAUL ARTAL MD, *Professor, Department of Obstetrics and Gynecology, University of Southern California School of Medicine, Los Angeles*

CHARLES A. BALLARD MD, *Professor and Chief, Division of Gynecology, Department of Obstetrics and Gynecology, University of Southern California School of Medicine, Los Angeles*

ARIEH BERGMAN MD, *Professor, Department of Obstetrics and Gynecology, University of Southern California School of Medicine, Los Angeles*

GERALD S. BERNSTEIN PhD, MD, *Professor, Department of Obstetrics and Gynecology, University of Southern California School of Medicine, Los Angeles*

HARBINDER S. BRAR MD, *Clinical Assistant Professor, Department of Obstetrics and Gynecology, University of Southern California School of Medicine, Los Angeles*

PAUL F. BRENNER MD, *Professor and Vice Chairman, Department of Obstetrics and Gynecology, University of Southern California School of Medicine, Los Angeles*

VAL DAVAJAN MD, *Professor, Department of Obstetrics and Gynecology, University of Southern California School of Medicine, Los Angeles*

ALAN FISHMAN MD, *Clinical Instructor, Department of Obstetrics and Gynecology, University of Southern California School of Medicine, Los Angeles*

T. MURPHY GOODWIN MD, *Assistant Professor, Department of Obstetrics and Gynecology, University of Southern California School of Medicine, Los Angeles*

JEFFREY S. GREENSPOON MD, *Director, Perinatal Intensive Care, Cedars Sinai Medical Center; Clinical Associate Professor, Department of Obstetrics and Gynecology, University of Southern California School of Medicine, Los Angeles*

DAVID A. GRIMES MD, *Professor and Vice Chairman, Department of Obstetrics, Gynecology and Reproductive Sciences, University of California San Francisco School of Medicine, San Francisco*

DEBRA K. GRUBB MD, *Clinical Instructor, Department of Obstetrics and Gynecology, University of Southern California School of Medicine, Los Angeles*

WILLIAM H. HINDLE MD, *Professor of Clinical Obstetrics and Gynecology, Department of Obstetrics and Gynecology, University of Southern California School of Medicine, Los Angeles*

ROBERT ISRAEL MD, *Professor, Department of Obstetrics and Gynecology, University of Southern California School of Medicine, Los Angeles*

THOMAS H. KIRSCHBAUM MD, *Professor, Department of Obstetrics and Gynecology, Albert Einstein College of Medicine, Bronx*

SIRI L. KJOS MD, *Assistant Professor, Department of Obstetrics and Gynecology, University of Southern California School of Medicine, Los Angeles*

KEE SENG KOH MD, *Clinical Professor, Department of Obstetrics and Gynecology, University of Southern California School of Medicine, Los Angeles*

BRUCE W. KOVACS MD, *Associate Professor, Department of Obstetrics and Gynecology, University of Southern California School of Medicine, Los Angeles*

ANNA S. LEUNG MD, *Clinical Instructor, Department of Obstetrics and Gynecology, University of Southern California School of Medicine, Los Angeles*

KIM R. LIPSCOMB MD, *Clinical Instructor, Department of Obstetrics and Gynecology, University of Southern California School of Medicine, Los Angeles*

ROGERIO A. LOBO MD, *Professor and Chief, Division of Reproductive Endocrinology and Infertility, Department of Obstetrics and Gynecology, University of Southern California School of Medicine, Los Angeles*

CHARLES J. MACRI MD, *Assistant Professor, Department of Obstetrics and Gynecology, Uniform Services University of Health Sciences, F. Edward Herbert School of Medicine, Bethesda*

CHARLES M. MARCH MD, *Professor, Department of Obstetrics and Gynecology, University of Southern California School of Medicine, Los Angeles*

ARNOLD L. MEDEARIS MD, *Associate Professor, Department of Obstetrics and Gynecology, University of Southern California School of Medicine, Los Angeles*

JORGE H. MESTMAN MD, *Clinical Professor, Department of Obstetrics and Gynecology and Internal Medicine, University of Southern California School of Medicine, Los Angeles*

GAIL MEZROW MD, *Assistant Professor, Department of Obstetrics and Gynecology, University of Southern California School of Medicine, Los Angeles*

LYNNAE K. MILLAR MD, *Clinical Instructor, Department of Obstetrics and Gynecology, University of Southern California School of Medicine, Los Angeles*

DANIEL R. MISHELL, Jr MD, *The Lyle G. McNeile Professor and Chairman, Department of Obstetrics and Gynecology, University of Southern California School of Medicine, Los Angeles*

MARTIN N. MONTORO MD, *Clinical Professor, Department of Obstetrics and Gynecology, University of Southern California School of Medicine, Los Angeles*

C. PAUL MORROW MD, *The Charles F. Langmade Professor and Chief, Division of Gynecologic Oncology, Department of Obstetrics and Gynecology, University of Southern California School of Medicine, Los Angeles*

LAILA I. MUDERSPACH MD, *Assistant Professor, Department of Obstetrics and Gynecology, University of Southern California School of Medicine, Los Angeles*

RICHARD H. PAUL MD, *Professor and Chief, Division of Maternal–Fetal Medicine, Department of Obstetrics and Gynecology, University of Southern California School of Medicine, Los Angeles*

RICHARD J. PAULSON MD, *Associate Professor, Department of Obstetrics and Gynecology, University of Southern California School of Medicine, Los Angeles*

LAWRENCE D. PLATT MD, *Chairman, Department of Obstetrics and Gynecology, Cedars-Sinai Medical Center; Professor, Department of Obstetrics and Gynecology, University of Southern California School of Medicine, Los Angeles*

CAROLINA REYES MD, *Clinical Instructor, Department of Obstetrics and Gynecology, University of Southern California School of Medicine, Los Angeles*

LYNDA D. ROMAN MD, *Assistant Professor, Department of Obstetrics and Gynecology, University of Southern California School of Medicine, Los Angeles*

SUBIR ROY MD, *Professor, Department of Obstetrics and Gynecology, University of Southern California School of Medicine, Los Angeles*

MARK V. SAUER MD, *Associate Professor, Department of Obstetrics and Gynecology, University of Southern California School of Medicine, Los Angeles*

JOHN B. SCHLAERTH MD, *Professor, Department of Obstetrics and Gynecology, University of Southern California School of Medicine, Los Angeles*

REUVEN SHARONY MD, *Clinical Instructor, Department of Obstetrics and Gynecology, University of Southern California School of Medicine, Los Angeles*

KATHRYN J. SHAW MD, *Assistant Professor, Department of Obstetrics and Gynecology, University of Southern California School of Medicine, Los Angeles*

ROBERT HURD SETTLAGE MD, *Professor, Departments of Obstetrics and Gynecology and Family Medicine, University of Southern California School of Medicine, Los Angeles*

DONNA SHOUPE MD, *Associate Professor, Department of Obstetrics and Gynecology, University of Southern California School of Medicine, Los Angeles*

LORRAINE STANCO MD, *Clinical Instructor, Department of Obstetrics and Gynecology, University of Southern California School of Medicine, Los Angeles*

FRANK Z. STANCZYK PhD, *Associate Professor of Research, Department of Obstetrics and Gynecology, University of Southern California School of Medicine, Los Angeles*

GEOFFREY STILES MD, *Attending Staff, Department of General Surgery, Sharp Memorial Hosptial, San Diego*

DENA TOWNER MD, *Clinical Instructor, Department of Obstetrics and Gynecology, University of Southern California School of Medicine, Los Angeles*

MICHAEL VERMESH MD, *Associate Professor, Department of Obstetrics and Gynecology, University of Southern California School of Medicine, Los Angeles*

Preface

The accumulation of new information, the development of new diagnostic and therapeutic equipment, and the revision of management plans and the formulation of new ones, continues to present the field of obstetrics and gynecology as one of the most challenging and dynamic in all of medicine. The refinement of fetal surveillance incorporating the assessment of amniotic fluid volume, the development of vaginal transducers as part of ultrasonography, color-flow Doppler studies, the medical management of persistent ectopic pregnancy, the loop electrosurgical excision procedure (LEEP) instrumentation for cervical tissue sampling, the Norplant contraceptive system, new tumor markers, pelviscopy, expanded use of gonadotropin-releasing hormone agonists and amino-infusion are just a few of the innovations new to the practice of obstetrics and gynecology since the second edition of *Management of Common Problems in Obstetrics and Gynecology* was published. All of these developments, as well as many others, have impacted positively on the obstetric and gynecologic care of patients.

Clearly, the care for the obstetric or gynecologic patient is not exclusively provided by the obstetrician–gynecologist. Every indication is that the family medicine physician, the internist, and the general practitioner will be asked to assume an even greater role in initially screening women with complaints and disorders of the reproductive organs. In addition the general surgeon and the emergency medicine physician may be involved in the management of these medical problems. This book is written for all physicians who as part of their clinical practice provide care for women with obstetric and/or gynecologic diseases. Each chapter incorporates the latest information into practical diagnostic and therapeutic management schemes used in obstetrics and gynecology.

The 49 contributing authors of the third edition of *Management of Common Problems in Obstetrics and Gynecology* are either current or former members of the Department of Obstetrics and Gynecology of the University of Southern California (USC) School of Medicine or medical staff at the Women's Hospital at Los Angeles County and University of Southern California Medical Center. This 340-bed hospital is the largest women's hospital in the United States. The diversity of clinical experience in this hospital includes 14 000 deliveries, 5000 gynecologic surgical procedures, and 46 000 emergency room visits annually. The large patient-population, and the diversity, acuity, and complexity of the medical problems with which these patients present, provide the medical staff with a broad exposure to clinical obstetrics and gynecology which is unique and unmatched in any other medical center in this country. It allows the staff the opportunity to develop and implement the most recent advances in obstetrics and gynecology in the care of these patients.

The authors would especially like to express their appreciation to the departmental secretaries who typed the chapters, and to the publishers for their advice and cooperation, which resulted in the completion of this work.

PART 1

Obstetrics

1

Heart disease in pregnancy

T. MURPHY GOODWIN & JEFFREY S. GREENSPOON

Maternal heart disease complicates the management of nearly 1% of pregnancies. The prevalence of rheumatic heart disease, the most common type of acquired heart disease among young adults, is decreasing in industrialized nations. However, the improved survival of the 0.8% of neonates with congenital cardiac disease has created an increasing demand for obstetric care as this cohort reaches reproductive age. In many urban centers congenital heart disease accounts for 50% or more of the cases of maternal heart disease seen in pregnancy.

Cardiovascular changes in pregnancy

Maternal pulse and cardiac output are significantly increased during the first trimester. The maternal pulse increases by 10–15 bpm from 70 to 85 bpm. Stroke volume increases from 63 to 70 ml/beat. Cardiac output has increased significantly over nonpregnant baseline by 30 weeks' gestation, and ultimately is increased by 30–50%, e.g., from 3.5 l/min to 6.0 l/min. Seventeen percent of cardiac output goes to the uterus.

Total blood volume increases 40–50% over prepregnant values, with the increase ranging from 20% to 100%. The plasma volume expands proportionately more than the red blood cell mass, accounting for the physiologically normal lower hematocrit in pregnancy. Twin pregnancy is marked by a larger increase in plasma volume, approximating 70%. Women with preeclampsia or chronic hypertension do not increase their plasma volume as much.

Maternal position, labor, and anesthesia can affect cardiovascular status. Prolonged standing with venous pooling decreases venous return to the heart and may provoke syncope. Supine hypotension occurs when the gravid uterus compresses the vena cava and impairs venous return to the heart, causing a fall in cardiac output and blood pressure. Uterine contractions in the supine position cause an increase in venous return, stroke volume, cardiac output, and a decrease in heart rate. Labor in the lateral recumbent position blunts the changes in these parameters associated with each contraction.

Normally, cardiac output increases during labor. The pain caused by uterine contractions can produce maternal tachycardia with unfavorable hemodynamic effects, reducing the diastolic flow time. Effective analgesia will minimize this effect. Epidural anesthesia without epinephrine is more effective than pudendal anesthesia in this regard. For nearly all types of cardiac disease, epidural anesthesia is preferred for vaginal or cesarean delivery.

During the second stage of labor, the maternal Valsalva maneuver, accompanying bearing-down efforts, reduces venous blood return to the heart by increasing intrathoracic pressure. When the straining is stopped, there is a rapid increase in cardiac output and blood pressure.

In the immediate postpartum period, the cardiac output has increased above the baseline seen at term prior to the onset of labor. This increase is 80% in patients receiving local analgesia and 60% in those receiving epidural anesthesia. The increase is due to reentry of blood to the central circulation, which previously was diverted to the uterus or pooled in the partially obstructed venous circulation of the lower extremities. Stroke volume is increased, and the heart rate reflexively falls.

The normal physiologic changes associated with pregnancy are well tolerated by a woman with a normal heart. Patients with cardiac disease who are unable to tolerate these antepartum or peripartum changes may decompensate and develop congestive heart failure.

Heart disease problems in pregnancy

Normal pregnant women frequently have symptoms and signs associated with heart disease in the nonpregnant state, such as dyspnea, increased fatigue, and lower-extremity edema. However, a normal pregnant woman can usually be distinguished from one with cardiac disease by a careful history, examination by a physician knowledgeable of the cardiovascular changes associated with pregnancy, and appropriately selected tests. A systolic flow murmur, S3, and occasionally S4 gallop are present in normal pregnant patients. Certain findings, however, deserve further evaluation. These are listed in Table 1.1.

If heart disease is suspected, a baseline electrocardiogram, chest

Table 1.1 Clinical cardiovascular findings that merit further evaluation

Symptoms
Dyspnea that limits activity
Progressive orthopnea or paroxysmal nocturnal dyspnea
Syncope with exertion
Angina pectoris
Hemoptysis

Signs
Pulse >100 or <50–60 bpm
Dysrhythmia
Diastolic murmur (exclude the mammary souffle and venous hum)
Systolic murmur grade 3/6 or louder
Signs of congestive heart failure
Cyanosis
Clubbing

radiograph (shielding the uterus from the radiation), and occasionally a baseline arterial blood gas are appropriate. Echocardiography can be used to diagnose anatomic abnormalities and intra- and extracardiac shunts, and to estimate valve orifice size. Echocardiography has reduced the

Table 1.2 Maternal risk of pregnancy for women with structural heart disease

Group 1: Slightly increased risk
Mild valvular stenosis
Moderate valvular regurgitation with normal chamber size and normal blood
   pressure

Group 2: Moderately increased risk
Moderate valvular stenosis
Significant valve regurgitation
Prosthetic heart valve with normal hemodynamic function

Group 3: Considerably increased risk
Severe valvular stenosis or regurgitation
Atrial fibrillation
Prosthetic heart valve with compensated heart failure

Group 4: Unacceptable risk
Symptoms with less than usual activity or at rest (NYHA class III or IV)
Congestive heart failure
Pulmonary hypertension
Eisenmenger syndrome
Marfan's syndrome with incompetent valve or aortic root dilation

need for cardiac catheterization in pregnancy. Monitoring for cardiac dysrhythmias may be done with a 24-h Holter monitor.

The New York Heart Association (NYHA) classification continues to be useful for management and prognostication:

Class I   Asymptomatic
Class II   Symptoms with greater than normal activity
Class III   Symptoms with normal activity
Class IV   Symptoms at bedrest

In general, the pregnancy prognosis is good for cardiac patients in classes I and II, although modifications in therapy may be required. For class III patients the prognosis is fair with therapy. Special attention during pregnancy and admission early in labor are recommended. Pregnancy is generally contraindicated for patients in class IV. Because this functional classification system relies heavily on subjective findings it is imperative to use other diagnostic tools to obtain objective information about the anatomic and physiologic abnormalities. Pregnancy risk may also be classified according to the specific cardiac defect (Table 1.2).

Preconception counseling and antepartum screening

Congenital heart disease occurs in approximately 8/1000 live births (Table 1.3). One-third of these, 2.6/1000 live births, have critical disease which will result in cardiac catheterization, cardiac surgery, or deaths in the first year of life. Due to improvements in care, 60% survive the first year.

Whittemore *et al.* found that 16% of women with a major heart defect had a fetus with a heart defect. Thus, all women with a congenital heart defect should undergo fetal echocardiography at 18–20 weeks. Fetal echocardiography employing a four-chamber view of the heart can identify many, but not all, of the common congenital lesions.

Women with cyanotic congenital heart disease have increased rates of

Table 1.3 Common types of congenital heart disease (CHD)

Dominant lesion	CHD (%)
Ventricular septal defect	10–30
Pulmonic stenosis	3–13
Patent ductus ateriosus	5–15
Atrial septal defect	3–10
Tetralogy of Fallot	4–10
Coarctation of the aorta	3–9

spontaneous abortion, preterm delivery, and small-for-gestational-age infants. The risk of worsening cardiac status during pregnancy is greater in cyanotic patients than in those without cyanosis (5% vs. 57%, respectively). Surgical correction, if possible prior to pregnancy, will improve obstetric outcome. Fifteen percent of patients with cardiac disease may develop pregnancy-induced or associated hypertension, compared to 4% in the general obstetric population.

Certain patients have an unacceptable risk of dying if pregnancy is attempted. This group includes patients with severe pulmonary hypertension of any cause, Eisenmenger syndrome, Marfan's syndrome and evidence of valvular incompetence or a dilated aortic root, and patients with congestive heart failure.

Antepartum management

Antepartum care of the pregnant cardiac patient should be done by a team including an obstetrician and cardiologist. Consultation with a geneticist if the disease is inheritable, a fetal echocardiographer, and dietitian is often appropriate. NYHA class I and II (cardiac status 1 and 2) patients may be seen every 2 weeks until the third trimester, then weekly. NYHA class III (cardiac status 3) patients should be seen weekly. NYHA class IV (cardiac status 4) patients are hospitalized for most of the pregnancy.

At each visit, weight gain, pulse, blood pressure, and pulse pressure are carefully noted. A pulse rate >100 bpm or rapid weight gain are often signs of impending heart failure. Pregnant patients with decompensated congestive failure should be hospitalized. Bedrest will reduce the demand for increased cardiac output by limiting oxygen consumption. Fetal growth and well-being may be monitored by serial ultrasound examinations and antepartum surveillance.

Patients with rheumatic heart disease should receive prophylaxis against recurrent group A β-hemolytic streptococcal infection which causes initial and recurrent attacks of rheumatic fever. The regimen is benzathine penicillin G 1.2 million Units intramuscularly given monthly. Alternative regimens include potassium penicillin V 125–250 mg orally twice daily or penicillin G 200 000 Units twice daily; the penicillin-allergic patient may use sulfadiazine 1 g daily. Patients allergic to both penicillin and sulfadiazine may use erythromycin 250 mg orally twice daily. The American Heart Association recommends that this regimen be continued until age 35 or until regular contact with children ceases.

Patients who require anticoagulation during pregnancy should be treated with subcutaneous heparin at 12-h intervals, rather than coumarin anticoagulant drugs. The most common reason for anticoagulation is chronic atrial fibrillation, which carries a lifetime risk of 30% for systemic thromboembolism in the untreated patient. The heparin dose is adjusted so that the activated partial thromboplastin time (or heparin levels, if available) is in the therapeutic range 6 h after the dose is given. Patients are advised to withhold heparin when labor begins so that they are not anticoagulated during labor and, thus, may receive epidural anesthesia. Digoxin or β-adrenergic blockers such as propranolol may be used to control the ventricular response to atrial fibrillation. Digoxin is also used for its positive inotropic effect in chronic congestive heart failure.

Patients in functional class I, II, or compensated III may await the onset of spontaneous labor at term. A maternal indication to deliver, e.g., preeclampsia or cardiac decompensation, or a fetal indication, e.g., intrauterine growth retardation or fetal distress, may require earlier delivery.

Intrapartum management

Intrapartum management of the cardiac patient is challenging. A team including obstetrician, anesthesiologist, and a critical-care nurse should be available. The patient should labor in the lateral recumbent position. Pain relief is best obtained with epidural anesthesia. Delivery should be planned at hospitals where an anesthetist skilled in this technique is available. If the patient has been recently anticoagulated, obtain an activated partial thromboplastin time before inserting an epidural catheter.

Endocarditis prophylaxis is given according to prescribed regimens (Tables 1.4 and 1.5).

We advise that it is not prudent to assume a delivery will be uncomplicated and prophylaxis for endocarditis should be given to all patients at risk for endocarditis. This includes patients with the conditions listed in Table 1.4. This opinion is due to the frequent use of instrumental delivery in cardiac patients, and a nonnegligible incidence of endometritis with bacteremia after cesarean delivery. Furthermore, 13% of women have a bacteremic episode when an intrauterine device is replaced.

The second stage of labor should be shortened if possible by employing forceps or vacuum when the application is easily achieved. The Sims position is desirable for spontaneous vaginal delivery. The lithotomy position is usually required for instrumental delivery, although the uterus should be displaced to the left side. Cesarean delivery is performed for obstetric reasons.

It is appropriate to use noninvasive monitoring equipment in all patients and invasive hemodynamic monitoring equipment in some cardiac patients in the peripartum period.

Table 1.4 Cardiac conditions and endocarditis prophylaxis

Endocarditis prophylaxis recommended
Prosthetic cardiac valves, including bioprosthetic and homograft valves
Previous bacterial endocarditis, even in the absence of heart disease
Most congenital cardiac malformations
Rheumatic and other acquired valvular dysfunction, even after valvular
   surgery
Hypertrophic cardiomyopathy
Mitral valve prolapse with valvular regurgitation

Endocarditis prophylaxis not recommended
Isolated secundum atrial septal defect
Surgical repair without residua beyond 6 months of secundum atrial septal
   defect, ventricular septal defect, or patent ductus arteriosus
Previous coronary artery bypass graft surgery
Mitral valve prolapse without valvular regurgitation
Physiologic, functional, or innocent heart murmurs
Previous Kawasaki disease without valvular dysfunction
Previous rheumatic fever without valvular dysfunction
Cardiac pacemakers and implanted defibrillators

Table 1.5 Regimens for genitourinary/gastrointestinal procedures

Drug	Dosage regimen
Standard regimen	
Ampicillin, gentamicin, and amoxycillin	Intravenous or intramuscular administration of ampicillin, 2 g, plus gentamicin, 1.5 mg/kg (not to exceed 80 mg), 30 min before procedure; followed by amoxycillin, 1.5 g, orally 6 h after initial dose; alternatively, the parenteral regimen may be repeated once 8 h after initial dose
Ampicillin/amoxycillin/penicillin-allergic patient regimen	
Vancomycin and gentamicin	Intravenous administration of vancomycin, 1.0 g, over 1 h plus intravenous or intramuscular administration of gentamicin, 1.5 mg/kg (not to exceed 80 mg), 1 h before procedure; may be repeated once 8 h after initial dose
Alternate low-risk patient regimen	
Amoxycillin	3.0 g orally 1 h before procedure; then 1.5 g 6 h after initial dose

Immediately postpartum, cardiac output increases. Patients with mitral stenosis characteristically develop pulmonary edema at this time. It can be avoided with careful attention to the patient's volume status by employing a pulmonary artery (Swan–Ganz) catheter during labor in patients with moderately severe and severe mitral stenosis.

Contraception in heart disease

Cardiac patients desiring sterilization who are well compensated can be considered for postpartum tubal ligation. In the poorly compensated cardiac patient, sterilization is usually best delayed until the cardiovascular system has returned to normal status at least 6 weeks postpartum. Many cardiac patients will not tolerate the pneumoperitoneum required for laparoscopic tubal ligation and will require a laparotomy under epidural anesthesia.

Patients with valvular heart disease or congestive heart failure are at increased risk for thromboembolic events. They should not be prescribed estrogen-containing contraceptives unless they are already anticoagulated. Norplant is an excellent alternative for these patients. Depo-Provera is also a suitable contraceptive for these patients, although it is not yet approved for this indication. The intrauterine device can be considered for patients who do not have high risk of bacterial endocarditis.

SUGGESTED READING

CLARK SL, PHELAN JP, GREENSPOON J, ALDAHL D, HORENSTEIN J. Labor and delivery in the presence of mitral stenosis: central hemodynamic observations. *Am J Obstet Gynecol* 1985;152:984.

DAJANI AS, BISNO AL, CHUNG KJ, *et al.* Prevention of rheumatic fever. *Circulation* 1988;78:1082–1086.

DAJANI AS, BINO AL, CHUNG KJ, *et al.* Prevention of bacterial endocardititis: recommendations of the American Heart Association. *JAMA* 1990;264:2919–2922.

DALEN JE, HIRSH J. National conference on antithrombotic therapy. *Chest* (Suppl) 1986;89:1S–106S.

ELKAYAM U. Pregnancy and cardiovascular disease. In: Braunwald E, ed. *Heart Disease*. 4th edn. Philadelphia: WB Saunders, 1992:1790–1809.

ELKAYAM U, GLEICHER N (eds). Cardiac problems in pregnancy. In: *Diagnosis and Management of Maternal and Fetal Disease*. 2nd edn. New York: Alan R. Liss, 1990.

SHIME J, MOCARSKI EJM, HASTINGS D, WEBB GD, McLAUGHLIN PR. Congenital heart disease in pregnancy: short and long-term implications. *Am J Obstet Gynecol* 1987;156:313.

WHITTEMORE R, HOBBINS JC, ENGLE MA. Pregnancy and its outcome with women with and without surgical treatment of congenital heart disease. *Am J Cardiol* 1982;50:641.

2

Bronchial asthma in pregnancy

HARBINDER S. BRAR

Asthma is characterized by an increased responsiveness of the tracheo-bronchial tree to a variety of stimuli. This is manifest clinically by reversible airway obstruction and eosinophilia. Approximately 3–5% of the population of the USA suffer from asthma; thus, between 0.7 and 1.4% of pregnant women are likely to have a history of asthma.

Etiology

Immunologic mechanisms appear to be involved in extrinsic (allergic) asthma. Serum levels of immunoglobulin E (IgE) may be elevated and have positive responses to provocative tests. Cases in which no specific cause is apparent are categorized as intrinsic. These persons often have a positive family history of asthma. Provocative skin tests are negative, and serum IgE levels are normal. In most cases the etiology of asthma is mixed. Although some patients may not fall clearly into a specific category, information obtained through the history will be helpful in categorizing patients and establishing the therapeutic approach. There are a variety of stimuli that provoke asthma, including the following: airborne allergens (e.g., pollen); aspirin, and related compounds; environmental (e.g., air pollution) or occupational (work-related irritants) factors; infections; exercise (particularly in cold air); and emotional stress. Asthmatics have an exquisite hyperirritability of both the large and small bronchi to these inhaled stimuli and also to several chemical mediators, including histamine, acetylcholine, serotonin, slow-reacting substance of anaphylaxis, bradykinin, and prostaglandins. This response is enhanced by β-adrenergic blockers (e.g., propranolol), which therefore should be avoided in asthmatics or persons with a history of asthma. It is postulated that overt clinical asthma may require both airway hyperreactivity and a trigger (an allergen or other stimuli).

Effects

There is some disagreement concerning the effect of pregnancy on asthma. Whereas some reports conclude that asthma worsens during pregnancy, others find that pregnancy has no effect, or that asthma improves during gestation. Some of the changes in pregnancy are beneficial for asthmatics, such as the smooth-muscle relaxant effect of progesterone, and increased levels of free plasma cortisol, which result in decreased airway resistance.

The effects of asthma on the fetus and the newborn are also controversial. Some studies have shown increased neonatal mortality, and others have found an increased incidence of preterm birth. Successful therapy can change the course of asthma and improve the outcome of pregnancy. Infants of asthmatic mothers seem to be at significant risk of developing asthma; 6–7% in the first year and 58% overall. If the father is also asthmatic, the risk for subsequent asthma is increased further (72%).

Treatment

In general, asthmatic patients are treated on the basis of subjective symptoms and physical findings. Wheezing and dyspnea are considered to be poor predictors of severity. Pulsus paradoxus is more reliable, but it is difficult to quantitate. Simple tests of pulmonary function (peak flow) can be performed easily at the bedside and are more reliable in evaluating the severity of the patient's condition and the anticipated efficacy of treatment.

Other conditions that also cause wheezing include upper airway obstruction (tumor, laryngeal edema), acute left ventricular failure, carcinoid tumors, recurrent pulmonary embolism, and chronic bronchitis, which must be entertained in the differential diagnosis.

The determination of the presence of blood and eosinophilia in the sputum (which can cause sputum to appear falsely purulent), while helpful diagnostically, is not specific. Chest X-rays may show hyperinflation (which is not diagnostic), or, rarely, a parenchymal infiltrate. Arterial blood gases will show mild hypoxemia and a decreased P_{CO_2} due to hyperventilation. A normal P_{CO_2} suggests incipient ventilatory failure, and an elevated value indicates the need for vigorous therapy that includes endotracheal intubation and mechanical ventilation.

Numerous drugs are used to treat asthma, which indicates that there is no single perfect agent. Most asthmatics are treated with a combination of drugs, and there is no marked superiority of one regimen over the others. In general, the treatment of asthma during gestation does not differ greatly from its treatment in nonpregnant asthmatics, except for some differences that will be discussed in this chapter. Although asthmatics are seldom reactive to just one allergen, avoidance or elimination of an allergen would be the most successful therapy. Immunotherapy or desensitization with extracts of the suspected allergens may be attempted in selected cases.

In mild asthma, a single oral agent may control the symptoms. The methylxanthines (e.g., theophylline) are the most widely used, but one of the newer sympathomimetics (e.g., terbutaline sulfate) can be equally effective. Theophylline produces bronchodilation by inhibiting the enzyme phosphodiesterase, which inactivates cyclic adenosine monophosphate (cAMP). Thus, cAMP increases intracellularly, producing relaxation of the smooth muscles. Combination tablets with theophylline and a sedative should be avoided. The usual oral dose of theophylline ranges between 800 and 1200 mg/day in divided doses. The airway response correlates with the blood level, and the therapeutic plasma concentration range is 10–20 µg/ml. The renal clearance of theophylline is small and constant, and pregnancy does not alter it significantly. Individualization of the drug dose is necessary because of individual variation in its metabolism. The half-life of theophylline is prolonged in liver disease and in the elderly but is shortened significantly in cigarette smokers. Side-effects include anorexia, nausea, vomiting, nervousness, headaches, tachyarrhythmias, and even seizures. Theophylline may reduce uterine motility, but it does so at higher doses than those required for the treatment of asthma.

During an acute exacerbation, intravenous aminophylline is widely used. A loading dose of 5–6 mg/kg iv, administered over 20–30 min, is followed by a constant infusion of 0.5–0.9 mg/kg per h. If the patient has taken oral theophylline intermittently, the loading dose is reduced by half. If the patient is receiving an adequate oral regimen, a loading dose of aminophylline should be avoided altogether, and the patient should begin with the maintenance intravenous dose.

An oral sympathomimetic agent (e.g., terbutaline) can be used as an alternative to a methylxanthine or in combination with theophylline if attacks continue despite treatment with a single agent. Only the β-agonists are useful in asthma and, ideally, one with just β_2 action should be used, which dilates airways without undesirable cardiac stimulation. Norepinephrine is not used because it is predominantly an α-agonist. Epinephrine has both α and β effects. It is useful in acute attacks and is given subcutaneously in doses of 0.3–0.5 ml of a 1:1000 solution every

20–30 min for two or three doses. Although considered safe, it may impair uteroplacental circulation. Isoproterenol has β action without α action and is the most potent bronchodilator of the group. It is usually given by inhalation (1:200 solution). Isoetharine is less potent than isoproterenol, but is more β_2-selective and causes much less cardiac stimulation. It is usually given as an aerosol (0.5 ml of a 1% solution) 4–6 times a day. The resorcinols and salinergins have more β_2 selectivity, somewhat longer action and, most importantly, they are active orally. The two available in the USA are metaproterenol and terbutaline (more widely used). The oral dose of terbutaline is 2.5–5 mg 3 or 4 times daily. It can also be given parenterally (0.25–0.5 mg sc) but by this route it has much less β_2 selectivity and causes tremor by its action on muscles. It may also be used as an aerosol by inhalation.

Ephedrine is also effective orally, but its usefulness is limited because it has both α and β stimulation. Many adrenergic stimulants are available for aerosol administration, which produces rapid bronchodilating action and fewer systemic side-effects. Despite the widespread use of intermittent positive pressure breathing devices to deliver bronchodilator aerosols, there is no sound evidence that they offer any advantage over simple, and much less expensive, hand-held nebulizers.

When asthma requires multiple drugs for control (e.g., theophylline + terbutaline + bronchodilator aerosol), a trial of chromolyn sodium should be considered. This drug is not a bronchodilator. It is not effective in the acute attack and should not be given during acute attacks. It inhibits degranulation of mast cells, thus preventing the release of chemical mediators of asthma. If it is not effective in 4 weeks, it should be discontinued and another form of therapy attempted. It is relatively nontoxic and administered by inhalation only. There are sporadic reports of its use during gestation in humans without evidence of teratogenicity, probably because it acts locally.

Use of corticosteroids is indicated when severe airway obstruction persists or worsens despite adequate bronchodilator therapy. Their chronic use is considered when the patient has frequent recurrences and progression of the illness despite an otherwise optimal regimen. The most widely used corticosteroid is hydrocortisone. It is administered as a loading dose of 4 mg/kg followed by a maintenance dose of 3 mg/kg every 6 h. Bronchodilator therapy must be continued, as the effect of corticosteroids is not immediate and takes 6 h or longer. After 2 or 3 days, the patient can be changed to oral prednisone, about 60 mg each morning and tapered gradually (5–10 mg reduction every 2 or 3 days). There is no evidence that higher doses are more beneficial except in the rare case when the patient may be "steroid-resistant," in which case the dose should be doubled. The synthetic steroids (prednisone, prednisolone)

Table 2.1 Suggested treatment protocol for asthma

Acute attack

1 Epinephrine 0.3–0.5 ml sc (1 : 1000 solution) or terbutaline, 0.25–0.5 mg sc every 20–30 min × 2–3 doses
2 Intravenous theophylline loading*: 5–6 mg/kg over 20–30 min
   Maintenance: 0.6–0.9 mg/kg per h
3 Sympathomimetic aerosol (hand nebulizer): Bronkosol, isoproterenol, terbutaline, 2 puffs every 3–4 h
4 Hospitalization if the above steps produce no improvement
5 In hospital:
   (a) continue steps 2 and 3;
   (b) obtain chest X-ray, ABG (serial), nasal oxygen, intravenous fluids, bedside spirogram, consider course of steroids
6 Steroids:
   (a) Short-term therapy
       Hydrocortisone   4 mg/kg bolus, 3 mg/kg q.i.d. maintenance × 2–3 days
       Prednisone   60 mg daily; taper by 5–10 mg every 2–3 days
   (b) Chronic use
       Betamethasone   inhaler, 100 mg (preferable) 2 puffs q.i.d.
       Prednisone   30–60 mg alternate days orally
7 Miscellaneous:
   (a) avoid sedatives, tranquilizers, β-blockers;
   (b) expectorants and mucolytics: little value; if used, avoid iodides;[†]
   (c) intravenous fluids to avoid dehydration;
   (d) intermittent positive pressure breathing: no advantage over hand nebulizers;
   (e) antibiotics: not routinely, for bacterial infections only;
   (f) nasal oxygen – keep PO_2 >60 mmHg

Chronic asthma

1 Avoid allergies if identified
2 Desensitization of known allergies
3 Drugs:
   (a) theophylline 800–1200 mg/day orally in divided doses
   (b) terbutaline 2.5–5.0 mg t.i.d. or q.i.d. orally

---

* Give half if history of intermittent use and void if on adequate oral theophylline.
[†] Large goiter in babies with high mortality rate (70%) due to asphyxia.
ABG, Arterial blood gas.

cause less sodium retention, and their use is preferred in pregnancy. If a need for chronic steroid therapy is indicated, every effort should be made to maintain an alternate-day dosage. Therefore, long-acting steroids (e.g., betamethasone, dexamethasone) should be avoided as they cause prolonged suppression of the pituitary–adrenal axis. The main complications of steroid aerosols are oropharyngeal candidiasis and hoarseness due to largngeal myopathy.

All sedatives, tranquilizers, opiates, etc., should be avoided because they depress alveolar ventilation. β-Adrenergic blockers (e.g., propranolol) should also be avoided. Expectorants and mucolytics are still used widely. Any preparation containing iodides must be carefully avoided as iodides are known to cause large goiters and hypothyroidism in infants; in turn this produces tracheal obstruction and high neonatal mortality (>70%) from asphyxiation. Intravenous fluids also are used to prevent dehydration and help to liquefy bronchial secretions. Antibiotics are not used routinely. When indicated, nasal oxygen should be given to maintain a $Po_2 > 60\,mmHg$. The inability to maintain a $Po_2 > 60\,mmHg$ is a criterion for intubation. The recommended treatment is shown in Table 2.1. For delivery, the vaginal route is preferable, and cesarean section is reserved for obstetric indications. Epidural anesthesia is preferred for asthmatic pregnant women. Breast-feeding is considered safe in women on antiasthma medication.

SUGGESTED READING

BAHNA SL, BJERKEDAL T. The course and outcome of pregnancy in women with bronchial asthma. *Acta Allergy* 1972;27:397.

BRAR HS. Medications for asthma in pregnancy. *Contrib Obstet Gynecol* 1986;28:145.

BRAR HS. Asthma therapy during pregnancy. In: Petrie RH, ed. *Perinatal Pharmacology*, vol 6. Oradell, NJ: Medical Economics Books, 1989:71–84.

CHERNJACK RM. Comprehensive approach to asthma. *Chest* (Suppl) 1985;87:94S.

DE SWIET M. Diseases of the respiratory system. *Clin Obstet Gynecol* 1977;4:287.

FELDMAN NT, MCFADDEN ER Jr. Asthma therapy, old and new. *Med Clin North Am* 1977;61:1239.

PATTERSON JW, WOOLCORK AJ, SHENFIELD GM. Bronchodilator drugs: state of the art. *Am Rev Respir Dis* 1979;120:1149.

SCHATZ M, PATTERSON R, ZEITZ S, *et al.* Corticosteroid therapy for the pregnant asthmatic patient. *JAMA* 1975;233:804.

3

Hypothyroidism in pregnancy

MARTIN N. MONTORO & ANNA S. LEUNG

Pregnancy in women with hypothyroidism is thought to be rare and is usually attributed to infrequent ovulation. In fact, until 1980, a review of the literature back to 1897 revealed only 36 reasonably well-documented cases. However, in most of those cases, the diagnosis of hypothyroidism was based solely on clinical grounds, and only in the more recent reports has clinical suspicion been confirmed by measurement of thyroid hormone levels. More recent data suggest that hypothyroidism during pregnancy is not so rare, now that more women are screened with more sensitive thyroid function tests.

Most of the obstetric and endocrinologic literature refers to older reports that describe frequent poor outcomes of the pregnancies that occurred in hypothyroid women: twice the average incidence of abortions, 20% perinatal mortality, a high incidence of congenital anomalies (10–20% or more) and, above all, impaired mental and somatic development in up to 50–60% of the surviving children. However, close scrutiny reveals that the exact thyroid status of the women cited in these reports is unclear. Diagnoses were generally based on what is described as hypothyroxinemia, or failure of the protein-bound or butanol-extractable iodines to increase as expected during pregnancy. Neither thyroid-stimulating hormone (TSH) concentrations nor other more accurate determinations of thyroid status were evaluated, and the authors did not suggest any explanations for the severe complications they observed.

More than 10 years ago we described a group of pregnant women (the largest series reported until that time) in which the diagnosis of hypothyroidism was unequivocally documented both clinically and by accurate determination of thyroid function. The outcome of these pregnancies was very favorable, even though conception, embryogenesis, and most of the fetal development occurred in the presence of hypothyroidism. The complications were not excessive (86% live births, 8% stillbirths, and 6% abortions), and much lower than usually reported. Davis *et al.* in 1988, described a high rate of maternal complications (preeclampsia, anemia, placental abruption, and postpartum hemorrhage) in a group of hypothyroid pregnant women but most of those women had other serious medical illnesses besides hypothyroidism.

Thus, the literature contains conflicting data on the effects of hypothyroidism on gestation and offspring. There are reports of reasonably well documented hypothyroidism without excessive complications and other reports of many complications; however, until now it has not been shown if these complications were caused by the hypothyroidism itself or if other factors were present as well.

A recent study

In order to elucidate the role of maternal hypothyroidism in the outcome of pregnancy, investigators at the University of Southern California studied 126 hypothyroid women who had no other illness. Women with other diseases, e.g., chronic hypertension, diabetes mellitus, etc., in addition to their hypothyroidism were excluded and will be reported on separately. This is the largest series reported to date regarding the outcome of pregnancy in hypothyroidism. In this study the patients were divided into four groups according to their initial thyroid function: 23 women had overt hypothyroidism (elevated TSH and low thyroxine (T4)), 45 women had subclinical hypothyroidism (elevated TSH but normal T4), 33 women became euthyroid with thyroxine replacement before pregnancy, and 25 women had goiters of various causes but were euthyroid without treatment. The last two groups had normal levels of both TSH and T4.

The only significant complications were related to pregnancy-induced hypertension which occurred in the overt hypothyroid and the subclinical hypothyroid women. The incidence of gestational hypertension was much greater in those women who were still hypothyroid at the time of delivery (30%) than in those who became euthyroid before delivery (8%). There was an increased incidence of low-birth-weight infants, but it occurred in those patients who were delivered before term because of hypertension. The only stillbirth occurred in a profoundly hypothyroid woman who developed eclampsia at 28 weeks. Another woman had an infant with club feet. No other adverse maternal, fetal, or neonatal outcomes were noted.

Therefore we conclude that the outcome of pregnancy in hypothyroid women without other concurrent illnesses can be quite favorable, particularly if the women are rendered euthyroid prior to pregnancy. If the diagnosis is made after conception, treatment should be instituted without delay, since normalization of thyroid function may decrease the incidence of gestational hypertension and its complications.

Our results are in agreement with current research. It is now well accepted that in humans the placenta is practically impermeable to T4, triiodothyronine (T3), and TSH. The fetal hypothalamic–pituitary–thyroid axis seems to develop and function independently and does not need maternal thyroid hormone for support. Some researchers have reported that in the rat there might be some placental passage of thyroid hormone, and that in this animal species even these small amounts may be important for fetal development. However, it does not seem that the information from those experiments can be extrapolated to humans. The fact that the infants of our hypothyroid mothers were euthyroid at birth supports that view. Several of the children followed for up to 3 years have remained euthyroid and continue to develop normally. Although longer follow-up of these children is needed, the information thus far justified optimism. Thus it appears that if maternal hypothyroidism affects the fetus at all, it must do so indirectly and in ways that have yet to be demonstrated. Based on our own data and on a few other well-documented cases, pregnant hypothyroid women should not be discouraged from carrying their pregnancies to term solely because of the hypothyroidism.

It should be noted that the above information does not apply to those mothers who are hypothyroid because of iodine deficiency. Those cases are found in areas of endemic goiter, which no longer exist in the USA. In the USA, the most common (up to 85%) causes of primary hypothyroidism during pregnancy are autoimmune thyroid disorders such as chronic thyroiditis or therapy for Graves disease (radioactive iodine ablation or thyroidectomy). The rest of the cases are due to thyroidectomy for various other disorders (benign and malignant tumors, toxic goiters, etc.). These causes are similar to those seen outside of pregnancy. The incidence of signs and symptoms of hypothyroidism is also similar to those reported for nonpregnant hypothyroid patients, with about one-fourth of the patients being essentially asymptomatic, one-half with several signs and symptoms, and the remainder with most of the classic, well-known signs and symptoms of hypothyroidism.

The diagnosis of primary hypothyroidism during pregnancy is no different than outside of pregnancy. The clinical history is very important, since in most patients the diagnosis is made prior to pregnancy. The most reliable test is the sensitive TSH. The total T4 level may not be as low during pregnancy because there is more T4-binding protein, and for this reason a free T4 index should also be obtained. Rarely, a true free T4 may be necessary. Thyroid autoantibodies are used outside of pregnancy, although some authors report that the titer may not be as elevated during pregnancy.

Based on the number of infants delivered at our institution (a referral center), the frequency of hypothyroidism is approximately 1:2000–3000 pregnancies. It may be lower in general obstetric practices based in community hospitals.

Thyroid replacement therapy

Treatment should be instituted without delay once the diagnosis is made, as in any patient with hypothyroidism. Because most pregnant women are young and without cardiovascular disease, therapy usually can be started with 0.075–0.1 mg of oral L-thyroxine. Equivalent doses of desiccated thyroid are also used by many physicians. However, the brand preparations of L-thyroxine are preferred, due to the numerous reports of unpredictable bioavailability with the various generic preparations. After 2 weeks, the dose can be increased to 0.125 mg or higher, depending on the patient's response and plasma levels of T4 and TSH.

In patients with severe hypothyroidism of long duration or associated cardiovascular disease, replacement should be instituted more slowly, as would be done in older patients. Therapy is started with 0.025–0.05 mg, increasing by 0.025 mg every 1–3 weeks until the desired replacement dose is reached, as indicated by the thyroid function tests.

Some women may require higher doses during pregnancy; to determine this, thyroid hormones and TSH levels should be monitored at regular intervals, at least once each trimester. Ideally, T4 should be kept in the upper-normal range, with the free T4 index and TSH levels returned to normal. Therapy should be continued during pregnancy in patients with a history of hypothyroidism who already are receiving adequate replacement. If there is any question about the diagnosis of hypothyroidism and the need for thyroid replacement, proper investigation should wait until after delivery.

SUGGESTED READING

BALEN AH, KURTIZ AB. Successful outcome of pregnancy with severe hypothyroidism. Case report and literature review. *Br J Obstet Gynaecol* 1990;97:536.

DAVIS LE, LEVNO KJ, CUNNINGHAM FG. Hypothyroidism complicating pregnancy. *Obstet Gynecol* 1988;72:108.

ECHT CR, DOSS JF. Myxedema in pregnancy: report of three cases. *Obstet Gynecol* 1963;22:615.

FISHER DA. Thyroid development and thyroid disorders in infancy. In: Van

Middlesworth L, ed. *The Thyroid Gland*. Chicago: Year Book Medical Publishers, 1986:111.

HENNESSEY JV, EVANL JE, TSENG YC, *et al*. L-Thyroxine dosage: a re-evaluation of therapy with contemporary preparations. *Ann Intern Med* 1986;105:11.

JONES WS, MAN EB. Thyroid function in human pregnancy: VI. Premature deliveries and reproductive failure of pregnant women with low butanol extractable iodine. *Am J Obstet Gynecol* 1969;104:909.

LEUNG AS, MONTORO M, MESTMAN JH. Perinatal outcome in hypothyroid pregnancies. *Am J Obstet Gynecol* 1992;166:306.

MONTORO M, COLLEA JV, FRASIER D, MESTMAN JH. Successful outcome of pregnancy in women with hypothyroidism. *Ann Intern Med* 1981;94:31.

PEKONEN F, TERAMO K, IKONEN E, *et al*. Women on thyroid hormone therapy: pregnancy course, fetal outcome and amniotic fluid thyroid hormone level. *Obstet Gynecol* 1984;63:635.

4

Hyperthyroidism in pregnancy

T. MURPHY GOODWIN & JORGE H. MESTMAN

Thyroid diseases are common in women of child-bearing age. The natural history of thyroid diseases may be affected by pregnancy and one of them (transient hyperthyroidism of hyperemesis of pregnancy) is peculiar to pregnancy. Therapy is directed by the knowledge of the interrelationship between fetus and mother and the role of the placenta. Neonatal outcome may be affected by the etiology of the thyroid pathology and the control of the disease during pregnancy. Therefore, a team approach in the care of these patients is highly recommended, with the participation of obstetricians, endocrinologists, anesthesiologists, and neonatologists.

Thyroid tests

The following tests are useful in selected situations.

Free thyroxine or its equivalent, free thyroxine index (FT4I)

The FT4I is easy and economically feasible in most commercial laboratories; in an outpatient setting it correlates very well with the actual determination of free thyroxine. It can be used as a first-line test. Normal values are not modified by pregnancy itself.

Free triiodothyronine or its equivalent, free triiodothyronine index (FT3I)

This test is useful once the diagnosis of hyperthyroidism is made, to follow and assess antithyroid therapy. On occasion, it may be elevated while the FT4I is within normal limits.

Serum thyroid-stimulating hormone (TSH)

The new tests (ultrasensitive, sensitive, second- or third-generation tests) are sensitive enough to detect low values and, as a consequence, minimal changes in thyroid pathology. A suppressed value is consistent with the diagnosis of hyperthyroidism and an elevated value is diagnostic of hypothyroidism due to intrinsic thyroid disease.

Thyroid antibodies (antimicrosomal (AMA) or antiperoxide (APO), and antithyroglobulin (ATA))

Presence of these antibodies in serum is diagnostic of autoimmune thyroid disease. They are useful in the elevation of goiter or hypothyroidism.

Serum thyroglobulin (Tg)

This test is used in following patients after ablation therapy for thyroid carcinoma. It is an early marker for recurrence of the disease.

TSH receptor antibody (TSHRAb)

This test is a marker of Graves disease. It is useful in patients with a past or present history of Graves disease. A significant elevation in maternal titer (>50%) may identify infants at risk for neonatal hyperthyroidism.

Transient hyperthyroidism of hyperemesis gravidarum (THHG)

In our experience, as many as 60% of patients with severe hyperemesis gravidarum (nausea and vomiting, >10% weight loss, large ketonuria) present with at least one thyroid test in the hyperthyroid range (i.e., suppressed TSH, elevated FT4I or, in 10–20% of cases, elevated FT3I). This is a self-limited abnormality and no specific antithyroid therapy is indicated. The differential diagnosis from hyperthyroidism due to autoimmune thyroid disease sometimes is difficult; the following points are helpful: no history or symptoms of thyroid disease preceding pregnancy, absence of goiter, negative thyroid antibodies, and resolution of symptoms and normalization of thyroid tests in 2–8 weeks.

Goiter

Goiter is defined as an enlargement of the thyroid gland; the normal thyroid gland weighs between 15 and 25 g, and in general is not palpable. In areas of normal dietary iodine ingestion, the thyroid gland enlarges minimally during pregnancy. Therefore, any enlargement detected by physical examination should be considered abnormal and deserves careful evaluation. The physician should be able to describe the size, consistency, symmetry, and tenderness, along with the presence of nodularity or adenopathy. The determination of FT4I and TSH will define the functional status of the goiter. The presence of thyroid antibodies is diagnostic of autoimmune thyroid disease as the etiology of the goiter. In the presence of a single thyroid nodule, fine-needle aspiration biopsy should be considered to rule out thyroid cancer, particularly before 20 weeks' gestation. Ultrasound of the nodule before biopsy may be helpful in separating solid from cystic lesions; the latter are usually benign if their diameter is <4 cm.

Hyperthyroidism

Hyperthyroidism complicates 0.5–2% of all pregnancies. In most cases symptoms precede pregnancy, although they may arise for the first time early in gestation or recur in a patient who has been in remission. Autoimmune thyroid disease may spontaneously recur or worsen during the first trimester or in the postpartum period, and may spontaneously improve in the second half of pregnancy.

The most common etiology of hyperthyroidism is Graves disease, accounting for over 85% of cases. Other causes include nodular goiter (single toxic nodule or multinodular), and chronic (Hashimoto's) thyroiditis. Hyperemesis gravidarum as a cause of biochemical hyperthyroidism was discussed previously.

Classical symptoms are weight loss, palpitations, nervousness, personality changes, irritability, heat intolerance, muscle weakness, insomnia, and frequent bowel movements. On physical examination a diffuse painless goiter is found in over 90% of cases; warm skin and moist palms, eye changes, tachycardia, wide pulse pressure, exaggerated deep tendon reflexes, and proximal muscle weakness are common findings. The diagnosis is confirmed by a suppressed serum TSH and an elevation in FT4I and/or FT3I.

The TSHRAb test is reserved for those patients with significant extrathyroidal manifestations (eye disease), those with large goiters and long-term history of Graves disease, and those women with a previous history of Graves disease treated with ablation therapy who present with unexplained fetal tachycardia. Fetal tachycardia, due to the passage of TSHRAb from mother to fetus, is recognized as early as 20–24 weeks' gestation.

Once the diagnosis is confirmed, drug therapy is the treatment of choice. Several guidelines are important in the management of patients with hyperthyroidism: (1) the minimum amount of medication to keep the patient clinically and biochemically euthyroid is used, since antithyroid drugs cross the placenta and may affect thyroid function in the fetus; (2) patients are seen every 2–3 weeks and changes in drug therapy are assessed (weight gain and pulse rate are two objective signs of improvement that correlate well with thyroid function tests); (3) β-blockers may be used at the time of diagnosis in very symptomatic patients and then are discontinued when symptoms improve; (4) antithyroid medication may be discontinued in the last 4–6 weeks of gestation in patients rendered euthyroid on a minimum amount of antithyroid therapy, especially those with small goiters and short duration of disease; (5) with few exceptions, tests for fetal well-being are limited to those situations in which fetal growth retardation or fetal tachycardia are detected, or in the presence of very high titers of TSHRAb; (6) patients are followed in the postpartum period since recurrences of hyperthyroidism are known to occur; and (7) infants of hyperthyroid mothers should be evaluated and followed by the pediatrician, since transient abnormalities may be present in 2–10% of these infants.

Propylthiouracil or methimazole are the drugs used in this country for the treatment of hyperthyroidism. Both are very effective in pregnancy and, contrary to some reports, both may be used in pregnancy. The initial dose of 200–400 mg of propylthiouracil or equivalent amounts of methimazole (20–40 mg) daily is given in two divided (b.i.d.) doses. Thyroid tests improve in 2–3 weeks and normalize in 3–6 weeks. The dose should be reduced by half as soon as the tests improve; adjustments are made every 2–3 weeks. Hypothyroidism must be avoided since it is an indication of overtreatment of mother and fetus. Therefore, the FT4I and the FT3I should be kept in the upper limits of normal. Serum TSH should not be repeated during pregnancy, since in the majority of cases it remains suppressed in spite of normalization of the other thyroid tests. The most serious side-effect is agranulocytosis, reported in 0.03% of patients. The patient should be advised to discontinue the use of antithyroid drug in the presence of sore throat, fever, or gingivitis and to consult her physician at once.

Complications seen in untreated or poorly controlled patients include premature delivery, small-for-gestational-age infants, gestational hypertension, and, on rare occasions, congestive heart failure and thyroid storm. Hospitalization should be reserved for patients with uncontrolled disease, poorly compliant patients, those seen for the first time in the third trimester, and those with fetal growth retardation or superimposed toxemia. If the mother is kept euthyroid during pregnancy, fetal mortality and morbidity are equivalent to normal pregnancies. Long-term follow-up of these infants indicates no significant sequelae.

Breast-feeding may be allowed when the total amount of medication is <200 mg of propylthiouracil or 20 mg of methimazole daily. The drug should be administered 4 times a day just after infant suckling. The pediatrician should be informed and the infant followed with appropriate thyroid function tests.

Postpartum thyroid dysfunction (PPTD) syndrome

Women with autoimmune thyroid disease frequently develop thyroid abnormalities within 1 year of delivery. The incidence of these abnormalities has been reported to be between 3 and 8% of all pregnancies. PPTD can be classified in three groups, of which two can be characterized by hyperthyroidism and will be discussed here. The first group consists of patients with a history of Graves disease who present with an exacerbation of hyperthyroid symptoms 1–3 months after delivery, occasionally later. The ^{131}I thyroid uptake is elevated, consistent with hyperthyroidism of Graves disease.

The second group comprises patients with chronic thyroiditis on no thyroid medication. Within 3 months of delivery these women may complain of enlargement of the thyroid gland and mild, nonspecific symptoms such as tiredness, fatigue, nervousness, heat intolerance, and personality changes. These symptoms are often attributed to postpartum "blues." Thyroid tests are in the hyperthyroid range and thyroid antibodies are positive, with titers greater than during pregnancy, if such information is available. Indeed, the presence of positive antibodies in the first trimester of pregnancy in a euthyroid woman is predictive of the development of the PPTD. If an ^{131}I thyroid uptake is obtained, it is low (below 5%), and serves to differentiate this condition from Graves disease. Without specific therapy, hypothyroidism ensues within a few months, frequently with few symptoms. Spontaneous recovery occurs within several months with normalization of thyroid parameters, but thyroid antibodies remain elevated. The goiter may decrease somewhat in size. Therapy with β-blockers is indicated for the occasional patient with significant hyperthyroid symptoms; conversely, thyroid hormone therapy may be necessary for some patients in the hypothyroid phase.

There can be considerable variability in the clinical course. Some patients may go into the hypothyroid phase without the hyperthyroid period. In an occasional patient the hyperthyroid phase is followed by complete recovery. Long-term follow-up of these patients indicates a significant incidence of permanent hypothyroidism.

SUGGESTED READING

CHERON RG, KAPLAN MM, LARSEN PR, *et al.* Neonatal thyroid function after propylthiouracil therapy for maternal Graves' disease. *N Engl J Med* 1981; 304:525.

DAVIS LE, LUCAS MJ, HANKINDS GD, *et al.* Thyrotoxicosis complicating pregnancy. *Am J Obstet Gynecol* 1989;1950:63.

GOODWIN TM, MONTORO M, MESTMAN JH. Transient hyperthyroidism and hyperemesis gravidarum: clinical aspects. *Am J Obstet Gynecol* 1992;167:648–652.

JANSSON R, DAHLBERG PA, KARLSSON FA. Post-partum thyroiditis. *Baillières Clin Endocrinol Metab* 1988;2:619.

KAMPMANN JP, JOHANSEN K, HANSEN JM, *et al.* Propylthiouracil in human milk. Revision of a dogma. *Lancet* 1980;1:736.

MESTMAN JH. Severe hyperthyroidism in pregnancy. In: Clark S, Phelan J, Cotton D, eds. *Critical Care in Obstetrics*. Oradell, NJ: Medical Economics, 1987: 262–279.

MESTMAN JH. Hyperthyroidism. *Contemp Ob/Gynecol* 1991;36:37–50.

5

Seizure disorders in pregnancy

REUVEN SHARONY

The most common serious neurologic problem during pregnancy is epilepsy, affecting 0.3–0.5% of all pregnant women. Epilepsy is a clinical syndrome characterized by recurrent seizure episodes, while a seizure is defined as a transient disturbance of neuronal synchrony. The diagnosis may often be difficult due to the episodic nature of the disease. A clear description of the attack by the patient and a witness, in addition to a thorough physical and neurologic examination, is of great value. The physician has to consider the differential diagnosis while emphasizing those conditions that are more common in pregnancy (Table 5.1).

Although the diagnosis is primarily clinical, an EEG may be very helpful both in terms of establishing the diagnosis and in specifying the seizure type. This specific diagnosis has an impact on the counseling process pertaining to the prognosis, relatives at risk, and the management of the patient. Epilepsy can be classified according to a number of criteria: etiology, age of onset, syndromes, and type of seizure. The most common way is by the seizure type, as was introduced by the 1981 Commission of the International League against Epilepsy (Table 5.2). However, it should be borne in mind that some patients might fit into more than one category or change their disease pattern with the passage of time.

The effect of the pregnancy on the natural history of epilepsy

Most studies agree that the effect of pregnancy on epilepsy varies from patient to patient and even during different pregnancies for the same

Table 5.1 Differential diagnosis of seizure disorders in pregnancy

Trauma	*Pregnancy*
Vascular disease	Eclampsia
Infections	Water intoxication
Toxic causes	Thrombotic thrombocytopenic
Metabolic and nutritional disturbances	purpura
Neoplasm	Cerebral venous thrombosis
Heredofamilial disorders	Amniotic fluid embolus

Table 5.2 A classification of epileptic seizures

Partial	*Generalized*
Simple (unimpaired consciousness)	Absence (petit mal)
Complex (impaired consciousness)	Myoclonic
Secondary generalized	Clonic
	Tonic
	Tonic–clonic
	Atonic

Table 5.3 Modifying factors of seizure frequency during pregnancy

Hormonal changes
Metabolic factors
Respiratory changes
Psychologic problems
Medication compliance problem
Altered pharmacokinetics of antiepileptic drugs

patient. In a review of 26 studies that included 2165 pregnancies, seizure frequency remained the same in approximately 50%, and the rest of the cases were divided almost equally between increased and decreased frequencies. Most of the seizures occurred during the first trimester. Most often the seizure frequency resumed its pregestational level after the pregnancy.

There are several factors which may alter the natural history of the disease during pregnancy; however, there is not yet a way to predict the course of epilepsy in a specific case, nor is there a reliable method to predict the onset of seizures during pregnancy. The various factors that may modify the frequency of seizures during pregnancy are summarized in Table 5.3. Among them, noncompliance and altered disposition of antiepileptic drugs (AED) seem to be the most important.

Hormonal changes

Estrogen has been shown to lower seizure threshold and thus to precipitate seizures in animals and humans. Progesterone and testosterone, on the other hand, lowered seizure threshold and caused a mild reduction in seizure frequency in animals. These hormonal influences are less important with partial seizures and differ from patient to patient. Most importantly, the described relationship is far more difficult to establish in the pregnant patient.

Metabolic factors

Weight gain and water retention have been associated in some studies with increased seizure frequency. Lower concentrations of sodium, potassium, calcium, and magnesium, as well as mild respiratory alkalosis, may also precipitate seizures in the nonpregnant patient. However, there is not conclusive data to establish these associations in pregnancy.

Psychologic aspects

A common fear of epileptic pregnant patients is that the newborn will have congenital anomalies or will inherit the maternal disease. As a consequence a psychogenic mechanism is believed to precipitate seizure activity. In addition, sleep deprivation may contribute to the increase in the number of seizures.

Noncompliance

As a result of the concern over the adverse effects of the antiseizure medication which is common to most epileptic patients during pregnancy, there is a tendency of patients to "forget" to take their medications or to lower the dosage.

Pharmacokinetics of antiseizure medication

Most studies agree upon the fact that plasma levels of the majority of the AEDs are lowered during pregnancy due to pharmacokinetic changes. These changes are dependent on the biochemical properties of the specific drug. The metabolic processing of the drugs by the liver enzymes is probably altered during pregnancy both by the hormonal changes and the interaction with other drugs (e.g., folic acid stimulates hepatic metabolism which leads to reduced plasma concentrations of diphenylhydantoin and phenobarbital). The absorption rate of AEDs is modified by the prolonged emptying time and the higher gastric pH. The secretion by the kidneys is probably unchanged since the tubular mechanism which is responsible for most AED excretion is unchanged. AEDs are protein-bound. Decreasing levels of the plasma proteins lead to an increased biologic effect of the nonprotein bound AEDs. The fall in plasma levels of AEDs in pregnancy are balanced by the increase in free AEDs in the peripheral circulation. Although some studies found a correlation between plasma levels of AEDs and seizure activity, it is not a persistent finding, and does not take into account the decrease in the protein-bound fraction of AEDs.

Lastly, approximately 10% of epileptic pregnancies start as gestational epilepsy (i.e., onset in the current pregnancy). This observation is not surprising since the age of onset of epilepsy and child-bearing age overlap in the general population. Only about 40% of women who first experience seizures during pregnancy remain true gestational epileptics. No association was found between the type of seizure, maternal age, or timing of the seizures during the pregnancy and the incidence of gestational epilepsy.

The effect of epilepsy on the pregnancy

Maternal complications

Pregnancy

There is approximately a twofold increase in the risk of vaginal bleeding throughout the pregnancy and about threefold increase in premature separation of the placenta (one study) in pregnant women with epilepsy. Some studies suggest that there is probably a twofold increase in the incidence of pregnancy-induced hypertension. The results of most of the studies do not reveal any increase in the risk for spontaneous abortions. Other pregnancy complications that were found in a higher incidence in epileptics than in nonepileptics are premature rupture of the membranes, polyhydramnios (one study), and patients on phenobarbital tend to have a higher incidence of abnormal contraction stress tests (one study).

Delivery

The incidence of cesarean section is increased approximately twofold over that in the general population. The higher incidence is explained by the increase in obstetric complications and the tendency among physicians to shorten the delivery process as much as possible in pregnant women with epilepsy. Abnormal presentations were also reported to be more frequent in epileptics than in the general population.

Fetal complications

The fetus of the epileptic mother is exposed to several types of risk. First is the effects of the maternal disease itself, including the risk of experiencing seizures during pregnancy. Second is the increased risk to the fetus to inherit epilepsy on a genetic basis. Third is the potential for teratogenic effects of the AED or the condition causing epilepsy in the mother.

Pregnancy

Microcephaly was reported to be associated with epilepsy even without medical treatment. A higher incidence of intrauterine growth retardation was also described in the fetuses of epileptic mothers, but social class, smoking, and alcohol abuse may be confounding factors. Perinatal mortality was reported to be elevated in every study published, with most of the stillbirths occurring in full-term babies. Among the reasons for this observation is the following: the epileptics belong to a lower social class than the general population, and there is a well-documented association between lower socioeconomic class and increased risk of perinatal death. Another reason is the increased incidence of congenital malformations among infants of epileptic mothers and the high incidence of mortality among this group. Prematurity is another complication that probably is iatrogenic due to a higher incidence of induction of labor among epileptic patients.

Congenital malformations

Children of treated epileptic mothers are at greater risk of malformations than children of untreated epileptic mothers, who are at greater risk than children of nonepileptic mothers. This may be related to the medication factor as well as to the indications for the treatment, such as the type of the epilepsy and the severity of the disease (Table 5.4).

Malformations may depend on the specific cause of the epilepsy. Epilepsy is a rather heterogeneous group of diseases with more than 50 clinically distinguishable types and a wide range of causes. The etiology may range from genetic syndromes to environmental causes such as head trauma or infection. Other factors that have to be considered in evaluating the differences in the type and incidence of malformation are duration of treatment, age at onset of the disease, and the maternal age during the pregnancy. A controversy exists among the studies that were designed to assess potential factors which affect malformation. However, the population in each study was too small to be evaluated separately and due to a wide variation in the characteristics of the patients it is impossible to perform a meta-analysis. There still remain several observations that

Table 5.4 Fetal anomalies associated with the usage of antiepileptic drugs

Drug	Frequently associated anomalies	Reported anomalies
Phenytoin	10% Fetal hydantoin syndrome: craniofacial dysmorphic features, minor limb defects, pre- and postnatal growth retardation, developmental delay (30% may have part of the syndrome)	Cardiac anomalies, genitourinary and CNS malformations, diaphragmatic hernia
Carbamazepine	NTD, smaller head circumference	Caraniofacial dysmorphic features, fingernail hypoplasia, developmental delay
Phenobarbital	"Phenytoin-like syndrome"	Cardiac defects
Valproate	NTD, limb malformations, craniofacial dysmorphic features	Cardiac defects
Ethosuximide	No specific anomaly known	
Trimethadione	Fetal trimethadione syndrome: developmental delay, growth retardation, craniofacial anomalies, irregular teeth, palatal anomalies	IUGR, cardiac defects, renal agenesis, club hand, meningomyelocele
Clonazepam	No specific anomaly known	

CNS, Central nervous system; NTD, neural-tube defects; IUGR, intrauterine growth retardation.

are pertinent to the search for the basis of the embryopathy seen in infants of epileptic mothers:

1 infants born to epileptic mothers have a two- to threefold increased risk of having congenital malformations;

2 epilepsy, itself, is associated with an increased risk for congenital abnormalities as suggested by the observation of increased malformed infants born to epileptic fathers;

3 there exists a common genetic tendency for epilepsy and congenital anomalies;

4 all AEDs are teratogenic in animals;

5 because neural tube defects have been associated with the use of carbamazepine and valproate, pregnant women receiving these medications in our medical center are screened with amniotic fluid α-fetoprotein.

Treatment

The goal of therapy offered to pregnant women with seizure disorders is to use the least number of drugs and the lowest dose of drug which is effective in preventing seizure activity. The known adverse effects associated with the use of AEDs should be discussed with every patient, before she conceives if possible, and the risks of AEDs should be evaluated in comparison to discontinuing the AEDs and the outcome of seizures during pregnancy. The common practice is to continue the treatment of those epileptic patients who have a confirmed diagnosis. If the diagnosis of epilepsy is uncertain, withdrawal of antiepileptic medication may be tried. If withdrawal of AEDs is being considered, it should not be attempted in a patient who has had a previous unsuccessful withdrawal of medication or who has predisposing factors for relapse of epilepsy during pregnancy. The relapse rate is about 40%, with most of the recurrences occurring during the first year following withdrawal. Known predisposing factors for relapse of seizures during pregnancy which have to be considered in evaluating the candidate for a trial of discontinuation are listed in Table 5.5. In general, it is preferred to continue the patient on the same protocol that has kept her asymptomatic.

New seizure disorders during the pregnancy should always be assessed in light of the specific causes related to pregnancy as well as the nonpregnant adult conditions which can cause seizures. Unless there is a known etiology, there is no need to treat first and short seizure episodes. Even in a recurrent or prolonged seizure episode, other etiologies of the seizure than epilepsy have to be ruled out.

Patients should be started on a small dose of a first-line drug appropriate for their seizure. Monotherapy is preferable (Table 5.7).

Drug levels should be obtained monthly during pregnancy and weekly after delivery. Unbound (free) drug levels have a better monitoring value, especially for phenytoin and valproic acid. However, their main benefit is

Table 5.5 Predisposing factors for relapse of epilepsy during pregnancy

Long-standing and severe disease
Anatomic abnormality
Neurologic deficit
Partial or secondary generalized seizures
Complex seizures (more than one type)
Onset before the age of 1 year
Short duration of treatment
Resistance to the treatment
EEG abnormality

Table 5.6 Evaluation of a a seizure episode

Evaluate vital signs

Resuscitate if necessary

Serum chemistry panel (glucose, calcium, magnesium, electrolytes, creatinine)

Drug levels (antiepileptic drugs, alcohol)

Urine toxicology screen

Administer 50 ml of 50% glucose bolus, and thiamine 100 mg im. If there is no response, AEDs can be started

Table 5.7 AED of choice for common seizure type

Type of seizure	Drug of choice
Generalized tonic–clonic	Carbamazepine, phenytoin, valproic acid
Generalized absence	Ethosuximide, valproic acid
Myoclonic epilepsy	Clonazepam, valproic acid
Partial with or without secondary generalization	Carbamazepine, phenytoin, valproic acid

as a check on compliance. Plasma levels are directly related to the dose, but they do not have a good correlation with the activity of the drug and its metabolites. Recently, measurement of the individual's ability to metabolize certain AEDs was introduced and a correlation was found between that genetic characteristic and the extent of the adverse effects of the drugs.

During and after delivery the infant should be closely watched for coagulation disorders, and treated with vitamin K at birth if necessary. Offspring of mothers on phenobarbital may experience a withdrawal syndrome starting about 1 week after delivery and lasting up to 4 months. The symptoms of the withdrawal syndrome include hyperexcitability, tremors, and feeding problems. The issue of whether or not to have epileptic mothers breast-feed their babies is not totally resolved. AEDs vary in their rate of transmission into breast milk (Table 5.8). However, it seems safe to note that with any one of these drugs, both the lactating mother and the physician have to be alert for the development of signs of drug effect in the newborn, and that an idiosyncratic reaction cannot be anticipated or avoided.

Table 5.8 Transmission rates of AEDs into the breast milk

Drug	Transmission rate (%)
Valproic acid	2
Phenytoin	30
Phenobarbital	40
Carbamazepine	45
Primidone	60
Ethosuximide	90

Status epilepticus

Prolonged seizure activity occurs in less than 1% of epileptics during pregnancy, which is about the incidence among the nonpregnant patients (around 1.5%). The diagnosis is made on the basis of one of the following criteria: a generalized motor seizure lasting for >30 min; recurrent generalized motor seizures without waking up for >30 min; three or more generalized motor seizures during 1 h; or 5 min of unresponsive generalized motor seizures. Status epilepticus may have an abrupt onset or may be heralded by an increasing number and severity of seizure attacks. It can occur during pregnancy, labor, delivery, and puerperium. There are two types of this condition: convulsive and nonconvulsive. The first type carries an increased risk for respiratory complications, metabolic acidosis, hyperthermia, fractures, rhabdomyolysis and renal failure, arrhythmias, and permanent neurologic deficits. However, it is the nonconvulsive type that is more difficult to diagnose. In both cases a complete differential diagnosis has to be considered, and a precipitating factor sought and eliminated or treated. A rapid diagnosis and treatment is a major factor in the prognosis of this emergency.

In a review of 29 reported cases, nine of the patients died and 14 of the fetuses died *in utero* or immediately postpartum. Based on the high mortality to the mother and the baby, many physicians tend to treat this complication aggressively without terminating the pregnancy.

SELECTED READING

COMMISSION OF GENETICS, PREGNANCY, AND THE CHILD, INTERNATIONAL LEAGUE AGAINST EPILEPSY. Guidelines for the care of epileptic women of childbearing age. *Epilepsia* 1989;30:409–410.

DELGADO-ESCUETA AV, JANZ D, BECK-MANNAGETTA G. Pregnancy and teratogenesis in epilepsy. *Neurology* 1992 (Suppl) 42:5.

FERDRICK J. Epilepsy and pregnancy: a report from the Oxford Record Linkage Study. *Br Med J* 1973;2:442–448.

GARDINER RM. Genes and epilepsy. *J Med Genet* 1990;27:537–544.

HART Y. The diagnosis and management of epilepsy. *Practitioner* 1990;234:160–163.

JAGODA A, RIGGIO S. Emergency department approach to managing seizures in pregnancy. *Ann Emerg Med* 1991;20:80–85.

JANZ D, BOOSI L, DAM M, HELGE H, RICHENS A, SCHMIDT D (eds). *Epilepsy, Pregnancy, and the Child*. New York: Raven Press, 1982.

SHARONY R, GRAHAM JM Jr. Identification of fetal problems associated with anticonvulsant usage and maternal epilepsy. In: Platt LD, ed. *Diagnostic Ultrasonography, Obstetrics and Gynecology Clinics of North America* 1991;18:933–951.

6

Acquired anemia in pregnancy

RAUL ARTAL

Pregnancy-associated anemia is undoubtedly the most common medical complication in pregnancy, affecting an excess of 50% of all pregnant women in the USA. The physiologic changes and cardiovascular adaptations to pregnancy lead to an increase in oxygen consumption, an increase in blood volume, and an increase in cardiac output by 30–50%. The increase in the blood volume is due to increases in both plasma volume and red cell mass. The mean plasma volume increase in pregnancy is 1075 ml or approximately 40–45% over the mean nonpregnant plasma volume. These changes are greater in twin pregnancy.

The disproportionate increase in blood volume in relation to the red cell volume results in a fall in erythrocyte count, hemoglobin, and hematocrit. The consequence of this process is a physiologic anemia or hydremia of pregnancy, which is not a disease, but rather a symptom that can be reversed in most instances.

Against the above background, the Centers for Disease Control have published guidelines for the diagnosis of anemia in pregnancy. In the first and third trimesters the lower limits for normality are 11 g/dl for hemoglobin and 33% for hematocrit. In the second trimester the lower limits are 10.5 g/dl for hemoglobin and 32% for hematocrit.

The etiology of anemia in pregnancy

The etiology of red cell and plasma volume changes in pregnancy is unknown and could only be speculated upon. However, it is imperative to rule out any potential underlying disease, of which anemia is only one

Table 6.1 Common types of anemia in pregnancy

Hypoproliferative (decreased production)
Iron-deficient erythropoiesis
Iron deficiency*
Relative (hemorrhage)*
Stem cell dysfunction
Erythrocyte aplasia or hypoplasia*

Ineffective
Folic acid deficiency*
Thalassemia

Hemolytic (increased destruction)
Hemolytic hemoglobinopathies*
Hereditary spherocytosis
Microangiopathies

---

*Could be acquired in pregnancy.

manifestation. In these conditions anemia will persist until the underlying disease has been treated.

The first step in recognizing the etiology of any anemia is to obtain the appropriate history, physical examination, and laboratory tests. This initial step will aid in the formulation of the differential diagnosis to distinguish between an acquired and genetically inherited anemia. In this chapter the acquired types of anemia in pregnancy will be described (Table 6.1).

By and large, pregnant women with anemia are asymptomatic in part because of the increase in blood volume. Furthermore, the physical examination is usually nondiagnostic. However, occasional diagnostic findings can be identified, such as glossitis (nutritional deficiencies), jaundice (hemolytic problems), petechiae (coagulopathies), skeletal abnormalities (hemoglobin sickle cell anemias) and others.

A review of the dietary habits is often helpful in identifying patients with iron deficiency in pregnancy or pica (including ingestion of starch, dirt, or ice). A detailed history will assist in distinguishing between an acquired and genetically inherited anemia.

The basic laboratory work-up includes a complete blood count, peripheral blood smear, iron studies, and urinalysis. Patients at risk for sickle cell anemia should also have a sickle cell screen. Rarely, a peripheral smear can be helpful in suggesting a diagnosis, and frequently additional tests will be required, for example, a hypochromic microcytic smear may be indicative of either an iron-deficiency anemia or a hemoglobinopathy (thalassemia or others). Additional tests will distinguish between these conditions (Table 6.2).

Table 6.2 Comparison of iron deficiency and β-thalassemia minor

	Mean cell volume (fl)	Iron reserves	Hematocrit (%)	Red cell distribution	HgbA$_2$
Iron deficiency	Variable	Low	<30	Elevated	Normal
β-Thalassemia minor	<80	Variable	Variable	Normal	Elevated

Iron-deficiency anemia

It appears that the most beneficial diagnostic laboratory tests in pregnancy are iron studies. The findings listed in Table 6.3 will be diagnostic of iron-deficiency anemia. The best laboratory test for iron deficiency is the measurement of the serum ferritin, which is directly related to stored iron. Twenty percent of pregnant women with a normal serum ferritin value may be iron-deficient. The definitive diagnostic test is bone marrow aspiration; staining for iron is a rarely indicated procedure.

The ideal body iron content in the adult woman is 3.5–4 g. Approximately 60–70% is contained in circulating hemoglobin; the remainder is stored iron in the form of ferritin and hemosiderin in the liver, spleen, and bone marrow.

Pregnancy requires an additional 700–1200 mg of iron. Of this, 200–300 mg is transferred to the fetus. Most of the iron requirements of pregnancy are in the second half of pregnancy, and they are approximately 5–6 mg/day. An average balanced diet will supply *only* 1–2 mg/day. Prophylactic iron supplementation in pregnancy is recommended by the World Health Organization and most experts. Daily supplementation with 300 mg ferrous sulfate (which contains 60 mg elemental iron) will satisfy the pregnancy requirements, when it is recognized that only 10–15% of the ingested iron is being absorbed. Women who enter pregnancy with adequate iron stores and receive prophylactic iron will not develop anemia, but most probably deplete their stores at the end of their pregnancy. Only approximately 300 mg is returned to the maternal stores following delivery. It is for this reason that iron supplementation should be recommended for at least 3 months postpartum and all through lactation. (See Table 6.4 for iron preparations.)

Table 6.3 Iron studies diagnostic of iron-deficiency anemia

Serum iron	<60 µg/dl
Iron-binding capacity	>300 µg/dl
Transferrin saturation	<15%

Table 6.4 Iron preparations

Preparation	Elemental iron content (%)	Dose containing 60 mg elemental iron (mg)
Ferrous sulfate	20	300
Ferrous fumanate	30	200
Ferrous gluconate	11	550

Table 6.5 Factors which contribute to or interfere with iron deficiency

Simultaneous intake of milk products
Nausea, vomiting, pica
Irregular intake
Gastrointestinal intolerance to oral iron, malabsorption
Bleeding (nasal, vaginal, rectal)
Multiple gestation

Once iron-deficiency anemia is identified, the treatment requires the administration of 900 mg of oral ferrous sulfate daily. On occasion some women will require parenteral iron therapy; the rapidity of response is the same as for oral iron. However, it is important to point out that there are a variety of factors that could contribute to or interfere with iron deficiency in pregnancy (Table 6.5).

A rise in hemoglobin concentration of 0.2 g/dl associated with an increase in reticulocytes indicates that the patient is responding to treatment.

Blood transfusion is seldom required – the potential risks are obvious (hepatitis, cytomegalovirus, human immunodeficiency virus); however, one must recognize that at hemoglobin levels of 4–6 g/dl there is a maternal risk for high-output cardiac failure and significant risk for fetal hypoxia and demise.

Anemia secondary to blood loss

Anemia secondary to blood loss can be divided into acute and chronic.

Acute blood loss in pregnancy is a relatively common obstetric complication and the different clinical entities have been described elsewhere in this text. It is important, however, to minimize blood loss at the time of delivery and, most significantly, not to underestimate this loss. Approximately 250 mg of iron is lost at the time of delivery. The amount of iron consumed at the time of lactation is relatively small – 1 mg/day – nevertheless, due to the intrapartum and postpartum blood loss, dietary iron supplementation is important during this period.

Chronic blood loss is a complicating factor of many disorders such as hemorrhoids, intestinal disorders, and parasite infections. Most of these anemias will not be eliminated without the initial treatment of the underlying disease.

In acute situations, fluid replacement and blood transfusion may be required. While contemplating administration of blood, the risk of hepatitis, cytomegalovirus, human immunodeficiency virus infection, and the possibility of sensitization to blood antigens should be considered. To restore blood volume, a patient with no hemodynamic changes and stable vital signs could be managed with other fluids and substances rather than whole blood or packed cells.

Megaloblastic anemia

Megaloblastic anemia is a nonspecific term utilized to describe hypo-proliferative disorders that have certain morphologic features, inadequate erythropoiesis, and hemolysis of red blood cells. Two such conditions may be acquired in pregnancy: pernicious anemia caused by vitamin B_{12} deficiency and folate deficiency. The biochemical defect is a deficiency in thymidylate formation, an essential rate-limiting step in DNA synthesis which requires tetrahydrofolic acid as a coenzyme. The vitamin B_{12} and folate deficiency delay DNA synthesis.

Pregnancy is a state of increased requirements for both vitamin B_{12} and folate that could result in megaloblastic anemia. Folic acid deficiency is the most common cause for megaloblastic anemia, while vitamin B_{12} deficiency is extremely uncommon during pregnancy.

Folic acid deficiency

The incidence of this complication has been reported to be between 1 and 30% of singleton pregnancies and 8 times more frequent in twin pregnancies. The folate requirements increase in pregnancy to 150–400 μg/day for singleton and in greater amounts for twin pregnancies.

In experimentally induced folic acid deficiency the following sequential events can be observed: decrease in serum folate in 3 weeks, hyperseg-mented neutrophils in 7 weeks, decrease in red cell folate in 18 weeks, megaloblastic bone marrow in 19 weeks, and anemia in 20 weeks.

The minimum daily requirement of folic acid in pregnancy is 100 μg/day. The recommended daily allowance during pregnancy is 0.5–1 mg/day. Higher doses have been recommended by the Centers for Disease

Control for women who had delivered infants affected with neural tube defects.

A variety of factors may precipitate folic acid deficiency: the fetus, multiple pregnancy, the expanding mass of red blood cells, inadequate diet, prolonged hyperemesis, chronic infection, ethanol, and drugs (nitrofurantoin, hydantoin).

The most prominent clinical features of megaloblastic anemias are roughness of the skin and glossitis. Diagnostic laboratory tests include the use of peripheral blood smears, hemoglobin values, red blood cell indices, and serum folate assay (normal folate values in pregnancy are 5–10 mg/ml). Different embryopathies have been associated with folate deficiency, such as neural tube defects and intrauterine growth retardation.

Hemolytic anemia in pregnancy

Extrinsic or intrinsic factors can lead to red cell defects and hemolysis.

The intrinsic factors include abnormal hemoglobins, enzyme deficiencies, and membrane abnormalities (spherocytosis and elliptocytosis). These patients usually reach the reproductive age and become pregnant after having undergone splenectomy. Their treatment in pregnancy includes folic acid supplementation.

The most common extrinsic acquired hemolytic anemia is drug-induced. It occurs in patients with an inherited enzyme glucose-6-phosphate dehydrogenase deficiency. About 2% of black women are heterozygous for this enzyme deficiency. Some of the common agents that could induce hemolysis in these patients are antimalarial agents, analgesics, and antipyretics (aspirin and phenacetin). This condition is diagnosed by the presence of predominantly immunoglobulin G antibodies on the red cell surface (positive direct Coombs test). When the antibodies are identified, other underlying diseases should be excluded: systemic lupus erythematosus, infections, and lymphoproliferative disorders.

The treatment of hemolytic anemia includes corticosteroids.

SUGGESTED READING

BELL W. Hematologic abnormalities in pregnancy. *Med Clin North Am* 1977;61:165.

CENTERS FOR DISEASE CONTROL. CDC criteria for anemia in children and childbearing age women. *MMWR* 1989;38:400.

CHESLEY LC. Plasma and red cell volumes during pregnancy. *Am J Obstet Gynecol* 1972;112:440.

COOLEY JR, KITAI DZ. Hematologic problems in pregnancy. Obstetric transfusion therapy. *Am J Obstet Gynecol* 1977;128:476.

DALIE JV. Autoimmune hemolytic anemia. *Arch Intern Med* 1975;135:1293.

GILES C. An account of 335 cases of megaloblastic anemia of pregnancy and the puerperium. *J Clin Pathol* 1966;19:1.

KITAI DZ. Folic acid deficiency in pregnancy. *Am J Obstet Gynecol* 1969;104:1067.

PERKINS RP. Inherited disorders of hemoglobin synthesis and pregnancy. *Am J Obstet Gynecol* 1971;111:120.

PITKIN RM. Nutritional influences during pregnancy. *Med Clin North Am* 1977; 61:3.

PRITCHARD JA, MASON RA. Iron stores of normal adults and replenishment with iron therapy. *JAMA* 1967;199:897.

PRITCHARD JA, WHALLEY PY, SCOTT DE. The influence of maternal folate and iron deficiencies on intrauterine life. *Am J Obstet Gynecol* 1969;104:388.

ROMSLO I, HARAM K, SAGEN N, *et al.* Iron requirement in normal pregnancy as assessed by serum ferritin, serum transferrin saturation and erythrocyte protomorphyrin determinations. *Br J Obstet Gynaecol* 1983;90:101.

ROSZKOWSKI I, WOJCICKA J, ZALESKA K. Serum iron deficiency during the third trimester of pregnancy: maternal complications and fate of pregnancy: maternal complications and fate of the neonate. *Obstet Gynecol* 1966;28:820.

WERNER EY, STOCKMAN JA. Red cell disturbances in the feto-maternal unit. *Semin Perinatol* 1983;7:139.

7

Deep venous thrombosis and pulmonary embolism in pregnancy: diagnosis

MARTIN N. MONTORO

Venous thromboembolism during pregnancy does not occur frequently, but it is potentially fatal. However, with a prompt diagnosis and appropriate treatment, a favorable outcome will result in many cases. Therefore a thorough knowledge of this disease entity is of the utmost importance for all of those involved in the care of pregnant women.

Pathophysiology

Pregnancy causes many changes in the coagulation and fibrinolytic systems: increased levels of factor VII, resulting in shortening of the prothrombin time (PT), and increased levels of circulating fibrinogen, just to name a few. These changes, however, have not been clearly associated with the risk of thrombosis during the gestational period itself.

There are several well-accepted risk factors for venous thrombosis (VT) and pulmonary embolism (PE) in the general population (trauma, surgery, immobilization, advancing age, obesity, previous thromboembolism, neoplasia) which, if present, also increase the risk of thromboembolism during pregnancy. There are other conditions known to increase the risk of thrombosis in the general population which will also increase the risk for pregnant women when present: these include deficiencies (usually hereditary and present in other family members) of antithrombin III, proteins C, S, and plasminogen, or the presence of the lupus anticoagulant (usually acquired, e.g., in systemic lupus erythematosus, and may be present before the other clinical manifestations of lupus appear). Except for the lupus anticoagulant which may prolong the partial thromboplastin time (PTT), none of the others can be detected by the standard coagulation screening tests and need to be specifically ordered when indicated, such as in patients with recurrent or unusually severe thromboembolism.

In most pregnant women (90–92%) with a single episode of VT or PE, no apparent underlying risk factors can be found, except that most cases tend to occur in the postpartum period, particularly after cesarean section or a traumatic delivery in overweight women. Only in 8–10% of the cases is a specific cause found, such as one of the hereditary or acquired coagulation disorders mentioned above.

Incidence

There have been wide discrepancies in the reported estimates in the literature. The reasons are probably varied, but are most likely due to the different requirements for documentation by objective auxiliary tests. According to those studies which required accurate objective documentation and our own experience at the University of Southern California (USC), the incidence is between 0.08 and 0.26%. A higher incidence in the immediate postpartum period than during pregnancy has been consistently reported by most authors.

PE continues to be reported as a common cause of maternal morbidity and mortality. At our institution for the period of 1957–1981, there were eight instances of maternal deaths due to PE, documented by autopsy, for the 308 509 deliveries during that period of time. However, since 1981 there have been only two episodes of fatal PE in patients without any obvious risk factors, except a cesarean delivery 2 days before. In the last several years, we have acquired a greater knowledge of the natural history of VT, as well as improved diagnostic techniques, particularly by noninvasive procedures. Both improved and standardized anticoagulant protocols have led to a safer and more effective therapy. The lower mortality rate from PE at USC suggests the effectiveness of the application of this knowledge.

Diagnosis

Diagnosis requires a high index of suspicion, good clinical judgment, as well as accurate interpretation of the appropriate objective tests. It is well known that the clinical signs and symptoms of both deep VT (DVT) and PE are, by and large, nonspecific, and that the diagnosis must always be confirmed by objective tests. Even when the clinical picture may seem very suggestive, we should not be tempted to initiate anticoagulant therapy without objective confirmation of the diagnosis. A missed diagnosis may result in a catastrophe which could have been prevented by accurate diagnosis and proper therapy in most cases.

The vast majority of thromboembolic events originate in the lower extremities or the pelvic veins. Recently, more cases of upper-extremity VT have been reported in drug addicts, particularly those using injectable cocaine in the arms. Therefore, more cases may be seen in the future in this population. Still, the overwhelming majority of cases will originate in the lower extremities, and the diagnostic procedures are based on this premise.

Superficial phlebitis

Superficial phlebitis rarely causes important clinical sequelae. It occurs more frequently in women with varicose veins. The diagnosis is clinically obvious (tenderness, erythema, palpable cord) and the treatment is usually symptomatic. Some of these patients may need investigations to exclude DVT, which would require more aggressive treatment, and some may need a brief course of anticoagulation until DVT is excluded.

Calf vein thrombosis

Studies in nonpregnant patients have shown a high incidence (20–30%) of postoperative calf thrombosis in patients who have undergone general surgery and even higher in those who have had orthopedic surgery. Since there are no prospective studies in pregnant women, many authors consider it reasonable to suspect that women undergoing cesarean sections are at a comparable risk. However, it has been suggested that the frequency of calf vein thrombosis (CVT) is probably lower after cesarean section than after abdominal surgery outside of pregnancy. Most of the CVT resolve spontaneously (75–80%) and have a benign course, except when the thrombus propagates into the proximal system (20–25%), in which case there is up to a 50% risk of pulmonary embolism.

The most sensitive test for CVT is the ^{125}I fibrinogen leg scan, which is contraindicated during pregnancy. Noninvasive testing (Doppler or plethysmography) is less sensitive. Contrast venography is the most sensitive test and can be performed safely during pregnancy (pelvic shielding limit exposure to the necessary minimum), but it cannot be performed serially. If the thrombus is confined to the calf, treatment can be withheld provided that the patient can be observed for propagation to the proximal veins. The importance of close observation should be stressed to the patient. Serial impedance plethysmography examinations (every 48–72h) are thought to be adequate to detect extension into the proximal veins. If extension has not occurred after 10 days of surveillance, subsequent extension and embolization are believed to be unlikely and treatment unnecessary. The cost of serial impedance plethysmography is about the same as that of a venogram.

Deep proximal vein thrombosis

DVT always requires confirmation by objective testing, since it has been shown in clinical trials that a diagnosis based on history and physical findings alone will be inaccurate in 50–70% of all cases. The initial examination should include Doppler or impedance plethysmography examinations. A normal test provides good evidence against DVT. Any abnormality can be further studied with colored-flow, real-time, high-resolution ultrasound, to exclude other conditions that may compromise venous return. Causes of false-positive tests when only Doppler or impedance plethysmography are done include: congestive heart failure, extrinsic compression on the deep venous system (e.g., term-size uterus), lower-extremity swelling of other causes, and excessive leg tension (e.g., inability to relax due to pain). The sensitivity of Doppler/impedance plethysmography alone for proximal DVT is reported at 83–93%, and when computerized colored-flow ultrasound is also performed, the sensitivity is even higher, equaling, if not surpassing, that of the venogram. Unlike venograms, they can allow serial evaluations and are noninvasive. Recent studies have reported that the use of real-time ultrasonic visualization of the deep venous system has a 95% sensitivity and 99% specificity in the detection of proximal DVT in symptomatic patients. However, the accuracy in asymptomatic patients is still reported to be much lower (e.g., screening in high-risk postoperative patients). This degree of accuracy has dramatically changed the diagnostic approach to suspected VT.

Only when the distinction between thrombosis and other causes of venous obstruction cannot be reliably made by noninvasive techniques should a venogram be performed to confirm or exclude the diagnosis. This is a rare occurrence at present. Magnetic resonance imaging and/or computed tomography scan have been used in an effort to diagnose pelvic vein thrombosis, with mixed success thus far.

Pulmonary embolism

The common signs and symptoms of PE (dyspnea, chest pain, tachypnea, tachycardia, hemoptysis, hypotension, cyanosis, syncope) are nonspecific and may be seen in patients with other conditions. Some patients may develop PE without specific symptoms or signs at first.

Data from the Urokinase Collaborative Study showed that 10–11%

of patients suffering a pulmonary embolus die within 1 h of the event. In those surviving the initial episode, if the diagnosis was again missed or delayed there was an additional 30% mortality. In great contrast, if the diagnosis was made and the appropriate treatment started in a timely fashion, the survival rate was 92–95%. This information greatly underscores the importance of prompt diagnosis and treatment in all cases of PE.

A high index of suspicion is needed for the diagnosis of pulmonary embolism; in patients with VT or risk factors for thromboembolism, one should always be on the alert. The clinical diagnosis alone is unreliable and confirmation by objective criteria is always necessary, either by lung scanning or pulmonary angiogram. Other tests (EKG, blood gases (hypoxia), etc.) may provide some information, but are not diagnostic. Pulmonary angiography is the most specific diagnostic test, but it is not usually recommended during pregnancy because of radiation exposure to the fetus and possible hazard of the test to the mother; however, if performed carefully and by experienced personnel, it is a relatively safe procedure. Therefore, during gestation the diagnosis of PE is highly dependent on the lung scan and its limitations must be thoroughly understood in order to make responsible management decisions.

Perfusion lung scans are very sensitive for the detection of PE, but they are not specific and a variety of other conditions must be excluded (e.g., pneumonia, atelectasis, pleural effusion, pulmonary edema, tumors). A chest X-ray must always be obtained before the lung scan is interpreted. In an effort to increase the specificity of the perfusion lung scan, a ventilation scan is frequently performed as well. (Ventilation/perfusion scans are usually abbreviated as *V/Q* scans). A normal perfusion scan and a normal chest X-ray exclude PE, and a ventilation scan is unnecessary. A segmental or a lobar perfusion defect which is clear on the X-ray and normally ventilated on the ventilation scan gives a high probability of PE. However, if both the ventilation and perfusion scans show "matched" defects, the likelihood of PE is decreased (low probability), although not completely excluded. Small perfusion defects are considered nonspecific, even if ventilation is normal; these small defects are abnormal, but not definitive for the diagnosis of PE.

There are patients whose scans are not definitively diagnostic, and management decisions may have to be made without a specific diagnosis. In these patients, obtaining additional data might be helpful (e.g., noninvasive studies for lower-extremity DVT, in an effort to find a source of PE). Nevertheless, in a small number of patients, the diagnosis cannot be definitively excluded or confirmed; in these cases, most physicians will choose to treat rather than proceed to a pulmonary angiogram while the patient is still pregnant, knowing that the diagnosis may not be completely accurate. In those patients who are already postpartum, a pulmonary angiogram can be performed if indicated, thus eliminating the need for unnecessary treatment if PE is not present. Outside of pregnancy, it has been very recently reported that patients with abnormal lung scans but "low probability" for PE, and negative serial testing for proximal DVT, can be safely followed and have a good prognosis without anticoagulant therapy (and without a pulmonary angiogram). Whether or not this management strategy can be also applied to pregnancy or the postpartum period remains to be seen.

SUGGESTED READING

BARNES RW, WU KK, HOAK JC. Fallibility of the clinical diagnosis of venous thrombosis. *JAMA* 1974;234:605–607.

BERGQUIST D, HEDNER U. Pregnancy and venous thromboembolism. *Acta Obstet Gynecol Scand* 1983;62:449–453.

BERGQUIST A, BERGQUIST D, HALLBOOK T. Deep vein thrombosis during pregnancy: a prospective study. *Acta Obstet Gynecol Scand* 1983;62:443–448.

DAVIDSON BL, ELLIOTT CG, LENSING AW. Low accuracy of color Doppler ultrasound in the detection of proximal leg vein thrombosis in asymptomatic high risk patients. *Ann Intern Med* 1992;117:735–738.

HUISMAN MV, BULLER HR, TEN CATE JW, VREEKEN J. Serial impedance plethysmography for suspected deep venous thrombosis in outpatients. *N Engl J Med* 1986;314:823–828.

HULL RD, RASKOB GE, COATES G, et al. A new non-invasive management strategy for patients with suspected pulmonary embolism. *Arch Intern Med* 1989;149:2549–2551.

LENSING AW, PRANDONI P, BRANDJES D, et al. Detection of deep vein thrombosis by real time B-mode ultrasonography. *N Engl J Med* 1989;320:342–345.

UROKINASE PULMONARY EMBOLISM TRIAL. A national cooperative study. *Circulation* (Suppl II) 1973;4:1–108.

WHITE RH, McGAHAN JP, DASCHBACH MM, HARTLING RP. Diagnosis of deep vein thrombosis using duplex ultrasound. *Ann Intern Med* 1989;111:297–304.

8

Deep venous thrombosis and pulmonary embolism in pregnancy: treatment

MARTIN N. MONTORO

Anticoagulant therapy

The diagnosis of venous thrombosis (VT) or pulmonary embolism (PE) must be firmly established prior to treatment, since anticoagulant therapy can be potentially dangerous. Heparin is the drug of choice for the pregnant woman because it is a large molecule and it does not cross the placental barrier. Unfortunately, it can only be administered parenterally. When there is a strong clinical suspicion of PE, heparin therapy should be initiated immediately, followed by the appropriate tests to confirm the diagnosis. In cases of VT alone, anticoagulant treatment is delayed until the diagnosis has been firmly established.

Oral anticoagulants (coumarin derivatives) have been shown to be dangerous to the fetus since they cross the placental barrier readily. Potential complications are warfarin embryopathy when given in the first trimester, which includes nasal hypoplasia, depression of the bridge of the nose, and epiphyseal stippling with irregular bone growth similar to chondrodysplasia punctata. Central nervous system and a variety of eye defects have been observed, irrespective of when warfarin is given, and fetal hemorrhage may occur following warfarin administration in the third trimester or during labor. Women who are on long-term anti-coagulant therapy should be converted to heparin, ideally prior to pregnancy. Some authors continue to advocate the safety of warfarin if given only during the second trimester. This recommendation still makes it necessary to change to heparin prior to pregnancy, then back to warfarin during the second trimester, and back to heparin for the third trimester.

This is complicated, requires more tests and, probably, hospitalizations. Above all, the safety of warfarin even when given only in the second trimester has not been established (probably due to fetal hemorrhage and subsequent scar formation).

Carefully monitored heparin therapy is very effective and safe during pregnancy. A measurable heparin concentration is needed to prevent propagation of thrombosis (0.2–0.4 U/ml). The response of the individual patient is variable and, consequently, monitoring is needed to maintain heparin levels within the therapeutic range. Heparin does not dissolve clots by itself (this is accomplished by the fibrinolytic system): it inhibits the coagulation process by binding to antithrombin III, which in turn facilitates its binding and the neutralization of thrombin and factors IXa, Xa, XIa, and XIIa.

The most accepted method of heparin administration is by continuous intravenous infusion; it produces a steady state of heparin concentration, a reduced incidence of major hemorrhagic events, particularly in those patients at higher risk of hemorrhage (recent surgery or other invasive procedures), and facilitates monitoring. The most commonly used test for monitoring heparin therapy is the activated partial thromboplastin time (aPTT). The therapeutic goal is to prolong it 2–2.5 times the control. Heparin levels are more sensitive, but at present they are not available in the USA except in research institutions. It is our hope that tests which measure heparin as antifactor Xa activity will be available soon, since it is reported that these tests are more sensitive than the aPTT. These tests are commercially available in many other countries.

Other drugs that are sometimes used outside of pregnancy are not safe or effective during gestation, e.g., aspirin, dipyridamole (Persantin), streptokinase, urokinase, TPA, etc. Dextran has been reported as somewhat effective in a few studies, but it is not widely used. Very seldom, interruption of the inferior vena cava to prevent recurrent pulmonary embolization might be considered in the face of failure or contraindication to anticoagulant therapy. Despite the relatively frequent reports of the use (outside of pregnancy) of inferior vena cava filters, there are no controlled studies and many questions remain about their indications, safety, and effectiveness. Their use during pregnancy should be considered only under exceptional circumstances.

Long-term anticoagulant therapy

After the initial treatment by continuous heparin infusion, anticoagulants should be continued to prevent recurrences. For calf vein thrombosis, 6 weeks is usually sufficient. For deep VT (DVT) or PE, anticoagulant therapy should be continued for at least 3 months or longer if there is a persisting underlying cause or risk factor. Oral anticoagulants can be used postpartum, even if the mother chooses to breast-feed, since they are reported to pass into breast milk in small amounts only. Measurement of the prothrombin time (PT) is used to monitor the anticoagulant effect of warfarin. Heparin therapy should be continued until the PT becomes prolonged to a therapeutic level – usually 1.5–2.5 the control. Periodic monitoring and adjustment of the dose is mandatory in order to minimize the risk of bleeding, which is the main danger of therapy with both warfarin and heparin.

Subcutaneous heparin is used during pregnancy because of the adverse effects of warfarin on the fetus. The daily requirements are the same as the 24-h intravenous amount that was required to produce full anticoagulation. It is then divided into two equal injections every 12 h subcutaneously. The heparin activity can be assessed by an aPTT 6 h after the injection, and the dose adjusted to achieve the desired effect (this is called adjusted subcutaneous heparin). Heparin levels can be used in a similar manner when available. The patient must learn the correct technique for subcutaneous injection, using disposable insulin or tuberculin syringes; we usually recommend concentrated heparin solutions of 20 000 U/ml. Therapy is stopped at the first signs of labor, and most of the time the effect of heparin will have disappeared by the time of delivery. Epidural anesthesia should be avoided if there is even the slightest risk of residual heparin effect (check coagulation tests!) and, therefore, bleeding. Rarely, neutralization of heparin with protamine might be required.

After delivery, intravenous heparin is resumed, anywhere from 6 to 24 h postpartum depending on the type of delivery, amount of bleeding, etc. For long-term therapy, either warfarin or adjusted-dose subcutaneous heparin can be used for continued secondary prophylaxis after delivery, and continued for as long as it is indicated.

Inadequate therapy for proximal DVT carries a 20–50% risk of recurrent DVT and PE.

It has recently been reported that certain heparin fractions of low molecular weight are as effective as unfractionated standard heparin in preventing VT and, in addition, they may cause less bleeding (perhaps by producing less inhibition of platelet function). There are no published studies to assess their efficacy during pregnancy, but they are likely to be as effective as when used in the nonpregnant state, and without danger to the fetus, because these heparin fractions are still large enough that they cannot cross the placenta.

Prevention of venous thrombosis

There is no uniform agreement as to which patients need prophylaxis, nor on the specific measures needed.

We recommend prophylaxis: (1) for patients with previous thrombosis, if there is evidence of residual symptomatology (e.g., chronic venous insufficiency or postphlebitic syndrome); (2) for those patients with a history of recurrent thrombosis; and (3) for those with a single episode but with lupus anticoagulant, anticardiolipin antibodies, antithrombin III deficiency, etc. present in their serum. Some investigators also recommend prophylaxis for any pregnant woman with a previous VT, even without residual symptoms, if it had occurred during a high estrogen exposure period, such as a previous pregnancy or while on birth control pills. In these cases, other authors recommend observation only during pregnancy and prophylaxis only for 4–6 weeks after delivery.

Small doses of heparin (5000 U every 12 h) are favored by some clinicians. There is no definite evidence that this method results in a reduction of VT during pregnancy. We prefer continuous surveillance without therapy in those women with a history of a single episode of thrombosis outside of pregnancy, without residual symptoms, with normal Doppler impedance plethysmography studies and negative serology (lupus anticoagulant, etc.). For those patients with definite risk factors (residual from old VT, history of recurrent thrombosis, etc.), adjusted-dose subcutaneous heparin should be given during pregnancy and postpartum. Recent reports from outside the USA describe the need to use less heparin when its activity is measured by the more sensitive method of antifactor Xa activity, rather than the aPTT, thus decreasing the risks of prolonged heparin treatment, such as bleeding, osteoporosis, thrombocytopenia and, not the least of all, expense.

Nondrug ways to reduce the risk of thromboembolism should also be used whenever possible: these include intermittent pneumatic leg compression during surgery, antiembolic stockings, leg elevation and early, postoperative ambulation.

SUGGESTED READING

BELL WE. Heparin-associated thrombocytopenia and thrombosis. *J Lab Clin Med* 1988;111:600–605.

DAHLMAN T, HELLGREN M, BLOMBACK M. Thrombosis prophylaxis in pregnancy with use of subcutaneous heparin adjusted by monitoring heparin concentration in plasma. *Am J Obstet Gynecol* 1989;161:420–425.

GINSBERG JS, KOWALCHUK G, HIRSH J, *et al*. Heparin therapy during pregnancy. Risks to the fetus and mother. *Arch Intern Med* 1989;149:2233–2236.

HELLGREN M, NYGARDS EB. Long-term therapy with subcutaneous heparin during pregnancy. *Gynecol Obstet Invest* 1982;13:79–89.

HOWELL R, FIDLER J, LETSKY E. The risk of antenatal subcutaneous heparin prophylaxis: controlled trial. *Br J Obstet Gynaecol* 1983;90:1124–1128.

HULL RD, RASKOB GE, PINEO GF, *et al*. Subcutaneous low-molecular weight heparin compared with continuous intravenous heparin in the treatment of proximal-vein thrombosis. *N Engl J Med* 1992;326:975–982.

ORME ML, LEWIS PJ, DESWIET M, *et al.* May mothers given warfarin breast-feed their infants? *Br Med J* 1977;1:1564.

RESEARCH COMMITTEE OF THE BRITISH THORACIC SOCIETY. Optimum duration of anticoagulation for deep-vein thrombosis and pulmonary embolism. *Lancet* 1992;240:873–876.

STEVENSON RE, BURTON OM, FERLANTO GJ, *et al.* Hazards of oral anticoagulants during pregnancy. *JAMA* 1980;243:1549–1551.

TENGBORN L, BERGQVIST D, MATZSCH T, *et al.* Recurrent thromboembolism in pregnancy and puerperium. Is there a need for thromboprophylaxis? *Am J Obstet Gynecol* 1989;160:90–94.

9

Urinary tract infections complicating pregnancy

LYNNAE K. MILLAR

Urinary tract infections (UTI) are among the most significant medical complications of pregnancy. There are three types of UTI: asymptomatic bacteriuria (ASB), cystitis, and pyelonephritis. Many of the normal physiologic changes that occur during pregnancy place the pregnant female at increased risk for symptomatic UTI, particularly acute pyelonephritis. Acute pyelonephritis occurs more frequently in patients with ASB antedating pregnancy, thus screening and treatment of ASB in pregnancy are important.

Asymptomatic bacteriuria

ASB is defined as persistent bacterial colonization of the urinary tract. Patients have no signs or symptoms of cystitis or pyelonephritis. Traditionally, ASB has been diagnosed in patients having >100 000 CFU/ml of a single uropathogen on two consecutive first-void clean-catch urine specimens. More recently, the isolation of >20 000 CFU/ml of a single bacterium has been associated with subsequent development of pyelonephritis. Urine samples obtained by urethral catheterization yielding a single uropathogen confirm bacteriuria but are usually unnecessary for the diagnosis of ASB unless repeatedly contaminated specimens are obtained and the diagnosis is in question.

ASB occurs in 2–10% of pregnant women. This is similar to the incidence in nonpregnant women, therefore pregnancy is not felt to be a predisposing factor in the development of ASB. If left untreated, 20–30% of pregnant females with ASB will develop pyelonephritis. Adequate antimicrobial treatment of ASB will reduce the development of pyelone-phritis to 3%. Therefore, an early urine culture will identify the majority of patients at risk for subsequent development of pyelonephritis in pregnancy.

The prevalence of ASB is inversely related to socioeconomic status, and is markedly elevated in the indigent population. Patients with diabetes mellitus and sickle cell trait or disease are also at increased risk.

The uropathogens most commonly isolated in ASB are similar to those isolated in cystitis and pyelonephritis. *Escherichia coli* is the primary pathogen in 70–80% of cases. Other pathogens include: *Klebsiella pneumoniae, Proteus mirabilis, Pseudomonas aeruginosa, Enterobacter* species, *Staphylococcus saphrophyticus, Enterococcus* and group B β-hemolytic *Streptococcus*. The identification of more than one species of bacteria in a urine culture, or the presence of *Propionibacterium* or *Lactobacillus*, usually indicates a contaminated specimen. If contamination is suspected the urine culture should be repeated.

Urine cultures are expensive and multiple other screening tests have been developed as alternatives to screen for ASB. The value and utility of these alternative tests vary depending on the method used. Before using a specific test, the clinician should understand the sensitivity, specificity, positive predictive value (PPV), and negative predictive value (NPV) of the test.

Currently at our institution all patients presenting for prenatal care are screened for ASB with a first-void clean-catch urine culture. If this is negative, a clean-catch urine specimen is obtained at each subsequent prenatal visit and is tested for the presence of nitrites and leukocyte esterase (Chemstrip LN test). Assessments of the sensitivity of the Chemstrip LN test vary from 50 to 92%. Specificity ranges from 65 to 95%. It is accurate at identifying patients without ASB (NPV = 99.2%). This test fails to identify patients with gram-positive ASB.

Patients with positive initial urine cultures are appropriately treated with antibiotic therapy. Urine cultures are obtained after completion of therapy to verify eradication of the bacteria. These patients are followed throughout their pregnancy with monthly urine cultures as there is a significant risk of recurrence of ASB. Regardless of the treatment chosen, or duration of therapy, approximately 30% of those women will develop recurrent bacteriuria during the course of their pregnancy.

Women who experience a relapse (same uropathogen) or reinfection (new uropathogen) should be treated with a second course of antibiotics. Patients with a third episode of bacteriuria should be suppressed for the duration of their pregnancy.

A fluorescein-tagged antiglobulin can be utilized to identify antibody-coated bacteria (renal in origin) in patients with ASB. Applying this

Table 9.1 Initial antibiotic choice for asymptomatic bacteriuria

Drug	Dosage	Schedule
Nitrofurantoin	100 mg	q.i.d. × 10 days
Ampicillin	500 mg	q.i.d. × 10 days
Cephalexin	250 mg	q.i.d. × 10 days
Sulfisoxazole	500 mg	q.i.d. × 10 days
Single-dose therapy		
Nitrofurantoin	200 mg	
Amoxycillin	3 g	
Cephalexin	2 g	
Sulfisoxazole	2 g	

technique it was demonstrated that approximately half of the bacteriuria was renal in origin and the other half was localized to the bladder. Relapses tend to occur in the first 2 weeks after completion of therapy and are more commonly associated with renal bacteriuria. Because renal bacteriuria is difficult to eradicate, relapses should be treated with a 2–3-week course of antibiotic therapy. Reinfections can be treated with a standard 10-day course of antibiotics.

It is indisputable that pregnant patients with ASB are at increased risk for the development of cystitis and pyelonephritis. However, recent studies have failed to confirm prior reports that untreated ASB is associated with an increased incidence of preterm birth and low birth weight. Similarly, ASB does not appear to be associated with preeclampsia or anemia.

A variety of antibiotics have been used to treat ASB and appear to be equally efficacious. Recommended initial treatment regimens can be seen in Table 9.1. Second courses of antibiotics for relapses or recurrences should be chosen based on urine cultures and sensitivities. Patients with persistent bacteriuria despite two courses of antibiotic therapy should be suppressed for the duration of their pregnancy and the first 2 weeks postpartum with nitrofurantoin 100 mg at bedtime.

Single-dose antibiotic therapy has been shown to be effective to treat ASB in nonpregnant women. These treatment regimens have not been adequately evaluated in pregnant women; however, studies to date show single-dose regimens to be equally efficacious as standard 10-day regimens in eradicating bacteriuria. Recommended single-dose therapies can be seen in Table 9.1. These types of antibiotic regimens may be particularly useful in noncompliant patients.

Before prescribing antibiotics the physician should be aware of complications and side-effects of the medications being utilized. Anaphylaxis to penicillins and cephalosphorins has been well documented. Sulfonamides prescribed in the third trimester can result in fetal kernicterus. Nitrofurantoin can cause hemolysis in patients or in the fetus with glucose-6-phosphate dehydrogenase deficiency. Trimethoprim–sulfamethoxazole is contraindicated in pregnancy due to potential teratogenic effects.

It has been demonstrated that most women with urinary tract infections have chronic bladder or renal anomalies. Many have historical and cystometric evidence of infrequent voiding resulting in a large bladder. Therefore all pregnant women with urinary tract infections should be encouraged to void frequently (at least every 3 h).

In summary, ASB occurs in 2–10% of pregnant women. Patients with untreated ASB are at increased risk for the development of pyelonephritis. Treating patients with ASB can prevent up to 80% of the cases of pyelonephritis that would occur without initial screening and treatment. Therefore all patients should be screened and treated for ASB in pregnancy.

Cystitis

Acute bacterial cystitis complicates 1–2% of pregnancies. The most common symptoms include dysuria, frequency, and urgency. Urine cultures are positive for >100 000 CFU/ml of a single uropathogen. Antepartum surveillance programs designed to eradicate bacteriuria have had no effect on the incidence of cystitis, therefore it appears most cases of cystitis arise *de novo*. Most women developing cystitis during pregnancy have negative screening cultures at initial prenatal evaluation, and cystitis is not associated with subsequent pyelonephritis. Fluorescein-coated antibody techniques have shown that most bacteria recovered from the urine of patients with acute cystitis are not antibody-coated, therefore most cases of cystitis arise from the bladder. The diagnosis of urethral syndrome should be considered in patients presenting with symptoms of cystitis and negative urine cultures. These patients should have urethral cultures sent for chlamydial culture.

The bacterium isolated from women with cystitis is similar to that isolated in patients with ASB or pyelonephritis. Treatment for acute cystitis is the same as that for ASB. Urine culture should be repeated following therapy and monthly throughout pregnancy.

SUGGESTED READING

DIOKNO AC, COMPTON A, SESKI J, VINSON R. Urologic evaluation of urinary tract infection in pregnancy. *J Reprod Med* 1986;31:23–26.

GERSTNER GJ, MULLER G, NAHLER G. Amoxicillin in the treatment of asymptomatic bacteriuria in pregnancy: a single dose of 3 gm amoxicillin versus a 4-day course of 3 doses 750 mg amoxicillin. *Gynecol Obstet Invest* 1989;27:84–87.

GOLAN A, WEXLER S, AMI TA, GORDON D, DAVID MP. Asymptomatic bacteriuria in normal and high-risk pregnancy. *Eur J Obstet Gynecol* 1989;33:101–108.

GORDAN MC, HANKINS GD. Urinary tract infections and pregnancy. *Compr Ther* 1989;15:52–58.

JAKOBI P, NEIGER R, MERZBACH D, PALDI E. Single-dose antimicrobial therapy in the treatment of asymptomatic bacteriuria in pregnancy. *Am J Obstet Gynecol* 1987;156:1148–1152.

LINDHEIMER MD, KATZ AI. The kidney in pregnancy. In: Brenner BM, Rector FC Jr, eds. *The Kidney*. 3rd edn. Philadelphia, PA: WB Saunders. 1986;2:651.

MCNEELEY SG. Treatment of urinary tract infections during pregnancy. *Clin Obstet Gynecol* 1988;31:480–487.

STAMM WE, COUNTY GW, RUNNING UR, *et al.* Diagnosis of culiform infection in acutely dysuric women. *N Engl J Med* 1982;307:463.

VANDORSTEN JP, BANNISTER ER. Office diagnosis of asymptomatic bacteriuria in pregnant women. *Am J Obstet Gynecol* 1986;155:777–780.

10

Pyelonephritis in pregnancy

LYNNAE K. MILLAR

Acute pyelonephritis occurs in 1–2% of all pregnancies and can result in marked maternal and fetal morbidity. Women with a history of pyelonephritis, urinary tract malformations, or calculi are at increased risk for the development of pyelonephritis and should be screened monthly with urine cultures. Eighty percent of pyelonephritis in pregnancy occurs antepartum and 20% occurs in the postpartum period.

Clinical signs and symptoms of acute pyelonephritis include: fever, shaking chills, flank pain, nausea and vomiting, costovertebral angle tenderness, and symptoms of cystitis. Diagnosis is confirmed by urine culture. Since the urine culture takes at least 24 h, the physician must rely on urinalysis for preliminary diagnosis. One or two bacteria/high-power field in an unspun catheterized urine specimen, or >20 bacteria/high-power field in spun urine correlates closely with >100 000 CFU/ml bacteria on urine culture. Pyuria is also common in pyelonephritis and the presence of white blood cell casts confirms the diagnosis.

Most patients with pyelonephritis are dehydrated and 15–20% have bacteremia. Hospitalization is recommended for intravenous hydration and strict monitoring of urinary output. A complete blood count, serum creatinine, and electrolytes should be obtained upon admission. Generally blood and urine cultures are obtained; however, this practice has been questioned as cultures are expensive and results seldom return in time to affect therapy. Currently at our institution urine and blood cultures are obtained, and patients with bacteremia are treated with a minimum of 5 days of intravenous antibiotic therapy.

Uropathogens isolated in pyelonephritis are similar to those in asymptomatic bacteriuria (ASB) and cystitis. The most common uropathogen is *Escherichia coli*. Historically ampicillin was the first-line treatment for pyelonephritis; however, it has fallen into disfavor as many uropathogens have become resistant to this antibiotic. Currently first-line antimicrobial therapy usually consists of a first-generation cephalosporin. Cefazolin 1 g every 8 h is the standard initial therapy at our institution. Unfortunately, *in vitro* antimicrobial resistance is now reported to some of the first-generation cephalosporins. This has not affected *in vivo* treatment efficacy at our institution to date, probably because high urinary tract concentrations of drug are achieved at recommended dosages, compared to minuscule doses of antibiotic tested against bacteria in the *in vitro* setting. The "extended-spectrum" penicillins, mezlocillin and piperacillin, have excellent coverage and could be considered as alternative antibiotics.

Patients appropriately treated for pyelonephritis usually respond within 48 h. Failure to improve clinically within 72 h suggests bacterial resistance to the antibiotic being utilized, urolithiasis, or urinary tract abnormalities. These patients should be reevaluated, cultures should be checked, and patients should be switched to an aminoglycoside. Gentamicin 80 mg every 8 h may be used provided the bacteria are sensitive to this antibiotic. Aminoglycoside levels should be monitored as renal dysfunction commonly occurs with pyelonephritis. Patients with recurrent pyelonephritis, or who fail to respond rapidly to an aminoglycoside, should have an intravenous pyelogram or a renal ultrasound done to look for renal calculi or urinary tract abnormalities. If an intravenous pyelogram is performed while the patient is pregnant, only one exposure at 20 min should be obtained to minimize radiation exposure to the fetus.

Intravenous antibiotic therapy should be continued until the patient is afebrile for at least 48 h; the patient can then be switched to oral antibiotic therapy. The complete course of antibiotics should last at least 2 weeks. After completion of antibiotic therapy a urine culture should be obtained to verify resolution of bacteriuria. Cultures should be obtained at monthly intervals for the duration of the pregnancy.

Some investigators have reported a decreased incidence of recurrent pyelonephritis in patients treated with nitrofurantoin suppression for the duration of their pregnancy. Other physicians feel monthly cultures are adequate to screen for recurrent bacteriuria. At our hospital all patients are placed on nitrofurantoin suppression 100 mg each night until they are 6 weeks postpartum.

Improved antibiotic regimens in recent years have decreased the incidence of low-birth-weight (LBW) and preterm delivery in patients with acute pyelonephritis. The incidence of LBW in the general population is 9%; the incidence of LBW with pyelonephritis ranges from 9 to 13%. Thus, pyelonephritis is not a significant cause of preterm delivery and LBW.

Patients with pyelonephritis often have anemia and decreased serum potassium levels, and can have elevated serum creatinine levels due to a transient decrease in creatinine clearance. Up to 25% of patients with pyelonephritis have seriously diminished glomerular filtration rates. These laboratory abnormalities do not usually require treatment and resolve spontaneously as the pyelonephritis resolves, although sometimes abnormal renal function and anemia can persist for weeks. Acute renal failure necessitating dialysis can occur but is extremely rare.

Thrombocytopenia and minimal elevation of fibrin split products have been identified in the serum of patients with pyelonephritis. This is seldom of clinical significance and resolves with treatment of the disease. The consumptive coagulopathy appears to be secondary to bacterial endotoxin release.

Septic shock is the most significant complication of pyelonephritis; however, it is seldom seen in recent years due to aggressive treatment with broad-spectrum intravenous antibiotic therapy. Women with septic shock appear seriously ill and frequently have multisystem failure. Endotoxemia causes capillary endothelial damage and severely diminished vascular resistance with low cardiac output. This hypotension fails to respond to intravenous fluids. These patients need to be admitted to the intensive care unit with careful observation of vital signs and urinary output. Antibiotics should be instituted immediately. Pulmonary artery catheterization is often required to manage the patient adequately. Dopamine may be necessary to maintain a systolic blood pressure of at least 90 mmHg. Respiratory insufficiency, toxic hepatitis, and disseminated intravascular coagulopathy are commonly seen in conjunction with septic shock.

Respiratory insufficiency is perhaps the most common serious complication of pyelonephritis. It has been estimated to occur in as many as 1 in 50 women with the disease. Bacterial endotoxin release alters the alveolar-capillary membrane permeability with subsequent pulmonary edema. In most patients the respiratory distress is transient and responds rapidly to oxygen; however, in a limited number of patients this complication can be life-threatening, ending in acute respiratory distress syndrome (ARDS). Patients with pulmonary injury will become symptomatic within 48 h of initiation of antibiotic therapy. Tachypnea in patients with pyelonephritis should be promptly investigated with chest X-ray and arterial blood gas analysis. Oxygen should be administered, and severely hypoxemic patients should be intubated and ventilated.

In summary, pyelonephritis is the most common serious medical complication in pregnancy. Patients should be hospitalized and intravenous antibiotic therapy should be initiated. Failure to respond to treatment in 48–72 h should prompt reevaluation of the patient. Patients should be monitored closely for the development of septic shock or ARDS as these are life-threatening complications of pyelonephritis. When afebrile for 48 h, patients may be switched to oral antibiotics. After the antibiotic course has been completed women should be followed with monthly urine cultures to monitor for recurrent bacteriuria for the duration of their pregnancy.

SUGGESTED READING

CUNNINGHAM FG. Urinary tract infections complicating pregnancy. *Bailliere's Clin Obstet Gynaecol* 1987;1:891–909.

CUNNINGHAM FG, LUCAS MJ, HANKINS GD. Pulmonary injury complicating antepartum pyelonephritis. *Am J Obstet Gynecol* 1987;156:797–807.

FARO S, PASTOREK JG, PLAUCHE WG, *et al.* Short-course parenteral antibiotic therapy for pyelonephritis in pregnancy. *Southern Med J* 1984;77:455.

GILSTRAP LC, CUNNINGHAM FG, WHALLEY PJ. Acute pyelonephritis in pregnancy: an anterospective study. *Obstet Gynecol* 1980;57:409–413.

HARRIS RE, GILSTRAP LC. Prevention of recurrent pyelonephritis during pregnancy. *Obstet Gynecol* 1974;44:637–641.

LENKE RR, VANDORSTEN JP, SCHIFRIN BS. Pyelonephritis in pregnancy: a prospective randomized trial to prevent recurrent disease evaluating suppressive therapy with nitrofurantoin and close surveillance. *Am J Obstet Gynecol* 1983;146:953–957.

MACMILLAN MC, GRIMES DA. The limited usefulness of urine and blood cultures in treating pyelonephritis in pregnancy. *Obstet Gynecol* 1991;78:745–748.

VANDORSTEN JP, LENKE RR, SCHIFRIN BS. Pyelonephritis in pregnancy. *J Reprod Med* 1987;32:895–900.

11

Diabetes in pregnancy: diagnosis, classification, and screening

SIRI L. KJOS & JORGE H. MESTMAN

Perinatal mortality in pregnancies complicated by diabetes is approaching that of the general population when major congenital anomalies are excluded. Improved outcome has resulted in part from several technologic advances: (1) improved surveillance of the fetus, utilizing antepartum testing, ultrasound estimation of gestational age and anomalies, maternal serum α-fetoprotein screening, and fetal lung maturation assessment; (2) home blood sugar monitoring, allowing euglycemic blood sugar control; and (3) improved neonatal care and resuscitation.

Classification of diabetes in pregnancy

The best known and most widely used classification of diabetes mellitus in pregnancy is the White classification (Table 11.1). This system is based on the patient's age and duration of disease. From a treatment standpoint it is more useful to group patients into three functional groups (Table 11.2):

1 gestational diabetes (patients developing diabetes for the first time during pregnancy);

2 preconceptional diabetes without diabetic sequelae (both insulin-dependent and noninsulin-dependent diabetes);

3 preconceptional diabetes with significant diabetic sequelae (nephropathy, advanced retinopathy, autonomic neuropathy, or coronary artery disease).

Table 11.1 White classification of diabetes in pregnancy

Class	Age at onset	Duration	Vascular disease	Therapy
A	Any	Any	0	A_1 – Diet A_2 – Insulin
B	>20 years	<10 years	0	Insulin
C	10–19 years	10–19 years	0	Insulin
D	10 or 20	10 or 20	Benign retinopathy	Insulin
F	Any	Any	Nephropathy	Insulin
R	Any	Any	Proliferative retinopathy	Insulin
H	Any	Any	Heart disease	Insulin

Table 11.2 Diabetes mellitus and functional classification in pregnancy

Gestational diabetes	Class A_1 Class A_2 (fasting and postprandial hyperglycemia)
Preconceptional diabetes Without complications	Type I (insulin-dependent) Type II (noninsulin-dependent)
With complications (type I or type II)	Advanced retinopathy Nephropathy Autonomic neuropathy Coronary artery disease

Gestational diabetes

Gestational diabetes is defined by the Third International Workshop Conference on Gestational Diabetes Mellitus as "carbohydrate intolerance of variable severity, with onset or first recognition during the present pregnancy." The majority of women with gestational diabetes are asymptomatic. The incidence varies between 2 and 13% of all pregnant women, being more frequent in certain ethnic groups, such as American Indians, Latinos and blacks. Controversy exists whether all pregnant women should be screened or only those with risk factors for diabetes mellitus (family history of diabetes, history of unexplained stillbirth, malformed or macrosomic infant, presence of maternal hypertension, obesity, or maternal age 30 years or above). The American College of Obstetricians and Gynecologists recommend screening these high-risk women between 24 and 28 weeks of gestation. The National Diabetes Data Group and the Society of Perinatal Obstetricians recommend screening all women with risk factors at their first prenatal visit and again between 24 and 28 weeks' gestational age if the initial screen was negative. Studies employing universal screening have demonstrated that almost half of women diagnosed with gestational diabetes had no risk factors and over half were <30 years old. At Women's Hospital we employ universal screening of all pregnant women.

The recommended screening for gestational diabetes, the random 1-h postglucose, measures the serum glucose 1h after the ingestion of a 50 g glucose solution at any time of the day. The patient need not be fasting. A serum glucose level of 140 mg/dl or greater mandates a glucose tolerance test. The glucose tolerance test recommended in pregnant women in the USA is the 3-h 100 g glucose tolerance test. After a 3-day diet rich in carbohydrates and an overnight fast, the patient ingests 100 g of glucose. Serum glucose levels are measured before and every hour for 3 h after the glucose load. Gestational diabetes is diagnosed when two or more values meet or exceed the following: fasting, 105 mg/dl; 1 h, 190 mg/dl; 2 h, 165 mg/dl and 3 h, 145 mg/dl. These patients are designated in the White classification as class A and account for 90% of diabetes in pregnancy. They are further subclassified by the American College of Obstetricians and Gynecologists according to the severity of intolerance into class A_1 and class A_2. Patients maintaining fasting serum glucose levels <105 mg/dl and 2-h postprandial glucose levels <120 mg/dl are designated class A_1, while those exceeding either of these levels are designated class A_2. The latter often will require insulin therapy to maintain euglycemia during pregnancy and have a much greater risk of developing overt diabetes after pregnancy.

Preconceptional diabetes

Women with preexisting diabetes prior to conception may have insulin-dependent (IDDM or type I) or noninsulin-dependent diabetes mellitus (NIDDM or type II). Although type II patients may be treated with diet therapy alone or may require additional oral hypoglycemic agents or insulin in the late stages of the disease, all pregnant women with preconceptional diabetes, both type I and II, require insulin during pregnancy. Progress in the treatment of diabetes has lessened the relationship of the severity of diabetic sequelae with the age and duration of disease. Although the White classification is still used, it is clinically more useful to categorize patients with preconceptional diabetes into those with and without significant medical complications. Pregnancy for the woman with diabetic sequelae is substantially more risky for both mother and fetus and requires close and highly specialized medical care. These complications include preproliferative or proliferative retinopathy, nephropathy, autonomic neuropathy, and coronary artery disease.

SUGGESTED READING

COUSTAN DR (ed). Diabetes in pregnancy. *Clin Obstet Gynecol* 1991;34:479–580.

GABBE SG. Management of diabetes mellitus in pregnancy. *Am J Obstet Gynecol* 1985;153:824.

MESTMAN JH. Outcome of diabetes screening in pregnancy and perinatal morbidity in infants of mothers with mild impairment in glucose tolerance. *Diabetes Care* 1980;3:447.

METZGER BE (ed). Proceedings of the third international workshop conference on gestational diabetes mellitus. *Diabetes* (Suppl 2) 1991;40:197.

12

Management of the pregnant diabetic: diet, insulin dosage, when and how to deliver

SIRI L. KJOS & JORGE H. MESTMAN

The goal in the management of all pregnant diabetic patients is to conclude a pregnancy with a healthy infant and mother. The cornerstone of therapy, whether treating gestational or preconceptional diabetes, is the maintenance of a euglycemic environment throughout pregnancy for proper fetal growth. This is achieved primarily through combinations of proper diet, insulin therapy, and home glucose monitoring. Antepartum fetal surveillance, utilizing ultrasound to monitor fetal growth and development and antepartum testing in the third trimester to monitor fetal well-being, are equally important tools. Diabetic pregnancy care requires a team approach, involving a perinatologist, endocrinologist, neonatologist, as well as a diabetic nurse specialist and nutritionist. The patient and her family are equally important members of the team and should be fully educated, instructed, and involved in her care.

Compliance with appropriately prescribed diet therapy is essential to control diabetic blood sugar. Elevated placental hormones result in peripheral insulin resistance with compensatory increased pancreatic secretion of insulin in all pregnant women. Clinically, this manifests itself as accelerated starvation, increased ketogenesis in the fasting state and elevated postprandial glucose levels in the fed state. Thus, the strategy of diet therapy in pregnant diabetic women is to utilize small frequent feedings to avoid ketogenesis and large glucose loads. Bedtime snacks are particularly important. Complex carbohydrates with high fiber are also avoided to prevent rapid high increases in glucose. Attention must be paid to proper total caloric prescription, timing, and content of meals in

Table 12.1 Diet therapy

Minimal caloric restriction: weight-maintaining diet
30–32 kcal/kg per day true body weight
25 kcal/kg per day true body weight in obese women
Lower limit: 1800 kcal/day
Upper limit: 2500 kcal/day

American Diabetes Association diet
50–55% carbohydrates (complex, high-fiber)
15–20% protein
25–30% fat (<10% saturated)

Caloric distribution during the day

Breakfast	15%
Morning snack	10%
Lunch	25%
Afternoon snack	10%
Dinner	30%
Bedtime snack	10%

---

order to achieve stable glucose levels and avoid large swings in serum glucose levels (Table 12.1).

Therapy strategies for different diabetic classes

Gestational diabetes

The first step in treatment of women with newly diagnosed gestational diabetes is to implement diet therapy. An exception to this is the presence of overt fasting hyperglycemia (>130 mg/dl) where insulin should be promptly instituted. Otherwise fasting (FSG) and postprandial (2HPP) glucose levels should be followed at least every 1–2 weeks. If these levels become elevated (FSG ≥ 105 mg/dl or 2HPP ≥ 120 mg/dl; class A_2), insulin therapy should be instituted and patients are treated similarly to preconceptional diabetic patients. Insulin use for patients with normal fasting glucose, but with elevated postprandial sugars, should be considered *vis-à-vis* management with diet alone. Often increased emphasis on diet counseling and compliance along with patient ambulation after meals is successful in controlling blood sugar. Again the goal is euglycemic blood sugar control.

Pregestational diabetes

Ideally, conception and embryogenesis in diabetic women should occur in a euglycemic environment (Table 12.2). Poorly controlled maternal

Table 12.2 Euglycemic blood sugar goals in pregnant diabetic women

Fasting	60–90 mg/dl
Preprandial	60–105 mg/dl
Postprandial	≤120 mg/dl
2–6 a.m.	60–90 mg/dl

diabetes during this time is associated with increased major congenital malformations (6–10% overall; up to 25% with very poor control). Recent animal and human studies strongly indicate that euglycemia at the time of conception and embryogenesis will reduce, and perhaps prevent, congenital malformations. Thus, euglycemic blood sugar control, using split-dose insulin and home glucose monitoring of pre- and postprandial blood sugars, must be instituted prior to attempting conception. In IDDM patients it is often necessary to reeducate the patient to institute tight control and monitoring, while NIDDM patients must be switched from diet and/or oral hypoglycemic agents to insulin. There is no place for oral antihyperglycemic agent therapy during pregnancy. If the patient is already pregnant, insulin therapy geared toward euglycemic control should be instituted as soon as possible.

Different dosing regimens, all utilizing split-dose therapy of insulin, are presented in Table 12.3. In most cases, adequate control is achieved by two or three daily injections. Initial insulin doses can be estimated based on gestational age and true body weight, although the final daily

Table 12.3 Insulin therapy required for all pregestational diabetics and gestational diabetics with persistent fasting or postprandial hyperglycemia (class A$_2$)

Example regimens: all are split-dose			
Breakfast	Lunch	Dinner	Bedtime
1 Reg + NPH	–	Reg + NPH	–
2 Reg + NPH		Reg	NPH
3 Reg	Reg	Reg	NPH

Guidelines for starting dosage of insulin
First trimester   0.5–0.6 total U/kg
Second trimester   0.7–0.8 total U/kg
Third trimester   0.9–1.0 total U/kg

Starting guidelines: twice-daily dosing
Give two-thirds total calculated dose in the morning: 2/3 NPH + 1/3 Reg
Give one-third total calculated dose in the afternoon: 1/2 NPH + 1/2 Reg

dose of insulin to achieve euglycemia may be two- to threefold higher. At our institution, insulin therapy is initiated in this fashion on an outpatient basis, with hospitalization reserved for women with medical complications or markedly elevated fasting hyperglycemia. There is a steady increment in insulin requirements in the latter half of pregnancy, which corresponds to the increased insulin resistance produced by increasing placental hormones. In some patients, the fasting glucose is elevated and a glucose level should be obtained at 03:00 h to rule out the possibility of the Somogyi reaction (rebound hyperglycemia). Blood sugar levels must be monitored with home glucose monitoring, 4–6 times a day, checking preprandial and postprandial glucose levels. Insulin and diet are adjusted accordingly.

Patients should be instructed to treat every hypoglycemic reaction promptly and should always carry carbohydrates with them. Mild hypoglycemic reactions are treated easily with oral carbohydrates in the form of nonfat milk or orange juice. Patients who are not responsive to this or are unconscious due to severe hypoglycemia require an injection of glucagon immediately. Pregnant diabetic women are particularly prone to hypoglycemia in the first half of pregnancy when morning sickness and the lack of the contrainsulin placental hormones make proper diet intake after insulin injection crucial. Maternal morbidity is unusual in well-controlled patients. Untreated or poorly controlled diabetes may result in ketoacidosis, which may occur at relatively low serum glucose levels and has a high perinatal mortality rate. Infections, particularly urinary tract infections, must be promptly treated. Lastly, the incidence of preeclampsia is increased in diabetic pregnancy. Early recognition and proper management are imperative. Liberal hospital admission is utilized for poor glucose control or the development of medical or obstetric complications.

Fetal evaluation

During the first trimester, elevated maternal hemoglobin A_{1c}, indicating poor maternal glucose control during embryogenesis, has been associated with increased major congenital anomalies, especially neural tube defects and cardiac anomalies. Therefore genetic consultation, maternal serum α-fetoprotein screening and a second-trimester ultrasound scan (18–20 weeks) to detect possible anomalies and to establish good dating criteria are indicated. Serial ultrasonography is helpful in assisting in the evaluation of fetal growth, macrosomia, and polyhydramnios.

In the third trimester, antepartum fetal surveillance should begin. In diabetic patients with medical or obstetric complications, the decision as to when to initiate antepartum testing is individualized and may be initiated as early as 27 weeks. Otherwise antepartum testing is generally initiated in well-controlled, noncomplicated preconception and class A_2 gestational diabetics in the 32nd–34th week of gestation. Antepartum testing in uncomplicated class A_1 patients (without any fasting hyperglycemia) is initiated at 40 weeks. The nonstress test, the contraction stress test, and the biophysical profile have all been successfully used in monitoring fetal well-being in diabetic pregnancies. Such testing has reduced the once high risk of third-trimester stillbirth in the diabetic almost to that of the general population. In patients in whom fetal evaluation is reassuring and blood sugar is well controlled, delivery can be delayed until term.

For high-risk patients with hypertension, mild nephropathy, poor glycemic control, or with a history of a previous stillbirth, elective delivery should be planned after 38 completed weeks of gestation if possible. In cases of poor pregnancy dating and poor glycemic control, fetal lung maturity should be documented by amniotic fluid lecithin:sphingomyelin ratio and/or the presence of phosphatidylglycerol.

Patients scheduled for labor induction or cesarean section should begin induction or surgery in the morning, withholding the morning insulin dose (Table 12.4). Patients should receive 5% intravenous glucose solutions at maintenance rates (125 ml/h) to avoid ketosis. When bolus hydration is required, such as administered during epidural anesthesia, plain normal saline solution should be used. During labor or induction of labor, blood sugar levels should be monitored every 1–2 h in insulin-requiring patients. Any hyperglycemia (above 110–120 mg/dl) should be controlled with insulin, preferably via continuous intravenous infusion. Most patients with A_2 gestational diabetes do not require insulin during labor, while those with IDDM do. The usual starting dose to begin insulin infusion for mild hyperglycemia is 0.5–1.0 U/h. The infusion rate

Table 12.4 Intrapartum maternal glycemic control via insulin infusion

---

Preferable to start induction in the morning
No morning insulin dose
Continuous glucose infusion (D_5 NS at 125 ml/h)
Insulin infusion via pump
    Type I: start at 0.5 U/h
    Most type II and class A_2: monitor venous/capillary BG
    Begin insulin p.r.n. BG >110–120 mg%
Titrate insulin to BG, usually beginning at 0.5–10 U/h
With marked hyperglycemia (>180 mg%) it is often necessary to give an
    intravenous bolus insulin of 2–10 U first
Individual insulin requirements vary and change during labor

BG, Blood gas; NS, normal saline.

is titrated to maintain a glucose level of 80–100 mg/dl. If continuous infusion is not available, or if a diabetic patient will be maintained on intravenous fluid without eating meals for a period of time, 10 U of regular insulin may be added to 1000 ml of solution with 5% glucose at an infusion rate of 100–150 ml/h. Hyperglycemia should be avoided at the time of labor and delivery, as glucose crosses the placenta and may produce severe hypoglycemia in the newborn due to endogenous insulin release. After delivery, the patient may not require insulin for 24–48 h. Postpartum, it is acceptable to keep serum glucose levels between 150 and 200 mg/dl.

Neonatal complications include macrosomia, hypoglycemia, respiratory distress syndrome, cardiomyopathy, polycythemia, and hyperbilirubinemia. Euglycemia blood sugar control throughout pregnancy can minimize these complications.

Counseling and family planning

All pregestational diabetics should be counseled to seek preconception care. They are at increased risk of congenital malformations (6–10%) which can be increased up to 25% when in poor glycemic control. The achievement of euglycemia, at conception and during the period of embryogenesis, has been shown substantially to reduce the risk of major congenital malformations (from 7.7 to 1.1%) in women with IDDM. The period of embryogenesis is usually completed by the seventh week of gestation. Safe and effective contraception is critical for all sexually active diabetic women of reproductive age who do not wish to conceive. Short-term use of low estrogen plus low progestin dose oral contraceptives may be used in diabetic women without vascular disease. Their past or current use, or duration of use, has been demonstrated not to have an effect on retinopathy or hypertension. Similarly their use has little effect on glucose control or serum lipid levels. Blood pressure, lipid, and glucose parameters must be followed regularly. Similarly, intrauterine devices, when used in diabetic women with low risk of sexually transmitted disease exposure (monogamous in a stable relationship, parous, and no history of recent sexually transmitted disease) have been shown to be safe and without increased risk of infection. Proper patient selection, regular follow-up, and careful patient education about early signs of pelvic infection are paramount. The diaphragm and condom should also not be ignored, and may be recommended for contraception and also have the added benefit of decreasing the exposure to sexually transmitted diseases and the human immunodeficiency virus. Thus many contraceptive options exist, but they should be prescribed with careful selection and close supervision. Once childbearing is complete, surgical sterilization should be seriously considered.

Table 12.5 Glucose tolerance testing in women with gestational diabetes after pregnancy

Nonpregnant 2-h oral glucose tolerance test
   3-day carbohydrate-rich diet preparation
   After overnight fast ingest 75 g glucose
   Serum glucose (SG) determinations performed at: fasting, 30, 60, 90, and
     120 min

Interpretation of nonpregnant 2-h oral glucose tolerance test
  1 Diabetes mellitus: a 30-, 60-, or 90-min SG ≥200 mg/dl *and* a 120- min SG
   ≥200 mg/dl
  2 Impaired glucose tolerance: a 30-, 60-, or 90-min SG ≥200 mg/dl *and* a
   120-min SG ≥140 mg/dl, <200 mg/dl
  3 Normal (previous abnormality of glucose tolerance)

Women with gestational diabetes should be tested 5–8 weeks postpartum for diabetes using a 75-g, 2-h oral glucose tolerance test (Table 12.5) to establish their nonpregnant glucose status as per the recommendation of the American College of Obstetricians and Gynecologists and the American Diabetes Association. Thereafter annual screening/testing for diabetes should be performed, as the incidence of overt diabetes by 10 years after delivery is over 50%. Counseling these patients to continue their diabetic diet, to achieve or maintain ideal body weight, and to engage in a regular program of exercise may reduce or delay the appearance of overt diabetes and is strongly encouraged. The short-term use of low estrogen plus low progestin oral contraceptives has been shown not to accelerate the development of diabetes or adversely affect serum lipid levels. Again, blood pressure, weight, lipids, and glucose tolerance testing should be monitored regularly. There is no contraindication to the use of intrauterine devices.

SUGGESTED READING

FREINKEL N (ed). Summary and recommendation of the second international workshop–conference on gestational diabetes. *Diabetes* (Suppl 2) 1985;34:123.

FUHRMAN K, REIHER H, SEMMLER K, GLUCKNER E. The effect of intensified conventional insulin therapy before and during pregnancy on the malformation rate in offspring of diabetic mothers. *Exp Clin Endocrinol* 1984;83:173.

GABBE SG. Management of diabetes mellitus in pregnancy. *Am J Obstet Gynecol* 1985;153:824.

KJOS SL, WALTHER FJ, MONTORO M, PAUL RH, DIAZ F, STABLER M. Prevalence and etiology of respiratory distress in infants of diabetic mothers: predictive value of fetal maturation tests. *Am J Obstet Gynecol* 1990;163:898–903.

KJOS SL, SHOUPE D, DOUYAN S, *et al.* Effect of low-dose oral contraceptives on carbohydrate and lipid metabolism in women with recent gestational diabetes:

results of a controlled, randomized, prospective study. *Am J Obstet Gynecol* 1990;163:1822.

KLEIN BEK, MOSS SE, KLEIN R. Oral contraceptives in women with diabetes. *Diabetes Care* 1990;13:895.

METZGEr B (ed). Proceedings of the third international workshop conference on gestational diabetes mellitus. *Diabetes* (Suppl 2) 1991;40:197.

MILLS JL, BAKER L, GOLDMAN AS. Malformations in infants of diabetic mothers occur before the seventh gestational week. *Diabetes* 1979;28:292.

SKOUBY SO, MOLSTED-PEDERSEN, KUHL C, *et al*. Oral contraceptives in diabetic women: metabolic effects of four compounds with different estrogen/progestogen profiles. *Fertil Steril* 1986;46:858.

13

Pregnancy in women with complications of diabetes mellitus

MARTIN N. MONTORO

Introduction

The overall outcome of pregnancy in diabetic women has greatly improved over the last few decades; however, the subgroup of diabetic women with vascular complications continues to show significantly elevated fetal and neonatal morbidity and mortality. Maternal morbidity and mortality may occur in some of these patients who have severe retinal, renal, and particularly ischemic cardiac disease. Nevertheless, advances in the medical treatment of diabetes and in obstetric and neonatal care also have improved the outcome in complicated diabetes. Until recently, these women frequently were advised to avoid pregnancy and undergo therapeutic abortion. Recommendation against pregnancy can now be made on an individual basis, as absolute contraindications are fewer and are limited to women with unusually severe complications, particularly ischemic heart disease.

Adequate and timely counseling and preconception control of diabetes are very important, as perinatal mortality due to congenital anomalies accounts for a large percentage (40–50%) of perinatal losses in this group. It should also be pointed out that many patients have multiple complications rather than the involvement of one organ system, and pregnancy outcome is usually worse in those with multiple organ involvement.

Retinopathy

The influence of pregnancy on the progression of retinopathy, or on its development if not present before gestation, remains controversial.

Several retrospective reports are conflicting, and several other more re-cent ones suggest either that pregnancy does not modify the course of retinopathy or that the changes are reversible postpartum. It also has been suggested that, rather than the pregnancy itself, the sudden institu-tion of strict diabetic control may be a factor in the worsening of reti-nopathy.

More recently published prospective studies using serial fluorescein angiography suggest that background retinopathy worsens during preg-nancy, even with minimal retinopathy and good metabolic control prior to pregnancy. The worsening is more obvious if the duration of diabetes mellitus is 5 years or longer. It remains to be seen whether these changes can regress after delivery, or if pregnancy will irreversibly affect the background rate of retinopathy. At present, it is believed that duration of diabetes, metabolic control, and blood pressure levels, not pregnancy, have the greatest impact on the overall long-term course of background retinopathy.

A recently published study has shown that the worsening of diabetic retinopathy is more severe in those women who develop pregnancy-induced hypertension, preeclampsia, or preeclampsia superimposed on chronic hypertension.

The influence of pregnancy on severe background retinopathy with preproliferative lesions or frank proliferative retinopathy also remains controversial. Some imply that most published studies are biased because of referral patterns to the specialized institutions reporting those studies.

It appears that even though some regression may occur postpartum in most (up to 80%) pregnant women, untreated proliferative retino-pathy will worsen during pregnancy. Treatment with photocoagulation prior to pregnancy may prevent progression during gestation. If pro-liferative retinopathy worsens during pregnancy, aggressive treatment may prevent further progression of retinopathy and preserve vision.

Proliferative retinopathy is no longer an absolute contraindication for pregnancy, given current treatment possibilities. These patients remain at high risk, however, and have to be monitored closely. They should be advised of their risk on an individual basis, if possible, prior to preg-nancy. General guidelines for the care of pregnant patients with retino-pathy are as follows:

1 Any patient with diabetes for longer than 5 years should be examined by an ophthalmologist at least once each trimester. If the diabetes has been present for fewer than 5 years, periodic ophthalmoscopic exams should be performed by the treating physician. If any changes are noted, the patient should be referred to an ophthalmologist.

2 Active proliferative retinopathy ideally should be treated prior to pregnancy. If it develops or worsens during pregnancy, it should be

treated aggressively. If it develops early in gestation (first trimester), and there is no positive response to photocoagulation, therapeutic abortion should be considered.

3   Vaginal delivery may be allowed for those patients with background or successfully treated proliferative retinopathy. The optimal route of delivery for those patients with active proliferative retinopathy has not been determined, since in nonpregnant patients vitreous hemorrhages may occur even during periods of inactivity. Vitreous hemorrhages have been observed during both cesarean sections and vaginal deliveries, but there is concern that they may occur more readily during the active expulsion phase. It is recommended that, in patients with active proliferative retinopathy, the mode of delivery be determined individually and in consultation with both the obstetrician and ophthalmologist.

Nephropathy

Until the late 1970s, pregnancy in women with diabetic nephropathy was strongly discouraged, and therapeutic abortions were recommended frequently. More recent reports have shown significantly improved perinatal outcome when good metabolic control is achieved and when current "state of the art" obstetric and neonatal care is available.

Diabetic nephropathy usually occurs in type I diabetes of 15 years' duration or longer, but it may occur also with shorter durations of diabetes and in patients with type II diabetes. All pregnant patients with diabetes should be evaluated for the presence or absence of nephropathy (class A_1, and A_2 gestational diabetics can be excluded) early in gestation and, ideally, prior to pregnancy. A 24-h urine specimen should be examined for protein and creatinine clearance; a renal biopsy is not absolutely needed for diagnosis.

Treatment should include strict diabetic control. If bedrest alone is insufficient, medical treatment of hypertension should be initiated. Frequent visits for close monitoring and liberal hospitalizations are recommended for worsening hypertension, deteriorating renal function, or fetal compromise. Periodic ultrasound examinations are useful for dating, detection of congenital anomalies, and assessment of fetal growth. In patients with vascular compromise, intrauterine growth retardation, rather than macrosomia, may be seen even if the diabetes is not well controlled. Fetal surveillance should be instituted as soon as the physician is willing to intervene for fetal distress. The mother should be carefully informed and her wishes taken into consideration.

Outpatient therapy is acceptable as long as the diabetes and hypertension are well controlled and renal function remains at an acceptable level; otherwise, hospitalization is strongly advised.

Delivery before term may be indicated for either maternal deterioration or fetal distress. For elective delivery prior to term, fetal lung maturity should be documented; patients with renal failure may experience accelerated fetal lung maturity, but this is not always the case. The route of delivery should be considered on an individual basis; many will require a cesarean section because of preterm delivery and fetal distress.

Improved neonatal care has allowed many of these premature infants to survive and has contributed significantly to the increasingly successful perinatal outcomes. Perinatal mortality in class F diabetics still is reported to be as high as 20% and pulmonary morbidity in the neonates up to 40%. A recent study reported a perinatal mortality of 12% and morbidity of 24% in a group of class F diabetics. The improvement of the outcome is most likely multifactorial and includes better control of diabetes and hypertension, fetal surveillance, and assessment of lung maturity prior to delivery as well as improved neonatal care.

Predictors of poor outcome are said to be: (1) massive proteinuria (3 g/day or more in the first trimester and 10 g/day in the third); (2) a serum creatinine of 1.5 mg or more; (3) hypertension at any time during pregnancy; (4) anemia (hematocrit of 25% or lower in the third trimester); and (5) patients with poor compliance.

Worsened renal function during pregnancy usually improves to pre-pregnancy levels postpartum but the improvement may take several weeks. However, some patients may continue to deteriorate to end-stage disease during pregnancy or postpartum. Hemodialysis has been used successfully during pregnancy in some cases.

Reports until 1977 showed that by the time children of women with diabetic nephropathy were 10 years old, 20% of those women had died. Whether or not the prognosis has improved since then is not yet known.

Pregnancy in patients on dialysis and after renal transplantation

Because the number of renal transplantations is increasing and also because of the strong desire for motherhood of some of these women, more pregnant patients with renal transplants will be seen in the future. About one-fourth of all patients on chronic dialysis or after renal transplantation are diabetic. Thus far, only a few cases of pregnancy in these patients have been reported.

In nine recently reported cases, there was one maternal death and six of the remaining eight patients developed hypertension. No transplant rejection occurred, although this complication has been reported in 10% of pregnant women posttransplant due to other kidney disease.

All infants were delivered prior to term, all by cesarean section due to fetal distress. There was one fetal death, and another infant had congenital anomalies. A surprisingly low rate of congenital anomalies has been observed with the use of steroids and azathioprine. Cyclosporine currently is being used more widely, and its effects on the fetus remain to be seen. Case reports of successful pregnancies in patients on chronic dialysis (both hemodialysis and continuous ambulatory peritoneal dialysis) have been reported as well. In all these patients, prepregnancy counseling and intensive monitoring in a tertiary-care facility are mandatory.

Coronary artery disease

There is little information available regarding pregnancy and ischemic heart disease in diabetic women. In the few cases reported, there was a maternal mortality of 75% due to myocardial infarction during pregnancy or early postpartum. The prognosis is slightly better if the myocardial infarction occurs prior to pregnancy or early in the first trimester. The perinatal mortality in the remaining potentially viable infants was 29%.

Women with coronary artery disease tend to be older and have longstanding diabetes. A detailed history, physical examination, electrocardiograph, and a stress test should be performed prior to pregnancy in any woman contemplating pregnancy if there is any suggestion of coronary insufficiency. Because of the high maternal mortality, pregnancy should be discouraged in this group of patients. However, if pregnancy occurs and termination is not accepted, these patients should be treated in the same manner as any patient with coronary insufficiency.

Diabetic ketoacidosis

There is little information on the current medical literature about diabetic ketoacidosis (DKA). A few case reports describe perinatal mortality ranging from 30 to 90% but no patient series has been available.

We recently reviewed the experience at Los Angeles County/University of Southern California Women's Hospital over 14 years (1972–1987). Twenty patients with DKA constitute the basis for the information below.

DKA is defined as an arterial pH of 7.30 or lower, serum bicarbonate of 15 mmol/l or lower, ketosis (serum acetone present at 1:2 dilution), and hyperglycemia (blood sugar 300 mg/dl or higher). It should be pointed out that in pregnant women DKA may occur with relatively low blood sugar levels, and the diagnosis should not be excluded because the blood sugar is "too low." Although the mean blood sugar in our patients was 526 mg/dl (range 156–1700 mg/dl), two patients had profound ketoacidosis despite blood sugars below 200 mg/dl (156 and 180 mg/dl, respectively).

DKA is life-threatening and a true medical emergency. Patients should be treated in an intensive care unit setting for general supportive care and intensive close monitoring. No maternal mortality occurred in our patients; but mortality in DKA, in general, is reported at about 10%.

Average fluid deficit is 5–6 liters, but it can be much higher. The first 3 l should be replaced in the first 2–3 h and the remainder in the following 12–15 h. Normal saline is used initially (first 1–2 liters), followed by 0.45 liters normal saline. Insulin is given by continuous intravenous infusion at a rate of 5–10 U/h and adjusted according to frequent (every 1–2 h) blood glucose measurements. Bicarbonate is not recommended unless the pH is 7.10 or lower, in which case only enough is given to bring the pH to that level. Electrolyte replacement (Na, K, P, Mg, etc.) is done according to serum levels and the status of renal function.

The search for a precipitating cause is mandatory. In our series, the most common factors were poor compliance (33%), infection (22%), and unrecognized new onset of diabetes (22%). If an infection is identified, it must be treated aggressively.

The perinatal mortality in our series was 35% but there were no fetal deaths once therapy was initiated. Improvement of fetal distress was seen in one fetus after correction of the maternal acidosis and hypovolemia. Fetal monitoring should be instituted in potentially viable fetuses. Aggressive treatment of the maternal condition may ameliorate fetal distress and allow postponement of intervention until the mother is less critically ill.

The patients with fetal losses included most patients with undiagnosed diabetes, those women whose gestational age was 30 weeks or beyond, and those with more severe dehydration and hypovolemia. These fetuses probably suffered from a more profound acidosis and placental hypoperfusion.

Because a significant proportion of DKA in this group occurred in patients not previously known to have diabetes (they accounted for 33% of the patients with DKA and 57% of the fetal demises), it is important to be attentive to the symptoms of uncontrolled diabetes. Common presenting symptoms include polyuria, polydipsia, nausea, vomiting, malaise, weakness, lethargy, abdominal pain, and headaches; less common are weight loss, visual disturbances, and leg cramps. Most of the precipitating factors are potentially preventable through closely supervised patient care and education, prompt recognition of uncontrolled diabetes, and implementation of screening programs.

Diabetic neuropathy

The peripheral neuropathy which is commonly seen in many diabetics is seldom of any consequence as far as pregnancy is concerned. Diabetic autonomic neuropathy on the other hand may pose serious difficulties for some pregnant women. It may be asymptomatic in the early stages and found only by specific examination. Symptoms may include loss of sweating in feet, bladder (urinary) dysfunction, abnormal cardiovascular reflexes (e.g., loss of beat-to-beat variability, postural hypotension, etc.), and in the more advanced states, sweat disturbances of the upper body, gastroparesis, diarrhea, and bladder atony.

Pregnancy may exacerbate gastroparesis and postural hypotension. Vomiting usually starts early in gestation but subsides postpartum. Those women whose autonomic neuropathy was asymptomatic prior to pregnancy have a better prognosis for resolution of the symptoms after delivery and a more benign course during pregnancy. Vomiting interferes with diabetic control and impairs the nutritional status of the mother (weight loss, ketone production, etc.) and the fetus (the main concern is growth retardation). Autonomic neuropathy may block the early "alarm" symptoms of the catecholamine phase of hypoglycemia, thus making these women very vulnerable to neuroglycopenia; this is particularly true when tight control of the diabetes is attempted, such as is commonly the case during pregnancy.

The therapeutic possibilities are limited for this condition in general and particularly during pregnancy. Antiemetics are seldom of value. Metoclopramide provides symptomatic relief in some patients. Other medications have been reported to be useful in other countries but are not yet available in the USA (domperidone, motilin, and others). Intravenous erythromycin (when given orally, it does not seem to be useful) has a motilin-like effect and has been reported to be useful in a group of nonpregnant patients. We have used this form of therapy in a few pregnant women after all other measures failed, with temporary improvement of days to weeks. Total parenteral nutrition should be started early and as soon as the other measures have proven ineffective.

SUGGESTED READING

JANSEENS J, PEETERS TL, VANTRAPPEN G, et al. Improvement of gastric emptying in diabetic gastroparesis by erythromycin. *N Engl J Med* 1990;32:1028.

KITZMILLER JL, BROWN ER, PHILLIPE M, et al. Diabetic nephropathy and perinatal outcome. *Am J Obstet Gynecol* 1981;141:741.

KLEIN BEK, MOSS SE, KLEIN R. Effect of pregnancy on progression of diabetic retinopathy. *Diabetic Care* 1990;13:34

MACLEOD AF, SMITH SA, SONKSEN PH, et al. The problem of autonomic neuropathy in diabetic pregnancy. *Diabetic Med* 1990;7:80.

MONTORO M, MYERS VP, MESTMAN JH, et al. The outcome of pregnancy in diabetic ketoacidosis. *Am J Perinatol* 1993;10:17–20.

NESLER CL, SINCLAIR SH, SCHWARTZ SS. Diabetic nephropathy and pregnancy. *Clin Obstet Gynecol* 1985;28:528.

OGBURN PL, KITZMILLER JL, HARE JW, *et al*. Pregnancy following renal transplantation in class T diabetes mellitus. *JAMA* 1986;225:911.

ROSSEN B, MIODOVNIK M, KRANIAS G, *et al*. Progression of diabetic retinopathy in pregnancy: association with hypertension in pregnancy. *Am J Obstet Gynecol* 1992;166:1214.

SILFEN SL, WAPNER RJ, GABBE SG. Maternal outcome in class H diabetes mellitus. *Obstet Gynecol* 1980;55:749.

SOUBRANE G, CANIVET J, COSCAS G. Influence of pregnancy on the evolution of background retinopathy. *Intern Ophthalmol* 1985;8:249.

14

Appendicitis in pregnancy

LORRAINE STANCO & GEOFFREY STILES

Introduction

Acute appendicitis is the most common nonobstetric condition requiring operation during pregnancy. Its incidence is variably reported from 1 in 1500 to 6600 pregnancies. There is approximately a 7% lifetime risk of appendicitis in the USA. Appendicitis is rare in infants, becomes increasingly common throughout childhood, and reaches its maximum incidence in the teens and 20s, corresponding to the child-bearing years. The incidence of appendicitis is neither increased nor decreased by pregnancy, with cases approximately equally distributed among the three trimesters.

As stated by Balber in 1908, "the mortality of appendicitis complicating pregnancy is the mortality of delay." Overall maternal morbidity is reported to be from 2 to 40% with a recent (since 1950) overall maternal mortality rate of 0.1–4%. Maternal mortality is associated with appendiceal perforation and third-trimester or puerperial cases. An overall fetal loss rate of 10.8% has been reported, but with gangrenous or perforated appendicitis fetal loss increases to 30–70%. Preterm delivery is reported to occur in up to 37% of cases.

Pathophysiology of appendicitis

Appendicitis occurs as a result of luminal obstruction. In about half of the cases this obstruction results from hyperplasia of submucosal lymphoid follicles in response to infection. In the other half of cases, obstruction is due to a fecalith, or rarely, a foreign body or parasite. Continued secretion along with increased bacterial replication in the static lumen causes significantly increased intraluminal pressure. Increased pressure in turn leads to obstruction of lymphatic drainage and venous outflow, producing edema and vascular congestion in the wall of the appendix. This is acute suppurative appendicitis.

As the process continues, arteriall insufficiency develops, leading to gangrene. Once gangrene has set in, luminal bacteria invade the wall of the appendix where they can potentially translocate to the serosal surface and spread intraperitoneally. If appendiceal wall infarction and necrosis develop, perforation will follow. Once perforation has occurred, the degree to which the omentum or other surrounding structures are able to wall off the infection (with possible abscess formation) determines whether diffuse peritonitis occurs. During the last two trimesters of pregnancy, the omentum is deflected upward by the enlarging uterus, and increased dissemination of bacterial infection and diffuse peritonitis may result. Gangrenous appendicitis is treated in the same way as perforated appendicitis, as both are associated with bacterial peritonitis.

Anatomy and clinical presentation

The location of the appendix is usually in the right lower quadrant of the abdomen at the inferior tip of the cecum. The three tenia coli of the cecum converge at the base of the appendix, forming a useful anatomic trail to follow to find the appendix during appendectomy. The position of the tip is, however, variable. Most commonly, the appendix lies behind the cecum but in an intraperitoneal location. Because the tip is within the pelvis or at the pelvic brim in one-third of cases, appendicitis may be confused with other pelvic pathology, especially in young women, even in early pregnancy.

As classically described by Baer *et al.* in 1932, the appendix is displaced superiorly and laterally by the enlarging uterus in pregnancy (Fig. 14.1). The tip also rotates counterclockwise so that, as term approaches, it commonly comes to lie over the right kidney. If adhesions exist or if the appendix is retrocecal, this migration may not occur.

Early in the course of appendicitis vague abdominal discomfort is centered in the periumbilical region. The initial pain is due to distention of the appendix associated with luminal obstruction. As the appendix is anatomically a midline-derived structure and the visceral innervation is autonomic, the pain is felt on both sides, centered on the umbilicus, and is often described as dull in nature. Anorexia, nausea, and vomiting may then follow.

As transmural inflammation of the appendix occurs, the partietal peritoneum (with somatic sensory innervation) adjacent to the appendix

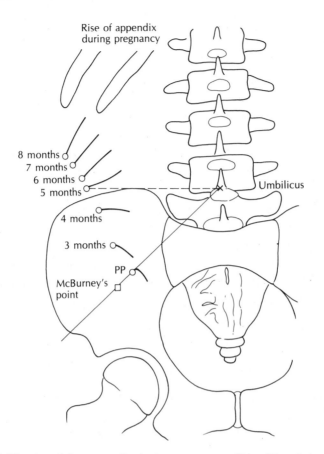

Fig. 14.1 The rise of the appendix during pregnancy. From Horwitz *et al.* 1985.

becomes irritated and causes localized pain, usually in the right lower quadrant. The migration and localization of pain often occur 1–12 h following the onset of symptoms. With perforation, bilateral lower quadrant or diffuse pain may develop.

Diagnosis in pregnancy

The above describes the typical progression of acute appendicitis. In the absence of pregnancy, only about 50% of cases are "typical," and with pregnancy this percentage is greatly diminished, especially in the latter two trimesters. Pain is the most common and reliable symptom of appendicitis in pregnancy. The pain becomes less characteristic, may be milder, and may be located in the right upper quadrant, entire right side, or right flank. Anorexia, nausea, and vomiting are all common complaints associated with pregnancy, and are often discounted. Vomiting, if present, may follow the onset of the pain in pregnant women with appendicitis. Up to 25% of patients will also complain of urinary tract symptomatology, including frequency and dysuria. Peritoneal irritation or bacterial peritonitis may lead to uterine contractions and preterm labor, which may further obscure the source of infection.

On examination, tenderness may be periumbilical or localized depending on the stage of the infection and the mediating effect of the enlarging uterus. Guarding and rebound tenderness are often present, although less often than in nonpregnant cases. Various signs have been described to differentiate pain and tenderness of uterine origin from appendicitis in pregnancy. Essentially, when the point of maximal tenderness does not shift as the gravid uterus is lifted away, the pain is not considered to be of uterine origin. If the appendix is within the pelvis, and if the cul-de-sac has not been diminished by the presence of fetal parts, right rectal wall tenderness may be elicited.

Fever and laboratory abnormalities are not reliably present with appendicitis during pregnancy. Temperature may be normal or only slightly elevated. Due to the leukocytosis of pregnancy, only a rising count or left shifts are useful in reaching a correct diagnosis. Urinalysis may reveal occasional pyuria if the appendix is near the ureter or in cases where peritonitis has developed, but bacteria are not typically present in the urine.

Further diagnostic tests are not consistently helpful in diagnosing appendicitis, and often lead to delay in appropriate management, leading to perforation, peritonitis, and increased morbidity and mortality. Plain abdominal films are generally of little help and are discouraged in pregnancy. Barium enema, while occasionally helpful, is frequently non-specific and requires multiple X-ray exposures, and is thus discouraged in pregnancy. Likewise, computed tomography, which is often inaccurate as well as costly, should not be employed in pregnancy. Ultrasound may be useful in pregnancy to rule out other etiologies of right lower quadrant pain and can also be employed to assess fetal status and viability in the event that premature labor or other obstetric complications arise.

The differential diagnosis of appendicitis in pregnancy includes other gastrointestinal etiologies (pancreatitis, cholecystitis, gastroenteritis, hepatitis), renal causes (nephrolithiasis, pyelonephritis, cystitis), adnexal etiologies (masses undergoing torsion, ruptured or leaking corpus luteum, ectopic gestation, salpingitis, round ligament syndrome), and uterine causes (contractions, infection, degenerating myoma).

Based upon clinical history, physical examination, and laboratory data, diagnostic accuracy for acute appendicitis ranges from 67 to 92%. An important corollary to that, however, is that those studies reporting a high diagnostic accuracy also have a high rate of perforation (30%). In the absence of pregnancy, a diagnostic accuracy of 80–85% overall appears optimal in terms of risk from either delay in operation or in performing a "negative appendectomy." In pregnancy because the diagnosis is more difficult and because morbidity and mortality are greatly increased with delayed diagnosis and perforation, a lower rate of diagnostic (64–72%) accuracy is acceptable as negative laparotomy is not associated with high fetal wastage (0–3%). Diagnostic accuracy is especially diminished in many series in the third trimester. In those reporting very high diagnostic accuracy (implying delayed diagnosis and increased perforation), fetal wastage and maternal morbidity and mortality were unacceptably high.

Management

Once a diagnosis of probable appendicitis has been established, the patient should be prepared for surgery as operative management is indicated. The technical aspects of appendectomy in pregnancy are no different than those for nonpregnant patients. A transverse skin incision over the point of maximal tenderness is best, as the position of the appendix is so variable in pregnancy. Following the skin incision, the external and internal oblique muscles are split in the direction of their fibers, enhancing both wound strength and postoperative healing. Uterine manipulation should be avoided if possible and a roll may be placed under the patient's right side to aid in deflecting the uterus away from the operative site. Irrigation of the entire abdomen should not be attempted as this serves only to distribute the infection throughout the abdomen. In the absence of gross purulence the skin is closed and drains are not required. Postoperative prophylactic tocolysis may be employed if practical, given the gestational age of the fetus.

In the first trimester when the diagnosis is uncertain some authors advocate a midline incision to facilitate surgical correction of nonappendiceal etiologies. This is largely unnecessary if a preoperative ultrasound rules out adnexal pathology and if the patient exhibits point tenderness on examination. If still uncertain, laparoscopy can be performed to aid in both diagnosis and choice of incision once a diagnosis has been reached.

Numerous studies have shown both fewer infectious complications and greater cost savings in patients with acute nonperforated appendicitis who are given perioperative antibiotic prophylaxis with a third-generation cephalosporin. In these cases, while postoperative therapy is commonly used, it is not necessary. Unquestionably, gangrenous or perforated appendicitis requires postoperative antibiotic therapy in conjunction with appendectomy. The most common aerobic organisms involved are *Escherichia coli*, *Streptococcus* (group D and *viridans*) and *Pseudomonas*. Of the anaerobic organisms, *Bacteroides* species, *Peptostreptococcus*, *Bilophilia* and *Lactobacillus* predominate, with many other species present, including *Clostridium*. To cover all these potential pathogens, triple antibiotic therapy is necessary. In pregnancy, a regimen of gentamicin, clindamycin, and ampicillin is commonly employed. Antibiotic therapy should be continued for at least 4 days postoperatively with a ruptured appendix and until the patient has been afebrile for 48 h. Gentamicin levels should be followed and adjusted appropriately.

Soft rubber or closed suction drains are advocated only in cases with a periappendiceal or pelvic abscess with significant gross pus present, and the skin should be left open. Occasionally in cases complicated by periappendiceal abscess or a severe inflammatory process noted at surgery, the general surgeon may elect to open the abscess cavity, establish drainage, and close. Interval appendectomy can be scheduled after the patient has recovered from the acute infection.

In the event that a normal appendix is found at the time of surgery, a systematic search to identify the source of illness should be carried out and the incision may need to be extended. In the pregnant female, adnexae should be palpated, although uterine manipulation should be minimized. If no source is found, appendectomy should be performed. The morbidity from this procedure is minimal, and it will simplify the search for other etiologies if the symptomatology persists postoperatively. Finally, cesarean delivery at the time of appendectomy should be considered for obstetric indications only.

SUGGESTED READING

BABAKINE A, PARSA H, WOODRUFF JD. Appendicitis complicating pregnancy. *Can J Surg* 1977;23:92.

BAER JL, REIS RA, ARENS RA. Appendicitis in pregnancy. *JAMA* 1932;98:1359–1364.

BALBER EA. Perforative appendicitis complicating pregnancy. *JAMA* 1908;51:1310.

BRANT HA. Acute appendicitis in pregnancy. *Obstet Gynecol* 1967;29:130–138.

CUNNINGHAM FG, McCUBBIN JH. Appendicitis complicating pregnancy. *Obstet Gynecol* 1975;45:415–420.

HOROWITZ MD, GOMEZ GA, SANTIESTEBAN R, BUNETT G. Acute appendicitis during pregnancy. *Arch Surg* 1985;120:1362–1367.

RICHARDS C, DAYA S. Diagnosis of acute appendicitis in pregnancy. *Can J Surg* 1989;32:358–360.

SAUNDERS P, MILTON PJD. Laparotomy during pregnancy: an assessment of diagnostic accuracy and fetal wastage. *Br Med J* 1973;3:165–167.

TAMIR IL, BONGARD FS, KLEIN SR. Acute appendicitis in the pregnant patient. *Am J Surg* 1990;160:571–576.

TOWNSEND JM, GREISS FC. Appendicitis in pregnancy. *Southern Med J* 1976;69:1161.

15

Abnormal labor

LYNNAE K. MILLAR & THOMAS H. KIRSCHBAUM

Labor is defined as a series of regular, coordinated contractile events of the uterus resulting in progressive dilatation of the cervix with descent and delivery of the products of conception within a reasonable time.

Prolonged labor – dystocia – is usually due to abnormalities in the contractile properties of the uterus. Dystocia can also occur secondary to cephalopelvic disproportion.

The graphic portrayal of cervical dilatation plotted against time was introduced in 1954 by Friedman. The use of the labor curve documented the similarity of the rate of cervical dilatation in multiparous and nulliparous women, especially during the active phase of labor. Once the expected pattern of cervical dilatation during normal labor was established, individual patients could be compared against a "normal labor curve," and abnormal patterns could be identified which would alert the physician to potential problems.

The labor curve is divided into two major parts, the latent phase and the active phase (Fig. 15.1). The latent phase begins with the onset of labor and ends with the active (acceleration) phase. During the latent phase the uterine contractions become coordinated, initiating at the uterotubal junction and flowing in an unbroken wave through the uterine wall. The cervix becomes softer and effaces due to disruption of collagen fibers, an increase in water content, and an increase in the content of proteoglycans in the cervical ground substance. The active phase begins with the upswing of the cervical dilatation curve, leading to the linear phase of maximum slope resulting in rapid dilatation. The mean duration of the latent phase is approximately 5.3 ± 4.1 h for multiparas and $8.6 \pm$

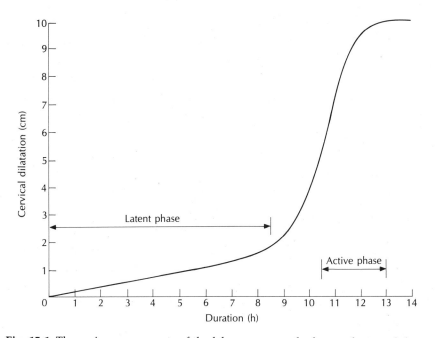

Fig. 15.1 The major components of the labor curve are the latent phase and the active phase. The active phase of labor is generally predictable and will follow the standard curve very closely. The latent phase is less predictable and may vary several hours within a normal range.

6.0 h for nulliparas. Using 2 SD from the mean to define prolongation of the latent phase, these data can be used to indicate that multiparas should not remain in the latent phase for more than 13.5 h, and nulliparas not more than 20.6 h.

Although prolongation of the latent phase is an abnormality of labor, Friedman reports that a prolonged latent phase is not associated with increased perinatal mortality and morbidity. Cesarean sections should not be performed for a prolonged latent phase. Excessive doses of narcotic analgesia and early epidural placement have been reported to prolong the latent phase beyond acceptable limits. The duration of the latent phase is unrelated to the duration of the active phase of labor.

There are two accepted methods of managing the latent phase. Friedman advocates expectant management. Prolongation of latent phase with a regimen of therapeutic rest. This employs the use of narcotic analgesics in large doses in an attempt to completely stop uterine contractions and provides 6–10 h of uterine rest. Good control is afforded with an initial dose of 10–15 mg of morphine sulfate given subcutaneously. The patient should be examined after 20 min to verify that her respirations are not suppressed and that her contractions have abated. If contractions are still perceived by the patient, but her cervical dilatation is unchanged, and there is no evidence of respiratory depression, an additional dose of 5–10 mg of morphine sulfate can be given subcutaneously. When patients awake in 6–10 h, 85% will have entered the active phase of labor. Ten percent will no longer experience contractions; in retrospect these women were in "false labor." The remaining 5% awaken and resume their ineffectual contractions. This group should then receive augmentation of their labor with oxytocin.

The other method of managing prolongation of the latent phase of labor is active intervention. O'Driscoll and Declan Meagher of the National Maternity Hospital in Dublin, state that the most important decisions are made during the first 2 h of labor and that many labor complications are the products of temporization. Active management consists of stimulating labor with oxytocin to shorten the latent phase so that active labor begins sooner, and the total duration of labor is shortened. In theory, a reduction in the duration of labor should benefit the patient by reducing the chances of infection, hemorrhage, and exhaustion. Outcomes seen at the National Maternity Hospital support this management protocol.

The active phase of labor begins at the onset of rapid cervical dilatation and ends with full cervical dilatation. The slowest normal rate of cervical dilatation in nulliparas is 1.2 cm/h, and in multiparas, 1.5 cm/h. In contrast, the average rate of dilatation in normal labor is 3.0 ± 0.08 cm/h for nulliparas and 5.4–6.8 cm/h for multiparas with a standard deviation varying from 0.22 to 0.78 which is directly proportional to parity. A protracted active phase is frequently associated with relative cephalopelvic disproportion, excessive sedation or analgesia, and conduction anesthesia.

Arrest of dilatation is defined as the cessation of progress of cervical dilatation during the active phase. This form of dystocia can occur due to abnormalities in presentation, size of the fetus or in the dimensions of the birth canal. Normal pelvic configuration can be assessed clinically by pelvic examination. X-ray pelvimetry should not be performed to assess adequacy of the pelvis except in the management of a breech presentation. Fetal size can be approximately ascertained with ultrasound and cesarean section should be performed for the mother with a macrosomic fetus and an arrest disorder.

If fetopelvic disproportion appears unlikely and uterine activity is less than optimal (contractions less frequent than every 2.5–3 min and their intensity less than 50 mmHg), uterine activity should be augmented with oxytocin. Adequate uterine activity generally corresponds to approximately 150–250 Montevideo units. Montevideo units represent the product of maximum intrauterine pressure in mmHg times the average number of contractions in a 10-min period.

Caution should be used when administering oxytocin since uterine sensitivity to a given dose can not be predicted. Oxytocin should be given intravenously in a dilute solution by controlled continuous infusion. The most commonly used concentration of oxytocin is 10 U (1-ml ampule) in 1000 ml of intravenous solution (usually dextrose in water). This provides a concentration of oxytocin of 1 mU for each 0.1 ml of intravenous solution.

The amount of oxytocin required to initiate or augment labor is much less than commonly employed in clinical practice. At term, required dosage is frequently as low as 2 mU/min and seldom exceeds 16 mU/min. An oxytocin concentration of 1 mU/0.1 ml will require an infusion rate of only 0.1–1.0 ml/min. Such low infusion rates require careful monitoring to prevent hyperstimulation. Prior to term, when the uterus is less responsive to oxytocin, larger doses may be required to stimulate uterine contractions.

The oxytocin should be given using a two-bottle (piggyback) technique. The oxytocin infusion is attached to the primary infusion near the point of administration to the patient. This allows more careful regulation of the oxytocin without restricting the amount of fluids the patient may receive from the primary infusion.

The half-life of oxytocin in the blood is quite short (about 4 min) but the half-life of its effect on uterine activity is 15–20 min. Therefore, at least 15–20 min should elapse between each increase in the oxytocin infusion rate to prevent a cumulative effect and hyperstimulation.

If a tetanic uterine contraction should occur, the oxytocin infusion should be discontinued immediately. The patient should be placed in the lateral position to prevent any pressure on the inferior vena cava. The tetanic contraction usually abates within minutes. If it persists, the patient should be delivered as expeditiously as possible. When the patient has no medical contraindications to β-mimetics, 125–250 μg of terbutaline sulfate can be given slowly by intravenous injection to treat tetanic uterine contractions.

Prostaglandins should not be utilized to treat abnormal labor, as they are not safe. They can be utilized for cervical ripening when labor needs to be induced in the patient remote from term.

Fetal descent begins when the labor curve has entered the phase of maximum slope. Once full cervical dilatation has been reached, descent occurs at rates exceeding 1 cm/h in nulliparas and 2 cm/h in multiparas. As long as progress is being made during the descent phase, labor can be allowed to continue. The prognosis for the fetus is good if there is no evidence of fetal compromise and if an operative vaginal delivery is avoided. Patients with an arrest of descent, for an hour or more, with adequate uterine contractions, should be delivered via cesarean section.

SUGGESTED READING

FRIEDMAN EA. The graphic analysis of labor. *Am J Obstet Gynecol* 1954;68:1568.

FRIEDMAN EA. *Labor: Clinical Evaluation and Management.* 2nd edn. New York: Appleton-Century-Crofts, 1978.

KNUPPEL RA (ed). Symposium on difficult labor and delivery. In: *Clinics in Perinatology*, vol 8. Philadelphia: WB Saunders, 1981;8:1–212.

O'DRISCOLL K, MEAGHER D (eds). *The Active Management of Labor.* London: WB Saunders, 1980.

16

Preterm labor:
background and prevention

T. MURPHY GOODWIN

Definitions and incidence

Preterm birth is defined as delivery occurring at less than 37 completed weeks' gestation (259 days from the last menstrual period). Low birth weight (LBW) is defined as the birth of an infant weighing less than 2500 g. In clinical settings where accurate dating of the gestation is difficult, there has been a tendency to rely on the birth weight as an indicator of prematurity, but there are important limitations. An LBW infant may not be premature, but growth-retarded. In fact, only half of the LBW infants are truly premature. Conversely, using birth-weight tables from populations at sea level, 2500 g is the mean weight for 35 weeks' gestation, not 37 weeks. The obstetrician and pediatrician should consult region-specific birth-weight tables. Combining obstetric dating criteria, birth weight and clinical and neurologic examination of the newborn allow the classification of any newborn, term or preterm, as small for gestational age (SGA), appropriate for gestational age (AGA) or large for gestational age (LGA).

Preterm birth is a major cause of neonatal morbidity and mortality in developed countries. In the USA, 75% of the neonatal deaths (excluding congenital malformations) result from preterm delivery. The overall incidence of premature delivery is 9% while the incidence of LBW is 7% and very low birth weight (VLBW, <1500 g) is 1.2%. These figures have not changed significantly since 1950.

Table 16.1 Approximate neonatal survival to discharge of preterm infants born in a tertiary-care center

Gestational age (weeks)	Birth weight (g)	Survivors (%)
24–25	500–750	55
26–27	751–1000	80
28–29	100–1250	93
30–31	1251–1500	96
32–33	150–1750	99
≥34	1751–2000	99+

Table 16.2 Approximate neonatal morbidity rates (%) by gestational age at birth

	Gestational age (weeks)						
	24–25	26–27	28–29	30–31	32–33	34	35
RDS	85	81	65	30	30	20	3
PDA	80	50	50	21	17	13	–
Sepsis	25	25	20	10	7	5	5
NEC	8	6	5	5	3	–	–
IVH grades III and IV	30	9	7	5	3	–	–

RDS, Respiratory distress syndrome; PDA, patent ductus arteriosus; NEC, necrotizing enterocolitis; IVH, intraventricular hemorrhage (Papille's classification).

Neonatal outcome after preterm delivery

Unless the gestational age is known with absolute certainty (as in assisted reproduction) both the estimated fetal weight and the estimated gestational age should be considered in anticipating neonatal survival. Table 16.1 shows a representative survival table compiled from LAC–USC and affiliated hospitals.

The principal conditions responsible for immediate morbidity in the intensive care nursery are respiratory distress syndrome, patent ductus arteriosus, intraventricular hemorrhage, necrotizing enterocolitis, and sepsis. Although incidence figures for these conditions can vary widely, approximate figures are shown in Table 16.2. Specific strategies to limit these morbidities are discussed in Chapter 17.

One of the principal concerns of parents and of care-givers is the potential for long-term major neurologic handicap (retardation, cerebral palsy, seizure disorder, blindness, deafness) in the VLBW infant who survives the neonatal intensive care unit. Data from the mid 1980s showed that such handicap was present in 26% of infants less than 800 g who survived, 17% of infants between 750 and 1000 g, and in 11% of infants weighing between 1000 and 1500 g. Knowledge of local or regional figures for neonatal morbidity and mortality is important for counseling and decision-making in preterm labor.

Etiology of preterm labor

Approximately one-third of premature delivery is due to maternal or fetal complications (hypertensive disorders, placental abruption, placenta previa, multiple fetal pregnancy, congenital malformations), one-third due to preterm premature rupture of membranes (PPROM, Chapter 18), and one-third due to "idiopathic" preterm labor with intact membranes. It is this latter group that is the principal focus of effort toward prevention and therapy. Although PPROM and preterm labor are often related clinically, they are different syndromes and should be analyzed separately.

Maternal infections outside the uterus (e.g., pneumonia, pyelonephritis, viral syndromes) are associated with 5–10% of preterm labor. The association of asymptomatic urinary tract infection with preterm labor is disputed but the weight of evidence favors this association.

Anatomic abnormalities of the uterus may account for between 3 and 15% of preterm labor with or without relative cervical incompetence. The important congenital anomalies include the septate and bicornate uterus, as well as those structural abnormalities associated with *in utero* diethylstilbestrol exposure.

Congenital anomalies of the fetus, especially those associated with fetal hydrops or severe oligohydramnios, can result in preterm labor. Uterine overdistention with severe polyhydramnios or multiple gestation is also associated with preterm labor. The high frequency of SGA infants among those delivered preterm supports the association of placental insufficiency of various causes and preterm labor. Trauma is an uncommon but well-documented cause of preterm labor.

Subclinical genital tract infection leading to intraamniotic infections by the ascending route has been postulated to cause as much as 30% of "idiopathic" preterm labor. It is not clear, however, to what extent the microbial invasion identified in these cases is a consequence of labor and cervical dilatation rather than a cause. If maternal and fetal complications and PPROM are excluded, the cause of approximately 50% of preterm labor remains uncertain; this is an area of active research.

Epidemiology of preterm labor

Socioeconomic and ethnic factors have important associations with preterm labor. The incidence of LBW is higher among the lower socioeconomic strata and certain ethnic groups. In the USA, for example, LBW
occurs in >12% of black women, 9% of Hispanic women, and 6% of
whites.

Maternal weight before pregnancy is related to the weight of offspring, as is lower than normal weight gain during pregnancy. Women
weighing <50 kg (112 lb) are three times as likely to deliver LBW babies as
are heavier mothers. Maternal smoking and extremes of age are also
associated with LBW. Work outside the house, especially that which
involves prolonged standing, has also been associated with LBW.

The highest risk for preterm birth exists among those women with a
history of a prior preterm delivery. Women with two or more preterm
births have a 50% chance of subsequent preterm delivery and a 20%
chance of delivery at <34 weeks gestation. A history of a single second-
trimester abortion or multiple first-trimester abortions is associated with
preterm birth.

Identification of patients at high risk for preterm delivery

Several different risk assessment schemes for preterm labor have been
devised based on the epidemiologic and etiologic factors described above.

Table 16.3 Risk factors in the prediction of spontaneous preterm labor

Major	Minor
Multiple gestation	Febrile illness
Diethylstilbestrol exposure	Bleeding after 12 weeks
Hydramnios	History of pyelonephritis
Uterine anomaly	Cigarettes – more than 10/day
Cervix dilated >1 cm at 32 weeks	Second-trimester abortion × 1
Second-trimester abortion ×2	More than two first-trimester abortions
Previous preterm delivery	
Previous preterm labor – term delivery	
Abdominal surgery during pregnancy	
History of cone biopsy	
Cervical shortening <1 cm at 32 weeks	
Uterine irritability	

The presence of one or more major factors and/or two or more minor factors
places the patient in the high-risk group.

An example of such a risk scoring scheme is shown in Table 16.3. The positive predictive value of such schemes is around 25%, while 40–60% of women are identified as high risk. Unfortunately, almost half of patients who deliver preterm are not identified as high risk. Nevertheless, in the absence of more precise markers, such assessment schemes may be useful.

Patient education in the warning signs and symptoms of preterm labor is now widely accepted as the minimum effort in preterm labor prevention. Such symptoms include rhythmic backache, a sensation of pelvic pressure, a change in vaginal discharge, vaginal spotting, and abdominal cramping. All patients should be encouraged to report these symptoms.

Assessment of cervical length on physical examination or by ultrasonography has been proposed as helpful in identifying patients at risk for preterm labor but neither approach has been widely applied in the USA. Investigators have searched in vain for a hormonal or biochemical predictor of preterm labor. Recently, the presence of cervicovaginal fetal fibronectin has been shown to have excellent predictive value for preterm labor in preliminary studies. Further studies are needed in this area.

SUGGESTED READING

EHRENHAFT PM, WAGNER JL, HERDMAN RD. Changing prognosis for very low birth weight infants. *Obstet Gynecol* 1989;72:528.

GIBBS RS, ROMERO R, HILLIER SL, *et al.* A review of premature birth and subclinical infection. *Am J Obstet Gynecol* 1992;166:1515–1528.

GOLDENBURG RL, NELSON KG, DAVIS RO, *et al.* Delay in delivery: influence of gestational age and the duration of delay on perinatal outcome. *Obstet Gynecol* 1984;64:480–484.

HACK M, HORBAR JD, MALLOY MH, *et al.* Very low birth weight outcomes of the National Institute of Child Health and Human Development Neonatal Network. *Pediatrics* 1991;87:587–597.

LOCKWOOD CJ, SENYEI AE, DISCHE MR, *et al.* Fetal fibronectin in cervical and vaginal secretions as a predictor of preterm delivery. *N Engl J Med* 1991;325:669–674.

LUANER LJ, VILLAR J, KESTLER E, *et al.* The effect of maternal work on fetal growth and duration of pregnancy. *Am J Epidemiol* 1984;119–309.

OWEN J, GOLDENBURG RL, DAVIS RA, *et al.* Evaluation of a risk scoring system as a predictor of preterm birth in an indigent population. *Am J Obstet Gynecol* 1990;163:873–879.

17

Preterm labor: management

T. MURPHY GOODWIN

Management of the patient at high risk to deliver preterm

Once a patient is identified as high risk for preterm delivery on the basis of a scoring system, cervical change, or increased uterine activity, education about preterm labor should be reinforced. Frequent pelvic examinations should be employed and consideration given to regular transvaginal assessment of the cervix, noting both the length and the character of the cervical internal os. Strenuous physical activity should be limited and the working environment modified, especially for women whose work regimen requires prolonged standing. Many such high-risk patients should stop work altogether. A change in the vaginal discharge, found to be associated with *Chlamydia*, group B *Streptococcus* (GBS) or bacterial vaginosis, should be treated aggressively. Coital abstinence should be recommended, especially for those patients who note increased uterine activity with orgasm.

Home uterine activity monitoring (HUAM) has been advocated as a tool to identify patients in preterm labor early in the process, thus leading to a higher rate of successful tocolysis. This tool combines telephone transmission of home external tocodynamometry signals with preterm labor awareness education. Although some studies have shown significant pregnancy prolongation with HUAM, others have not. The precise role of this technique in prematurity prevention is still debated and should be considered investigational. Prophylactic tocolytics or antibiotics have been recommended by some investigators for the high-risk patient. The benefits of such interventions are not clearly established as yet.

Diagnosis of preterm labor

The strict definition of preterm labor requires evidence of cervical change in response to regular uterine contractions. Nevertheless, in clinical practice tocolytic therapy is commonly started on the basis of persistent contractions alone, out of concern for difficulty in stopping advanced labor. If the diagnosis is based on uterine contractions alone, at least 50% of patients will be falsely diagnosed. In a patient without documented cervical change, a period of several hours of bedrest and hydration with monitoring may clarify the situation. If cervical change occurs, tocolytic therapy may be considered. If contractions persist at a rate >1 every 10 min, further observation is warranted, at a minimum.

This observation period should be used to evaluate the mother and the fetus for conditions that may play a role in the onset of labor (e.g., premature rupture of membranes, hydramnios, multifetal gestation, trauma) and/or preclude inhibition of labor (e.g., fetal demise, fetal anomaly incompatible with life, maternal hemorrhage, severe hypertensive disease, amnionitis, or evidence of fetal maturity). A history and physical examination, urinalysis, complete blood count, and cervical culture for GBS, gonorrhea, and *Chlamydia* should be performed. A complete ultrasound examination should be performed as well. If intrauterine infection is suspected, amniocentesis for gram stain, culture, and cell count is indicated.

Approach to tocolytic therapy

In a patient who presents in preterm labor, two conditions must be met before tocolytic therapy is instituted: (1) the patient must meet minimum criteria for the diagnosis of labor; and (2) the fetus should benefit from the delay of delivery. For this reason the gestational age is evaluated with sonography. Evidence of intrauterine growth retardation, which may be seen frequently in patients with preterm labor, should be sought carefully. Tocolytic therapy is usually restricted to gestations between 24 and 34 weeks. Prior to 24 weeks and between 34 and 37 weeks, therapy may be individualized. In the latter gestational age group, amniocentesis to document fetal lung maturity should be considered prior to instituting tocolytic therapy.

The use of antenatal steroids to enhance pulmonary maturity has been studied extensively and the weight of evidence favors a beneficial effect, which includes a reduction in necrotizing enterocolitis and intraventricular hemorrhage. Commonly used regimens include betamethasone, 12 mg intramuscularly given twice, 24 h apart, or dexamethasone, 5–8 mg given twice daily for a total of four doses. The beneficial effect appears to extend from 24 h of initiation of the regimen up to 7 days.

Once the decision is made to treat with tocolytics, the agents employed in the USA are the β-mimetics (ritodrine, or terbutaline) and magnesium sulfate. Only ritodrine is approved by the Food and Drug Administration for the indication of preterm labor and there is little clinical experience with the latter agent. The β-mimetics (ritodrine in particular) have been subjected to the most serious study. The only unequivocal effect noted

Table 17.1 Tocolytic protocols using intravenous magnesium sulfate or ritodrine

---

Hydrate with 500 ml isotonic crystalloid over 20 min
Maintain strict input and output
Solution: 10 g $MgSO_4$ in 100 ml
Loading dose: 4 g bolus/20 min
Start constant infusion 2 g/h
Increase infusion rate 0.5 mg every 20 min until tocolysis is achieved
Continue infusion at the lowest effective dose for 12 h once tocolysis is
    achieved
VS every 15 min during loading and every 1 h while on maintenance
Check DTR every 1 h while on maintenance
Discontinue infusion and call the doctor if:
    There are no DTRs
    Respirations are less than 12/min
    Chest pain or tightness
    Urine output less than 30 ml/h
Dose of $MgSO_4$ above 3 g/h requires physician reevaluation, placement of
    cardioscope and serum Mg levels every 6 h

Intravenous ritodrine
Hydrate with 500 ml isotonic crystalloid over 20 min
Maintain strict input and output
Place patient on cardioscope*
Solution: 150 mg ritodrine in 500 ml 0.45% NS
Start infusion at 0.1 mg/min
Increase dose by 0.05 mg/min every 10 min until tocolysis is achieved
Continue infusion at the lowest effective dose for 12 h after tocolysis is
    achieved
Discontinue infusion if:
    Maternal pulse >140 bpm
    Systolic blood pressure >180 mmHg
    Diastolic blood pressure <40 mmHg
    Fetal heart rate >200 bpm
    >6 maternal or fetal PVCs per min
    Evidence of respiratory impairment
    Persistent chest pain

---

*Some investigators recommend a baseline EKG.
DTR, Deep tendon reflexes; NS, normal saline; PVC, premature ventricular contractions; VS, vital signs.

from the more than 18 randomized controlled trials of ritodrine is a delay in delivery of 48 h. There is less information available for magnesium but the effect appears to be comparable. Though these results have not met expectations, most clinicians feel that there may be a subset of patients who benefit from a given tocolytic regimen. Furthermore, tocolytics in conjunction with steroids or other agents to enhance fetal maturity may confer greater benefit. This latter area has not been thoroughly investigated.

Tocolysis with magnesium sulfate

Because of its comparable efficacy to ritodrine and fewer side-effects, the first-line drug for tocolysis at Los Angeles County–University of Southern California (LAC–USC) is magnesium sulfate. The only absolute contraindication to its use is maternal myasthenia gravis. Relative contraindications include renal insufficiency, asthma, and cardiac disease. The most common complaints (chest pain, severe nausea, flushing drowsiness, or weakness) are seen in less than 5% of patients. Magnesium toxicity which can result in respiratory arrest is counteracted immediately by the administration of one ampule (10 ml) of 10% calcium gluconate. This should be kept readily available. Fluid intake and output should be monitored closely to insure adequate renal excretion of magnesium and to prevent pulmonary edema. A serum concentration of 5–8 mg/dl is desirable. The protocol for the administration of magnesium for tocolysis at LAC–USC is shown in the upper panel of Table 17.1.

Tocolysis with β-mimetics

Contraindications to β-mimetic therapy are listed in Table 17.2. Therapy is usually begun by the intravenous route, although some practitioners prefer subcutaneous administration. The protocol for intravenous usage at LAC–USC is shown in the lower panel of Table 17.1. Maternal complications of parenteral β-mimetic tocolytic therapy include hypokalemia and hyperglycemia, although these are rarely significant in nondiabetic patients. Shortness of breath and chest pain occur in 5–15% of patients, while cardiac dysrhythmias, ischemic changes on EKG, and pulmonary edema occur in 1–5% of patients. The occurrence of the latter complication is more common in multiple gestations and can be reduced by using hypotonic fluids and restricting intake while limiting the total dose and length of β-mimetic therapy. The risk of pulmonary edema may be increased with combined magnesium and parenteral β-mimetic therapy.

Additional tocolytic agents are now available but there are insufficient data to allow recommendation for general use. The subcutaneous terbutaline pump has been advocated, based on the theory that down-

Table 17.2 Contraindications to the administration of β-mimetic agents

---

Maternal cardiac disease (structural disease, ischemia, dysrhythmias)
Hyperthyroidism
Poorly controlled diabetes mellitus
Uncontrolled hypertension
Severe hypovolemia
Any contraindication to tocolysis in general

---

regulation of β-receptors can be diminished with continuous low-dose administration of the drug, combined with intermittent boluses at times of peak uterine activity. Unfortunately, this regimen has been studied insufficiently to document safety and efficacy.

Antiprostaglandins, such as indomethacin, can be given orally or rectally and appear to have efficacy comparable to intravenous agents. Questions of their safety for the fetus are not resolved. It is our custom to use indomethacin (25–50 mg orally or per rectum every 6 h) as a third-line tocolytic between 20 and 32 weeks for not more than 48 h. Calcium channel blockers, such as nifedipine, have been subjected to several studies in humans and appear promising, but a clear demonstration of their safety and efficacy awaits further studies.

Delivery in the preterm infant

Special conditions apply to the delivery of the preterm especially the VLBW, infant. Survival rates for preterm infants born in tertiary-care centers are higher than those of equivalent birth weights transported after delivery. Thus transport to a tertiary-care center prior to delivery should be undertaken if this can be done safely. In the case of the extremely premature infant (500–650 g estimated fetal weight, 23.5–25 weeks estimated gestational age), decisions about what estimated fetal weight and estimated gestational age will require intervention in the event of fetal distress are critical. The obstetrician, neonatologist, and family members should all participate in the decision-making process which should be guided, as much as possible, by local survival and morbidity statistics. Infants erroneously judged to be previable have worse outcomes than gestational-age- and weight-matched controls.

Because of the risk of head entrapment, nonvertex presentations should be delivered by cesarean section if the ultrasound-estimated fetal weight is less than 2000 g. A low vertical or classical uterine incision may be required, especially if labor is not well established. For the vertex premature infant of any weight there is no clearly established benefit for cesarean delivery in the absence of evidence of fetal compromise. A controlled delivery over a generous episiotomy to reduce pressure on the head is recommended. In the event that a recent cervical culture negative for GBS is not available, intravenous ampicillin should be administered during the intrapartum period to reduce the risk of vertical transmission of GBS to the neonate. There is preliminary evidence that the risk of fetal/neonatal intraventricular hemorrhage may be reduced by intrapartum administration of phenobarbital to the mother.

SUGGESTED READING

AHN MO, KWANG YC, PHELAN JP. The low birth weight infant: is there a preferred route of delivery? *Clin Perinatol* 1992;19:411–423.

BENEDETTI TJ. Maternal complications of parenteral beta-sympathomimetic therapy for premature labor. *Am J Obstet Gynecol* 1983;145:1.

CANADIAN PRETERM LABOR INVESTIGATORS GROUP. Treatment of preterm labor with the beta-adrenergic agonist ritodrine. *N Engl J Med* 1992;327:308–312.

COLLABORATIVE GROUP ON ANTENATAL STEROID THERAPY. Effect of antenatal dexamethasone administration on the prevention of respiratory distress syndrome. *Am J Obstet Gynecol* 1981;141:276.

GRIMES D, SCHULT KF. Randomized controlled trials of home uterine activity monitoring: a review and evaluation. *Obstet Gynecol* 1992;79:137–142.

HOLLANDER DI, NAGEY DA, PUPKIN MJ. Magnesium sulfate and ritodrine hydrochloride: a randomized comparison. *Am J Obstet Gynecol* 1987;156:631–637.

MOU SM, SUNDERJI SG, GALL S, *et al.* Multicenter randomized clinical trial of home uterine activity monitoring for detection of preterm labor. *Am J Obstet Gynecol* 1991;165:851.

PAUL RH, KOH K, MONFARED A. Obstetric factors influencing outcome in infants weighing from 1001 to 1500 grams. *Am J Obstet Gynecol* 1979,133:503.

TASLIMI MM, SIBAI BM, AMON E, *et al.* A national survey on preterm labor. *Am J Obstet Gynecol* 1991;160:1352–1360.

18

Premature rupture of the membranes

RAUL ARTAL

Premature rupture of the membranes (PROM) remains one of the most controversial topics in obstetrics, posing numerous clinical questions. PROM is defined as "spontaneous rupture of the chorioamniotic membranes at any time prior to the onset of labor," regardless of the stage in gestation. Term rupture of membranes (TROM) should be distinguished as a separate clinical entity with different management problems from preterm (prior to 37 weeks) rupture of membranes (PREROM). The latent period is part of this clinical equation that could significantly impact the outcome of the pregnancy. The interval from rupture of the membranes to the onset of uterine contractions is defined as the latent period. This period is frequently focused upon to determine clinical decisions.

Incidence

The incidence of PROM ranges from 3 to 18%, with a higher incidence in term patients. Prior to 34 weeks' gestation, this complication occurs in only 3–4% of the total births. As many as 30% of these patients may have prolonged rupture of membranes (PROROM) with a latent period in excess of 7 days.

Etiology

The etiology of PROM is multifactorial. At this time, the possible mechanisms for PROM can only be speculated upon. The known clinical conditions associated with PROM may be caused by different etiologic factors, among them:

1 cervical incompetence;

2 overdistended uterus (multiple pregnancies, polyhydramnios);

3 inherited membrane defect (genetic conditions, low maternal serum copper, vitamin C deficiency);

4 exogenous effects on the biomechanical properties of the membranes (by proteolytic enzymes produced by mycoplasma, *Escherichia coli*, *Streptococcus* B and D, and by the release of collagenase-like enzymes present in seminal fluid).

The following is a possible mechanism leading to PROM: the chorio-amniotic membranes that lack vascularization following premature dilatation of the cervix and/or detachment of the chorioamniotic membranes from the site of uterine implantation undergo a process of devitalization, necrotize, and eventually burst. The same process may be accelerated by infection and/or structural deficiency. The biomechanical strength of the membrane is primarily dependent upon the structural changes in the collagen matrix, the main structural strength being derived from the basement membrane of the amnion. The histologic structure of the chorion reflects a supportive nutrient supplier function rather than a biomechanical function. Events leading to alterations in the membrane structure may also be part of a natural process of aging of the collagen matrix.

Diagnosis

Rupture of membranes is easily diagnosed in the majority of cases, and is confirmed by either clinical findings or tests that include pooling of amniotic fluid, a ferning nitrazine test, or staining of fetal cells. The history is usually typical, with the patient reporting fluid escaping from the vagina. On occasions it is important to determine the nature of the fluid; it could be urine lost as a result of urinary stress incontinence.

The initial examination is critical for its subsequent clinical implications and potential adverse outcome and should be limited to a *sterile* speculum examination. The examination should be performed by a skilled individual in order to avoid excessive pelvic manipulation, a significant factor in precipitating subsequent infections. The amniotic fluid sample is obtained from the posterior vaginal vault. False-positive tests may result when the amniotic fluid sample is mixed with blood, cervical mucus, urine, talc, or lubricants. Fetal lung profile determinations and cultures could be obtained from the fluid collected. Cultures for β-*Streptococcus* should also be obtained from the introitus and rectum.

Evaluation

The first evaluation of the patient includes an ultrasound evaluation and fetal heart monitoring. Preterm deliveries are known to occur with a higher frequency in infants with congenital malformations; therefore, an attempt should be made to rule out such malformations. An evaluation of the amniotic fluid volume could predict potential changes in the fetal status secondary to cord compression. A search for easily accessible pockets of amniotic fluid is undertaken in the attempt to perform an amniocentesis to rule out the occurrence of chorioamnionitis and to evaluate the fetal lungs. The presence of bacteria in the amniotic fluid has been associated with a 75% subsequent development of chorioamnionitis. In the very rare case where there is doubt whether the patient has ruptured membranes, a dye (such as indigo carmine) can be instilled into the amniotic sac under ultrasound guidance and recovered vaginally to confirm the diagnosis of PROM (Fig. 18.1).

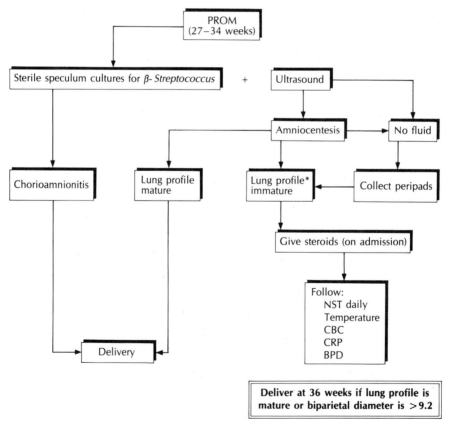

*If in labor, consider tocolytics for 24–48 h

Fig. 18.1 Management of premature rupture of membranes (PROM). NST, nonstress test; CBC, complete blood count; CRP, C-reactive protein; BPD, biparietal diameter.

When unable to perform an amniocentesis, C-reactive protein (CRP) levels can be monitored to predict developing chorioamnionitis. CRP is produced in the liver and is present in healthy pregnant women at concentrations ranging from 0.3 to 0.8 mg/dl (the upper 95% confidence limit in pregnancy is 2 mg/dl). CRP rises significantly following injury and inflammation. Because of this latter association, its serum measurement can aid in the management of patients with PROM. The positive predictive value for CRP in predicting chorioamnionitis is somewhat higher than that of other, commonly utilized nonspecific tests (such as complete blood count, temperature course, etc.). The clinical importance in CRP determinations is its negative predictive value, i.e., a CRP of lower than 2 mg/dl will indicate an absence of infection for approximately an additional 24 h in 98% of cases. Conversely, elevated CRP in the absence of uterine contractions will predict chorioamnionitis in 82% of cases. The elevation in CRP will precede other common signs of chorioamnionitis: maternal fever by 21–34 h, uterine activity by 17–28 h, and an increase in white blood cells by 16 h. It is also important to point out that corticosteroid administration does not affect the CRP levels, in contrast to other tests. In the event that amniotic fluid cannot be obtained via amniocentesis for fetal lung profile determinations, the patient's peripads may be collected, refrigerated and squeezed to obtain a few millimeters necessary for lung profile determinations. On those occasions, the only valid parameter is phosphatidylglycerol, since vaginal secretions could affect the validity of the remainder of the fetal lung profile.

Management

The principle guiding the management of patients with PROM emphasizes judicious clinical attempts to prolong pregnancy until fetal lung maturity is attained or chorioamnionitis is diagnosed or suspected. The reported incidence of chorioamnionitis has decreased in recent years; however, its consequences include significant complications for both mother and fetus. Prolonging pregnancy is an option only in the absence of chorioamnionitis – its diagnosis becomes an absolute indication for the termination of pregnancy, regardless of gestational age. About 10–15% of patients with PROM will develop chorioamnionitis; of them, only 15% will become critically ill and septic. The reported incidence of infections in the neonates is much higher. As many as 50% of neonatal deaths have evidence of a preceding infection. With the advent of newer broadspectrum antibiotics, serious complications can be lessened or prevented.

From the neonatal point of view, surveys of the literature still indicate that neonatal morbidity and mortality due to prematurity exceed complications due to infection.

These facts dictate an initial approach of expectant management for patients with PROM. Hence, maternal transport to a tertiary-care center is an important factor where delivery of a preterm baby is best accomplished. In such instances, during the transfer, uterine tocolytic agents may be administered. In case of the appearance of a solitary presumptive sign of infection, clinical judgment determines the therapeutic approach.

In the absence of chorioamnionitis, the clinical approach varies, depending on the gestational age and may be grouped as follows: when membranes rupture at: (1) >36 weeks; (2) 32–36 weeks; (3) 26–32 weeks; and (4) <26 weeks.

It is generally accepted that the patient should be delivered as soon as fetal lung maturity is documented. In the absence of diabetes mellitus, patients at a gestational age >36 weeks with ruptured membranes should be delivered; the risks outweigh the benefits. Fetal lung maturation is occasionally delayed in the infant of diabetic mothers, and an amniocentesis should be considered to determine if the fetal lungs are mature.

It has been reported that when a patient ruptures her membranes at term, induction of labor should be delayed 8–12 h. In the absence of infection and/or fetal distress prolongation of the latent period will result in a lower incidence of cesarean section; however, a relatively higher incidence of resulting endometritis has been observed. This latter approach of delaying the induction of labor appears also to benefit patients at 32–36 weeks' gestation. At 32–36 weeks, delaying the induction of labor by at least 16 h may significantly reduce the incidence of respiratory distress syndrome in the neonate. There is no benefit to be gained by prolonging the pregnancy further at this gestational age if estimated fetal weight exceeds 2000 g. Therefore, after 16 h has elapsed, labor should be induced if it has not begun spontaneously.

Controversy surrounds the management of patients with PROM at 26–32 weeks. In some cases, successful outcome is possible at gestational ages as low as 26 weeks or less. It is encouraging that improved neonatal care of low-gestational-age infants has reduced neonatal mortality significantly. However, long-term morbidity and neurologic deficit for the surviving infants is a significant factor for which there are no solutions as yet. In patients managed expectantly, daily nonstress tests, CRP, temperature, and white blood cell counts are monitored. If the nonstress test is nonreactive, a biophysical profile should be performed. Some 30–40% of patients with PROM at <34 weeks will develop spontaneous contractions within the first 24 h. Tocolysis of uterine contractions may be selectively attempted only after chorioamnionitis has been ruled out, preferably by an amniocentesis. A 48-h delay of labor could benefit the fetus; during this time corticosteroids may be administered to promote secretion of surfactant by the immature fetal lungs. It is important to recognize that the literature is equally divided between those claiming beneficial fetal effects from maternal steroid administration and those who deny any such effect. Administering steroids only in selected patients in whom infection has been ruled out and in whom fetal lung immaturity has been documented may be a judicious approach. In such events, intramuscular betamethasone, 12 mg, is administered at 24-h intervals for a total of two doses. Maximum therapeutic effect is obtained 72 h after administration and wanes 7 days later. Repeat treatment should be considered. One should be aware that the patient's immunoresponse will be suppressed during such treatment and she should be closely monitored for signs of infection. Monitoring CRP levels is reliable and not influenced by steroids.

The most difficult clinical decision pertains to patients who rupture their membranes between 16 and 26 weeks' gestation. Only 25% of such pregnancies will reach viability: the remainder will be lost because of either premature delivery or the development of an infection. A few of these fetuses may develop significant limb and other deformities while approximately 10% will not survive because of lung hypoplasia. Up to 90% of surviving extremely-low-birth-weight infants demonstrate moderate to severe neurologic impairment at 20 months of age and later. Therefore, a decision has to be made with the parents as to the desire to terminate or to attempt to prolong the pregnancy.

Delivery

Once the decision is made to deliver the patient, attempts should be made to carry out a vaginal delivery. Should infection develop, there is no need to expedite the delivery. Cesarean section should be reserved for obstetric indications only. Broad-spectrum antibiotic therapy should be initiated in the form of ampicillin in combination with gentamicin for patients with infection. Newer cephalosporins such as Cefizox may provide some benefit since, in addition to covering a broad spectrum, they cross the placenta readily. The use of prophylactic antibiotics in patients with PROM with no sign of infection remains investigational at this time. Their administration is reserved for patients at risk for postpartum endometritis and in whom concurrent medical disorders such as diabetes or heart disease are present. However, it appears that they may delay the onset of infection, thereby prolonging pregnancy, and also reduce maternal and neonatal morbidity.

Summary

In patients with PROM, one must balance the risk of developing infection in the mother and fetus if undelivered versus the risk of delivering a premature infant who may develop significant morbidity and mortality. If there is no evidence of chorioamnionitis, patients can be managed expectantly, consequently lowering the incidence of respiratory distress syndrome and other morbidity in the neonates.

SUGGESTED READING

ARIAS F, TOMICH P. Etiology and outcome of low birth weight and preterm infants. *Obstet Gynecol* 1982;60:277.

ARTAL R, SOKOL RJ, NEWMAN M, *et al*. The mechanical properties of prematurely and non-prematurely ruptured membranes. *Am J Obstet Gynecol* 1976;125:655.

ARTAL R, BURGERSON R, FERNANDEZ FJ, *et al*. Fetal and maternal copper levels in patients at term with and without premature rupture of membranes. *Obstet Gynecol* 1978;53:608.

ARTAL R, BURGERSON RE, HOBEL CI, *et al*. An *in vitro* model for the study of enzymatically mediated biomechanical changes in the chorioamniotic membranes. *Am J Obstet Gynecol* 1979;133:656.

COLLABORATIVE GROUP ON ANTENATAL STEROID THERAPY. Effect of antenatal dexamethasone administration on the prevention of respiratory distress syndrome. *Am J Obstet Gynecol* 1981;141:276.

CROWLEY P, CHALMERS I, KEIRSE MJ. The effects of corticosteroid administration before preterm delivery: an overview of the evidence from controlled trials. *Br J Obstet Gynaecol* 1990;97:11.

DAIKOKU NH, KALTREIDER F, JOHNSON TRB, *et al*. Premature rupture of membranes and preterm labor. Neonatal infection and perinatal mortality risks. *Obstet Gynecol* 1981;53:417.

EVANS MI, HAJJ SN, DEVOE LD, *et al*. C-reactive protein as a predictor of infectious morbidity with premature rupture of membranes. *Am J Obstet Gynecol* 1980;138:648.

GARITE TJ, FREEMAN RK. Chorioamnionitis in the preterm gestation. *Obstet Gynecol* 1982;54:539.

GARITE TJ, FREEMAN RK, LINZEM EM, *et al*. Prospective randomized study of corticosteroids in the management of premature rupture of membranes and the premature gestation. *Am J Obstet Gynecol* 1981;141:508.

GIBBS RS, BLANCO JD. Premature rupture of membranes. *Obstet Gynecol* 1982; 60:671.

GOLDSTEIN AS, MANGURTEN HH, LIBRETTI JV, *et al*. Lecithin/sphingomyelin ratio in amniotic fluid obtained vaginally. *Am J Obstet Gynecol* 1980;138:232.

GUNN GC, MISHELL DR, MORTON DG. Premature rupture of the fetal membranes. A review. *Am J Obstet Gynecol* 1970;106:469.

HERSCHEL M, KENNEDY JL, KAYNE HL, *et al*. Survival of infants born at 24 to 28 weeks' gestation. *Obstet Gynecol* 1982;60:154.

JOHNSON JWC, DAIIKOKU NH, NIEBYL JR, *et al*. Premature rupture of the membranes and prolonged latency. *Obstet Gynecol* 1981;57:547.

JONES MD JR, BURD LI, BOWES WA Jr, *et al*. Failure of association of premature rupture of membranes with respiratory distress syndrome. *N Engl J Med* 1975;292:1253.

KOH KS, CHAN FH, MANFARED AH, *et al*. The changing perinatal and maternal outcome in chorioamnionitis. *Obstet Gynecol* 1979;53:730.

MORALES WJ, DIEKEL ND, LATER AJ, ZADROZNY D. The effect of antenatal dexamethasone administration on the prevention of respiratory distress syndrome in preterm gestations in the premature rupture of the membranes. *Am J Obstet Gynecol* 1986;154:591.

NAEYE RL. Factors that predispose to premature rupture of the fetal membranes. *Obstet Gynecol* 1982;60:93.

NAEYE RL, PETERS EC. Causes and consequences of premature rupture of fetal membranes. *Lancet* 1981;1:192.

NELSON LH, MEIS PJ, HATJIS CG, *et al*. Premature rupture of membranes: a prospective, randomized evaluation of steroids, latent phase and expectant management. *Obstet Gynecol* 1985;66:55.

OHLSSON A. Treatments of preterm premature rupture of the membranes: a meta analysis. *Am J Obstet Gynecol* 1989;160:890.

ROMEM Y, ARTAL R. C-reactive protein in pregnancy in the postpartum period. *Am J Obstet Gynecol* 1985;151:380.

ROMEM Y, ARTAL R. C-reactive protein as a predictor for chorioamnionitis in cases of premature rupture of the membranes. *Am J Obstet Gynecol* 1984;150:546.

ROMEM Y, GREENSPOON J, ARTAL R. Clinical chorioamnionitis – analysis of the incubation period in patients with preterm premature rupture of membranes. *Am J Perinatol* 1985;2:314.

ROMERO R, QUINTERO R, DYARZUM E, *et al*. Intraamniotic infection and the onset of labor in preterm premature rupture of the membranes. *Am J Obstet Gynecol* 1988;159:661.

SCHREIBER J, BENEDETTI T. Conservative management of preterm premature rupture of the fetal membranes in a low socioeconomic population. *Am J Obstet Gynecol* 1980;136:92.

SPERLING RS, RAMAMORPHYR S, GIBBS RS. A comparison of intrapartum versus immediate postpartum treatment of intraamniotic infection. *Obstet Gynecol* 1987;70:861.

WEBB GA. Maternal death associated with premature rupture of the membranes. An analysis of 54 cases. *Am J Obstet Gynecol* 1967;98:594.

19

Chorioamnionitis: significance and treatment

KEE SENG KOH

Chorioamnionitis is an acute inflammation of the fetal membranes. The likely causative organisms are usually the endogenous cervicovaginal flora. Although retrospective analyses showed an incidence of 0.5–1% of all pregnancies, recent prospective studies suggest a prevalence rate of 4.3–10.5%. Despite the potential seriousness of this complication to the mother and fetus, it presents a considerable diagnostic and therapeutic dilemma for the obstetrician.

Etiology

Intraamniotic infection is a mixed aerobic–anaerobic polymicrobial infection. The infecting microorganisms may enter the amniotic cavity by: (1) ascending infection, either via intact membranes or, more commonly, after the membranes have ruptured; (2) transplacental infection by the hematogenous route. This is particularly the case with *Listeria monocytogenes* and group A streptococci; or (3) diagnostic and therapeutic procedures such as amniocentesis, cordocentesis, and cervical cerclage.

The predisposing factors include: prolonged rupture of membranes (infection occurs in 3–25% of women whose membranes have ruptured for more than 24 h); frequent vaginal examinations; prolonged labor, and internal fetal monitoring.

Many patients with chorioamnionitis experience dystocia. The incidence of chorioamnionitis is higher in patients of low socioeconomic status.

Clinical features

The clinical features of chorioamnionitis are often difficult to detect even in the presence of established infection. A high index of suspicion is the cardinal rule in the diagnosis of chorioamnionitis. From the practical point of view, the presumptive diagnosis is usually based on the following factors.

1 A temperature above 38°C or 100.4°F in the absence of any other obvious causes of fever, including dehydration.

2 Purulent or malodorous amniotic fluid. This is not commonly observed.

3 Presence of bacteria with or without leukocytes in a gram-stained specimen (unspun sample at 100× magnification) of the amniotic fluid. The specimen may be obtained by transabdominal amniocentesis or through an intrauterine pressure catheter, provided that the first 10 ml of aspirated fluid is discarded.

Additional clinical features may include:

1 uterine tenderness;

2 maternal tachycardia;

3 fetal tachycardia;

4 maternal leukocytosis (>12 000–15 000 white blood cells per μl) with a left shift. A progressive rise in white blood counts on serial complete blood counts is an important warning sign.

It is often difficult to correlate the clinical picture of intrauterine infection with the findings of bacteriologic and histologic studies of the placenta, umbilical cord, and fetal membranes after delivery. Occult chorioamnionitis (intraamniotic bacterial colonization detected by transabdominal amniocentesis) has been associated with 15–25% of preterm labor with intact membranes and is refractory to tocolytic therapy. Using a research laboratory, Watts *et al.* detected occult amniotic fluid infection in 19% of gravida in idiopathic preterm labor with intact membranes between 23 and 34 weeks; 65% of the positive cultures occurred before 30 weeks. The frequency of positive cultures was inversely related to gestational age. *Fusobacterium* and *Bacteroides* were commonly isolated before 30 weeks and *Ureaplasma* was frequently found after 30 weeks. Forty percent of patients with positive cultures for bacteria determined by the research laboratory had negative cultures performed by the hospital's clinical laboratory. Clinical characteristics did not differentiate between women with and without positive cultures. Only an elevated C-reactive protein and a positive amniotic fluid gram stain were sensitive indications of amniotic fluid infection.

It would seem appropriate to consider an amniocentesis in patients in preterm labor at <30 weeks' gestation. Similarly, patients in preterm labor who failed to be tocolyzed by one agent should be considered for an amniocentesis before a second tocolytic is begun.

Perinatal complications

The presence of chorioamnionitis does not indicate that fetal or neonatal infection is present, but suggests that such infection may occur. The outcomes of newborns of mothers with chorioamnionitis are related to gestational age at delivery and birth weight. The premature and the dysmature fetuses are the most vulnerable. The possible consequences are:

1 no clinical effects, only signs such as newborn bacterial colonization;
2 premature birth, with the usual risks of premature newborns, especially respiratory distress syndrome and intracranial hemorrhage;
3 perinatal infection, particularly involving the lungs, gut, blood stream, meninges, and brain;
4 intrauterine death.

Maternal complications

Maternal mortality is exceedingly rare. Chorioamnionitis and postpartum endomyometritis, when untreated, can progress to chronic pelvic inflammatory disease with subsequent risk of infertility, ectopic pregnancy, and menstrual disturbances.

With recent advances in obstetric care, intrapartum biophysical and biochemical fetal monitoring, neonatal intensive care, safer blood transfusion, better anesthesia, and modern antibiotics, the maternal and perinatal outcomes in cases of chorioamnionitis have improved considerably when compared with older published data.

Management

The best treatment of chorioamnionitis is prevention of its occurrence. If premature rupture of membranes occurs at term, labor should be induced in a cephalic presentation if it has not started within 6–12 h.

Current antibiotic trials draw no definite conclusion as to the efficacy of antibiotics in prolonging pregnancy in patients with either preterm labor or preterm premature rupture of membranes.

Early diagnosis and prompt treatment remain the cornerstones of management. Evacuation of the uterus, regardless of fetal maturity, is mandatory. In the face of infection, spontaneous labor usually ensues; if not, oxytocin induction is usually commenced. Close monitoring of maternal vital signs, urine output, and continuous fetal heart rate monitoring are mandatory.

A thorough septic work-up is indicated before commencing antibiotic therapy. It includes complete blood count, blood culture, SMA 18, urinalysis and culture, and amniotic fluid culture if possible. A gram stain of the amniotic fluid may guide initial therapy.

Full doses of broad-spectrum antibiotics should be given. The combination of ampicillin (2 g iv every 6 h) and gentamicin (80 mg iv every 8 h) is administered until the patient is afebrile for 48 h. Erythromycin (500 mg iv every 6 h) or a first-generation cephalosporin (Ancef 1 g iv every 6 h) is substituted for ampicillin in the penicillin-allergic patient. For the postcesarean section patient, the regimen of clindamycin (900 mg iv every 8 h) and gentamicin (80 mg iv every 8 h) is recommended in view of the increased amount of devitalized tissues which favor anaerobic infection. The parenteral antibiotics should be continued until the patient is afebrile for 48 h and oral antibiotic treatment is unnecessary following intravenous antibiotic therapy. Single-agent antibiotic therapy has been proposed with various third-generation cephalosporins and ureidopenicillins, but their relative safeties and efficacies have not been firmly established. Such alternatives may be useful in patients susceptible to the toxicity of aminoglycosides.

Vaginal delivery is preferred in the patient with chorioamnionitis. Cesarean section is performed only if there is an obstetric indication, since it carries an increased risk of septic pelvic thrombophlebitis and wound infection. Extraperitoneal cesarean section and cesarean hysterectomy are not indicated today because of the availability of effective antibiotics. No optimal diagnosis-to-delivery interval has been defined to minimize maternal or perinatal morbidity or mortality. At delivery, aerobic and anaerobic cultures should be obtained from the placental membranes.

Not all neonates born out of a septic intrauterine environment require antibiotics. Care should be individualized. The premature and the symptomatic newborns should be aggressively treated with antibiotics. Careful examination and investigation of newborns should lead to better means of determining who will require antibiotics. Aids to the early diagnosis of newborn infection are:

1   total and differential white blood count;
2   blood culture: aerobic and anaerobic;
3   urine: gram stain, culture, and antigen screen for *Escherichia coli*, group B streptococci, and *Haemophilus influenzae*;
4   chest X-ray, especially in the presence of respiratory distress;
5   cerebrospinal fluid: gram stain, cell count and culture if the newborn is clinically septic, urinary antigen-positive or blood culture-positive.

Examination of the gastric aspirate is of little value since it merely reflects ingestion of the amniotic fluid contents.

The common antibiotic regimen used is a combination of ampicillin (100–200 mg/kg per 24 h iv in two or three divided doses) and gentamicin (2 mg/kg per 24 h iv once daily for newborns weighing less than 1500 g;

3.5–4.0 mg/kg per 24 h in two divided doses for newborns weighing between 1500 and 2500 g; and 4.5–5.0 mg/kg per 24 h in two divided doses for newborns weighing more than 2500 g). This regimen covers a wide range of organisms, yet limits potential toxicity of the initial therapy. The choice of antibiotics may be altered when the culture results become available. The duration of antibiotic therapy will depend on the clinical findings and the response to therapy. If the newborn is clinically asymptomatic and all cultures are negative, the antibiotics may be discontinued after 3 days. For gram-negative septicemia, the antibiotics are usually given for 10–14 days, and for meningitis, the antibiotics are usually given for 2–3 weeks.

SUGGESTED READING

GIBBS RS, ROMERO MD, HILLIER SL, *et al*. A review of premature birth and subclinical infection. *Am J Obstet Gynecol* 1992;166:1515–1528.

KOH KS, CHAN FH, MONFARED AH, *et al*. The changing perinatal and maternal outcome in chorioamnionitis. *Obstet Gynecol* 1979;53:730–733.

MERCER BM, MORETTI ML, PREVOST RR, *et al*. Erythromycin therapy in preterm premature rupture of the membranes: a prospective, randomized trial of 220 patients. *Am J Obstet Gynecol* 1992;166:794–802.

ROMERO R, MAZOR M, MORROTTI R, *et al*. Microbial invasion of the amniotic cavity in spontaneous rupture of membranes at term. *Am J Obstet Gynecol* 1992;166:129–133.

WATTS DH, KROHN MA, HILLIER SL, *et al*. The association of occult amniotic fluid infection with gestational age and neonatal outcome among women in preterm labor. *Obstet Gynecol* 1992;79:351–357.

WAX JR, JOHNSON TRB. The etiology, diagnosis, and management of acute chorioamnionitis. *Female Patient* 1992;17:15–20.

20

Meconium during labor: significance and management

CHARLES J. MACRI

Introduction

Meconium is a dark-green, mucilaginous material in the intestine of the full-term fetus. It is a mixture of the secretion of the intestinal glands and amniotic fluid. There have been several hypotheses to explain meconium passage *in utero*. Walker measured umbilical vein oxygen saturation in the presence of meconium and found lower levels when compared to those in whom meconium was absent. Saling proposed that fetal hypoxia leads to vasoconstriction in the fetal gut, which results in increased peristalsis, sphincter relaxation, and meconium passage. Hon studied fetal heart rate (FHR) patterns associated with meconium. He suggested that cord compression and vagal activation, not hypoxia, may lead to meconium passage. Meconium passage may be a normal physiologic response, especially in the mature fetus.

Meconium passage and alterations in the FHR have been described as signs of fetal distress. The mere presence of meconium in the amniotic fluid during labor is not considered either a sensitive or specific indicator of intrauterine fetal distress, and may simply indicate the maturing fetal vagal system provoked by fetal stress. However, its presence may be a sign of oligohydramnios, postdates gestation, or FHR abnormalities. Even when meconium passage is not associated with fetal stress, it may be associated with meconium aspiration syndrome in the neonate.

Risk factors

The consistency of meconium has been shown to be a useful indicator of risk to the fetus. We now understand that the consistency of meconium is inversely related to the amniotic fluid index (AFI). Thus, the presence of thick meconium reliably predicts oligohydramnios. Postdate pregnancies are at risk for both oligohydramnios and meconium passage. The reported perinatal mortality rate with meconium passage varies widely; from 1 to 13.5% when no other signs of fetal distress are found. In 1955, Resnick reported a perinatal mortality rate of 8% when thin meconium was present with an abnormal FHR, and 32% when thick meconium was present with an abnormal FHR. The association of higher rates of fetal morbidity and mortality associated with thick meconium has been confirmed by more recent studies.

The presence of meconium and an abnormal FHR pattern may indicate fetal acidosis. Hobel found a good correlation between fetal scalp blood pH below 7.25 and a 1-min Apgar score under 7, if signs of fetal distress as demonstrated by meconium and/or abnormal FHR were present. Fetal acidosis was identified earlier in labor if meconium was present, than if meconium was absent. When meconium was absent, even when FHR abnormalities were seen, acidosis developed later in labor. Finally, infants with thin meconium with or without FHR abnormalities had similar 1- and 5-min Apgar scores when compared to controls. Those with heavy meconium with or without FHR abnormalities had the lowest 1- and 5-min Apgar scores of all those studied.

In 1975, Miller *et al.* studied and reported 366 high-risk patients with singleton, vertex pregnancies who were prospectively studied during labor. In this group of patients, FHR and intrauterine pressure were continuously monitored, and fetal scalp blood samples were performed during early labor, at 5 cm dilatation, and at delivery. Umbilical artery and venous blood samples were performed after delivery and analyzed for pH, P_{O_2}, P_{CO_2}, and base deficit. The incidence of meconium in the amniotic fluid was 29%. While this is higher than the general obstetric population, it reflects the high-risk obstetric population at Los Angeles County–University of Southern California. They found that there was no apparent difference in the incidence of FHR deceleration patterns between the meconium and nonmeconium groups. If late decelerations were present with less than 10% of the contractions, there was no statistical difference in the incidence of low Apgar scores between the meconium and nonmeconium groups. However, if late decelerations were present with more than 10% of the contractions, the patients with meconium were statistically more likely to have low Apgar scores than the nonmeconium patients. Thus, meconium without late decelerations did not predict fetal acidosis. However, neonates born after meconium staining may be at increased risk for meconium aspiration even when no abnormalities of the FHR are noted.

When meconium is identified in labor, a careful reevaluation of the pregnancy record and labor should be performed. A review of the medical record will identify the postdates fetus, intrauterine growth retardation, hypertension, or other disorders that may be associated with placental dysfunction. Postdate pregnancy is associated with a higher incidence of macrosomia, shoulder dystocia, oligohydramnios, and meconium passage. Identification of the postdates fetus with oligohydramnios and thick meconium, especially when associated with an abnormal FHR pattern, is important. Breech presentation may not have been recognized at the initial examination and should be excluded. Labor abnormalities can be excluded by graphic analysis of labor, clinical pelvimetry, and estimation of fetal size. An intrauterine pressure catheter can be used to quantify uterine pressure. Fetal well-being can be evaluated using electronic FHR monitoring and fetal scalp blood sampling. Ultrasound examination should be used to evaluate amniotic fluid volume (AFI), and can aid in fetal weight estimation. When oligohydramnios is identified, amnioinfusion should be considered.

Oligohydramnios

Rutherford and Phelan described the increased risk for adverse perinatal outcome in the presence of oligohydramnios in labor. Oligohydramnios was defined as an AFI of 5.0 cm or less. Patients with oligohydramnios were at increased risk of FHR abnormalities, meconium passage, and cesarean delivery for fetal distress. Sarno confirmed that the fetus with an abnormal response to fetal acoustic stimulation and oligohydramnios was at increased risk for FHR abnormalities in labor and meconium passage.

Strong *et al.* determined that prophylactic amnioinfusion in patients with oligohydramnios in labor led to a decreased incidence of: (1) meconium passage; (2) FHR abnormalities; and (3) cesarean delivery for fetal distress. Amnioinfusion decreases cord compression, often associated with oligohydramnios. In the presence of thick meconium, amnioinfusion may dilute the meconium and decrease the incidence of cord compression.

Management: amnioinfusion

Amnioinfusion has been shown to decrease dramatically the incidence of meconium aspiration in fetuses with a normal FHR pattern, and should be considered in every case of thick meconium with a normal FHR. We have found that thick meconium is a reliable predictor of oligohydramnios. In patients with thick meconium and oligohydramnios, in which the FHR is normal, prophylactic amnioinfusion was associated with a decreased incidence of FHR abnormalities during labor, cesarean delivery for fetal distress, and meconium below the vocal cords. There were no cases of meconium aspiration syndrome in the neonates when amnio-infusion was performed. DeLee suction of the oropharynx and naso-pharynx was performed in all cases. Furthermore, all neonates were evaluated by pediatricians in the delivery room, and underwent intuba-tion and endotracheal suctioning after birth.

Meconium aspiration

Currently, there are conflicting theories about when meconium aspiration occurs, and what circumstances lead to respiratory distress and mecon-ium aspiration syndrome in the neonate. There have been several reports of meconium aspiration in neonates born by elective repeat cesarean section, before labor and in early labor, in which the FHR was normal. Because meconium aspiration can occur *in utero*, it appears that preven-tion is not always possible. We do recommend amnioinfusion in labor as described, and also recommend DeLee suction at delivery, as well as pediatric evaluation of these neonates in the delivery room.

Several neonatologists believe that routine intubation and endotra-cheal suctioning is not necessary to prevent meconium aspiration syn-drome, and may be potentially harmful because of increased risk of barotrauma, upper airway trauma, depression, and apnea. However, this viewpoint is not universally accepted. Larger prospective studies should be done before eliminating routine intubation and endotracheal suction-ing for the neonate, especially those exposed to thick meconium *in utero*. Authorities at each institution may wish to determine their own policy while awaiting definitive data.

Summary

When meconium is present in the amniotic fluid a careful review of the pregnancy and labor should be performed to identify etiologic factors. In all cases when meconium is present in the amniotic fluid, continuous electronic FHR monitoring should be performed during labor. If any abnormal FHR changes are identified, further evaluation of the fetus by fetal scalp blood sampling for acid–base analysis is indicated.

Amnioinfusion in patients with thick meconium has been shown to decrease the incidence of FHR abnormalities, decrease the incidence of meconium below the vocal cords, and to decrease the incidence of cesarean delivery for fetal distress. Prophylactic amnioinfusion has been shown to decrease the incidence of meconium passage when performed in pregnancy complicated by oligohydramnios.

Oligohydramnios and meconium are frequently present in postdates pregnancies. These pregnancies may also be associated with macrosomia. Extreme care should be taken to avoid difficult or traumatic delivery, fetal hypoxia, maternal hypotension, and uterine hyperstimulation. At delivery, DeLee suction of the airway should be performed. Evaluation of the neonate by a pediatrician or other qualified personnel in the delivery room should be considered, especially when thick meconium with or without FHR abnormalities is present. While routine examination of the trachea by laryngoscopy followed by suction in all neonates born with meconium may not be required, skilled personnel and equipment should always be available in the delivery room.

SUGGESTED READING

CARSON BS, LOSEY RW, BOWER WA, SIMMONS MA. Combined obstetric and pediatric approach to prevent meconium aspiration syndrome. *Am J Obstet Gynecol* 1976;126:712.

HOBEL CJ. Intrapartum clinical assessment of fetal distress. *Am J Obstet Gynecol* 1971;110:336.

HON EH. The fetal heart rate. In: Carey HM, ed. *Modern Trends in Human Reproductive Physiology*. London: Butterworth, 1963:245.

KATZ VL, BOWES WA. Meconium aspiration syndrome: reflections on a murky subject. *Am J Obstet Gynecol* 1992;166:171–183.

MACRI CJ, SCHRIMMER DB, LEUNG A, GREENSPOON JS, PAUL RH. Amnioinfusion improves outcome in pregnancies complicated by thick meconium and oligohydramnios. *Am J Obstet Gynecol* 1992;167:117–121.

MEIS PJ, HALL M, MARSHALL JR, HOBEL CJ. Meconium passage: a new classification for risk during labor. *Am J Obstet Gynecol* 1978;131:509.

MILLER FC, SACKS DA, YEH SY, *et al.* Significance of meconium during labor. *Am J Obstet Gynecol* 1978;122:573.

RESNICK L. Fetal distress: a comparison of fetal mortality in relation to meconium staining of the liquor amnii postmaturity. *S Afr Med J* 1955;29:857.

RUTHERFORD SE, PHELAN JP, SMITH CV, JACOBS N. The four-quadrant assessment of aminotic fluid volume: an adjunct to antepartum fetal heart rate testing. *Obstet Gynecol* 1987;70:353–356.

SALING EW. *Foetal and Neonatal Hypoxia in Relation to Clinical Obstetric Practice*. London: Edward Arnold, 1968:117.

SARNO AP, AHN MO, PHELAN JP, PAUL RH. Fetal acoustic stimulation in early intrapartum period as a predictor of subsequent fetal condition. *Am J Obstet Gynecol* 1990;162:762–767.

STRONG TH, HETZLER G, SARNO AP, PAUL RH. Prophylactic intrapartum amnioinfusion: a randomized clinical trial. *Am J Obstet Gynecol* 1990;162:1370.

WALKER J. Meconium staining and lower umbilical vein oxygen saturation. *J Obstet Gynecol Br Empire* 1954;61:162.

WENSTROM DK, PARSONS MT. The prevention of meconium aspiration in labor using amnioinfusion. *Obstet Gynecol* 1989;73:707.

21

Intrapartum amnioinfusion: indications and techniques

CHARLES J. MACRI & JEFFREY S. GREENSPOON

Introduction

Intrapartum amnioinfusion is a procedure used to restore the amniotic fluid volume to normal by instilling normal saline into the amniotic cavity via a transcervical intrauterine catheter. This procedure will reduce the rate of cesarean delivery for fetal distress. Amnioinfusion will improve neonatal outcome as measured by umbilical artery pH and will decrease the rate of meconium aspiration in pregnancies complicated by the presence of thick meconium.

Among patients who had amnioinfusion for thick meconium, the cesarean delivery rate was 29% in the control (not amnioinfused) patients and halved to 15% in the patients who received amnioinfusion. When amnioinfusion was performed prophylactically for oligohydramnios, the rates of operative delivery for fetal distress decreased from 26 to 14% in the control group compared to the amnioinfusion group.

Indications

Amnioinfusion has been demonstrated to be beneficial in the following clinical situations: oligohydramnios (amniotic fluid index (AFI) $\leqslant 5$ cm, or the deepest vertical pocket <3 cm); prolonged or repetitive variable decelerations; thick meconium; and preterm premature rupture of membranes (Table 21.1).

We do not exclude patients undergoing vaginal birth after cesarean delivery from amnioinfusion. We administer amnioinfusion in labors

Table 21.1 Criteria for amnioinfusion (must have rupture of membranes and be able to pass intrauterine pressure catheter)

One or more indications are present:
    Oligohydramnios (amniotic fluid index ≤5 cm, or the deepest vertical
       pocket <3 cm)
    Prolonged or repetitive variable decelerations
    Thick meconium
    Preterm premature rupture of membranes
Singleton pregnancy in vertex presentation
Patient must be a candidate for trial of labor

---

complicated by intraamniotic infection if an indication for amnioinfusion is present. We have observed few adverse effects of the amnioinfusion but have encountered increased uterine activity with prolonged deceleration. No controlled studies have demonstrated untoward side-effects or adverse neonatal outcome associated with intrapartum amnioinfusion.

Contraindications to amnioinfusion

Amnioinfusion should be used cautiously in patients with existent fetal distress or in arrest disorders likely to require operative delivery. The contraindications are listed in Table 21.2.

Complications

When amnioinfusion is administered correctly, complications are extremely rare. We have not observed significant complications when the protocol described below has been followed. Amnioinfusion, as described below, does not increase uterine pressure in a clinically significant way. However, excessive rates and/or volumes infused have led to elevated intrauterine pressure and fetal bradycardia.

Table 21.2 Contraindications to amnioinfusion

Multiple gestation
Malpresentation
Uterine anomalies
Undiagnosed third-trimester bleeding
Fetal distress
    Late decelerations
    Fetal scalp pH <7.20
    Persistently nonreactive fetal heart rate pattern unless pH ≥7.20
Imminent delivery

Table 21.3 Guidelines for amnioinfusion of normal saline

Infuse 500 ml over 20–30 min by gravity infusion
Reassess the amniotic fluid index 4 h after completing the initial infusion
Reassess AFI if fetal heart rate abnormalities recur
Reinfuse if:
     AFI ≤5 cm – reinfuse 500 ml
     AFI 5.1–10 cm – reinfuse 250 ml

AFI, Amniotic fluid index.

Methods

The infusion fluid is normal saline. The fluid may be at room temperature for term pregnancies, and warmed to 37°C for preterm pregnancies. At the University of Southern California we follow a modification of the protocol originally described by Miyazaki and Nevarez. The initial infusion of 500 ml of normal saline is infused into the intrauterine catheter over a time interval of 20–30 min by gravity flow, with the intravenous fluid at a height 90 cm (36 in) above the patient.

The tocodynamometer or a double-lumen catheter can be used to monitor uterine activity during the infusion. The infusion is discontinued if uterine hyperstimulation, excessive uterine contractions, or fetal heart rate abnormalities occur.

The AFI is measured prior to the amnioinfusion when oligohydramnios is suspected. It is not mandatory to measure the AFI prior to the infusion if an acute indication, prolonged or repetitive variable decelerations, or thick meconium is encountered. Our experience suggests that when thick meconium is observed, the AFI is usually <5 cm. The length of time before reinfusion is required has been noted to be >3 h, thus a reevaluation of the AFI at 4 h after infusion seems reasonable. If variable or prolonged decelerations recur, the AFI can be reassessed at that time (see Table 21.3 for guidelines for reinfusion).

An alternate method of amnioinfusion is that described by Nageotte *et al.* This method does not require periodic reassessment of the amniotic fluid index. The initial infusion is 300 ml over the first hour, followed by a continuous infusion at the rate of 180 ml/h until delivery.

Possible future applications

Ogita and associates have described amnioinfusion via a specially designed transcervical catheter to administer fluid and antibiotics during the expectant management of pregnancy complicated by preterm premature rupture of membranes. This application is experimental until further data regarding safety and efficacy are available.

Conclusion

Amnioinfusion is a procedure that can reduce the rate of cesarean delivery for fetal distress and improve neonatal outcome when used for established indications. In addition to the active management of labor, three procedures — external cephalic version, vaginal birth after cesarean delivery, and amnioinfusion — are now part of the obstetrician's armamentarium which, when properly used, will decrease the rate of cesarean birth.

SUGGESTED READING

IMANAKA M, OGITA S, SUGAWA T. Saline solution amnioinfusion for oligohydramnios after premature rupture of the membranes. A preliminary report. *Am J Obstet Gynecol* 1989;161:102–106.

MACRI CJ, SCHRIMMER DB, LEUNG A, GREENSPOON JS, PAUL RH. Amnioinfusion improves outcome in pregnancies complicated by thick meconium and oligohydramnios. *Am J Obstet Gynecol* 1992;167:117–121.

MIYAZAKI FS, NEVAREZ F. Saline amnioinfusion for relief of repetitive variable decelerations: a prospective randomized study. *Am J Obstet Gynecol* 1985;153:301–306.

NAGEOTTE MP, FREEMAN RK, GARITE TJ, DORCHESTER W. Prophylactic intrapartum amnioinfusion in patients with preterm rupture of membranes. *Am J Obstet Gynecol* 1985;153:557–562.

POSNER MD, BALLAGH SH, PAUL RH. The effect of amnioinfusion on uterine pressure and activity: a preliminary report. *Am J Obstet Gynecol* 1990;163:813–818.

SCHRIMMER DB, MACRI CJ, PAUL RH. Prophylactic amnioinfusion as a treatment for oligohydramnios in laboring patients: a prospective randomized trial. *Am J Obstet Gynecol* 1991;165:972–975.

SIVAN E, SEIDMAN DS, BARKAI G, ATLAS M, DULITZKY M, MASHIACH S. The role of amnioinfusion in current obstetric care. *Obstet Gynecol Survey* 1992;47:80–87.

STRONG TH, HETZLER G, SARNO AP, PAUL RH. Prophylactic intrapartum amnioinfusion: a randomized clinical trial. *Am J Obstet Gynecol* 1990;162:1370–1375.

22

The incompetent cervix

RAUL ARTAL

The incompetent cervix is one of the most controversial topics in obstetrics and gynecology. Controversy surrounds every aspect, from definition and diagnosis to treatment. The entity has been classically described to be a condition whereby progressive painless dilatation of the cervix in the second trimester or early in the third trimester of pregnancy leads to premature rupture of the membranes. In the true anatomic sense, the internal cervical os is not a sphincter, although it fullfills such a function.

The conditions leading to cervical patency and spontaneous abortion when cervical incompetence occurs have been described as follows: the patient experiences an uneventful first trimester of pregnancy. In the mid or late second trimester, there is bloodless and relatively painless effacement and dilatation of the cervix. A watery vaginal discharge, accompanied by spotting and vague abdominal pressure, is noticed. Then a sudden rupture of the membranes occurs. Most patients do not experience any uterine contractions until the last moment of membrane rupture, though some perceive regular contractions similar to menstrual cramping prior to rupture. Soon after, the products of conception are aborted.

Etiology

Most of the confusion and subsequent controversy arise from the fact that no randomized prospective studies have proven the unequivocal value of cervical cerclage. The main criticism of the studies published relates to the fact that all comparisons were made with the study subjects' reproductive history serving as their own control. The treatment and the successful outcome of the pregnancy are held as the ultimate confirmation of the initial diagnosis. The reality is that, in some instances, recognizing painless dilatation of the cervix and providing appropriate treatment do not always lead to a successful outcome. Conversely, other patients may experience a "painful" dilatation of the cervix but are treated as if they had an incompetent cervix and may have a successful pregnancy. It appears that patients with either anatomic or structural changes are the ones who best fit the clinical description and benefit most from the treatment. The primary disorder is a disruption of the sphincteric mechanism, secondary to either abnormalities in the muscular isthmus or a disruption of the cervical fibrous tissue.

The etiology of the incompetent cervix can be divided into three categories, traumatic, hormonal, and congenital factors. The reported incidence varies from 1:1930 to 1:140 pregnancies. Cervical iatrogenic trauma is the most common cause for cervical incompetence. It is frequently caused by lacerations that occur during labor or delivery secondary to precipitous labor or breech delivery through an incompletely dilated cervix. First-trimester termination of pregnancy is a significant risk factor if mechanical cervical dilatation is done without prior use of laminaria.

Hormonal factors are postulated to affect the cervicoisthmic junction. High levels of relaxin or low levels of progesterone have been implicated as a cause of cervicoisthmic relaxation.

The congenital etiology could be a result of several causes. A cervical distribution of muscle fibers could cause cervical incompetence. Under the influence of progesterone and relaxin, the laxity of the muscular content will lead to cervicoisthmic laxity. A more common form of congenital incompetency is caused by *in utero* exposure to diethylstilbestrol. Cervicovaginal abnormalities are present in 25–50% of these patients. Patients exposed to diethylstilbestrol with or without cervical abnormalities have an increased incidence of preterm labor and delivery.

Diagnosis

There are no specific diagnostic tests to confirm the accurate diagnosis of incompetent cervix. The most important diagnostic criterion is a careful obstetric history. The classic history includes one or multiple spontaneous abortions or deliveries between 16 and 28 weeks' gestation, preceded by premature rupture of the membranes without bleeding, and with few or no uterine contractions. Many, but not all, women with an incompetent cervix report such a history. In the vast majority of cases, there has been previous cervical trauma from surgical manipulation, traumatic delivery,

Table 22.1 Causes for second-trimester pregnancy loss

Idiopathic
Incompetent cervix
Uterine factors
 Congenital anomalies
 Intrauterine septi
 Leiomyomas
Medical disorders, i.e., lupus, etc.
Infectious factors, local and generalized
Immunologic factors
Chromosomal abnormalities

therapeutic abortion, diagnostic dilatation and curettage, or placenta previa.

Any history of second-trimester abortion in successive pregnancies strongly suggests the diagnosis of incompetent cervix. Serial vaginal examinations indicating rapid effacement of the cervix in the second trimester of pregnancy may confirm the diagnosis (cervical effacement usually occurs over 6–8 days). However, once cervical dilatation occurs, it is rapid and usually recognized too late to permit therapeutic intervention. It is certainly crucial to exclude other possible causes for second-trimester losses and to ascertain that there are no intercurrent causes. A thorough work-up should exclude the other causes, listed in Table 22.1.

In the nonpregnant patient, the hysterogram and Hegar test are specific but not sufficiently sensitive as diagnostic tests. A luteal-phase hysterogram demonstrating that the width of the internal os is 1 cm or greater when intrauterine pressure does not exceed 100 mmHg is suggestive of incompetent cervix. If a number 8 Hegar dilator can be passed beyond the internal os without resistance, or a pediatric Foley catheter with a 3-ml inflated bulb can be withdrawn through the internal os without resistance, the diagnosis may also be advanced. The main difficulty with these procedures is that neither cervical anatomy nor physiology is the same in the pregnant state as in the nonpregnant state. Not every dilated cervix in the nonpregnant state means subsequent incompetent cervix in pregnancy or, conversely, not every undilated cervix in the nonpregnant state excludes the occurrence of incompetent cervix in the subsequent pregnancy.

Early serial vaginal ultrasound examinations can add to our diagnostic abilities. Progressive dilatation of the cervix (beyond 1.5–2 cm) in pregnancy is suggestive of the development of cervical incompetence. But, again, not every dilated cervix results in spontaneous abortion or premature delivery.

Management

The incompetent cervix can be managed surgically or by nonsurgical means. In the absence of visual anatomic defects, either treatment remains controversial because there is no .objective scientific evidence to prove its efficacy. Conversely, preterm delivery has been reported to occur with higher frequency among patients who had a cervical cerclage. The various techniques of cervical cerclage are now summarized: the Lash procedure is a preconceptual procedure rarely used. It causes permanent scarring of the cervix, occasionally resulting in infertility, and most of the time those patients require cesarean section. Maternal death has been reported as a complication associated with this procedure.

A variety of procedures to be performed during pregnancy have been described. The Shirodkar procedure originally utilized strips of fascia lata. The fascia was tunneled submucosally above the vesicovaginal fascia of the cervix at the level of the internal os, and then tied. The fascia lata has been replaced subsequently by a variety of suture materials from silk to steel wires and, most recently, by Mersilene bands. The McDonald cerclage procedure is currently the most commonly used transvaginal method. With the availability of improved suture materials, such as Mersilene bands, the modified McDonald procedure has a clear and distinct advantage. Compared with the Shirodkar procedure, it is simpler, faster, and less traumatic. In the McDonald procedure the suture material is inserted in the submucosa of the cervix at the level of the internal cervical os. I prefer not to empty the bladder and, if necessary, fill it with saline. A full bladder displaces the uterine corpus and minimizes the chance of penetrating the amniotic sac. Furthermore, it allows a more caudal placement of the suture closer to the internal cervical os. In a modification of the McDonald procedure we recommend tying the knot posteriorly. Anterior placement of the knot has been reported to result in severe abrasions and ulcerations of the anterior vaginal wall, including the urethra. The suture should be tied snugly to the surface of the cervix. Excessive strangulation of the cervix could result in the formation of cervical lacerations (fenestrations) and frequently results in uterine irritability. After the procedure the tightness of the cervix should not be tested by inserting the finger in the endocervical os, as is sometimes recommended. This practice may disrupt the cervical mucus and promote infection and failure of the procedure.

Transabdominal cervicoisthmic cerclage should be reserved only for rare cases in which the procedure technically cannot be carried out transvaginally. This would be for patients who have an extremely short or amputated cervix or multiple cervical lacerations or defects.

Timing of the surgical procedure

Timing of the procedure is extremely important: the earlier the procedure is done, the more successful it is. The optimal time for cerclage is between 12 and 14 weeks' gestation. By 12 weeks, first-trimester spontaneous abortions caused by chromosomal abnormalities have already occurred, and the possibility of performing a cerclage on a genetically defective pregnancy is markedly reduced. With the advent of high-resolution ultrasound one could perform early scans and detect congenital mal-formations that would contraindicate the procedure. If performed later than 20 weeks, the success of cerclage is very limited.

Emergency cerclage procedures have been performed with various degrees of success up to 26 weeks' gestation. On all occasions an ultra-sound examination should be performed to verify fetal viability and to rule out congenital anomalies. During an emergency cerclage several procedures could improve the chance of success. Protruding membranes could, on occasion, be reduced by placing the patient in the Trendelenburg position. In addition, the urinary bladder can be filled with up to 500 ml of 0.45% saline. Transabdominal amniocentesis would reduce the in-traamniotic cavity volume and pressure. Should the membranes still protrude, they could be gently reduced by utilizing a gauge sponge on a ring forceps covered by a finger cot.

Contraindications, absolute or relative, to surgical cerclage are given in Table 22.2. Complications of surgery include puncture of the chorio-amniotic membranes during surgery, premature labor, amnionitis, and cervical lacerations from the suture. Occasionally, patients will have increased uterine irritability necessitating treatment. Both magnesium sulfate and ritodrine hydrochloride have been found to be very effective for the control of uterine contractility. Following the Shirodkar procedure, about 50% of patients experience vaginal infections that require treat-ment. The incidence appears to be lower following McDonald cerclage.

Postoperative precautions

Following surgery, the patient should remain at bedrest for at least 24 h, and should be observed for signs of infection or threatened abortion.

Table 22.2 Contraindications to and complications of surgical cerclage

Hyperirritability of the uterus with bulging membranes
Cervical dilatation >4 cm
Suspected fetal malformations
Suspected intrauterine fetal death
Premature rupture of the membranes

Following the procedure, patients are advised to abstain from intercourse for 1–2 weeks and to avoid strenuous physical activity for the remainder of the pregnancy. Patients are seen at frequent intervals, and a careful speculum examination is performed on the first return visit. The frequency of examinations is determined by patient complaints, such as uterine contractions, bleeding, or cervical effacement. Vaginal or abdominal ultrasound exams can be very helpful in assessing the cervical status.

Excessive uterine irritability is the predominant cause for failure of the surgical cerclage. In the absence of infection, uterine activity can be suppressed with magnesium sulfate or ritodrine. Patients exhibiting uterine irritability, when evaluated after delivery, may or may not have anatomic uterine defects. The McDonald cerclage procedure is successful in 75% or more of properly selected patients, when performed at the correct gestational age.

The surgical procedure

As simple as the procedure appears, the success is naturally linked to its correct performance. It is not within the scope of this chapter to describe surgical procedures; however, it is important to recognize the most common pitfalls.

The most common one is the tendency to tie the suture too tight. This will inevitably lead to tissue necrosis, irritability, and cervical lacerations. Another common pitfall is inserting a finger in the cervix while performing the cerclage. This procedure not only disrupts the cervical mucus plug and environment, but may dislodge the chorioamniotic membranes and cause their necrosis and eventual rupture. Puncture of the chorioamniotic sac is another complication that can be prevented in those patients with a short cervix by directing the placement of the needle into the cervix under direct ultrasound visualization.

Careful selection of patients and correct surgical approaches will maximize the surgical success.

Suture removal

In the past, it was suggested that the cervical sutures should be left in place for future pregnancies, with elective cesarean sections performed to effect delivery. This approach should be abandoned. The simplicity of the McDonald procedure and the benefits of vaginal delivery outweigh the risks associated with abdominal delivery. Other possible complications linked to leaving the sutures in place include granulomatous changes with foreign-body tissue reactions. Their consequences are unknown.

We advocate elective suture removal at 38–39 weeks' gestation. This approach allows a planned delivery and avoids possible lacerations of the dilating cervix prior to the removal of the cerclage.

Once the suture is removed, one-third of the patients go into immediate labor (any patient showing cervical dilatation >4 cm will go into labor immediately after suture removal). In the other two-thirds, pregnancy usually continues to term. This is explained by the formation of a fibrotic band that mechanically serves the function of the cerclage.

Labor and delivery following suture removal

Each stage of labor is usually shortened in these patients. The deceleration phase is absent, and the acceleration phase is shorter than usual. A prolonged latent phase may occur in patients with a fibrotic band in the cervical matrix. The cervix will usually remain dilated to 3–4 cm for 6–8 h. Then the acceleration phase and delivery will occur suddenly, within a period of 30 min. The incidence of complications and cesarean section is no greater than in control populations.

Alternatives to surgical cerclage

Synthetic gestagens were used in the past because they may have a quiescent effect on the uterus. They are no longer utilized and are considered contraindicated in early pregnancy. Smith–Hodge pessaries have also been used. They usually shift the axis of intrauterine pressure from the cervix to the lower uterine segment, preventing cervical dilatation. Another therapeutic approach is prolonged bedrest, but the preferred treatment today for cervical incompetence is surgical cerclage.

None of the treatments, surgical or nonsurgical, has withstood scientific scrutiny and been proven to be unequivocably effective. However, careful selection of patients for each has been individually beneficial, and this approach will probably persist.

SUGGESTED READING

Artal R, Shachar Y, Insler V, Serr DM. Course of delivery following cerclage for cervical incompetence. *Harefuah* 1971;81:65.

Artal R, Shachar Y, Insler V, Serr DM. Course of pregnancy following cerclage for cervical incompetence. *Harefuah* 1971;81:63.

Haning RV Jr, Steinetz B, Weiss G. Elevated serum relaxin levels in multiple pregnancy after menotropin treatment. *Obstet Gynecol* 1935;66:42.

Hortenstive JS, Witherington R. Ulcer of the trigone: a late complication of cervical cerclage. *J Urol* 1987;137:109.

Kirkley WH, Gilbert JC, McDaniel GC. Pathologic examination of a postpartum uterus containing Dacron used for cerclage. *Obstet Gynecol* 1962;20:626.

LASH AF, LASH SR. Habitual abortion: the incompetent internal os of the cervix. *Am J Obstet Gynecol* 1950;59:68.

MCDONALD IA. Suture of the cervix for inevitable abortion. *J Obstet Gynaecol Eur* 1957;64:346.

RAPHAEL SI. Incompetent internal os of the cervix. *Obstet Gynecol* 1966;28:438.

SCHULY KF, GRIMES DA, GATES W Jr. Measures to prevent cervical injury during suction curettage abortion. *Lancet* 1983;1:1182.

SHIRODKAR VN. Long term results with operative treatment of habitual abortion. *Triangle* 1967;8:123.

VARMA TR, PATEL RH, PILLAI U. Ultrasonic assessment of cervix in "at risk" patients. *Acta Obstet Gynaecol Scand* 1986;65:147.

23

Postterm pregnancy

KATHRYN J. SHAW

The postterm pregnancy continues to be a problem in modern obstetrics. The purpose of this chapter is to discuss the management of the postterm gestation in terms of the associated complications, methods of antepartum surveillance, and indications for delivery versus expectant management.

Definition and incidence

The definition of postterm pregnancy varies, but by strict criteria it implies a gestation that has progressed to or beyond 42 completed weeks (294 days) from the first day of the last menstrual period (LMP). In the clinical setting, a pregnancy is often considered postterm at the completion of 41 weeks. The terms postdates, prolonged, and postterm pregnancy are often used interchangeably. In contrast, the term postmature is not synonymous and should be reserved for the postterm pregnancy resulting in the birth of a dysmature infant secondary to relative placental insufficiency.

The incidence of postterm pregnancy ranges from 3 to 12%, depending on the definition used, the population, and the dating criteria used. Calculation of the gestational age (GA) according to the LMP is based upon Naegele's rule and the assumption that ovulation occurs 14 days after the first day of the LMP. Many earlier studies describing the incidence of postterm pregnancy were based upon LMP-derived GA, coupled with early physical examination. In a large prospective study addressing this topic, 3000 patients with a pelvic examination confirming GA prior to 13 weeks were followed. Patients with irregular menses or any medical or obstetric complications were excluded. In this group, the incidence of postterm gestation was 11.4%. The inherent inaccuracy in relying solely on the LMP and the value of an early ultrasound have been demonstrated in several reports. When the diagnosis of postterm pregnancy was made based only upon LMP, the incidence was 11%, compared to an incidence of 2–6% when based upon an early ultrasound between 16 and 18 weeks. The differing incidence of postterm pregnancies is likely due in part to erroneous LMP or variable timing of ovulation. Thus, it is probable that as many as half of supposed postterm pregnancies actually have not gone beyond 294 days.

A postterm gestation should be further described as poor dates versus good dates, referring to accuracy of dating. The criteria for good obstetric dates include the following: (1) positive pregnancy test by 6 weeks from the first day of the LMP; (2) bimanual exam in the first trimester that confirms the GA; (3) fetal heart tones (FHT) heard by DeLee stethoscope by 20 weeks' GA or 22 weeks or more of auscultated FHTs; and (4) confirmatory ultrasound prior to 26 weeks.

A pregnancy is considered well dated if any of the above criteria are met.

Significance

The postterm pregnancy is one that often creates anxiety in both the physician and patient. Generally, this is a complication of pregnancy considered to be associated with considerable risks for both the fetus and the mother. Early reports demonstrated a significant increase in perinatal mortality. McClure-Brown reported a doubling of the perinatal mortality rate after 42 completed weeks, a tripling after 43 weeks, and after 44 completed weeks the rate had quadrupled. More recent reports have continued to show an increased perinatal morbidity, but have not shown an increase in the perinatal mortality rate compared to the term gestation. The improvement in the perinatal loss rate is likely due to the development of antepartum surveillance, intrapartum monitoring, and improved neonatal care. The persistent greater perinatal morbidity is attributable to the complications described below.

Macrosomia

Numerous reports have described an increase in the frequency of macrosomic infants (>4500 g) in postterm gestations. Twenty-five percent of postterm infants will weigh more than 4000 g; 2–5% will weigh more than 4500 g, compared to 0.8% in term infants. Macrosomic infants at any GA experience increased birth trauma (11 versus 2% in normal-sized infants), shoulder dystocia (14 versus 0.3%), and require more cesarean section births (35 versus 17%). In the extreme case of shoulder dystocia, severe perinatal asphyxia and death may result.

Oligohydramnios

Oligohydramnios is clearly more common in the postterm gestation. While various research methods exist for quantitation of amniotic fluid volume, clinical use of the amniotic fluid index (AFI) is highly reliable and easy to perform. This is accomplished by dividing the maternal abdomen into four quadrants, using the umbilicus and the linea nigra. The ultrasound transducer is placed along the patient's long axis, perpendicular to the floor. The deepest vertical pocket is measured in each quadrant. The AFI is the sum derived from these measurements. Using the AFI, amniotic fluid volume has been shown to increase up until 30 weeks, and then plateau until term. The AFI has been shown to decrease by as much as 30% between 40 and 42 weeks. Measurement of the deepest vertical pocket in any given quadrant is another assessment of amniotic fluid volume. Oligohydramnios is generally defined as an AFI <5 cm, or deepest vertical pocket <3 cm. The primary complication associated with oligohydramnios is that of umbilical cord compression and resultant fetal distress.

Meconium

Meconium passage – an event more common as the fetus matures – is reported in 25–30% of postterm patients. While meconium passage may occur as a response to fetal distress, the finding of meconium is neither a sensitive nor specific predictor of fetal compromise. Of more relevance is the finding of thick (3–4+) meconium. This is uniformly associated with oligohydramnios. The primary concern related to meconium is the risk of meconium aspiration syndrome, which is more common in the postterm gestation and with thick as opposed to thin meconium. Meconium aspiration syndrome is associated with significant neonatal morbidity and mortality. Recognition of meconium in the amniotic fluid requires active oropharyngeal suctioning at the time of delivery to minimize the risk of meconium aspiration.

Postmaturity syndrome

An infrequent but significant morbidity associated with the postterm gestation is the occurrence of the postmaturity syndrome. Synonyms for this finding include placental dysfunction and dysmaturity syndrome.

The latter term is preferable because this syndrome may occur at any gestational age. Dysmaturity probably results from subacute placental dysfunction/insufficiency. Features of dysmaturity unclude failure of fetal growth, loss of subcutaneous tissue, dry, wrinkled skin, and a high incidence of meconium aspiration syndrome. Postnatally, these infants often experience hypothermia or hypoglycemia, secondary to decreased fat and glycogen stores. Older literature suggests the incidence of the dysmaturity syndrome is 3% at term, compared to 10–20% in the postterm pregnancy. More recent reports indicate the incidence to be less in postterm gestations, likely due to aggressive antepartum surveillance. The long-term significance to infants exhibiting the syndrome in terms of developmental sequelae is controversial, but several studies have demonstrated developmental delay in children who had dysmaturity at birth.

Management

There is little disagreement that the postterm pregnancy presents a high-risk situation with increased maternal and perinatal risks. Given this, the question arises as to the optimal management approach for these patients. The two primary options include routine labor induction versus expectant management, coupled with induction for specific indications. The concept of inducing all postterm patients at 294 days and beyond was promoted in 1963 by McClure-Brown who reported the increase in perinatal morbidity and mortality in postterm pregnancies. Currently, with the widespread availability of antepartum surveillance, improved neonatal care, and a better understanding of the pathophysiology associated with postterm pregnancy, the use of routine induction is probably neither necessary nor prudent. A significant proportion of these pregnancies (40–50%) are not postterm and thus would be needlessly induced. The majority of studies addressing the option of inducing all postterm pregnancies have demonstrated a significant increase in cesarean section rate and no discernible decrease in perinatal morbidity. A more appropriate approach is to individualize and assess the pregnancy for any features that would contraindicate expectant management.

Expectant management

When a gestation has reached 41 completed weeks, a management plan should be made that takes into consideration the following:
1   accuracy of GA (good dates?);
2   cervical examination (inducible?);
3   maternal or fetal conditions postentially worsened by continuation of pregnancy.

If the pregnancy is well dated and the cervix is inducible (Bishop score >6), elective induction is recommended. If the cervix is inducible but the dating criteria are poor, then elective induction is not usually conducted unless there is evidence of fetal maturity, either by ultrasound criteria (biparietal diameter >9.2 cm, femur length >7.3 cm) or determination of the lecithin: sphingomyelin ratio. If the cervix is not inducible, a thorough search for maternal or fetal contraindications to expectant management should be made. These would include any medical illness potentially worsened by pregnancy, such as hypertension, renal disease, or diabetes mellitus. Obstetric factors such as a prior cesarean section or abnormal lie would also be contraindications to expectant management. Additionally, evaluation of the fetal status is necessary and should include ulrasound esimate of fetal weight, and some form of antepartum testing. Options for antepartum surveillance include the nonstress test, contraction stress test, biophysical profile, and amniotic fluid volume assessment.

At the Los Angeles County–University of Southern California Medical Center (LAC–USC Medical Center) we use a modified biophysical profile, including the nonstress test and assessment of the AFI. Oligohydramnios is diagnosed if the AFI is <5 cm. If there are no maternal or obstetric contraindications, and antepartum fetal testing is reassuring, expectant management is appropriate. This should include weekly clinical examinations to assess cervical status, and to be alert to evidence of macrosomia, or the development of any complications such as preeclampsia. Twice-weekly antepartum testing is also instituted as a part of this approach. Expectant management should be terminated and delivery effected in the

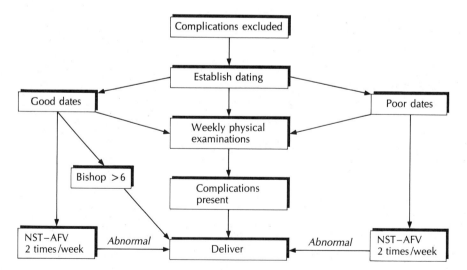

Fig. 23.1 The management scheme used for postterm pregnancy at the Los Angeles County–University of Southern California Medical Center. NST, Nonstress test, AFV, amniotic fluid volume.

following instances: evidence of fetal jeopardy on antepartum testing, estimated fetal weight >4000 g, inducible cervix, or if any maternal complications develop. The management scheme in use at LAC–USC Medical Center is shown in Fig. 23.1. This approach in the properly screened patient has been very successful and associated with perinatal outcome comparable to patients at term.

Intrapartum management

Regardless of whether labor is spontaneous or induced for maternal or fetal indications, the postterm fetus is at high risk for complications during labor. Initial assessment should be ultrasound evaluation of fetal weight and amniotic fluid volume. Although a firm rule cannot be made regarding at what weight a cesarean section should be performed, the risks of macrosomia and associated birth trauma should be strongly considered if the estimated fetal weight is >4500 g. The decision to allow a trial of labor or proceed to cesarean birth must take into account a number of factors, including past obstetric history, assessment of clinical pelvimetry, presence of diabetes mellitus, and maternal consent. If vaginal birth is to be attempted in this setting, the obstetrician should be well prepared to handle a shoulder dystocia if it should occur. Additional specific intrapartum concerns include the increased incidence of meconium passage with risk of aspiration, oligohydramnios with associated umbilical cord compression, and uteroplacental insufficiency. If either oligohydramnios, with or without variable fetal heart rate decelerations, or thick meconium is noted, we recommend prophylactic amnioinfusion, which has been shown significantly to reduce the number of cesarean sections performed for fetal distress. This can be accomplished after adequate cervical dilatation once a intrauterine pressure catheter is in place. Five hundred milliliters of normal saline at 37°C is infused by gravity flow at a rate of 15–20 ml/min. Ultrasonography is performed after the infusion to reassess the AFI and to confirm adequate replacement of the intrauterine fluid volume, the goal being an AFI >10. If this has not been achieved, placement of the catheter should be confirmed and a repeat infusion performed.

Summary

In conclusion, the postterm pregnancy continues to be a significant management dilemma. Controversy remains regarding what constitutes the ideal management. Rather than adopting any rigid protocol, it is more appropriate to individualize treatment for each patient. In a well-dated postterm pregnancy with a favorable cervix, an elective induction can be done. In patients with a noninducible cervix, and no medical or obstetric contraindications, expectant management is a reasonable and safe approach.

SUGGESTED READING

AMERICAN COLLEGE OF OBSTETRICIANS AND GYNECOLOGISTS. *Diagnosis and Management of Postterm Pregnancy*. ACOG Technical Bulletin 130. Washington, DC: ACOG, 1987.

BEISCHER NA, EVANS JH, TOWNSEND L. Studies in prolonged pregnancy. I. The incidence of prolonged pregnancy. *Am J Obstet Gynecol* 1969;103:476.

DYSON DC. Fetal surveillance vs labor induction at 42 weeks in postterm gestation. *J Reprod Med* 1988;33:262.

LAGREW DC, FREEMAN RK. Management of postdate pregnancy. *Am J Obstet Gynecol* 1986;154:8.

MCCLURE-BROWN JC. Postmaturity. *Am J Obstet Gynecol* 1963;85:573.

PERSSON PH, GENNSER G. Benefits of ultrasound screening of a pregnant population. *Acta Obstet Gynaecol Scand* (Suppl) 1978;78:5.

RUTHERFORD SE, PHELAN JP, SMITH CV, JACOBS N. The four-quardrant assessment of amniotic fluid volume: an adjunct to antepartum fetal heart rate testing. *Obstet Gynecol* 1987;70:353.

SAITO M, YAZAWA K, HASHIGUCHI A, KUMASAKA T, NISHI N, KATO K. Time of ovulation and prolonged pregnancy. *Am J Obstet Gynecol* 1972;112:31.

SCHRIMMER DB, MACRI CJ, PAUL RH. Prophylactic amnioinfusion as a treatment for oligohydramnios in laboring patients: a prospective, randomized trial. *Am J Obstet Gynecol* 1991;165:972.

WARSOF SL, PEARCE JM, CAMPBELL S. The present place of routine ultrasound screening. *Clin Obstet Gynecol* 1983;10:445.

WEINSTROM KD, PARSONS MT. The prevention of meconium aspiration in labor using amnioinfusion. *Obstet Gynecol* 1989;73:647.

24

Diagnosis and management of intrauterine growth retardation

ARNOLD L. MEDEARIS

The evaluation of normal fetal growth and the clinical diagnosis and management of abnormal growth is a significant component of the care required for all pregnant patients. Intrauterine growth retardation (IUGR) represents a significant cause of adverse perinatal outcome. Besides an increased incidence of fetal and neonatal death and the immediate complications of asphyxia, recent data suggest a significant reduction in both physical and mental development of children affected by IUGR when compared with normal controls at age 12.

Normal fetal/neonatal growth

Fetal growth depends upon a balance between the natural growth potential of the fetus and the fetal environment. Normal fetal growth is assessed by comparing the neonatal evaluation of birth weight or birth length at a specific gestational age to established growth charts. The measurement of birth weight and length is the traditional method of pediatric evaluation for the neonate. These measurements are plotted against gestational age to assess the neonatal risk of complications secondary to IUGR. Generally, birth weights below the 10th percentile for gestational age are considered small-for-gestational-age (SGA) and identify neonates at risk for complications associated with IUGR. Birth weight and length are used in the Ponderal index (birth weight (g) $\times$ 100/(crown heel length)^3) to evaluate symmetry in the neonate. Asymmetric neonates are more likely to have complications secondary to uteroplacental insufficiency. Neonatal assessment, however, is an incomplete evaluation of fetal growth because it is limited to a single observation made after the delivery and restrospectively evaluates intrauterine growth events. Curves for evaluation of premature infants are based on information from abnormal pregnancies, or they would not have been born premature. Growth curves before 34 weeks do not represent a normal population and underestimate the incidence of abnormal fetal growth.

A more contemporary approach in evaluating fetal growth is to measure intrauterine fetal structures or to use a combination of measurements to calculate intrauterine fetal weight using diagnostic ultrasound. Measurement of the fetal head (biparietal diameter and head circumference), the abdomen (circumference), and the femur (length) with ultrasound is the best method for the obstetrician to evaluate normal growth of individual fetal structures and calculate fetal weight during pregnancy. Normal graphs for all standard structures used for the assessment of fetal growth are available (Fig. 24.1). The abdominal circumference is the single measurement that contributes the most to formulas used for estimating fetal weight. Measurement of the abdominal circumference is the most sensitive measurement for assessing fetal growth. Intrauterine weight calculation using multiple measurements of fetal structures is the closest estimate to actual birth weight (delivery is within 5 days). When calculated, fetal weight is compared to the neonatal growth chart; this technique is the most specific method for the assessment of growth.

Using a concept of risk assessment in which a patient with normal fetal growth is treated differently from a patient with decreased fetal growth, we are extremely confident that the techniques of antepartum testing used can prevent fetal compromise. Because antepartum fetal surveillance can prevent compromise in a fetus or neonate considered at risk for IUGR, we use growth of less than the 10th percentile to identify a population that is monitored with increased testing.

Factors associated with abnormal fetal growth

The factors associated with IUGR can be divided into maternal, placental, and primary fetal categories.

Maternal factors

The influences of small maternal stature, poor maternal weight gain, low prepregnancy weight, cigarette smoking, and low socioeconomic class on fetal growth are well recognized. Many studies have shown that all of the above factors, working individually or in combination, are associated with a reduction in birth size. Often the common denominator is socioeconomic class. Because of the multiple problems experienced by patients in lower

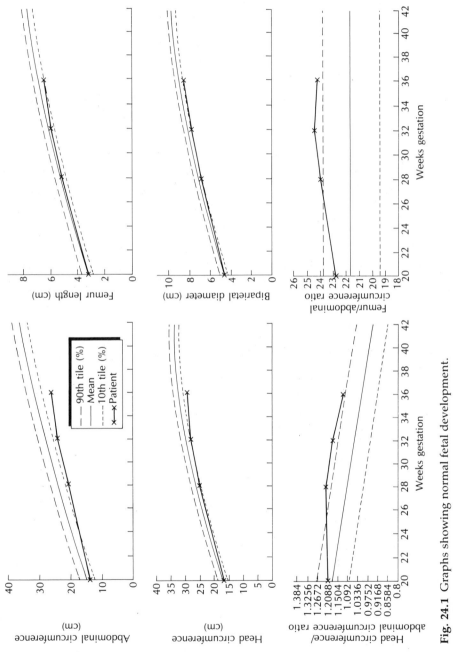

Fig. 24.1 Graphs showing normal fetal development.

socioeconomic populations, they are considered at risk for IUGR. Severe maternal malnutrition has been associated with IUGR but, in most of these cases, caloric intake was less than 500 kcal/day. Such poor diets are rare in industrialized societies.

Maternal medical complications are associated with fetal growth retardation. The most common for these conditions includes moderate to severe hypertension, especially in the presence of proteinuria; advanced-class diabetes mellitus when complicated by vascular problems; and collagen vascular disorders (systemic lupus erythematosus or lupus-like circulating anticoagulants). These diagnoses and other maternal medical conditions are associated with abnormal fetal growth because of abnormal placental function. The pattern of IUGR seen is asymmetric with fetal complications (antepartum demise, abnormal antepartum fetal surveillance, intrapartum fetal death, intrapartum fetal distress, neonatal compromise, or neonatal death) occurring secondary to uteroplacental insufficiency.

Asymmetric growth retardation occurs later in pregnancy. Patients with asymmetric IUGR secondary to uteroplacental insufficiency are intrinsically normal. Under these circumstances, total cell number is not affected. Fetal growth potential is inhibited by failure of the placenta to deliver sufficient nutrients and oxygen. If significant antepartum and intrapartum compromise can be prevented with antepartum surveillance, intrapartum fetal monitoring or, in severe cases, preterm delivery, these neonates when they receive adequate nutrition will achieve full potential. Therefore, it is important to prevent the complications of asphyxia. In most of the cases, if preterm delivery is indicated it is after 28–30 weeks of gestation and the complications of prematurity can be managed without long-term residual effects.

Placental factors

Placental damage because of partial separation may occur at any stage of pregnancy. If it is an early event, the regenerative capability of the placenta will enable full function to be restored. However, such damage occurring later in pregnancy over a significant period of the gestation as in a chronic abruption may permanently reduce the efficiency of the placenta and give rise to IUGR similar to that seen with uteroplacental insufficiency.

Fetal factors

Congenital fetal anomalies and the primary fetal effects of drug and infectious teratogens are associated with IUGR in over 10% of cases. IUGR is found in almost all cases of trisomy 18 seen in the third trimester.

Abnormal growth is seen in varying frequencies in many other combinations of aneuploidy. In addition, it has recently been shown that IUGR is found in cases in which the placenta is mosaic for normal and aneuploid cell lines. Abnormal growth can also be a component of many specific fetal/neonatal genetic syndromes.

The importance of medications, drugs, and intrauterine infection (particularly viral infections) that affect the fetus at the cellular level should not be underestimated. These conditions are significant because they represent a group of patients that exhibit symmetric growth retardation. Symmetric growth retardation appears early in pregnancy, initially around 18–20 weeks. It appears that there is a reduction in total cell number. "Head-sparing" growth is not apparent. After birth, these babies have a higher incidence of mental handicaps and grow into physically smaller children. Symmetric IUGR does not have an increased incidence of antepartum, intrapartum, or neonatal complications. However, the long-term residual effects with major and minor deficits seen in these patients are a burden to families and society. Alcohol is the most common teratogen with a primary fetal influence. Maternal alcohol use in pregnancy has been estimated to cause as high as a 10% incidence of IUGR in certain populations. Intrauterine cytomegalovirus infection can leave the affected child with significant residuals. These conditions cause irreversible damage and offer the obstetrician and pediatrician very few, if any, options to improve long-term outcome.

Diagnosis

The clinical diagnosis of IUGR depends upon historical and developing problems, physical examination, and the establishment of an accurate assessment of the menstrual (gestational) age of the pregnancy. The most important aspects of the historical and developing problems involve the factors mentioned previously. The mother's social history, including her diet, habits (smoking, drinking, drugs), and type of habitation are important. Elucidation of the previous obstetric history with particular reference to birth weights, gestational ages, and neonatal development is also essential. An initial careful assessment of gestational age in all patients is required. The diagnosis and management of IUGR is impossible without this information. Clinical examination of the patient, including ultrasound evaluation, should be performed before 20 weeks' gestation, in cases judged to be at risk for IUGR. Ultrasound in these pregnancies should be repeated at regular intervals. It has been shown that IUGR is diagnosed in only 30–40% of cases by clinical assessment alone. The obstetrician may improve the diagnostic rate by assessing fetal growth in every patient examined. The simple measurement of fundal height using the McDonald technique (measurement from the symphysis to the top of the fundus with a centimeter tape between 20 and 36 weeks correlates 1 cm for each week of gestation) can identify over 50% of growth-retarded fetuses when a decrease of greater than 4 cm is used to initiate further evaluation with ultrasound.

The use of ultrasound in obstetrics has brought a new perspective to the diagnosis of IUGR. Clinically, we use graphic representation of growth to evaluate the fetal risk for delivery of an infant that is SGA. Representative graphs of abdominal circumference, femur length, biparietal diameter, and head circumference are seen in Fig. 24.1. The first determination that must be made is the menstrual/gestational age of the fetus. After the gestational age is decided, measured fetal values are plotted. If the estimate of the age of the fetus is accurate, then the measurements can quickly be determined to be normal, increased, or decreased. The single most important structural measurement to use in the assessment of fetal growth is the abdominal circumference, which accounts for approximately 80% of the explained variance in fetal weight prediction models. Under the described conditions, if this measurement is below the normal limit, then the fetus is probably growth-retarded.

This initial assessment of measurements (Fig. 24.1a–d) should include ratios of the head:abdominal circumferences and femur length:abdominal circumference (Fig. 24.1e,f). If there is the need to evaluate a fetus on multiple occasions we examine the fetus at 28, 32, and 36 weeks' gestation. The clinician must look at the interval growth of the fetus compared with normal mean growth. When interval ultrasound growth is parallel to the mean, the fetus is growing normally. An example of asymmetric IUGR is plotted in Fig. 24.1.

Management

Since the diagnosis of IUGR is difficult and the etiology is multifactorial, it is impossible to devise a single management/treatment scheme. Treatment of symmetric growth-retarded fetuses, even when identified, is unlikely to be helpful. Because of the association with chromosomal malformations in fetuses with symmetric IUGR, consideration should be given for amniocentesis or percutaneous umbilical blood sampling. If chromosomal malformations are identified, an unnecessary cesarean section may be avoided.

Management after the identification of asymmetric IUGR is not simple. Frequently the treatment depends on the presence or absence of fetal maturity. Fetal lung maturation as assessed by the lecithin:sphingomyelin ratio is often accelerated in IUGR. However, there often is decreased amniotic fluid that cannot successfully be obtained, even with ultrasound guidance. If the patient is near term or the examination of the amniotic fluid obtained by amniocentesis suggests fetal lung maturation, it may be prudent to consider delivery of the fetus. Always, close monitoring of these patients in whom induction of labor is performed is necessary. One-third of patients with IUGR will display fetal distress in labor. Conversely, if lung maturation is not present, or the patient is early in the pregnancy, the patient should stop working, be placed on complete bed-rest, lying most of the time on her left side. Fetal status should be evaluated regularly with frequent antepartum fetal heart rate testing and amniotic fluid assessment. In many cases, individualization must occur because corticosteroid administration with subsequent delivery might prove beneficial. In the presence of fetal distress the fetus should be delivered even without lung maturation.

Our current antenatal testing protocol uses the nonstress test with amniotic fluid assessment twice weekly for evaluating the fetus at risk for IUGR. In patients with nonreactive nonstress tests, usually secondary to fetal immaturity, we use the full components of the biophysical profile to evaluate the pregnancy and allow the fetus to remain *in utero* if the profile components are reassuring. Scoring of the biophysical profile is assessed with the summation of two points assigned for the presence of each of the five components. Scores of 8 and 10 are reassuring. A score of 6 is equivocal. Values of 0, 2, and 4 require immediate clinical assessment, with delivery being strongly considered. In the growth-retarded fetus with these latter values and with a high likelihood of fetal maturity, delivery is the best method of management. After 36–37 weeks' gestation, when fetal maturity is attained, if the cervix is inducible and the clinician is confident of the diagnosis of IUGR, delivery is recommended.

The timing of the initiation of antepartum testing depends on the clinical diagnosis. No testing is started until after fetal viability and ultrasound diagnosis. There are clinically justifiable exceptions for delaying the initiation of testing when there is a decreased likelihood of disease, for example when the diagnosis is made early in the third trimester using sensitive criteria. In the patient with no known risk factors for IUGR and an abdominal circumference measurement below the 10th percentile at 30 weeks, testing may be delayed until after an interval growth examination in 4 weeks or at 35–36 weeks' gestation. Patients with a symmetric ultrasound structural examination, questionable pregnancy dating, and a medical and obstetric history free of risk factors for IUGR may only need antepartum testing once a week. Conversely, we pay close attention to those patients with biometric evidence of decreased fetal growth and who are at high risk of developing IUGR.

Neonatal outcome

The immediate neonatal period is a time of great risk for the growth-retarded infant. Studies have shown that the first 72 h following birth are particularly critical. Because of intrauterine malnutrition, stores of glycogen and fat are low. This can lead to both hypoglycemia attacks and a failure of temperature control. Blood glucose levels below 40 mg% may cause cerebral damage. Hypocalcemia and hyponatremia may be present; the former is often diagnosed after the baby has become "jittery" or convulsed. Polycythemia and increased blood viscosity may cause sludging in the capillaries, possibly resulting in cerebral, pulmonary, and peripheral damage. Necrotizing enterocolitis, sometimes seen in IUGR infants, may have a similar etiology.

The long-term prognosis of IUGR has not been entirely assessed. Many studies have failed to distinguish between symmetric and asymmetric patterns of growth retardation. The outcome in these two groups is likely to be very different. There is some evidence that with asymmetric head-sparing growth retardation, subsequent neurologic development is normal. Once these infants are delivered from the growth-inhibiting environment in which they existed, they grow rapidly, usually attaining their potential growth percentile within 6 months. However, when growth retardation is symmetric, these small children may have lower intelligence quotients and are more likely to manifest other neurologic deficits later in life.

Summary

IUGR is an important complication of pregnancy. Diagnosis is difficult; once it is made, management depends on the type and degree of growth retardation and fetal maturity. Asymmetric IUGR represents a subgroup of fetuses in which obstetric management can significantly improve prenatal outcome. Current antenatal testing with twice-weekly nonstress testing and amniotic fluid assessment, backed up with assessment of fetal breathing movements, fetal movement, and fetal tone, is considered adequate to produce an acceptable perinatal morbidity rate. The neonatal course can be precarious in the immediate postdelivery period. The long-term effect on the outcome in these children is unclear. It would appear that symmetric growth-retarded infants are more likely to display some level of cerebral dysfunction.

SUGGESTED READING

MANNING FA, PLATT LD, SIPOS L. Antepartum fetal evaluation – development of a fetal biophysical profile. *Am J Obstet Gynecol* 1980;135:787.

MEDEARIS AL. The evaluation and interpretation of ultrasonic assessment of fetal growth. *Semin Perinatol* 1988;12:31.

MEDEARIS AL. Detection and management of intrauterine growth retardation: an American approach. *Ultrasound Obstet Gynecol* 1993;2:1437.

MEDEARIS AL, BEAR MB, HIRATA GI, PLATT LD. Statistical materials and methods in the evaluation of fetal growth. *Ultrasound Q* 1989;7:191.

PLATT LD, PAUL RH, PHELAN J, WALLA CA, BROUSSARD P. Fifteen year experience with antepartum fetal testing. *Am J Obstet Gynecol* 1987;156:1509.

25

Multiple gestations

BRUCE W. KOVACS

Although multiple gestations account for less than 1% of all births, their contribution to perinatal morbidity and mortality is disproportionately large. Perinatal mortality in twin gestations ranges between three and six times that of singleton gestations and higher yet in pregnancies with more than two fetuses. Accordingly, multiple gestations are high-risk pregnancies and involve unique considerations due to the presence of multiple fetuses. The major cause of excess morbidity and mortality is prematurity but birth trauma, growth disorders, congenital anomalies, and fetal death also contribute.

Incidence

The incidence of multiple gestation varies with various demographic characteristics relative to the patient population. On average, twins occur in 1:90 births. Triplet births occur about once every 8000 births. Clinically, the incidence of multiple conceptions exceeds that of multiple births, as reflected by a higher pregnancy loss rate. Based on early sonographic examinations there appears to be a very early attribution rate of at least 50% in twin conceptions which often goes unrecognized.

Dizygotic births occur more frequently than monozygotic births, at a rate of about 7.5:1000 varying with age, parity, race, and family history. Monozygotic births occur at a rate of about 3.5:1000, and do not vary with those factors. It follows that about 70% of twins are dizygotic (nonidentical), though this will vary slightly with population samples, and about 50% of these will be of the same sex. These figures apply only to conceptions occurring as a result of spontaneous ovulatory cycles. Stimulation of ovulation and extracorporeal fertilization increase the rate of multiple gestations, due to increases in multizygotic conceptions. In pregnancies induced by clomiphene the incidence of multiple gestation is about 8% and higher yet when gonadotropins are used. The increased risk of multiple gestations makes routine early ultrasonographic fetal examinations in such pregnancies mandatory.

Diagnosis

The accuracy of antenatal diagnosis of twin gestations varies from nearly 100% in populations who are routinely screened with ultrasound examinations to slightly more than 50% in large clinic services without routine screening. Most multiple gestations can be diagnosed antenatally by maintaining an index of suspicion and liberally using ultrasonography. Importantly, however, some caution is advised when patients are advised of the diagnosis of twins based on an early ultrasound examination because of the relatively common loss of one twin.

Later in gestation, a fundal height greater than expected for gestational age is usually the first indication of a twin gestation. However, a uterine size greater than dates is not routinely detected before the 24th week. Less often, auscultation of two fetal heart tones leads to an earlier diagnosis. In either case, these findings should be further evaluated by a complete ultrasonographic examination. Special attention should be directed toward documenting the presence of a dividing membrane, determining fetal sizes and sex and amniotic fluid volume, and verifying normal fetal anatomy.

The advent of routine maternal serum α-fetoprotein (MSAFP) testing in some areas has resulted in a marked increase in the early diagnosis of multiple gestations. We use a value for MSAFP of >2.5 multiples of the mean (MOM) as a level at which ultrasonographic evaluation should be performed. However, it is important to be aware that values of MSAFP are higher in multiple gestations than in singletons of the same gestational age. Therefore, values used in screening for neural tube defects (NTDs) need to be adjusted upward with twin pregnancies. Our current policy calls for diagnostic evaluation of NTDs (and other anomalies) at levels greater than 4.5 MOM in documented twin gestations.

Antenatal care

The antenatal course of multiple gestations is more likely to be encumbered by complications than are singleton gestations. Thus, one of the primary goals in antenatal management is the prevention and early identification of maternal complications. Our experience at Los Angeles County–University of Southern California Women's Hospital has shown that 70% of twin gestations will be complicated by preterm labor, pregnancy-induced hypertension, or intrauterine fetal death. Other complications such as anemia, gestational diabetes, and pyelonephritis also occur; however, their incidence does not appear to be significantly increased over that found in single gestations.

Optimal prenatal care includes increasing caloric intake by at least 300 kcal/day, and supplementation of vitamins, iron, and other minerals. Even in the absence of complications, more frequent prenatal visits are indicated and patients are advised of the extra physiologic burden that these gestations impose. We schedule routine visits every 3 weeks until 28 weeks, and every 2 weeks thereafter until 34 weeks when weekly visits are started. Our current management protocol calls for ultrasonographic examinations every 3 weeks after 21 weeks with assessment of fetal growth and amniotic fluid volume. Special attention is given to determining the degree of size discordance between each fetus based on estimated fetal weight. We have found that size discordance >20% is associated with a significant increase in perinatal morbidity and mortality. When this occurs we begin conducting more detailed fetal evaluations consisting of a biophysical profile on a more frequent basis. The efficacy of routine bedrest in twin gestations remains controversial and has not been shown to be beneficial in resolving significant growth discordance or in reducing preterm labor. However, bedrest may reduce the incidence of a suboptimal outcome in some other complications such as premature rupture of membranes or mild pregnancy-induced hypertension. A prudent approach in uncomplicated multiple gestations would be to encourage increased periods of rest rather than insisting on forced full-time bedrest.

Birth defects occur more frequently in fetuses of multiple gestations than in those of single gestations. For the most part, the etiologies of these defects are the same as that in singletons. However, some anomalies are particular to twins, such as conjoined twins. Birth defects are more common in monozygotic than in dizygotic twins and can occur in one or both fetuses. Genetic amniocentesis is indicated in multiple gestations for the same reasons as it is in singletons; however, the procedure is complicated by the need to sample both amniotic sacs. We perform amniocentesis under direct ultrasound guidance, aspirating 15–20 ml from one sac, followed by instillation of 2 ml of 0.1% indigo carmine dye. The amniocentesis is then performed on the second sac and its success is verified by the absence of a blue color in the fluid. The procedure is repeated if more than two fetuses are present. Methylene blue should not be substituted for indigo carmine as adverse outcomes have been associated with its use. In addition to routine karyotype and AFP determinations, we also advocate the use of molecular genetic fingerprinting of a portion of the fluids to determine zygosity in cases where sex is found to be the same in the fetuses.

Preterm labor occurs in slightly less than half of all multiple gestations and represents the single most important factor in the increased fetal morbidity and mortality. Unfortunately, several large studies have shown that little, if anything, is efficacious in preventing preterm labor. Most importantly, oral or subcutaneous prophylactic tocolysis has not been shown to be effective in preventing either premature labor or preterm delivery and cannot be advocated. Continuous or periodic home uterine activity monitoring also does not prevent preterm labor; however, it has been advocated by some in preventing preterm birth. Currently, we do not routinely use this modality in our outpatient clinic.

When premature labor without coincident rupture of membranes occurs, management is determined by assessing causation and amount of cervical dilatation, and evaluating fetal maturity and status. As in single gestations, fetuses compromised by chorioamnionitis or fetal distress should not undergo tocolysis. In the absence of contraindications, tocolysis should be instituted, with magnesium sulfate as the primary agent. Tocolysis with a β-sympathomimetic is associated with an increased potential for maternal complications, including pulmonary edema, and is not generally advised. Tocolysis with other agents such as indomethacin has not been studied enough in multiple gestations to be recommended. Importantly, tocolysis will seldom be successful when cervical dilatation is >4 cm and should not be aggressively pursued. In addition, tocolysis can only be recommended in the absence of documented fetal maturity, as determined by analysis of the lecithin:sphingomyelin ratio in amniotic fluid.

Lecithin:sphingomyelin ratios of 2.0 or greater may be used to predict pulmonary maturity in the absence of diabetes. Caution is advised in extrapolating the lecithin:sphingomyelin ratio of one fetus to its twin. When a smaller fetus is caused by a growth disorder it is likely that the lecithin:sphingomyelin ratio will be greater in the smaller infant than in its larger twin. However, not all small fetuses result from this process. When fetal weight appears small due to constitutional factors or ultrasonographic measurement error, it cannot be assumed this phenomenon will occur. When possible, the fluid from both sacs should be evaluated for lung maturity.

Ongoing fetal evaluation is an integral part of antenatal care. The nonstress test, combined with ultrasonographic evaluation of the fetal status, is the best general indicator of fetal status. The same criteria for fetal well-being apply to twin gestations as to singletons. Ultrasonographic evaluation of fetal growth is also very important; however, it is often complicated by suboptimal fetal visualization. Several criteria have been described for determination of fetal weights by ultrasonographic measurements. In twin gestations, caution should be exercised in employing a single determination to diagnose growth discordance. Serial measurements are of greater value to determine differences in fetal size caused by a compromised fetal environment.

Discordance of 20% or greater in estimated fetal weights is cause for concern and requires more intensive surveillance. Although differences in biparietal diameter >5 mm alone can be used to suggest the presence of significant discordance, determination of estimated fetal weights using abdominal circumference with biparietal diameter provides the best method. When such measurements indicate consistently divergent growth or pronounced decreases in growth rates of both fetuses, delivery is advised as soon as maturity is documented. Prior to lung maturity, serial biophysical profile determinations are recommended as a good method to follow fetal well-being. Clinically significant twin-to-twin vascular communication is uncommon in twin gestations but is an important (albeit uncommon) cause of size discordance. Thus, in cases of significant size or amniotic fluid volume discordance, twin-to-twin transfusion should be considered in the diagnostic work-up. Doppler studies may be useful for this purpose and can be performed to help evaluate fetal blood flow in cases of twin-to-twin transfusions, if required.

Fetal death of one or both twins occurs on the average in about 4% of these gestations. In multifetal gestation of greater than two, the incidence may be higher. The demise of one twin in the antenatal period is a particularly difficult circumstance. Importantly, the death of one twin *in utero* may or may not have an effect on the outcome of the survivor. The factors which influence the surviving twin's outcome are: chorionicity, gestational age at death, and cause of death. Our experience has shown that most often no untoward outcome occurs with a single intrauterine death and this is particularly true when the fetal death occurs before 20 weeks and when dichorionicity exists. This is also true in cases of selective fetal reductions in twin gestations and in cases with more than two fetuses.

In our experience we have not noted any cases of coagulopathy occurring in this group of patients. However, later in pregnancy in monozygotic gestations with monochorionic membranes there is a significant possibility of embolization of toxic products through vascular anastomoses and these pregnancies require specialized and frequent evaluation. Because 30% of twin gestations are monozygotic and 70% of these monochorionic, it holds that about 20% of all twin gestations are monochorionic. In recent years there has been an increasing number of reports of the surviving twin suffering from thromboembolism and central nervous system damage and greater concern is warranted in monochorionic gestations. Thus, when the membrane type is known (e.g., opposite-sex twins are dichorionic), counseling and management are predicated on risks to the surviving fetus. In dichorionic twin gestations, only when the cause of fetal death is due to maternal complications or a hostile intrauterine environment is the surviving twin in danger. However, when chorionicity is unknown, increased fetal surveillance should be instituted. Lastly, prudence and sympathy for parental anxiety warrant that in some twin gestations with a single fetal death, the surviving twin should be delivered as soon as pulmonary maturity can be documented.

Intrapartum care

Spontaneous labor occurs earlier on average in multiple gestations than in singleton pregnancies and its onset is inversely proportional to the number of fetuses present. Only in unusual circumstances should multiple gestations be allowed to continue past 40 completed weeks of gestation. Patients presenting in labor or for induction of labor should have an ultrasonographic examination to document the fetal positions. Pharmacologic labor induction and augmentation in twin gestation are not contraindicated and follow the same guidelines as in singleton gestations.

Intrapartum electronic fetal heart rate monitoring is essential in the management of labor of multiple gestations. Both fetuses should be simultaneously monitored and the same criteria applied to interpretation of the fetal heart rate pattern as with singletons. Difficulty arises in situations where only the second fetus demonstrates an abnormal pattern and cannot be further evaluated. If no assurance of fetal well-being can be obtained, immediate delivery is advised.

The route of delivery is predicted on presentation, estimation of birth weights, experience of the obstetrician, and the compliance of the patient. In the majority of situations (73% in our experience) the first twin will present by the vertex and a trial of vaginal delivery may be selectively attempted. When both twins present by the vertex a trial of vaginal delivery should be attempted regardless of the estimated fetal weights. In situations where presentation of the second twin is not vertex and its estimated fetal weight is >2000 g, a trial of vaginal delivery may be undertaken with either subsequent external or internal version of the second twin. Hazards of this routine involve relative inexperience of the obstetrician, lack of patient acceptance, and lack of appropriate immediate surgical back-up. In cases of a nonvertex second twin with estimated fetal weight <2000 g, cesarean section has been advocated to prevent increased morbidity and mortality of vaginally delivered breech fetuses in this weight range. The option of careful external cephalic version and subsequent vaginal trial also remains a viable one for those experienced in the method.

Cesarean section is advised in the circumstance of first twins presenting other than vertex regardless of second twin presentation and in cases of monoamnionic twin gestations. It should be noted that cesarean section may, on occasion, be required for delivery of second twins only, most commonly as a result of fetal distress. The same criteria of cesarean section for documented fetal distress or failure to progress in labor are applied to remaining second twins as would be applied to singleton gestations. Exceptions can be made when there is an ability to perform a prompt, atraumatic delivery through the fully dilated cervix. Judicious augmentation of labor for second twins is often useful, since a period of relative uterine dysfunction sometimes occurs after delivery of the first twin. Given good indicators of fetal status and progress of labor there is no arbitrary time limit for delivery of second twins. Decisions on cesarean sections in twin gestations should be tempered with reasonable estimates of fetal survivability.

Summary

Multiple gestations are high-risk pregnancies with high incidences of perinatal morbidity and mortality. Some antenatal complications occur more frequently in twin gestations than singleton gestation. Optimal care requires liberal use of ultrasonography, antenatal fetal hart rate monitoring, and aggressive treatment of preterm labor in the absence of fetal maturity. A trial of vaginal delivery is advocated depending on presentation of first twin, estimate of fetal weights, obstetric experience, and patient compliance.

SUGGESTED READING

ANDREWS WW, LEVENO KJ, SHERMAN ML, et al. Elective hospitalization in the management of twin pregnancies. *Obstet Gynecol* 1991;77:826–831.

ARNOLD C, MCLEAN FH, KRAMER MS, USHER RH. Respiratory distress syndrome in second-born versus first-born twins. A matched case-control analysis. *N Engl J Med* 1987;317:1121–1125.

BEBBINGTON MW, WITTMAN BK. Fetal transfusion syndrome: antenatal factors predicting outcome. *Am J Obstet Gynecol* 1989;160:913–915.

BENIRSCHKE K, KIM CK. Multiple pregnancy. *N Engl J Med* 1973;288:1276–1284.

BERKOWITZ RL, LYNCH L, CHITKARA U, et al. Selective reduction of multifetal pregnancies in the first trimester. *N Engl J Med* 1988;318:1043–1047.

D'ALTON ME. In: Creasy RK, Warshaw JB, eds. *Seminars in Perinatology.* 1986; 10(1):2–91.

D'ALTON ME, DUDLEY DK. The ultrasonographic prediction of chorionicity in twin gestation. *Am J Obstet Gynecol* 1989;160:557–561.

MAHONY BS, PETTY CN, NYBERG DA, *et al.* The "stuck twin" phenomenon: ultrasonographic findings, pregnancy outcome, and management with serial amniocenteses. *Am J Obstet Gynecol* 1990;163:1513–1522.

NANCE WE, ALLEN G, PARISI P (eds). *Twin Research: Biology and Epidemiology.* New York: AR Liss, 1978.

SHAH YG, GRAGG LA, MOODLEY S, WILLIAMS GW. Doppler velocimetry in concordant and discordant twin gestations. *Obstet Gynecol* 1992;80:272–276.

TESSEN JA, ZALTNIK FJ. Monoamniotic twins: a retrospective controlled study. *Obstet Gynecol* 1991;77:832–834.

WENSTROM KD, TESSEN JA, ZLATNIK FJ, SIPES SL. Frequency, distribution, and theoretical mechanisms of hematologic and weight discordance in monochorionic twins. *Obstet Gynecol* 1992;80:257–261.

WINN HN, GABRIELLI S, REECE EA, *et al.* Ultrasonographic criteria for the prenatal diagnosis of placental chorionicity in twin gestations. *Am J Obstet Gynecol* 1989;161:1540–1542.

26

Management of breech presentation

CAROLINA REYES

Management of breech presentation is surrounded by controversy. On the one hand, we have patients demanding perfect babies. On the other, we have obstetricians in fear of litigation. Breech deliveries are associated with an increase in perinatal morbidity and mortality, therefore the management has generally been conservative with delivery by cesarean section. The discussion of managing breech presentations has focused on what constitutes a safe delivery for both mother and baby. Many obstetricians highly trained in the mechanical art of breech delivery, and concerned about the maternal complications associated with cesarean deliveries, favor vaginal delivery. Others who have a concern for the perinatal risks associated with a vaginal breech delivery favor cesarean section. This chapter will discuss the maternal and fetal risks associated with breech presentation and management of a breech delivery.

Incidence and etiology

Breech presentations represent a small proportion of the total deliveries. The incidence of breech presentation varies with the gestational age. At 28 weeks or less, the incidence is 25%. At term, the incidence of breech presentation decreases to 3–4%.

Factors that predispose to a breech presentation include uterine and fetal malformations, polar placentation, multiple gestation, a previous breech presentation, and oligohydramnios. Because congenital and other abnormalities are found more often in the breech presentation, when this presentation is suspected, a sonographic evaluation of the uterus and fetus is highly recommended.

Prematurity is more common among fetuses presenting breech (20–30%) than the vertex (6–8%). Prematurity is the leading cause of perinatal mortality in obstetrics today. The overall prematurity rate in our institution is about 8–10%, but the rate of prematurity in the breech presentation is as high as 25%. This is probably a result of the higher incidence of breech presentation in the early third trimester. The delivery of a premature breech is much more conservative than the mature breech. Duenholter *et al.* compared the delivery of the premature breech by cesarean section versus vaginal delivery and found the perinatal mortality rate increased from 2.3% when the fetus presenting breech is delivered abdominally to 15.9% when delivered vaginally. This is due to premature babies having a narrower margin for oxygen desaturation, a greater propensity to hypoxic lung injury, interventricular hemorrhage, infections, and long bone fractures. The premature fetus presenting breech is at great risk for umbilical cord prolapse, nuchal arm, and head entrapment. Until 35 weeks, the head circumference is greater than the abdominal circumference and a small body can pass through a cervix before it is completely dilated, therefore trapping the larger after-coming head. If the premature fetus presenting breech is nonviable, then a vaginal delivery is recommended.

Term breech presentations are also associated with umbilical cord prolapse. The incidence varies with the type of breech. The overall rate of umbilical cord prolapse in the vertex presentation is approximately 0.5–0.9% and only slightly higher in the frank breech presentation. In contrast, the overall incidence of cord prolapse in complete and incomplete breech presentations is 5% and up to 10% in the footling breech presentation. Cord prolapse primarily occurs during the second stage of labor or during delivery, but it can occur at any time and is considered a true obstetric emergency.

Management considerations in the breech presentation

Management has focused on selection criteria to be used for safe vaginal delivery or on the use of routine cesarean birth. At our institution, women with a breech presentation who are candidates for an attempted vaginal delivery must meet strict criteria in order to minimize perinatal morbidity. The criteria include a term pregnancy with an estimated fetal weight between 2000 and 4000 g. Macrosomic babies with an estimated fetal weight >4000 g have a 10 times greater risk of perinatal death. So a fetal weight limit of 3800 g allows a 10% error by ultrasound on estimation of fetal weight. Other criteria include a compliant patient who is well informed and consents to the procedure; the type of breech presentation – fetal head attitude must be flexed and <105° between the mandible and cervical spine; X-ray pelvimetry must meet the 10, 11, 12 rule (interspinous diameter ⩾10 cm; anteroposterior diameter of the inlet ⩾11 cm; transverse diameter of the inlet ⩾12 cm); and a well-organized delivery team. A fetus in the breech position is not a one-person delivery. To ensure better control and avoid possible trauma at delivery, one person stands by the maternal abdomen guiding the body, the fetal head is maintained in a flexed position, Piper forceps should be considered for the delivery of the after-coming head, and a generous second-degree episiotomy should be performed. If patients qualify for a trial of labor, they undergo continuous fetal monitoring during labor, and an epidural during the active phase is readily placed. The trial of labor is aborted, using the same guidelines as for a vertex presentation.

Using this approach, randomized studies performed at this institution by Collea *et al.* in the frank breech presentation and Gimovsky *et al.* in the nonfrank breech presentation have shown that vaginal breech delivery is a reasonable consideration. In those investigations, the most common reason for not undertaking a trial of labor was an inadequate pelvis as determined by X-ray pelvimetry (40%). Of the remaining 60% who underwent a trial of labor, 75% achieved a vaginal delivery. The chances of a successful vaginal delivery were greater in the frank breech (82%) than in the nonfrank breech (50%). Overall, 44% of the women with a breech presentation delivered vaginally. Both groups concluded that, if a breech delivery was appropirately evaluated, the perinatal morbidity rate was not statistically different from vertex vaginal births. However, in the study by Collea *et al.*, complications occurred in three vaginal breech deliveries, all with a nuchal arm, which led to brachial plexus palsy in two infants without residua.

Although the use of strict criteria for a vaginal breech delivery can reduce the perinatal morbidity outcome, it is not completely eliminated. On the other hand the corrected perinatal mortality rate in the uncomplicated breech presentation at term, delivered by cesarean section, is almost zero. Routine cesarean birth for breech presentation prevents umbilical cord prolapse, birth injury, and birth anoxia associated with a vaginal delivery. Cesarean section does not eliminate the perinatal risks associated with prematurity or congenital abnormalities. Nonetheless, cesarean birth is a major operative procedure with its own inherent risks to the mother. The risks and benefits of the method of delivery for both the mother and the fetus should be given careful consideration.

Prevention of breech presentation

At term, the spontaneous conversion rate of a breech presentation to a vertex presentation is 15–20%. After 40 weeks' gestation, the spontaneous conversion rate is negligible. One solution to reducing the incidence of breech presentation at term is the use of external cephalic version (ECV) under tocolysis. Three randomized clinical trials by Van Dorsten *et al.*, Brocks *et al.*, and Hofmeyr *et al.* showed a reduction in the incidence of breech presentation at birth and in the cesarean delivery rate using ECV. Weiner performed a metaanalysis of four randomized trials examining the effect of ECV on the overall cesarean section rate. He concluded that there was not a significant decrease in the cesarean section rate with the use of ECV when the four studies (comprising 815 patients) were combined in a single analysis. However, if a trial of labor for any breech fetus was not allowed, ECV did decrease the cesarean section rate. At this institution, a randomized clinical trial by Wallace *et al.* [8] showed a success rate of 77% using ECV. In the successful group, 95% presented vertex when labor began. The cesarean section rate was 25% in the successful-ECV group and 87% in the failed-ECV group.

At this institution, candidates for ECV include patients expected to have a term fetus of 36–40 weeks' gestation, a normal real-time ultrasound with an adequate amniotic fluid index, and a reactive nonstress test. A patient who meets the above criteria for version is given a β-mimetic − ritodrine hydrochloride by infusion pump at 100 μg/min or magnesium sulfate by infusion pump at 4 g over 20 min, then 2 g/h to relax the uterus. When the uterus is relaxed, an ECV is attempted with monitoring of the fetal heart rate. The likelihood of success is 70–80%. Of those with a successful version, approximately 95% remain vertex. Of those who fail version, none spontaneously convert.

A fetal heart rate tracing should be obtained after the procedure. The reported incidence of fetal heart rate changes associated with version is 40%; most of the time these changes are transient. Less than 1% may require immediate admission to the hospital for prolonged decelerations. There is a 3–4% risk of a fetal−maternal bleed and RhoGAM (300 μg) should be administered to the Rh− patient. After the procedure, fetal surveillance using the nonstress test is recommended until the patient is delivered.

Summary

In summary, when a breech presentation is suspected, a careful real-time ultrasound should be performed to rule out uterine, fetal, or placental abnormalities. Vaginal breech delivery is a reasonable approach for a term or near-term fetus if appropriately evaluated and a well-organized team is available for the delivery. Given the maternal risks of cesarean section, a routine elective cesarean should not be the primary option. One method of reducing the incidence of breech presentation is by performing ECV.

SUGGESTED READING

BRUCKS V, PHILIPSEN T, SECHER WJ. A randomized trial of external cephalic version with tocolysis in late pregnancy. *Br J Obstet Gynecol* 1984;91:653.

COLLEA JV, CHEIN C, QUILLIGAN EJ. The randomized management of term frank breech presentation. A study of 208 cases. *Am J Obstet Gynecol* 1980;137:235.

DUENHOELTER JH, WELLS CE, REISH RSS, JIMENEZ JM. A paired control study of vaginal and abdominal delivery of the low-birth-weight breech fetus. *Obstet Gynecol* 1979;54:310.

GIMOVSKY ML, WALLACE RL, SCHIFRIN BS, *et al.* Randomized management of nonfrank breech presentation at term: a preliminary report. *Am J Obstet Gynecol* 1983;146:36–40.

GIMOVSKY MO, PETRIE RH, TODD WD. Neonatal performance of the selected term vaginal breech delivery. *Obstet Gynecol* 1980;46:687.

HOFMEYER GJ. Effect of external cephalic version in late pregnancy on breech presentation and cesarean section rate: a controlled trial. *Br J Obstet Gynecol* 1983;90:392.

LUTEKORT M, PERSSON P, WELDNER B. Maternal and fetal factors in breech presentation. *Obstet Gynecol* 1984;64:55.

PHELAN JP, BETHEL M, DEVORE G, *et al.* Use of ultrasound in the breech presentation with hyperextension of the fetal head: a case report. *J Ultrasound Med* 1984;148:223.

PHELAN JP, STINE LE, MUELLER E, *et al.* Observations of fetal heart rate characteristics related to external cephalic version and tocolysis. *Am J Obstet Gynecol* 1984;149:658.

RAMNEY B. The gentle art of external cephalic version. *Am J Obstet Gynecol* 1973; 116:239.

SCHEER K, NUBAR J. Variation of fetal presentation with gestational age. *Am J Obstet Gynecol* 1976;125:269.

STINE LE, PHELAN JP, WALLACE RH, *et al.* Update on external cephalic version at term – its clinical usefulness and safety: a continuing experience at LAC/USC Medical Center. *Obstet Gynecol* 1985;65:642.

VANDORSTEN JP, SCHIFRIN BS, WALLACE RL. Randomized control trial of external cephalic version with tocolysis in late pregnancy. *Am J Obstet Gynecol* 1981;141:417.

WALLACE RL, VANDORSTEN JP, EGLINGTON GS, MUELLER E, McCART D, SCHIFRIN BS. External cephalic version with tocolysis: observations and continuing experience at the Los Angeles County/University of Southern California Medical Center. *J Reprod Med* 1984;29:745.

WEINER CP. Vaginal breech delivery in the 1990s. *Clin Obstet Gynecol* 1992;35:1559.

27

Hydrocephalus

DENA TOWNER

Hydrocephalus is defined as an abnormal accumulation of fluid in the cranial vault. One of the more commonly encountered congenital anomalies, hydrocephalus occurs with an incidence of 1:2000 births. Congenital hydrocephalus is associated with numerous conditions, representing a range of etiologies, ultrasound characteristics, and prognoses. Hydrocephalus is generally due to an obstruction in cerebrospinal fluid (CSF) flow, but may be secondary to increased production. Hydrocephalus can be diagnosed prenatally as large collections of CSF are readily visualized on ultrasound examination.

There are many etiologies for congenital hydrocephalus, including neural tube defects and other central nervous system (CNS) malformations, *in utero* vascular accidents, infections, and genetic disorders. The most common association is with neural-tube defects, accounting for 30% of cases. CNS malformations, such as agenesis of the corpus callosum, Dandy–Walker malformation, and holoprosencephaly, can also be associated with hydrocephalus. Genetic causes include X-linked aqueductal stenosis, Meckel–Gruber syndrome, Walker–Warburg syndrome, and certain skeletal dysplasias (osteogenesis imperfecta, achondrogenesis, and thanatophoric dysplasia). Rarely, trisomy 13, 18, and 21 have been associated with hydrocephalus. Congenital cytomegalovirus and toxoplasmosis have been implicated as an etiology of hydrocephalus by causing aqueductal stenosis via inflammatory scarring. Intracranial tumors can lead to hydrocephalus by preventing normal CSF flow. Intracerebral hemorrhage can also occur, leading to obstructed CSF flow or cavitation, with resultant porencephalic cysts filled with CSF.

The prenatal diagnosis of hydrocephalus is made by ultrasound examination of intracranial structures. One can evaluate the lateral ventricles by determining the ratio of the lateral ventricular width (LVW) to the lateral hemispheric width (LHW) in a plane immediately cephalic to the plane for measuring the biparietal diameter. LVW is measured from the falx in the midline to the lateral aspect of the ventricle and LHW is measured from the midline to the inner side of the distal parietal bone. Through 18 weeks' gestation the normal ratio is <70%, after 18 weeks <50%, and from 24 weeks to term <33%. Another clue to the presence of hydrocephalus is the appearance that the choroid plexus dangles in the dilated ventricle. Periventricular calcifications may be noted and are suggestive of congenital infection. Irregular CSF-filled cavities suggest porencephaly secondary to an intracerebral bleed or infarction. Occasionally an old blood clot can be seen in the porencephalic cyst, thus aiding in its diagnosis. A fluid-filled cystic cavity in the posterior fossa is suggestive of Dandy–Walker malformation. A crescent-shaped fluid collection without midline structures is classic for alobar holoprosencephaly.

Once hydrocephalus is diagnosed by ultrasound examination, other structural anomalies must be sought. Another anomaly is found in 70–85% of cases, of which 50–60% are concurrent CNS malformations. There is a correlation between an increased number of anomalies and poorer prognosis and increased likelihood of a fetal chromosomal anomaly. A key structure to evaluate fully is the spine, as neural tube defects represent the most commonly associated defects. The face should be evaluated for clefts and hypotelorism, which are frequently seen with holoprosencephaly. Limbs should be evaluated for evidence of skeletal dysplasias. However, any organ system may be found to be abnormal.

An amniocentesis should be offered for karyotypic analysis, determination of α-fetoprotein level, and assessment for acetylcholinesterase. Late in gestation and between 22 and 24 weeks, fetal blood sampling may be indicated for rapid karyotyping. Maternal antibody titers for cytomegalovirus and toxoplasmosis should be evaluated. If fetal blood is sampled, immunoglobulin M levels and a complete blood count should be obtained in addition to karyotype. The complete blood count should include a platelet count to exclude alloisoimmune thrombocytopenia, which frequently causes intracranial hemorrhages.

Thorough counseling must be given to the patient and her family as to the natural history and prognosis of the defect, not only in the neonatal period but throughout life. Neonatal mortality is generally 70–80% if there are other anomalies and 40% in isolated cases of hydrocephalus. Neurologic outcome in the survivors is poor, with normal neurologic development ranging from 10 to 50% depending on the study and severity of the hydrocephalus.

If the diagnosis is made prior to 24 weeks, termination of the pregnancy should be offered. If the pregnancy is more advanced or termination is not an option, then the physician and patient should have a detailed discussion about delivery plans. All plans should be tailored to the specific etiologic category and should consider the predicted long-term outcome. In general a vaginal delivery should be anticipated with a cesarean delivery only for the usual indications. Fetuses with neural tube defects, however, may benefit from abdominal delivery to protect the nerve function at the level of the defect. Should a cesarean be done for fetal distress? Some authors claim that a fetus with as much as 1 cm of cortical tissue can have a relatively normal outcome. Most perinatologists use this criterion as the cut-off point for when intervention is offered for fetal reasons. When a fetus is considered nonviable and there is an obstructed vaginal delivery due to the hydrocephalus, cephalocentesis should be performed. This can be done vaginally when the fetus is vertex or transabdominally for a breech presentation. An 18-gauge spinal needle is introduced into the dilated ventricular system and CSF drained, usually with low suction. Rarely is a fetus liveborn after this procedure.

In the past it was thought that *in utero* shunting of CSF would prevent sequelae of long-standing hydrocephalus. However, this does not appear to be the case and in fact such procedures may cause more harm than nonintervention.

After delivery a thorough genetics evaluation should be undertaken, including autopsy, X-rays, and toxoplasmosis, rubella, cytomegalovirus, and herpes titers on cord blood if a definitive diagnosis was not made prior to delivery. This enables the physician to determine the cause of the hydrocephaly and provide informative counseling regarding the recurrence risk to the parents and other family members. Referral to support groups even prior to delivery may be advantageous for some patients, especially if the hydrocephalus is isolated and mild.

SUGGESTED READING

NYBERG DA, MAHONY BS, PRETORIUS DH. *Diagnostic Ultrasound of Fetal Anomalies: Text and Atlas*. St Louis, MO: Mosby-Year Book, 1990.

ROMERO R, PILU G, JEANTY P, GHIDINI A. *Prenatal Diagnosis of Congenital Anomalies*. San Mateo, CA: Appleton & Lang, 1988.

28

Pregnancy-induced hypertension

KATHRYN J. SHAW

Introduction

Hypertension of any type in pregnancy is well recognized as a significant risk for both the mother and the fetus. Hypertensive disorders remain one of the three leading causes of maternal mortality, along with hemorrhage and pulmonary embolism. In a 10-year review recently conducted at Women's Hospital at the Los Angeles County–University of Southern California Medical Center, hypertension was the number one cause of maternal death. Significant maternal morbidity is also common. Perinatal morbidity and mortality are similarly increased with this disease, often as a result of a necessary premature delivery, intrauterine fetal growth retardation, or placental accidents such as placental abruption.

Normal pregnancy is associated with a variety of physiologic changes that affect the cardiovascular and renal systems, which should be kept in mind when caring for patients with hypertension. Plasma volume increases early in gestation by as much as 40–60%. Renal blood flow increases as does the glomerular filtration rate, resulting in a decrease in the serum blood urea nitrogen and creatinine. Cardiac output is elevated, while systemic and pulmonary vascular resistances are decreased. Compared to prepregnancy values, both systolic and diastolic blood pressure decrease, the latter to a greater degree than the former. The nadir of this decline is between 18 and 22 weeks. Blood pressures subsequently return to the prepregnancy values as term approaches. This pattern is noted in both normotensive and hypertensive patients. In fact, in patients with moderate to severe chronic hypertension prior to pregnancy, the blood pressure may decrease into the normal range by the midtrimester. This may lead to misidentification of this patient as normotensive if the prior history is not known.

Another important observation in pregnancy is the development of a blunted sensitivity to vasopressors, best described with angiotensin II. This is evident by the second trimester. The angiotensin sensitivity test demonstrates that pregnant women require a greater dose of angiotensin II to achieve a given blood pressure increase compared to the nonpregnant patient.

Definitions

A variety of terminologies exist for hypertension in pregnancy, creating some confusion. It is important to distinguish preexisting hypertension from that which develops during pregnancy as the etiologies are presumed to be different. A practical classification scheme is that described in *Williams' Obstetrics*:

1   pregnancy-induced hypertension (PIH) – hypertension that develops as a consequence of pregnancy, appearing after 20 weeks' gestational age (GA) and regressing postpartum:

    (a) hypertension alone (no evidence of proteinuria or pathologic edema) – gestational hypertension;

    (b) hypertension + proteinuria and/or pathologic edema – preeclampsia;

    (c) eclampsia – occurrence of seizures in the setting of PIH;

2   chronic hypertension – hypertension diagnosed prior to pregnancy or evident prior to 20 weeks' GA;

3   chronic hypertension with superimposed PIH –

    (a) superimposed preeclampsia;

    (b) superimposed eclampsia.

Diagnosis and incidence

PIH is a multisystem disorder. A variety of organs may be affected, including the central nervous, renal, hepatic, cardiovascular, and coagulation systems. The diagnosis is based primarily upon clinical findings. Unfortunately no specific test exists to distinguish chronic hypertension from that developing as a consequence of pregnancy. The patient group that develops apparent gestational hypertension (no sign of preeclampsia) may indeed have other unrecognized causes for hypertension. In the absence of preconceptional records or early prenatal care, it is often impossible to make a definitive diagnosis when hypertension is evident at the first prenatal visit, if this is in the third trimester. As noted above, even the patient with significant hypertension prior to pregnancy may be normotensive in the second trimester. As the third trimester progresses, this patient's blood pressure will return to prepregnancy hypertensive values. If the history of chronic hypertension is not known, this patient would be misdiagnosed as having PIH. In this setting, the correct diagnosis would be evident postpartum, since PIH will resolve and chronic hypertension would persist.

The diagnostic criteria for PIH in a patient without a history of hypertension or renal disease are as follows:

1 hypertension
    (a) blood pressure ≥ 140/90 mmHg or;
    (b) blood pressure increase over baseline: systolic 30 mmHg, diastolic 15 mmHg (this should be documented at least twice, 6 h apart);
2 proteinuria
    (a) random specimen 1+ or greater on urine dipstick;
    (b) >300 mg/24-h collection;
3 nondependent edema (especially face or hands).

If proteinuria and/or significant edema are present, the diagnosis of preeclampsia is made. A word of caution should be given with regard to the finding of blood pressure elevation above baseline. This can lead to overdiagnosis of PIH, if one uses a second-trimester blood pressure as the baseline, since blood pressure is at its nadir at this point. Ideally, the baseline should be blood pressure prior to pregnancy, which is often not available.

PIH is classified as either mild or severe. The diagnosis of severe PIH is made if *any* of the following is present:

1 blood pressure ≥160/110 mmHg taken twice, 6 h apart;
2 proteinuria ≥5 g/24 h or 3–4+ on random collection;
3 oliguria (<20–30 ml/h or <500 ml/24 h);
4 significant visual symptoms or headache;
5 HELLP syndrome:
    *h*emolysis;
    *el*evated liver enzymes;
    *l*ow *p*latelets;
6 eclampsia;
7 pulmonary edema.

The incidence of PIH ranges between 5 and 10% in the general population, with a significant increased incidence in certain patient groups, including:

1 primagravidas;
2 multiple gestations;
3 diabetes mellitus;
4 preexisting hypertension of any etiology;

5 underlying renal disease;
6 collagen vascular disease;
7 gestational trophoblastic disease (GTD);
8 family history (sister, mother);
9 PIH in prior pregnancy.

In the first three groups, PIH will occur in 15–20% of patients; with preexisting hypertension, or collagen vascular disease, the incidence of PIH will depend to some degree on the extent of the underlying disease. It is important to remember that if there is severe preexisting hypertension, vascular or renal disease or GTD, signs may rarely appear prior to 20 weeks' GA. Chesley demonstrated the genetic predisposition associated with PIH, noting that daughters of women who had PIH carried a 25% risk of developing the disease themselves. This pattern was in turn described in the granddaughters as well.

Management

Management decisions for PIH must take into consideration various factors, such as GA, disease severity, and maternal and fetal status. As with any disease, it is important to individualize treatment. Information to consider includes maternal symptoms, physical and laboratory findings, and indicators of fetal status (ultrasound and fetal heart rate monitoring). Definitive treatment for PIH is delivery, yet in many instances this jeopardizes the premature fetus. Management decisions must weigh the risks to the mother of prolonging pregnancy versus the risks to the fetus if delivery occurs.

In the patient at term with PIH, whether mild or severe, there is little to gain by prolonging pregnancy. Adequate observation and laboratory assessment should occur to confirm the diagnosis. Once confirmed, delivery should be effected. If the patient is not in labor, induction should be considered depending on patient stability. The GA at which one elects to deliver versus temporize will depend on certainty of the GA. In most instances, mild PIH presenting with a GA >35 completed weeks should be delivered.

Mild PIH presenting preterm is usually amenable to some form of expectant/temporizing management. Initially, hospitalization should be considered for complete evaluation, which must include laboratory and fetal assessment. Laboratory tests should include assessment of renal, hepatic, and hematologic function. Fetal status should be evaluated from the standpoint of fetal growth, amniotic fluid, and fetal heart rate pattern. The compliant patient who demonstrates good blood pressure response to bedrest and lacks features of preeclampsia (i.e., has gestational hypertension only) may be managed as an outpatient. In this case the patient can often be instructed in monitoring her blood pressure and at a minimum should check for proteinuria daily. If proteinuria or other signs of preeclampsia develop, hospitalization is preferable since disease deterioration can be rapid. Expectant management as an inpatient or outpatient should include frequent laboratory studies, antepartum surveillance twice weekly, and serial ultrasound to assess fetal growth. If mother and fetus remain stable, evaluation of fetal lung maturity and cervical status should be done at 35–36 weeks to allow planning of delivery.

The presentation of severe PIH remote from term presents a difficult management dilemma. Treatment options must weigh the risks imposed upon the mother if pregnancy is prolonged for the benefit of the fetus versus the risks to the fetus if premature delivery is effected for the benefit of the mother. Several studies have addressed the expectant (temporizing) management of severe PIH in the preterm patient. Although the results of these studies vary somewhat, the majority indicate that delaying delivery offers little benefit to the fetus while significantly increasing maternal morbidity and mortality. Occasionally, parameters designating disease severity may improve on bedrest, allowing for administration of betamethasone to enhance fetal lung maturity. Any attempt to prolong the pregnancy for the benefit of the fetus should be fully discussed with the mother to inform her of the risks involved, and requires extremely close monitoring. This option should only be undertaken in rare circumstances, as delivery is necessary in the vast majority of cases of severe PIH.

The development of eclampsia at any GA requires delivery, once the diagnosis is confirmed and other possible causes for seizures have been excluded. If the antecedent clinical picture is consistent with PIH, and focal neurologic findings are absent, radiologic evaluation is not indicated (i.e., computed scan, tomography or magnetic resonance imaging).

The route of delivery for patients with pregnancy-induced hypertension, whether mild or severe, or eclampsia will depend on maternal and fetal status, and cervical status. If the maternal condition is critical in the setting of an unfavorable cervix or if there is acute fetal compromise, a prolonged induction should be avoided, and a controlled cesarean delivery performed. If the maternal and fetal status are stable, even in the case of severe PIH or eclampsia, labor and vaginal delivery should be attempted. The duration allowed to achieve vaginal delivery must be decided on an individual basis, depending upon disease status.

All patients with PIH receive magnesium sulfate for seizure prophylaxis. This may be administered either intravenously or intramuscularly. In our institution, magnesium sulfate is given as a 4-g iv load, followed by 2 g/h, aiming for serum levels 4–8 mmol/dl. Magnesium clearance is primarily by the kidney, thus renal function and urine output must be evaluated. Magnesium toxicity is evidenced by muscular paralysis resulting in respiratory arrest. The earliest sign of toxicity is the loss of deep tendon reflexes, which can be easily monitored.

In general, antihypertensive drugs are not used in the management of PIH, unless blood pressure is >160/110 mmHg. With this degree of hypertension, delivery is usually indicated, thus antihypertensive therapy is short-term. While the greatest experience is with intravenous hydralazine, other options are also available, including intravenous labetolol and sublingual nifedipine. Use of the latter is usually reserved for the postpartum period. Hydralazine intravenous is given as a 5 mg initial dose. Blood pressure should be evaluated after 10 and 20 min. If an adequate response is not achieved, subsequent 5 mg dose may be repeated at 20 min intervals, up to a total dose of 30 mg. Intravenous labetolol is begun with a 10–20 mg initial dose and blood pressure response evaluated after 10 min. If the blood pressure remains elevated further doses of 20–40 mg every 10 min may be given, up to a maximum of 300 mg. The majority of patients will respond to initial efforts and if hypertension is resistant, further evaluation including central hemodynamic monitoring may be required. Persistent hypertension postpartum is less often a problem, but can be treated with a wide variety of agents.

Much discussion has occurred regarding the use of central hemodynamic monitoring in cases of severe PIH. While this should not be taken lightly, it is important to understand the accepted indications, which include:

1 oliguria, unresponsive to limited (500–1000 ml) intravenous fluid challenge;

2 hypertension unresponsive to pharmacologic maneuvers;

3 pulmonary edema.

In each of these settings, cardiac function and fluid status cannot be definitively ascertained (i.e., over- or underhydrated) and a simple central venous line is not adequate.

Conclusion

In spite of many advances in obstetrics, hypertensive complications of pregnancy remain a major cause of both maternal and fetal morbidity and mortality. Diagnosis is often difficult and management must weigh maternal versus fetal risks. Expectant management is an option as long as close observation continues for signs of deterioration. If severe PIH is evident, delivery is usually the safest option for mother and fetus alike.

SUGGESTED READING

CHESLEY LC. Hypertension in pregnancy: definitions, familial factor, and remote prognosis. *Kidney Int* 1980;18:234–240.

CLARK SL, COTTON DB. Clinical indications for pulmonary artery catheterization in the patient with severe preeclampsia. *Am J Obstet Gynecol* 1988;158:453–458.

EDEN RD, WILLIAMS AY, GALL MA, GALL SA. Pregnancy-induced hypertension and postpartum maternal morbidity. *Obstet Gynecol* 1986;68:86–90.

FERRAZZANI S, CARUSO A, DE CAROLIS S, MARTINO IV, MANCUSO S. Proteinuria and outcome of 444 pregnancies complicated by hypertension. *Am J Obstet Gynecol* 1990;162:366–371.

FRIEDMAN SA. Preeclampsia: a review of the role of prostaglandins. *Obstet Gynecol* 1988;71:122–138.

IMPERIALE TF, PETRULIS AS. A meta-analysis of low-dose aspirin for the prevention of pregnancy-induced hypertensive disease. *JAMA* 1991;266:260–264.

KORNBLITH PL, CANTU RC, WILKINSON HA, SANTAMARINA BAG. Syndrome of temporal lobe herniation in pre-eclampsia. *Am J Obstet Gynecol* 1969;104:923–924.

NOVA A, SIBAI BM, BARTON JR, MERCER BM, MITCHELL MD. Maternal plasma level of endothelin is increased in preeclampsia. *Am J Obstet Gynecol* 1991;165:724–727.

PIRCON RA, LAGREW DC, TOWERS CV, DORCHESTER WL, GOCKE SE, FREEMAN R. Antepartum testing in the hypertensive patient: when to begin. *Am J Obstet Gynecol* 1991;164:1563–1570.

REISS RE, TIZZANO TP, O'SHAUGHNESSY RW. The blood pressure course in primiparous pregnancy: a prospective study of 383 women. *J Reprod Med* 1987;32:523–526.

ROBERTS JM, TAYLOR RN, MUSCI TH, RODGERS GM, HUBEL CA, McLAUGHLIN MK. Preeclampsia: an endothelial cell disorder. *Am J Obstet Gynecol* 1989;161:1200–1204.

SIBAI BM. Pitfalls in diagnosis and management of preeclampsia. *Am J Obstet Gynecol* 1988;159:1–5.

SIBAI BM. Eclampsia: VI. Maternal–perinatal outcome in 254 consecutive cases. *Am J Obstet Gynecol* 1990;163:1049–1055.

SIBAI BM, McCUBBIN JH, ANDERSON GD, DILTS PV. Eclampsia: treatment and referral. *South Med J* 1982;75:267–269.

SIBAI BM, SPINNATO JA, WATSON DL, HILL GA, ANDERSON GD. Pregnancy outcome in 303 cases with severe preeclampsia. *Obstet Gynecol* 1984;64:319–325.

SIBAI BM, TASLIMI M, ABDELLA TN, BROOKS TF, SPINNATO JA, ANDERSON GD. Maternal and perinatal outcome of conservative management of severe preeclampsia in midtrimester. *Am J Obstet Gynecol* 1985;152:32–37.

SIBAI BM, EL-NAZER A, GONZALEZ-RUIZ A. Severe preeclampsia–eclampsia in young primigravid women: subsequent pregnancy outcome and remote prognosis. *Am J Obstet Gynecol* 1986;155:1011–1016.

VAN DAM PA, RENIER M, BAEKELANDT M, BUYTAERT P, UYTTENBROECK F. Disseminated intravascular coagulation and the syndrome of hemolysis, elevated liver enzymes, and low platelets in severe preeclampsia. *Obstet Gynecol* 1989;73:97–102.

29

Rhesus erythroblastosis fetalis: diagnosis and management

ARNOLD L. MEDEARIS & LAWRENCE D. PLATT

Introduction

Rhesus (Rh) erythroblastosis fetalis represents one of the greatest success stories in the fields of hematology, genetics, immunology, neonatology, and maternal fetal medicine. It is the prototype disease process in which a multiple disciplinary approach over the last 50 years has led to the discovery of a blood group, the identification of the effects of immunologic incompatibility during pregnancy, development of techniques of neonatal treatment, population screening for pregnancies at risk, development of fetal assessment and subsequent intrauterine therapy, and the development of a successful plan of prevention of sensitization in mothers at risk. In an era of rapidly expanding knowledge of the molecular basis of disease, the study of Rh incompatibility will continue to be a classic example of the importance of progressive applications of technology and therapy in reducing the incidence and impact of a genetic condition.

History

Erythroblastosis fetalis was probably first recorded by Hippocrates in 400 BC. However, its etiology remained without convincing elucidation until the discovery of the Rh blood group system in 1940 by Landsteiner and colleagues. Shortly after that, Levine and coworkers demonstrated the central role of Rh antigen incompatibility in a reported pregnancy complicated by maternal transfusion reaction that ended in hydropic stillbirth. A modern concept of maternal immunologic intolerance for a foreign fetal blood-cell antigen then emerged. Despite conceptual insight, however, perinatal mortality remained at 40–50%.

Wallerstein in 1946, introduced the use of exchange transfusion, which nearly halved the neonatal mortality. His original use of the sagittal sinus for transfusion was later modified by Dimond, who successfully used umbilical vessels for cannulation.

The actual relationship between hyperbilirubinemia from fetal hemolysis and subsequent newborn kernicterus was demonstrated by Allen in 1950. This helped to explain how exchange transfusion improved neonatal outcome.

Despite these advances, there still remained no help for the erythroblastotic infant doomed to die of hydrops fetalis before term. Starting in 1954, induction of labor at as early as 32 weeks gestation was instituted, based on either high maternal Rh-antibody titers or the poor outcome of previously affected pregnancies. Mortality rates were reduced further to <20%. However, prediction of actual severity of disease, based on titer and history alone, was accurate only 62% of the time.

Critical work by Bervis in 1956, using spectrophotometric analysis of fluids obtained by amniocentesis, established the inseparable relationship between amniotic fluid bilirubin concentration and the severity of the disease *in utero*. This observation provided the first reliable tool for antenatal assessment of potentially hydropic fetuses. Complications of prematurity were significant with this approach.

The understanding of the pathophysiology again increased in 1957 when Kleihauer and Betke developed a differential straining technique to identify and quantify fetal red blood cells in the maternal circulation. Beyond its immediate clinical applicability, this technique served to cement the thesis of transplacental passage of fetal red blood cells. In addition, various clinical conditions could be studied to find the risk of fetal to maternal hemorrhage.

Using established techniques of spectrophotometric analysis, in the early 1960s Liley developed a graphic means of evaluating normal versus abnormal amniotic fluid bilirubin trends (change in optical density at 450 wavelength; Δ OD 450) in samples obtained by amniocentesis from affected pregnancies. He then reported the first successful intrauterine transfusion: after accidentally puncturing the fetal abdomen during amniocentesis, he injected blood into the fetus. With the assessment of hemolysis from the evaluation of amniotic fluid and the utilization of intrauterine transfusion, the total perinatal mortality from Rh sensitization dropped to nearly 10%.

The next major achievement in Rh incompatibility came in the area of prevention. Based on a thoroughly investigated pathogenetic model for erythroblastosis fetalis, and data obtained using Kleihauer–Betke straining that detected most fetal cells passing into maternal circulation, independent American and British teams set forth to develop preventive, passive immunization for Rh sensitization. In 1966, the successful prevention of sensitization by administration of an anti-Rh antibody preparation following delivery was reported. This preparation was released for general use in 1968, under the trade name of RhoGAM.

With the utilization of postpartum RhoGAM the incidence of Rh sensitization was significantly reduced. A further reduction of maternal sensitization was achieved by prophylactic administration of Rh immunoglobulin in the late second and early third trimester of pregnancy. Recently, this treatment at 28 weeks' gestation has become the standard of practice in the USA.

In the late 1970s and 1980s the use of diagnostic ultrasound fetoscopy and percutaneous umbilical blood sampling opened new vistas in the diagnosis and management of Rh disease. Fetal blood sampling showed a strong association between the amniotic fluid assessment and the neonatal hematocrit. However, there is an imprecise correlation between Δ OD 450 and fetal hemoglobin in many cases when the fetal hematocrit is obtained. This lack of correlation between fetal hemoglobin levels and hydrops fetalis has made management difficult at times.

With the development of diagnostic ultrasound and, in particular, real-time ultrasound in 1975, intrauterine ultrasound assessment of the fetus played an increasing role in the conservative management of the Rh-sensitized pregnancy. Signs of hydrops fetalis (scalp edema and ascites) can be readily seen *in utero*. Fetal echocardiography is a specific application of ultrasound that we have used to improve the management of patients with Rh sensitization. Using state-of-the-art ultrasound equipment, an M-mode echocardiogram can be obtained through the four-chamber view of the heart to evaluate the fetus. Bilateral ventricular dilatation and the presence of minimal pericardial effusion can be used in the early recognition of hydrops.

The experience gained with fetoscopic blood sampling and ultrasound led in 1981 to direct intrauterine fetal blood transfusion. This technique has now replaced intraperitoneal transfusion and is the preferred method of treatment in the anemic or hydropic fetus remote from delivery. Percutaneous umbilical blood sampling under ultrasound guidance for transfusion or the assessment of anemia has allowed the evaluation and treatment of the potentially compromised fetus with a more physiologic technique.

In summary, after a short period of distinguished efforts, the enigma or erythroblastosis fetalis has been unraveled and in the majority of cases the successful prevention of sensitization has been achieved. The newer discoveries about pathogenesis, which became the basis for the development of prevention of Rh sensitization, are summarized in three prerequisite principles: (1) the existence of a maternal–fetal red cell antigen incompatibility; (2) the maternal ability to develop a specific and potentially destructive antibody against this foreign antigen; and (3) the entrance of this maternal antibody into the fetal circulation, causing hemolysis and subsequent hydrops.

Sensitization and incidence

In the classic case, the unsensitized Rh− pregnant woman is exposed to Rh+ cells by fetal transplacental hemorrhage. The Kleihauer–Betke technique has provided a sensitive method for detecting its incidence and relative amount. Nearly 50% of studied cases show evidence of transplacental hemorrhage during pregnancy or immediately postpartum. Recently investigations have revealed that all pregnancies have a very low level of transplacental passage of fetal cells.

The frequency and amount of fetal–maternal hemorrhage may be increased with antepartum bleeding, external cephalic version, cesarean section, manual removal of the placenta, tumultuous labor, mid-forceps delivery, and toxemia. Significant fetal to maternal hemorrhage may occur with ectopic pregnancy and abortion. Invasive prenatal diagnostic procedures are not without risk. Aminocentesis, chorionic villi sampling, and percutaneous umbilical cord sampling can lead to increased fetal–maternal hemorrhage. Besides pregnancy-related events, sensitization can occur from incompatible transfusion of blood or blood products, or immunizations when human serum is used.

The amount of transplacental hemorrhage influences the risk of isoimmunization. Eight percent of Rh− women are sensitized within 6 months postpartum after the first Rh+, ABO-compatible pregnancy. Most often, primary exposure to the foreign antigen during pregnancy results in minimal antibody production, but significant immunologic memory. A subsequent Rh-incompatible pregnancy will usually provoke an anamnestic response, and carry an additional risk of 8%. Thus, the overall risk is 16%. As parity increases, the anamnestic response may diminish, reaching an acme of risk of 50% by the fifth Rh-incompatible pregnancy. Finally, the incidence of sensitization prior to delivery is 2%. This incidence was determined from the number of first Rh+ pregnancies in Rh− women developing sensitization during gestation or within 3 days postpartum.

It is important to realize that not all patients receiving Rh-incompatible blood will develop sensitization. Only 33% of patients receiving an incompatible transfusion of 40 ml of whole blood will develop an immunologic response. Many of these initial responders will fail to develop significant titers with subsequent exposures. However, other patients may develop marked anamnestic response on as little as 0.1 ml of blood.

In patients who develop an immune response, immunoglobulin G (IgG), which crosses the placenta, is produced after a short period of IgM production.

An additional alteration in the incidence of sensitization occurs when there is maternal–fetal ABO incompatibility. In this instance the Rh+ fetus confers some protection against sensitization, probably by somehow interfering with immunologic recognition of Rh antigen sites on the red blood cell membrane. Here, the total risk is reduced to nearly 2%.

Prevention

Since the availability of Rh immunoglobulin, the incidence of Rh isoimmunization has fallen dramatically. The protective effect is dose-dependent. A single dose of 300 μg appears to suppress the immune response produced by 30 ml of whole Rh+ blood or 15 ml of packed cells. Transplacental hemorrhage greater than this amount occurs in approximately 1:300 pregnancies at risk, leading to a net failure rate of only 0.3%. The Kleihauer–Betke or Feraldex stain may be used to help assess suspected large transplacental hemorrhages. Both of these techniques identify fetal blood in the maternal circulation either by alcohol denaturation or an acid hydrolysis technique.

Since the Rh antigen has been detected in the fetus as early as 38 days after conception, the risk of sensitization from abortion in the first trimester or following a first-trimester chorionic villi sample is real and estimated to range from 2 to 4%. The presence of a Rh antigen group variant Du in an Rh– mother may protect her from sensitization. Du+ Rh– patients rarely develop anti-D antibodies. However, because there still is a risk of the development of sensitization, RhoGAM is administered to Du+ patients without evidence of sensitization.

In our institution, indications for Rh immunoglobulin administration include: (1) completion of any term pregnancy in which the mother lacks both Rh and D antigens, has no history of sensitization, and the infant is Rh+ and/or D+ with a negative direct Coombs test; (2) ectopic pregnancies in Rh– women; (3) chorionic villi sampling or amniocentesis performed on a Rh– woman; (4) abortion in the Rh– woman; (5) antepartum transplacental hemorrhage proven by the Kleihauer–Betke technique (a patient with simple hemorrhage without a positive Kleihauer–Betke technique is typically not given RhoGAM); and (6) incompatible blood transfusions of Rh+ blood or blood products. It should be emphasized that the Rh– mother with atypical antibodies, such as anti-Kell, Duffy, etc. is still a Rh immunoglobulin candidate. Naturally, previous exposure and sensitization make any attempt at prophylaxis useless.

Reduced doses of Rh immunoglobulin have been successfully used in preventing sensitization from abortion. However, if bleeding is excessive, quantitative straining techniques should be done and extra Rh immunoglobulin given as indicated. Rh immunoglobulin should be administered within the first 72 h postpartum or upon indication.

Recent studies have shown the efficacy of antenatal prophylaxis with Rh immunoglobulin. It has now become the recognized standard of practice to administer 300 µg at 28 weeks and then again postpartum. The benefactors of this administration are those few unsensitized women developing antibodies during the gestation. It should be remembered that women treated antepartum will have a positive antibody titer if tested after the administration of RhoGAM and before or immediately after delivery. In spite of a positive antibody screen after antepartum Rh immunoglobulin, RhoGAM should still be administered postpartum in these patients. While Rh immunoglobulin is a blood product, it is prepared by a technique that removes risk of contracting any blood-borne medical diseases.

Detection of the affected pregnancy

Management of isoimmunization is critically dependent upon identifying mothers at risk and detecting sensitization. The first prenatal visit requires a blood sample for blood grouping and antibody screening. Approximately 17% of a mixed Caucasian population will lack the Rh antigen. In sharp contrast, most Orientals are Rh+. All Rh− women with negative antibody screens are at risk for isoimmunization during pregnancy.

It is essential to learn both the identity and nature of any blood group antibody. Although 98% of reported cases of erythroblastosis fetalis involve either ABO or Rh incompatibilities, there are at least 30 other irregular blood group antigens associated with the disease. Thus, the presence of a non-Rh antibody does not preclude the development of hydrops fetalis.

Rh+ patients deserve to be rescreened at least once during each pregnancy to eliminate any possible laboratory error. In confirmed Rh+ patients with no irregular antibodies, only normal prenatal follow-up is required.

Rh− mothers without detectable Rh or irregular antibodies require monthly antibody screening after 22 weeks to rule out developing sensitization. Patients without detectable antibodies should be expected to deliver without complication at term. The development of a detectable maternal Rh-antibody titer indicates sensitization and requires further diagnostic attention. Rh+ mothers with detectable nonRh-associated antibody should be treated with equivalent precautions.

The reported titer is often dependent upon laboratory technique and may vary between different centers. The obstetrician must become familiar both with the methods used and the significance of values reported by the laboratory doing the testing.

In our own laboratory, in a first sensitized pregnancy, or in subsequent pregnancies when prior pregnancies did not require transfusion, an albumin titer of eight or less has not been associated with a stillbirth. With a titer of 16 or greater, or a previous history of affected fetuses, the risk of hydrops becomes very real.

Management of the affected pregnancy

Detection of fetal status and the relationship to fetal hemolysis has changed during the past few years. Traditional fetal assessment was based on analysis of bilirubin in the amniotic fluid. Bilirubin, a normal breakdown product of fetal hemoglobin, is an indirect assessment of the amount of fetal hemolysis. Using antibody titers in maternal serum, when the critical level was reached (in most laboratories 16 or greater) or there was a history of an affected fetus or neonate (fetal or neonatal loss, required transfusion or preterm or term delivery of a severely affected neonate), the clinician performed an amniocentesis to find the bilirubin content. The first procedure typically was done around 20–24 weeks' gestation. This is the gestational age at which intrauterine transfusion was feasible. With improved methods, including real-time ultrasound, transfusion became possible earlier in the second trimester. Therefore, new graphs measuring bilirubin content have been created for second-trimester analysis.

Fortunately, most patients, even with elevated titers, do not require invasive fetal therapy. Despite their antibody titer, women with a previous stillborn, prior intrauterine transfusion, or the need for multiple neonatal exchange transfusions require amniotic fluid analysis earlier in pregnancy. In attempts to identify patients at greatest risk for the need of fetal therapy, a combination of techniques using ultrasound and percutaneous umbilical blood sampling has been developed over the past few years. This discussion will focus first on the traditional methods, using amniocentesis as the primary method of surveillance, and subsequently on the newest assessment schemes using the combination of ultrasound, fetal echocardiography, and percutaneous umbilical blood sampling.

In all sensitized pregnancies it is important to obtain the genotype of the father of the child. Occasionally, even in the presence of a maternal antibody, the father of the child may be Rh− and the fetus is not at apparent risk for erythroblastosis fetalis. At other times the father of the child may be a heterozygote for the Rh antigen. This fetus has a 50%

chance of being Rh−. With the use of ultrasound we can now find the fetal blood type by obtaining an umbilical blood sample.

Once amniocentesis is decided to be necessary, the procedure should be carried out under ultrasound guidance. This involves continuous ultrasound during the procedure. Any amniocentesis not done by this approach compromises the ability to obtain a clear specimen and is an inherent risk to the fetus.

Once the fluid is obtained it is placed in a brown bottle or bag to prevent photooxidation of the bilirubin. In the laboratory the fluid is centrifuged and filtered to remove debris. A separate aliquot is typically set aside for pulmonary maturity studies. This is particularly important later in pregnancy when, in the presence of a mature leicithin:sphingomyelin ratio, the fetus has a higher chance of survival following early delivery than remaining *in utero* and being exposed to antibody. Using a spectrophotometer, optical densities are then measured over a range of 350–700 μm and recorded on graph paper (Fig. 29.1). Normally, a smooth sloping curve appears with increasing absorbancy of incident light at shorter wavelengths. Affected pregnancies show a characteristic rise or hump in optical density, peaking at 450 μm, secondary to bilirubin and associated hemoglobin breakdown products. The deviation from normal is then quantitated by drawing a straight line tangent to the curve, connecting points at 375 and 525 μm and measuring the vertical distance (in units of optical density) between the lines and the peak of the hump at 450 μm. The value obtained is called the Δ OD 450. Using the Liley method, the Δ OD 450 is plotted on a graph where the vertical axis is logarithmic and in units of Δ OD 450, while the horizontal axis is linear and in units of weeks' gestation. Thus, successive Δ OD 450 measurements are plotted against estimated gestational age, which is best obtained by ultrasound measurements early in pregnancy.

The graph is divided into three oblique zones of prognostic significance with downward sloping parallel lines from left to right. Values falling in the upper zone (zone III) are usually ominous and signify significant fetal hemolysis. Those falling in the intermediate zone (zone II) usually suggest moderate disease. Values in the upper 80% of zone II and those that plateau in zone II are worrisome. Lower values are more reassuring. Values falling in the lower 20% of zone II or in zone I may reflect an infant requiring therapy after delivery. Bilirubin is a normal component of amniotic fluid in early pregnancy and gradually decreases in concentration toward term. Therefore, some fetuses will be Rh−. Unfortunately, recent work has shown a poor correlation between absolute hemoglobin levels obtained at time of fetoscopy and Δ OD 450. This observation has led to new and innovative methods of assessing the fetus.

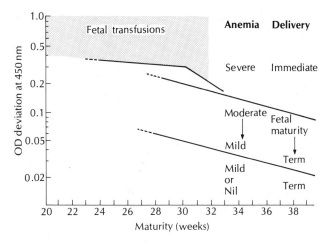

Fig. 29.1 Modified Liley curve. From *Management of Common Problems of Obstetrics and Gynecology*, 2nd edn.

Although single values on the Liley graph may be predictive, a series of examinations and plotting on the graph establish a valuable trend. The trend suggests the course of intrauterine disease more reliably than an individual value. Until percutaneous umbilical blood sampling was introduced, ultrasound-guided amniocentesis was repeated in 4 weeks if the plots were in zone I, 2 weeks in low zone II, 1 week in high zone II with a downward trend and sooner with a rising trend in high zone II. A plot in zone III is ominous and requires an immediate decision of either percutaneous umbilical sampling and possible intrauterine transfusion or delivery of the fetus.

Newer techniques

Using the Liley curve and the previously described management approach, the reduction of perinatal morbidity and mortality seen is striking. However, following the application of this methodology, clinicians became able to assess early signs of fetal hydrops with ultrasound. It is well recognized that once the fetus is hydropic the perinatal mortality rate increases. However, with high-resolution, real-time ultrasound and M-mode echocardiography it is now possible to assess and identify early ultrasound markers of impending hydrops. Since amniotic fluid Δ OD 450 is only an indirect assessment of fetal hemolysis, this method of looking at early signs of fetal hydrops has been encouraging. The ultrasound is directed to the four-chamber view of the heart and careful analysis of the pericardial sac is carried out. An M-mode line can be placed at the atrial–ventricular junction, which is an early point of development of pericardial effusion. We have found this method useful in following sensitized patients and do not perform an amniocentesis when pericardial effusion is absent. This reduction in the number of amniocentesis has been followed by a reduction in the incidence of fetal maternal hemorrhage. We now perform only an occasional amniocentesis for the management of Rh sensitization. We use ultrasound of the fetal heart as our primary method of fetal evaluation to decide the timing of delivery or intrauterine transfusion.

Antepartum and intrapartum management

Patients in zone I or low zone II with a normal fetal cardiac examination are generally allowed to progress to at least 38 weeks' gestational age. Obviously, any rise of titer should dictate earlier assessment of fetal pulmonary maturity with the lecithin:sphingomyelin ratio. When the trend is rising to high zone II, or a pericardial effusion exists, the presence of a mature lecithin:sphingomyelin ratio dictates delivery.

The combined use of the Liley curve and ultrasound to identify the fetus at risk has led to the more liberal use of percutaneous umbilical blood sampling. Under ultrasound guidance a needle is advanced to the umbilical vein and a fetal blood sample obtained. The hematocrit is assessed. When fetal anemia is identified, an intrauterine transfusion can be carried out. The blood sampled can be used for a type and cross-match. Then type-specific blood can be given to the fetus during future therapy. Conversely, an O− cross-match against the mother can still be used. With experience it is felt that percutaneous umbilical blood sampling carries with it a risk only slightly greater than that of amniocentesis.

When performing intrauterine transfusions, ultrasound-directed intravascular transfusions are used exclusively. A transfusion is performed to produce a fetal hematocrit of approximately 45%. The earliest transfusion performed in our center is at 16 weeks with the last transfusion performed at 32 weeks. After transfusion, we have chosen to use assessment by ultrasound 3 times a week for evaluation of pericardial effusion. If pericardial effusion is absent we will perform another percutaneous umbilical blood sample in 2–3 weeks and transfuse dependent upon the level of fetal hemoglobin.

After transfusion, delivery is dependent upon the number of interrelated variables, including pulmonary maturity, gestational age, the outcome of previously affected pregnancies, and the presence or absence of hydrops. Traditional antenatal assessment with both the nonstress test and fetal biophysical profile is used in these patients. Sinusoidal heart rate patterns are a reflector of fetal anemia. The combination of the sinusoidal heart rate pattern and variable decelerations is an ominous predictor of perinatal outcome. If necessary, the contraction stress test can also be used in the management of these patients.

Consideration is given to whether vaginal delivery might adversely influence an affected fetus. In cases in which severe hydrops is present we have elected to deliver these patients by cesarean section to insure optimal conditions in pediatric attendance and availability at delivery and an atraumatic delivery. Vaginal delivery is reasonable, in the absence of fetal distress, for a fetus without severe hydrops.

Adequate preparation for delivery demands communication with an alerted pediatric team and available frozen, type-specific or type O Rh−, buffy-coat-free, packed red blood cells cross-matched with the maternal serum in case neonatal transfusion is needed in a delivery suite. Alternately, irradiated cells can be used for the frozen blood. Both these techniques help remove lymphocytes from the blood and reduce the incidence of graph-versus-host reactions.

Atypical blood group antibodies with a history of significant adverse perinatal outcome are generally managed in a protocol similar to Rh-sensitized patients.

Conclusion

The use of exchange transfusion, early delivery, prenatal assessment, and finally intrauterine transfusion cut the staggering mortality in Rh erythroblastosis fetalis from 50% to less than 10%. With the introduction of Rh immunoglobulin, along with a heightened clinical consciousness, the sensitized woman is fortunately becoming an infrequent clinical problem in patients receiving modern obstetric care. Given the high mortality of fetal hydrops in early pregnancy, the morbidity of intrauterine transfusions and fetal therapy, and the inherent inaccuracies of present modes of prediction, including the risks of fetal blood sampling, further reduction of total mortality from erythroblastosis fetalis must come mainly through the eradication of Rh isoimmunization. While the elimination of erythroblastosis is possible, because of failures in utilization of Rh immunoglobulin, it is unlikely to occur in the next decade. The responsibility is for every clinician who is associated with the health care of women to strive individually to prevent this immunogenetic disorder.

SUGGESTED READING

AMERICAN COLLEGE OF OBSTETRICIANS AND GYNECOLOGISTS. *Prevention of D Isoimmunization*. ACOG Technical Bulletin 147. Washington DC: ACOG, 1990.

AMERICAN COLLEGE OF OBSTETRICIANS AND GYNECOLOGISTS. *Management of Isoimmunization in Pregnancy*. ACOG Technical Bulletin 148. Washington DC: ACOG, 1990.

BOWMAN JM. Hemolytic disease (erythroblastosis fetalis). In Creasy RK, Resnik R, eds. *Maternal–Fetal Medicine: Principles and Practice.* 2nd edn. Philadelphia: WB Saunders, 1989.

BRANCH DW, SCOTT JR. Isoimmunization in pregnancy. In Gabbe SG, Niebyl JR, Simpson JL, eds. *Obstetrics: Normal and Problem Pregnancies.* New York: Churchill Livingstone, 1986.

30

Nonimmune hydrops fetalis

ARNOLD L. MEDEARIS

Hydrops fetalis occurs when there is a pathologic increase in interstitial fluid and total fetal body water. The diagnosis of hydrops fetalis requires the detection of fluid in at least two fetal compartments. The compartments evaluated are the serous cavities (pleural, pericardial, intraperitoneal) and fetal soft tissue edema. To establish the diagnosis of nonimmune hydrops fetalis there must be no evidence of isoimmunization, i.e., fetal–maternal blood group incompatibility, detected as a cause of hemolysis and anemia leading to the hydrops fetalis.

Incidence

Nonimmune hydrops fetalis is reported in between 1:1500 and 1:4000 deliveries. Hydrops can occur at any time during gestation. In the first trimester, hydrops is occasionally seen with spontaneous abortion. First- and second-trimester hydrops is associated with fetal death. Polyhydramnios is frequently the presenting diagnosis in third-trimester hydrops. Most often a specific etiology for nonimmune hydrops cannot be found. The incidence of specific clinical conditions associated with nonimmune hydrops varies with patient populations. α-Thalassemia is a common cause of fetal hydrops in patients from southeast Asia, southern India, and eastern Mediterranean descent. Syphilis can be an important cause of hydrops. During seasonal epidemics, parvovirus may be the cause of a significant number of cases of nonimmune hydrops. Other genetic etiologies may be seen in varying frequencies depending on the patient population.

Pathology

Hydrops fetalis occurs when there is alteration in hydrostatic pressure or colloid osmotic pressure leading to fluid collection in various fetal compartments. Common causes include cardiac failure, chronic anemia, hypoproteinemia, decreased venous return, infections, and malformations.

Intrauterine cardiac failure is probably the most common cause of nonimmune hydrops fetalis in our patient population. Abnormalities associated with the cardiac conduction system or cardiac malformations, vascular anomalies, intracardiac tumors, myocardial dysfunction, and premature closure of the foramen ovale or the ductus arteriosus may give rise to hydrops fetalis.

Marked fetal anemia, particularly in association with abnormal hemoglobinopathies (most commonly α-thalassemia, glucose-6-phosphate dehydrogenase deficiency), pure red cell aplasia, or chronic fetal blood loss may be the cause of hydrops. Decreased venous return from thoracic and pulmonary diseases, intraabdominal tumors and gastrointestinal disorders, placental abnormalities, skeletal dysplasia, and metabolic disorders have also been documented as causes in nonimmune hydrops. Intrauterine infections, including syphilis and cytomegalovirus and parvoviruses, which affect red cell precursors, additionally may be responsible for hydrops in the fetus.

Diagnosis

The intrauterine diagnosis of nonimmune hydrops is easily made with diagnostic ultrasound. Fluid collections can be readily seen. Ascites and pleural effusion are seen as echo-free (dark) areas in the abdomen and pleural cavity of the fetus. Examination of the fetus can demonstrate marked skin edema. Pericardial effusion may be grossly detected or may be visualized using M-mode ultrasound examination. To establish the diagnosis of hydrops fetalis more than one site of fluid collection must be seen on ultrasound. Polyhydramnios, diagnosed when the amniotic fluid index is ⩾24, is seen in 50–75% of the cases of nonimmune hydrops. Occasionally, oligohydramnios is present.

Diagnostic procedures

The diagnostic procedure of choice for evaluating the fetus with nonimmune hydrops has been percutaneous umbilical blood sampling. Sampling allows the analysis of blood to determine if there is fetal anemia, to obtain blood chemistries (including liver enzymes), as well as DNA analysis for infection, and possibly further testing as to etiology of an anemia. In addition, chromosomal studies may be rapidly performed on the sample.

Prognosis

It is our experience that the best predictor of perinatal outcome in the fetus with nonimmune hydrops is the presence of a normal biventricular outer diameter during systole obtained from an M-mode ultrasound. At our institution, those cases that have resolution of hydrops or survived with hydrops have had normal cardiac dimensions. Spontaneous resolution has occurred in a small number of fetuses. Patients with abnormal cardiac size have had a perinatal or neonatal death.

Management

It is difficult to discuss intrauterine therapy and prenatal management without knowledge of the initial evaluation. Many known causes of nonimmune hydrops are not candidates for therapy. Therapeutic measures in a fetus with normal chromosomes include primarily intrauterine fetal transfusion for anemia in the absence of a diagnosis of a hemoglobinopathy. Antepartum surveillance of the hydropic fetus includes interval evaluation of status and size of the fluid collections, evaluation of fetal cardiac dimensions, and antepartum testing with nonstress testing and the biophysical profile. Initiation of testing and the choice of specific techniques for assessment are individualized in each case.

The route of delivery in the patient with nonimmune hydrops is dependent upon the gestational age at delivery, the degree of fetal edema or ascites, and the general prognosis of the fetus based on cardiac examination. A vaginal delivery is recommended in the previable fetus, the fetus with a markedly abnormal cardiac examination, or the fetus with edema or ascites sufficient to obstruct delivery.

Summary

Nonimmune hydrops represents a complex condition caused by many different known and unknown clinical conditions. Nonimmune hydrops involves the abnormal location of fluid in two fetal compartments (pericardial, pleural, intraperitoneal, or skin) and can be readily diagnosed by ultrasound examination. The prognosis is dependent on the etiology of the hydrops and the degree of fetal cardiac involvement. Evaluation should include fetal blood sampling to determine anemia, biochemistry, the possibility of fetal infection, and fetal chromosomes. There are multiple modalities of treatment depending on the etiology of the hydrops and the physical findings of the affected fetus that are individualized in each clinical case.

SUGGESTED READING

CARLSON DE, PLATT LD, MEDEARIS AL, HORENSTEIN J. Prognostic indicators of the resolution of nonimmune hydrops fetalis and survival of the fetus. *Am J Obstet Gynecol* 1990;163:1785–1787.

HANSMAN M. ARABIN B. Nonimmune hydrops fetalis. In: Cervenak FA, Isaacson GC, Campbell S, eds. *Ultrasound in Obstetrics and Gynecology,* 2nd edn. Boston: Little, Brown, 1993.

HOLZGREVE W. The fetus with nonimmune hydrops. In: Harrison MR, Golbus MS, Filly RA, eds. *The Unborn Patient: Prenatal Diagnosis and Treatment,* 2nd edn. Philadelphia: WB Saunders, 1991.

SHAH YP, HADLOCK FP. Hydrops and ascites. In: Nyberg DA, Mahony BS, Pretorius DH, eds. *Diagnostic Ultrasound of Fetal Anomalies: Text and Atlas.* St Louis, MO: Mosby-Year Book, 1990.

31

Hyperemesis gravidarum

PAUL F. BRENNER & T. MURPHY GOODWIN

Hyperemesis gravidarum is one of those medical entities for which a well-defined definition based on a universally accepted set of diagnostic criteria does not exist. Generally, if a pregnant woman experiences nausea and emesis in the first half of her pregnancy to the extent that there is documented significant weight loss, dehydration, and metabolic alterations leading to hospitalization, the diagnosis of hyperemesis gravidarum is applied.

As many as 85% of women in early pregnancy experience symptoms of nausea and vomiting. For most of these women the symptoms are relatively mild, tend to diminish in the second half of pregnancy, and their pregnancy proceeds to term without any serious sequelae to the mother or fetus. The symptoms of nausea and vomiting are usually more frequent in the morning, giving rise to the lay diagnosis of morning sickness. While nausea and emesis are usually more severe in the morning and tend to abate as the day goes on, for some women these symptoms may persist for the entire day. These symptoms occur most commonly between the 6th and 16th week of pregnancy, although some women report nausea and vomiting being present throughout their entire pregnancy. Nausea and emesis during the first half of pregnancy severe enough to require hospitalization is uncommon, with a reported incidence of hyperemesis gravidarum of 3–16 cases per 1000.

Nausea and vomiting are experienced so frequently by pregnant women that it is very tempting to "go where the money is" and diagnose all gravid women with these mild symptoms as having morning sickness or, if the symptoms become more severe, as having hyperemesis gravi-

Table 31.1 Causes of excessive vomiting not related to pregnancy

Hepatic/gastrointestinal
Gastroenteritis
Cholecystitis
Pancreatitis
Peptic ulcer disease
Acute appendicitis
Inflammatory or obstructive bowel disease
Hepatitis
Hiatal hernia

Genitourinary
Pyelonephritis
Renal calculi
Ovarian torsion
Degenerating fibroid

Miscellaneous
Drug toxicity
Metabolic disorders
Hyperthyroidism
Central nervous system lesions
Vestibular disorders

darum. It is important to diagnose conditions which may contribute to hyperemesis such as multiple gestations or hydatidiform mole. Other surgical and medical complications of pregnancy which may be expressed clinically as nausea and vomiting are summarized in Table 31.1.

Frequent and copious emesis can result in the inability to retain required nutrients in the diet. Starvation leads to weight loss, acidosis, and anemia. Fluids, hydrochloric acid, and electrolytes are lost in vomitus. Depletion of fluids, hydrochloric acid and potassium, sodium and chloride may lead to dehydration, oliguria, hemoconcentration, constipation, and hypokalemic alkalosis. Serum amylase levels can be up to $2\frac{1}{2}$ times normal in 10% of patients. Impaired liver function with elevation of liver enzymes and slight jaundice can occur in more than 40% of patients. The evaluation of gravid women with sustained nausea and vomiting includes the medical history and physical examination. Weight loss and signs of dehydration help to establish the severity of the symptoms and the need for hospitalization. Adjunctive laboratory tests should include serum electrolytes, liver function tests, amylase, glucose, complete blood count with a differential, and an urinalysis. Thyroid function tests may be abnormal but their value in management is not established.

Urinalysis and urine diastase should be obtained. An abdominal ultrasound scan is performed to assess fetal viability, and the presence of a multiple gestation or a hydatidiform mole.

The prognosis is excellent for both the mother and fetus if prompt and appropriate treatment is initiated. There are some increased maternal and fetal risks if therapy is delayed for a long period of time or is inadequate. Maternal complications that result from persistent emesis include electrolyte depletion, acid–base imbalance, aspiration pneumonia, dental erosions, and, very rarely, hemorrhagic retinitis, rupture of the esophagus, and encephalopathy. Biochemical hyperthyroidism occurs in as many as 60% of women with hyperemesis gravidarum. It is transient and does not require specific antithyroid treatment. A slight increase in fetal malformations has been found by some investigators but the association is still in doubt.

Most of the time the symptoms of nausea and vomiting during pregnancy can be treated on an outpatient basis. Changing eating patterns to smaller meals at more frequent intervals, discontinuing oral iron supplements, and avoiding specific foods which seem to precipitate these symptoms is often beneficial. Oral antiemetics are prescribed as needed. Prochlorperazine (Compazine) 5–10 mg, trimethobenzamide hydrochloride (Tigan) 100–250 mg, or promethazine (Phenergan) 25–50 mg may be taken 3 times a day. Doxylamine succinate plus pyridoxine (Bendectin) is no longer available in the USA to treat nausea and vomiting of pregnancy. Litigation has linked an increased risk of fetal malformations *in utero* to the maternal use of Bendectin, even though there are several medical prospective studies which have failed to find any evidence of teratogenicity with Bendectin.

Gravid women with frequent and copious emesis require hospitalization if they have ketonuria, electrolyte imbalance, dehydration, weight loss, or hepatic and renal damage. The goal of inpatient therapy is to hydrate the patient, restore electrolyte balance, and provide adequate calories and nutrition for the mother and the fetus. Initially it is imperative to place the patient at complete gastric rest (nothing by mouth) and administer intravenous fluids while monitoring in a precise manner the patient's intake and output. Electrolytes, lactate or bicarbonate, glucose, and water replacement are administered parenterally in amounts necessary to correct fluid and electrolyte imbalance. To relieve the nausea the patient is given an initial dose of 10 mg prochlorperazine by intramuscular injection and then trimethobenzamide hydrochloride 200 mg rectal suppositories every 6 h as needed. When emesis has been eliminated and the patient's desire for food returns, a clear liquid diet is started and slowly advanced as tolerated by the patient. The patient is eligible for discharge from the hospital when the ketones are cleared from her urine and she is tolerating her diet. The patients are usually given an antiemetic to take home with them. In some women with severe nausea and vomiting in early pregnancy, parenteral nutrition has been used successfully. With the availability of parenteral nutrition it is rarely necessary to terminate a pregnancy because of severe hyperemesis gravidarum.

For some women with hyperemesis gravidarum there is a very significant psychologic component. Inadequate support systems for the unwed mother, marital conflict, and desire for pregnancy termination in the face of religious or family constraints are examples of a psychologically stressful environment. Women with hyperemesis gravidarum associated with strong emotional or psychologic factors characteristically show dramatic improvement when they are hospitalized and freed from their stressful environment, only to relapse when they are discharged and returned to their emotional conflicts. These women benefit greatly from psychologic and social counseling.

SUGGESTED READING

CHIN RKH. Hyperemesis gravidarum and fetal growth retardation. *Am J Obstet Gynecol* 1990;162:1349.

GODSEY RK, NEWMAN RB. Hyperemesis gravidarum. A comparison of single and multiple admissions. *J Reprod Med* 1991;36:287–290.

GOODWIN TM, MONTORO M, MESTMAN JH. Transient hyperthyroidism and hyperemesis gravidarum: clinical aspects. *Am J Obstet Gynecol* 1992;167:648–652.

GOODWIN TM, MONTORO M, MESTMAN JH, et al. The role of chorionic gonadotropin in transient hyperthyroidism of hyperemesis gravidarum. *J Clin Endocrinol Metab* 1992 (in press).

GREENSPOON JS, MASAKI DI, KURZ CR. Cardiac tamponade in pregnancy during central hyperalimentation. *Obstet Gynecol* 1989;73:465–466.

GROSS S, LIBRACH C, CECUTTI A. Maternal weight loss associated with hyperemesis gravidarum: a predictor of fetal outcome. *Am J Obstet Gynecol* 1989;160: 906–909.

LEVINE MG, ESSER D. Total parenteral nutrition for the treatment of severe hyperemesis gravidarum: maternal nutritional effects and fetal outcome. *Obstet Gynecol* 1988;72:102–107.

RAYBURN W, WOLK R, MERCER N, ROBERTS J. Parenteral nutrition in obstetrics and gynecology. *Obstet Gynecol Surv* 1986;41:200–214.

WEIGEL MM, WEIGEL RM. Nausea and vomiting of early pregnancy and pregnancy outcome. An epidemiologic study. *Br J Obstet Gynaecol* 1989;96:1304–1311.

32

Vaginal delivery following
cesarean birth

DEBRA K. GRUBB

For most of this century, the maxim, "Once a cesarean, always a cesarean," was the rule in the USA. Because of concern about rupture of the uterine scar, women with a prior cesarean delivery almost uniformly underwent elective repeat cesarean delivery in all subsequent pregnancies. However, many large studies done since the 1970s have shown that a trial of labor after a prior cesarean delivery may be undertaken without increased risk of maternal or fetal morbidity. With documentation of the safety of vaginal birth after cesarean (VBAC), the standard practice of electively performing repeat cesarean in all cases has slowly begun to change.

Cesarean birth has become the most common hospital-based procedure performed in the USA, with cesarean delivery rates >30% in many communities. Approximately 50% of the increase in cesarean birth rates is due to performance of elective repeat cesarean delivery. Considerable attention has been focused on reducing the cesarean delivery rate by identifying women who may be candidates for vaginal delivery. Since studies have demonstrated the safety of a trial of labor after a prior cesarean birth, the American College of Obstetricians and Gynecologists has recommended that women with one prior cesarean birth be counseled to undergo a trial of labor in a subsequent pregnancy. Implementation of this recommendation has proceeded very slowly, but more and more women with a prior cesarean birth are choosing a trial of labor each year. This trend has substantial implications for reduction of both maternal morbidity secondary to cesarean delivery and health-care costs.

Risks and benefits of a trial of labor should be discussed with every patient with a prior cesarean delivery before labor begins. The likelihood of a successful vaginal delivery, the risks of uterine rupture or dehiscence, and the risks of maternal and fetal morbidity and mortality in both vaginal and abdominal deliveries should be considered.

The likelihood of a successful trial of labor is approximately 80% overall. The indication for the first cesarean birth affects the likelihood of success of the trial of labor. Patients with a prior cesarean performed for breech presentation have the highest probability of successful vaginal delivery (91%), while those whose prior cesarean was for dystocia have the lowest (77%). Of those women whose prior indication for cesarean delivery was dystocia, 33% delivered a larger infant during a subsequent trial of labor.

The risk of separation of the uterine scar during labor should also be considered when deciding upon a trial of labor. Separations of the uterine scar may be divided into dehiscences and ruptures. Dehiscence is generally considered to be an asymptomatic separation of the scar, usually not extending through the overlying uterine serosa. Uterine rupture, on the other hand, is a separation associated with significant hemorrhage or with fetal distress, and usually extends through the serosa into the peritoneal cavity, into the broad ligament, or into the urinary bladder. The incidence of scar separation is not significantly increased by trial of labor compared to the incidence of separation found at elective repeat cesarean delivery. There are no reported cases in the literature of maternal mortality associated with rupture of a uterine scar. Although fetal deaths associated with uterine scar separation have been reported in up to 56% of cases of uterine rupture, almost all of those occurred prior to the use to electronic fetal heart rate monitoring.

The relative incidences of overall maternal and fetal morbidity in VBAC and elective repeat cesarean delivery should also be considered when deciding upon a trial of labor. Maternal morbidity associated with trial of labor is significantly less than that associated with elective repeat cesarean birth. The difference is due to lower incidences of febrile morbidity and peripartum hysterectomy in patients undergoing VBAC. However, patients undergoing a failed trial of labor have a higher incidence of febrile morbidity compared to those undergoing elective repeat cesarean.

Management of a trial of labor should follow established guidelines published by the American College of Obstetricians and Gynecologists. These include:

1 routine counseling to undertake a trial of labor in women with one prior cesarean birth unless a specific contraindication to labor exists;

2 women with two prior cesarean births should not be discouraged from attempting vaginal delivery;

3 decisions should be individualized in the cases where risks are unknown;

4   a prior classical uterine incision is a contraindication to labor;

5   resources should be available to respond to obstetric emergencies within 30 min, as with any other laboring patient;

6   normal activity should be encouraged during latent phase;

7   a physician capable of evaluating labor and performing a cesarean delivery should be available.

A number of controversial issues regarding management of a trial of labor during VBAC have been raised, and some have been addressed in the literature. Some of these issues include the use of oxytocin augmentation, the use of epidural anesthesia, and the suitability of trial of labor in patients with low vertical uterine incisions, those with breech presentations, and those with multiple gestation.

The use of oxytocin to augment or induce labor in women undergoing a trial of labor has been studied retrospectively. No increase in the risk of uterine scar separation or fetal distress has been found in patients receiving oxytocin appropriately. However, if oxytocin is required, the risk of unsuccessful trial of labor is increased threefold.

The use of conduction anesthesia was once felt to be contraindicated in women undergoing a trial of labor because the pain associated with uterine rupture would be masked. However, subsequent studies have shown that characteristic pain is a very rare sign of uterine rupture, and epidural anesthesia is a safe option in trial of labor.

Insufficient data exist to determine the magnitude of risks associated with trial of labor in patients with a low vertical uterine incision, in those with breech presentation, and in those with twins. These patients may be offered a trial of labor if no contraindication exists and the patient wishes to attempt a vaginal birth. However, more information is needed regarding risks in these groups.

During a trial of labor, continuous electronic fetal monitoring should be available, as well as typed and cross-matched blood and intravenous access. An intrauterine pressure catheter is probably unnecessary, since a change in intrauterine pressure is not a useful indication of uterine rupture.

Controversy exists regarding the need routinely to examine the uterine scar after every successful VBAC, since laparotomy to repair a scar separation is not indicated in the stable patient with no vaginal bleeding or hematuria. However, some authorities believe that patients with an asymptomatic scar separation should be counseled not to undergo another trial of labor. In this case, manual examination of the uterine scar after each VBAC will provide additional information regarding management of the patient's next pregnancy.

The patient with evidence of a uterine ruture requires immediate laparotomy. The most common sign of uterine rupture is fetal distress secondary to extrusion of fetal parts or umbilical cord through the rupture, leading to cesarean delivery. Other signs include postpartum hemorrhage, sudden-onset severe lower abdominal pain, loss of station of the presenting part, and hematuria.

In summary, a trial of labor after a prior cesarean delivery should be recommended to women with one low transverse uterine scar and no contraindications to vaginal delivery, and may be offered to many other women with prior cesarean births. Up to 80% of these trials of labor will produce successful vaginal deliveries, resulting in reductions in maternal morbidity and considerable savings in health-care costs.

SUGGESTED READING

ACOG COMMITTEE OPINION. Guidelines for vaginal delivery after a previous cesarean birth. Number 64, 1988.

BEALL M, EGLINTON GS, CLARK SL, *et al.* Vaginal delivery after cesarean section: the unknown uterine scar. *J Reprod Med* 1984;19:31.

BOUCHER M, TAHILRAMANY M, EGLINTON GS, *et al.* Maternal morbidity related to a trial of labor after previous cesarean delivery: a quantitative analysis. *J Reprod Med* 1984;29:12.

FLAMM BL, LIM OW, JONES C, *et al.* Vaginal birth after cesarean section: results of a multicenter study. *Am J Obstet Gynecol* 1988;158:1079.

HORENSTEIN JM, PHELAN JP. Previous cesarean section: the risks and benefits of oxytocin usage in a trial of labor. *Am J Obstet Gynecol* 1985;151:564.

MARTIN JN, HARRIS BA, HUDDLESTON JF, *et al.* Vaginal delivery following previous cesarean birth. *Am J Obstet Gynecol* 1983;146:255.

PHELAN JP, CLARK SL, DIAZ F, *et al.* Vaginal birth after cesarean. *Am J Obstet Gynecol* 1987;157:1510.

PORRECO RP, MEIER PR. Trial of labor in patients with multiple previous cesarean sections. *J Reprod Med* 1983;28:770.

33

Placenta previa

KATHRYN J. SHAW

Placenta previa is defined as the implantation of the placenta over the cervical os. This entity is further classified as *complete* if the placenta totally covers the os, *partial* if only a portion of the os is covered, and *marginal* if the placental edge extends up to but not over the cervical os. If the implantation site is in the lower uterine segment but the placenta does not reach the cervix, this is termed a low-lying placenta, which is not a form of placenta previa. Complete placenta previa is evident in 50–60% of cases, with the remainder of cases divided equally between partial and marginal placenta previas.

The incidence of placenta previa is 1:200 deliveries. The occurrence is increased in association with prior cesarean section, in proportion to the number of prior incisions. Clark *et al.* reported a 0.26% incidence of placenta previa in the unscarred uterus, compared to 0.65, 1.8, and 3.0% with one, two and three prior cesarean sections respectively. In the patient with four or more prior cesarean sections, the incidence of placenta previa was 10.0%. Other reported risk factors for placenta previa include cigarette smoking, increasing maternal age, and parity.

Clinical presentation and diagnosis

The classic presentation of placenta previa is painless vaginal bleeding in the third trimester, yet 20% may have associated uterine contractions or irritability. Ten percent of cases will not have any antepartum bleeding and will be diagnosed either at the time of cesarean section being performed for other indications, or during ultrasound evaluation. The primary means of diagnosis in the symptomatic patient is transabdominal ultrasound, which has a diagnostic accuracy of 90%. Most errors will be made in those cases of posterior placentation where the leading edge of the placenta cannot be clearly identified. Vaginal probe ultrasound has been described in the setting of placenta previa and appears to be a safe procedure. The use of magnetic resonance imaging (MRI) in the diagnosis of placenta previa is also reported to be highly accurate. While abdominal ultrasound examination remains the most frequent means of diagnosis, vaginal probe ultrasound and/or MRI may be helpful in cases of partial or posterior placenta previa.

With the widespread use of prenatal ultrasound, diagnosis in the asymptomatic patient is not infrequent. Placenta previa has been identified in 5% of patients undergoing ultrasound examination between 16 and 18 weeks. Follow-up in the third trimester reveals that 90% of these placentas were no longer described as previa in location. This has been referred to as placental migration. It is clear that the placenta in these cases does not detach and relocate; rather, differential growth in the lower uterine segment results in the placental implantation site no longer being in the proximity of the cervix. Thus, the diagnosis of placenta previa should be reserved for gestations beyond 24 weeks. If earlier ultrasound identifies an apparent placenta previa, it is best to describe the findings, and schedule a follow-up ultrasound examination after 24 weeks. If the patient at this point is asymptomatic with no bleeding, it is not necessary to modify lifestyles based upon a mid-trimester ultrasound, pending reevaluation after 24 weeks.

Pregnancies complicated by placenta previa are associated with an increase in both maternal and perinatal morbidity and mortality. Abnormal fetal lie (breech, transverse lie) will be identified in 30% of cases. This will not likely affect the route of delivery since the majority of cases of placenta previa require cesarean delivery. More importantly, this association should be kept in mind such that when abnormal fetal lie is identified, placenta previa should be ruled out. Delivery prior to 36 weeks' *gestational* age will be necessary in two-thirds of cases of placenta previa, with complications of prematurity the primary causes of neonatal mortality. Presentation with the first bleeding episode prior to 20 weeks significantly increases the risk for premature delivery. A significant number of infants (10–20%) will be anemic at birth. This reflects the fact that the bleeding associated with placenta previa is due to placental separation in the developing lower uterine segment, thus being a type of placental abruption. In this setting the blood lost may be either maternal or fetal. The risk of neonatal anemia is directly correlated with the degree of maternal hemorrhage and rate of maternal transfusion.

Maternal morbidity and mortality are primarily related to hemorrhage and operative complications. Prolonged hospitalization is often necessary. Some 30–50% of patients will require antepartum blood transfusion. The majority of cases will necessitate cesarean delivery. In addition to the complications associated with any cesarean delivery, these patients are at a marked increased risk for intraoperative hemorrhage, mostly due to uterine atony and placenta accreta. Uterine atony is increased, primarily because of the poorly contractile lower uterine segment. Additionally, placenta previa is associated with an increased risk for placenta accreta, defined as an abnormal adherence of the placental villi to the uterine myometrium, resulting from an absent decidual layer. The risk for a placenta accreta in the setting of a placenta previa is especially increased if there has been a prior cesarean delivery. Clark *et al.* reported a 5% incidence of placenta accreta with a placenta previa in the unscarred uterus. They also noted that, as the number of prior cesarean sections increases, so does the risk of placenta accreta, describing a 24 and 48% incidence of accreta with one and two or more prior cesarean deliveries, respectively, when associated with a placenta previa. When placenta accreta is histologically confirmed, the placental implantation site is noted to be over the cesarean scar. In cases complicated by placenta accreta, 75% require hysterectomy because of intractable hemorrhage. Needless to say, this carries with it a significant increase in need for blood product replacement and maternal morbidity.

Management

In the patient who presents with third-trimester bleeding, the first step is to determine if this is due to placenta previa. If the diagnosis is confirmed, usually by ultrasound examination, the subsequent management will be dictated by maternal and fetal stability and gestational age, with the two options being that of immediate delivery versus expectant management. Stabilization of the mother is critical, as is the establishment of adequate intravenous access and assurance of blood product availability. Immediate delivery should be implemented in the following settings, regardless of gestational age: (1) persistent hemorrhage, especially if multiple transfusions are required; (2) persistent uterine contractions unresponsive to tocolysis; (3) coagulation defect; and (4) fetal distress with a viable fetus. Delivery should be strongly considered in patients who present at or beyond 36 weeks, even if clinically stable. Assessment of fetal lung maturity should be made in these cases if gestational dating is in question, or if the gestation is less than 37 weeks. In the patient who presents in labor with a partial or marginal placenta previa, consideration can be given to performing a "double set-up" examination. The patient should be taken to the operating room, and fully prepped for cesarean section with surgeons and anesthesiologist available. A gentle speculum exam should be done to determine if placental tissue can be seen in the cervical os. If this is negative, a vaginal examination is performed. The fornices should be palpated to determine if fullness and a spongy consistency of placenta are evident adjacent to the cervix. If neither approach demonstrates placental tissue in or immediately adjacent to the cervix, one can consider allowing a trial of labor, assuming immediate cesarean section is feasible, if needed. If the placenta appears on ultrasound examination to be a complete previa, a double set-up exam is not indicated.

In the patient who is hemodynamically stable, the option of expectant management exists. This assumes normal fetal heart rate pattern and a normal maternal coagulation profile. Expectant management consists of: (1) strict bedrest in the hospital; (2) maintenance of hematocrit greater than 30%; (3) availability of blood products; and (4) RhoGAM if the patient is Rh−. In those patients who present with an immature fetus and evidence that delay of delivery will be short-lived, administration of beta-methasone should be considered, in the hope of reducing the risk of respiratory distress syndrome. Patients who show signs of preterm labor should be tocolyzed if the bleeding is not severe. $MgSO_4$ is the first choice; if $MgSO_4$ is not effective, use of β-mimetics may be considered. While not absolutely contraindicated, β-mimetics may cause tachycardia and hypotension, creating a dangerous, confusing picture and thus should not be used in the setting of maternal hypovolemia. If bleeding ceases on bedrest with no uterine activity, limited ambulation can be attempted. If the patient remains asymptomatic, discharge to home can be considered. This option requires a reliable patient with a home environment conducive to rest and close proximity to the hospital.

Fetal evaluation should include ultrasound every 2–3 weeks to assess growth. We do not routinely recommend antepartum fetal heart rate testing unless other indications are present or if there is concern for chronic placental abruption. This approach has been highly successful, with the most recent review of 99 cases of placenta previa at Los Angeles County–University of Southern California Medical Center revealing no intrauterine deaths. When the pregnancy reaches 35–36 weeks, assessment of fetal lung maturity should be undertaken via amniocentesis.

Summary

Placenta previa remains a leading cause of third-trimester bleeding. Optimal outcome depends on prompt diagnosis, rapid blood product replacement as needed, and tocolysis of labor if maternal status allows. Especially important is the awareness of the risks associated with placenta previa in the setting of a prior cesarean section. With this combination one should anticipate and be prepared for the possibility of placenta accreta and the associated surgical complications.

SUGGESTED READING

ARIAS F. Cervical cerclage for the temporary treatment of patients with placenta previa. *Obstet Gynecol* 1988;71:545–548.

CLARK SL, KOONINGS P, PHELAN JP. Placenta previa/accreta and prior cesarean section. *Obstet Gynecol* 1985;66:89–92.

COTTON DB, READ JA, PAUL RH, QUILLIGAN EJ. The conservative aggressive management of placenta previa. *Am J Obstet Gynecol* 1980;137:687–695.

D'ANGELO LJ, IRWIN LF. Conservative management of placenta previa: a cost–benefit analysis. *Am J Obstet Gynecol* 1984;149:320–326.

FARINE D, FOX HE, JAKOBSON S, TIMOR-TRITSCH IE. Vaginal ultrasound for diagnosis of placenta previa. *Am J Obstet Gynecol* 1988;159:566–569.

FARINE D, PEISNER DB, TIMOR-TRITSCH IE. Placenta previa – is the traditional diagnostic approach satisfactory? *J Clin Ultrasound* 1990;18:328–330.

LIM BH, TAN CE, SMITH APM, SMITH NC. Transvaginal ultrasonography for diagnosis of placenta praevia. *Lancet* 1989;25:444–445.

MCSHANE PM, HEYL PS, EPSTEIN MF. Maternal and perinatal morbidity resulting from placenta previa. *Obstet Gynecol* 1985;65:176–182.

POWELL MC, BUCKLEY J, PRICE H, WORTHINGTON BS, SYMONDS EM. Magnetic resonance imaging and placenta previa. *Am J Obstet Gynecol* 1986;154:565–568.

RIZOS N, DORAN TA, MISKIN M, BENZIE RJ, FORD JA. Natural history of placenta previa ascertained by diagnostic ultrasound. *Am J Obstet Gynecol* 1979;133:287–291.

SAUER M, PARSONS M, SAMPSON M. Placenta previa: an analysis of three years experience. *Am J Perinatol* 1985;2:39–42.

SILVER R, DEPP R, SABBAGHA RE, DOOLEY SL, SOCOL ML, TAMURA RK. Placenta previa: aggressive expectant management. *Am J Obstet Gynecol* 1984;150:15–22.

34

Placenta accreta

KATHRYN J. SHAW

In this chapter the definition, incidence, and risk factors for placenta accreta will be discussed, as well as the clinical presentation and findings. Additionally, more recent reports suggesting a role for ultrasound in the antenatal diagnosis of placenta accreta will be reviewed. Finally, the management options for dealing with this serious obstetric complication will be considered.

Definition and incidence

Placenta accreta is defined clinically as an abnormal adherence of the placenta to the uterine wall, and histologically by the invasion of the chorionic villi up to or into the myometrium. A common finding in all cases is either an absence of, or a poorly formed decidual layer. Placenta accreta is further classified, depending on the depth of invasion noted on histologic review. The term *placenta accreta*, in addition to collectively referring to all forms of this abnormality, is applied to the least invasive form, where the chorionic villi penetrate only the inner third of the myometrium. *Placenta increta* refers to invasion by the chorionic villi into the outer third of myometrium. *Placenta percreta* is that form in which the chorionic villi have extended out to, or through, the uterine serosa. On histologic examination, it has been noted that all degrees of invasion may be noted in one uterus, yet in the majority of cases (78%) the invasion is limited to the inner third of the myometrium (accreta). The more invasive forms are much less frequent, with placenta increta accounting for 17% of cases and placenta percreta 5% of cases.

In early reports, the incidence of placenta accreta was 1:30 000 deliveries. With each decade the incidence has steadily increased as follows: 1930–1950 1:30 739; 1950–1960 1:19 000; 1960–1970 1:14 780. A more recent report by Read from Los Angeles County–University of Southern California reviewed 22 cases from 1975 through 1979, noting an incidence overall of 1:2562 deliveries. This included cases that were managed conservatively without hysterectomy being required, and therefore are based only upon clinical diagnosis. When only cases with histologic confirmation were considered, the incidence in this report was 1:4027 deliveries, which still represents a significant increase from prior reports. As noted before, this increase is probably at least in part due to the increased rate of cesarean section.

Etiology and risk factors

The pathologic findings of placenta accreta have been well described. A common finding in all cases is the absence or poor formation of the decidua basalis, allowing the villi to come into direct contact with the underlying myometrium. The remainder of the decidua, the decidua parietalis, may be normal but more often is partially or completely deficient. Although invading into the myometrium, the chorionic villi are normal, lacking any evidence of trophoblastic abnormalities or hyperplasia. Any event that may impair decidual development would predispose the patient to placenta accreta.

A variety of risk factors have been identified. Increasing maternal age and gravidity are associated with increased risk for placenta accreta. The risk associated with increased age is, at least in part, due to the fact that this is a complication primarily of multiparous patients. In fact, placenta accreta is unusual in a primigravid patient, with 88–95% of cases occurring in multiparous women. In Fox's study of 622 cases, only 34 women were primigravid; of these, 74% had other risk factors for placenta accreta, such as prior curettage or placenta previa.

Obstetric history is also important. Prior retained placenta requiring manual removal, and/or curettage, is associated with increased risk of placenta accreta in future pregnancies. In Fox's study, 10% of patients with placenta accreta gave this history. One-third of these patients had required manual removal with two or more previous pregnancies. The need for manual removal of the placenta invariably had occurred in the most recent pregnancy preceding that complicated by placenta accreta. It is quite probable that the manual removal itself did not lead to poor decidualization in the next pregnancy, but rather was a reflection of some degree of abnormal placental adherence.

One of the more common associated factors with placenta accreta is a history of uterine surgery. While the most frequent previous surgery is a cesarean section, other procedures such as prior curettage, myomectomy, and cornual resection for ectopic pregnancy also increase the risk for placenta accreta. Approximately 25% of cases will have a history of at least one prior cesarean section. In many of these cases, a placenta previa is also present, which places the implantation site directly in the area of the uterine scar. In and of itself, a placenta previa is also a risk factor for placenta accreta. Clark *et al.* reported a 5% incidence of placenta accreta in the setting of placenta previa. Even the low-lying placenta that does not encroach upon the cervical os is a risk factor. This finding is due to the poor decidual reaction noted in the lower uterine segment. The combination of placenta previa and prior cesarean section is now well recognized as a major risk factor for placenta accreta. In Clark's study, the occurrence of placenta accreta in association with placenta previa increased with the number of prior cesarean sections, from 5% in the unscarred uterus, to 24% with one prior uterine incision, to 48% with two or more prior cesarean sections.

Presentation and diagnosis

Definitive diagnosis of placenta accreta can only be made at the time of delivery, although prenatal diagnosis with ultrasound has been reported and is discussed below. The majority of these patients are asymptomatic up until delivery. In those cases associated with placenta previa, antepartum bleeding is not unusual but is not likely due to the placenta accreta itself. In cases with placenta percreta, presentation with an acute abdomen and hemoperitoneum has been reported. Findings at delivery vary. In some instances the diagnosis of placenta accreta is obvious at the time of cesarean section prior to delivery, with the placenta being visible through the serosa or the thinned uterine wall. In the case of a cesarean delivery, an attempt to remove the placenta is often associated with immediate profuse hemorrhage, especially if the entire placental bed is involved. In cases of only focal accreta the bleeding may be much less. If delivery is by vaginal route, spontaneous separation and delivery of the placenta do not occur and manual removal is required. As with cesarean section, it is usually at the time of removal that the hemorrhage occurs.

There are several reports in the literature that describe ultrasound findings strongly consistent with placenta accreta. In normal placentation ultrasound demonstrates a subplacental echo-free space, with an average thickness of 9.5 mm. It is believed that this area corresponds to the decidua basalis and underlying myometrium. Multiple reports describe an absence of this subplacental echolucent zone in patients who were subsequently found to have placenta accreta. In the reports describing this sign, there is no comment regarding the false-positive rate of this finding. Similarly, since not all patients with placenta accreta have had antenatal ultrasound, it is not possible at this time to state that this is a uniform finding. In patients at high risk for accreta, it is prudent to perform an ultrasound exam, and evaluate the placental attachment site for evidence of this echolucency. If absent, then one should be alert to the possibility of placenta accreta, and prepared accordingly.

Management

The finding of placenta accreta at the time of delivery is truly an obstetric emergency. As noted, the hemorrhage can be massive in a matter of moments. In the report of Read *et al.* from this institution, the mean blood loss at delivery and in the immediate postpartum period was nearly 4000 ml, with patients receiving an average of 8 U of blood replacement products. Coagulation abnormalities were evident in 18%. Clinical findings consistent with placenta accreta require rapid attention. Prior to 1950, immediate hysterectomy was considered the only option because of the high maternal mortality associated with more conservative therapy. Given the advances in blood banking, blood product availability, and antibiotics, a more conservative approach may be feasible. In more recent reports, authors have described fertility-conserving approaches including curettage, oversewing of the area involved, and hypogastric, or uterine artery ligation. In Read's report, conservative attempts were made in 12 of 22 patients and were successful in eight of these 12 women, giving a required hysterectomy rate of 64%. The decision as to whether to proceed to hysterectomy or to attempt conservative measures will be dictated by the estimated blood loss and by the patient's wish for future fertility. One must be ready to abandon conservative attempts if not rapidly successful in halting the hemorrhage. A special comment should be made regarding the patient who has the unfortunate combination of placenta previa and prior cesarean section. In this setting, cesarean section should be scheduled with the complication of accreta in mind. Surgery should be performed electively with ample blood products available and with an experienced surgical assistant. If placenta accreta requiring hysterectomy is evident, every atempt to perform a total hysterectomy should be made. Since the lower uterine segment and often the cervix are involved, a subtotal procedure is often associated with persistent hemorrhage and need for a second surgery.

Summary

The incidence of placenta accreta clearly appears to have increased, in part due to the simultaneous increase in cesarean births. Certain clinical characteristics identify patients at highest risk, namely the presence of a placenta previa and/or history of a prior cesarean section. While both maternal and perinatal mortality have drastically improved, hemorrhage and associated coagulopathy remain the gravest threats. Optimal outcome demands an awareness of this complication, rapid recognition, and institution of therapy.

SUGGESTED READING

CLARK SL, KOONINGS PP, PHELAN JP. Placenta previa/accreta and prior cesarean section. *Obstet Gynecol* 1985;66:89–92.

COX SM, CARPENTER RJ, COTTON DB. Placenta percreta: ultrasound diagnosis and conservative surgical management. *Obstet Gynecol* 1988;71:454–456.

DE MENDOONCA LK. Sonographic diagnosis of placenta accreta: presentation of six cases. *J Ultrasound Med* 1988;7:211–215.

FOX H. Placenta accreta, 1945–1969. *Obstet Gynecol Surv* 1972;27:475–490.

HOLLANDER DI, PUPKIN MJ, CRENSHAW MC, NAGEY DA. Conservative management of placenta accreta: a case report. *J Reprod Med* 1988;33:74–78.

READ JA, COTTON DB, MILLER FC. Placenta accreta: changing clinical aspects and outcome. *Obstet Gynecol* 1980;56:31–34.

TABSH KMA, BRINKMAN CR, KING W. Ultrasound diagnosis of placenta increta. *J Clin Ultrasound* 1982;10:288–290.

TRETIN JCH, KOENIGSBERG M, RABIN A, ANYAEGBUNAM A. Placenta accreta: additional sonographic observations. *J Ultrasound Med* 1992;11:29–34.

35

Abruptio placentae

KATHRYN J. SHAW

Definition

Third-trimester bleeding occurs in approximately 4% of pregnancies and is a potential cause of significant maternal and perinatal morbidity. Thirty percent of third-trimester bleeding is due to abruptio placentae, defined as the premature separation of a normally implanted placenta prior to delivery of the fetus. The degree of separation may be partial or complete, and its occurrence may be chronic or acute. Placental abruption has further been classified into three grades, based upon clinical and laboratory findings.

Grade 1 abruption is associated with minimal clinical symptoms, both mother and fetus being stable. The amount of bleeding is slight, uterine activity mild, and there is no evidence of coagulopathy.

In a *grade 2* placental abruption, the symptoms are more marked. Vaginal bleeding is of moderate quantity and uterine activity is present with possible tetanic contractions. Maternal vital signs may reflect significant blood loss and there is usually evidence of fetal distress. Laboratory evidence of a mild, early coagulopathy is present.

Grade 3 placental abruption is an emergency situation. The degree of hemorrhage is severe and hypovolemic shock is often present. Painful, tetanic uterine contractions are typical. Fetal distress is uniform and intrauterine fetal demise common. Coagulopathy is obvious with decreasing clotting factors and thrombocytopenia.

Incidence

The incidence of abruptio placentae varies from 0.8 to 1.2%, but this obstetric complication accounts for as much as 15–20% of perinatal mortality. Grade 1 placental abruption is demonstrated in 40% of cases, grade 2 in 45%, and grade 3 placental abruption is evident in approximately 15% of cases. Eighty percent of all cases will present before the onset of labor.

Etiology and risk factors

Although the precise cause of placental abruption is unknown, various risk factors have been identified. Earlier reports suggested an increasing risk for abruptio placentae with advancing maternal age and parity, yet more recent studies have been unable to confirm this association. A large population-based study using birth certificate data from the state of Washington similarly found no relationship between maternal age, parity, and the risk for abruption. Significant risk was demonstrated in the presence of hypertension, either preexisting or pregnancy-asociated, and maternal diabetes. Hypertension of any sort has been described in 20–25% of all cases of placental abruption, but the association is particularly strong with grade 3 abruption, being reported in 40–50% of these cases. It is important to keep in mind that hypertension may not always be obvious at the time of presentation, due to the degree of hemorrhage, and may only be evident once blood volume is replaced. Maternal trauma is actually a rare cause of placental abruption (2%), but this complication should always be considered when dealing with accident victims, as clinical signs may be subtle initially. An increased risk has also been suggested with cocaine use, and is thought to be related to the known hypertensive and vasoconstrictive effects of this drug. A past history of placental abruption is very important, with a recurrence rate of 11%. If two prior pregnancies have been complicated by abruption, the recurrence rate is as high as 25%. Other reported risk factors include cigarette smoking, rapid decompression of the uterus as might occur with amniotomy in the setting of hydramnios or twins, and short umbilical cord.

Clinical presentation

While traditionally abruptio placentae is viewed as a complication of the third trimester, ultrasound has demonstrated signs of subplacental bleeding prior to 20 weeks. The typical history is that of acute onset of vaginal bleeding associated with crampy or constant abdominal pain. The degree of bleeding is highly variable; in 15–20% of cases the hemorrhage is concealed, meaning no bleeding is seen from the vagina. This occurs when edges of the placenta remain attached to the uterine wall, containing the hemorrhage in the retroplacental space. In this setting, the developing hematoma may rupture in the amniotic sac, with bloody fluid noted at the time of amniotomy. The patient may present with tachycardia and in hypovolemic shock. This is especially true with concealed abruption, when there is no external evidence of bleeding causing the patient to seek medical attention. Uterine tenderness is very common and the degree of uterine activity variable depending on the extent of the abruption. The uterus may be quiet in cases of mild abruption. Uterine irritability or preterm labor may also be evident. In more severe abruptions the uterus may be hypertonic with an elevated resting tone.

Diagnosis

The diagnosis of placental abruption must always be considered in patients with antepartum hemorrhage. In most cases, this is a diagnosis based upon the typical clinical presentation as described above. The role of ultrasound in the diagnosis of third-trimester bleeding is most important to rule out placenta previa. Ultrasound, unfortunately, is much less reliable in identifying placental abruption, with initial reports noting that ultrasound made the diagnosis in only 2% of cases. Given the enhanced resolution available with the newer ultrasound equipment, the ability to diagnose placental abruption has improved.

Complications

The most common complication of placental abruption is maternal hemorrhage. The blood loss can be significant, especially in cases of grade 3 abruption where the average is 2000–2500 ml. Equally important is the risk for disseminated intravascular coagulation (DIC). Placental abruption is the most frequent cause for DIC in pregnancy, and is evident in 30% of those cases presenting with a fetal demise. The DIC associated with placental abruption is not due to the consumption of clotting factors in the retroplacental clot, but is thought to be due to the release of a tissue factor that activates the extrinsic coagulation cascade. Since placental abruption results in a disruption of the maternal--fetal exchange surface, fetal distress is common, occurring in 50–60% of all cases. Another well-recognized complication of placental abruption is the Couvelaire uterus, which is encountered in 8% of patients who undergo cesarean section. This is the result of extravasation of blood into the myometrium creating the classic blue-purple discoloration of the uterus. Uterine atony has been described in association with a Couvelaire uterus but is actually more the exception than the rule, as most of these uteri will contract well following delivery.

Management

Once the diagnosis of placental abruption has been made, certain steps must be undertaken immediately. These include establishment of secure intravenous access, blood product availability, and ongoing assessment of maternal hemodynamic status. Urine output is a sensitive barometer of tissue perfusion and should be maintained at 30 ml/h or greater. Because of the likelihood of fetal distress, continuous fetal monitoring is necessary if the fetus is deemed viable.

Laboratory assessment of coagulation status is critical and should include the following:

1 hematocrit and hemoglobin;
2 platelet count;
3 prothrombin time;
4 fibrinogen;
5 fibrin split products (FSPs).

A clot lysis test should also be performed, which can provide a rapid estimate of the fibrinogen level. Blood collected in the absence of anticoagulants or preservatives is allowed to clot. If a clot does not form within 6 min or if it forms and then lyses within 30 min, a coagulation defect is probable and suggests a fibrinogen level <150 mg%, normal being >350 mg%.

In the preterm gestation with suspicion of only a mild abruption (grade 1), expectant management can be considered. The feasibility of this will depend upon a variety of factors including maternal hemodynamic status, coagulation profile, fetal status, and gestational age. If uterine irritability or premature contractions are present in this type of patient, tocolysis is reasonable. Given the potential for hemodynamic compromise should the abruption expand, β-mimetics are best avoided. Magnesium sulfate is an alternative without the cardiovascular complications associated with β-mimetics.

Expectant management is usually not an option for the majority of patients, delivery being indicated because of maternal and/or fetal condition. The issue to be decided in these cases is whether time will allow labor and vaginal delivery. Again the acuity of the situation is important in determining the route of delivery. In the setting of fetal compromise at a viable gestational age or severe hemorrhage regardless of the gestational age, prompt delivery via cesarean section should be undertaken, allowing for maternal stabilization if possible. If the patient is in labor and maternal and fetal status is stable, labor may be allowed to progress with frequent (every 2–3 h) assessment of coagulation profile. Evidence of a coagulopathy should prompt blood product replacement, not necessarily surgical intervention if the coagulopathy responds to therapy. In the setting of severe hemorrhage, whole blood is ideal. Unfortunately this is often not available and component therapy is necessary. While the presence of fetal demise indicates a severe abruption, this does not in and of itself neccesitate cesarean section.

Summary

Abruptio placentae is an obstetric emergency associated with significant maternal and perinatal morbidity and mortality. Optimal outcome demands a high index of suspicion and rapid assessment of both mother and fetus. The decision to proceed with expectant management versus delivery will depend upon the severity of the abruption and its complications. A specific time limit for labor cannot be provided. As long as maternal coagulation function and volume status are stable and fetal distress absent, labor may be safely undertaken.

SUGGESTED READING

ABDELLA TN, SIBAI BH, HAYS JM, ANDERSON GD. Relationship of hypertensive disease to abruptio placentae. *Obstet Gynecol* 1984;63:365–370.

HURD WW, MIODOVNIK M, HERTZBERG V, LAVIN JP. Selective management of abruptio placentae: a prospective study. *Obstet Gynecol* 1983;61:467–473.

KROHN M, VOIGT L, MCKNIGHT B, DALING JR, STARZYK P, BENEDETTI TJ. Correlates of placental abruption. *Br J Obstet Gynaecol* 1987;94:333–340.

NYBERG DA, MACK LA, BENEDETTI TJ, CYR DR, SCHUMAN WP. Placental abruption and placental hemorrhage: correlation of sonographic finds with fetal outcome. *Radiology* 1987;164:357–361.

SHOLL JS. Abruptio placentae: clinical management in nonacute cases. *Am J Obstet Gynecol* 1987;156:40–51.

TOWNSEND RR, LAING FC, JEFFREY RB. Placental abruption associated with cocaine abuse. *Am J Radiol* 1988;150:1339–1340.

36

Uterine atony

HARBINDER S. BRAR

Uterine atony is the principal cause of postpartum hemorrhage and is associated with a number of factors, including prolonged labor, oxytocin augmentation of labor, overdistention of the uterus by twins or hydramnios, general anesthesia, chorioamnionitis, malnutrition, grand multiparity, fetal macrosomia, uterine apoplexy, and dystocia. Diagnosis is made early by palpation of a relaxed uterine fundus, followed by careful vaginal inspection to rule out coexisting cervical or vaginal lacerations, and manual exploration of the uterus to rule out retained placental fragments or membranes and uterine rupture. Whenever the possibility of uterine atony can be anticipated, advance preparations should include establishing an intravenous line using a large-bore needle or cannula and cross-matching of the patient's blood.

Initial management of atony includes establishment of an infusion of 5% dextrose in lactated Ringer's solution or normal saline containing 20–40 U of oxytocin. Cross-matched blood (2–4 U) should be available. Then the placenta and membranes are removed manually, and the fundus is elevated and massaged through the abdominal wall.

If the initial response is unsatisfactory, 0.2 mg of ergonovine (Ergotrate) can be given either intramuscularly or slowly intravenously; to minimize the risk of drug-induced hypertension. As an alternative, 10 U of oxytocin (Pitocin, Syntocinon) can be injected into the cervix. If available, 0.25 mg of 15-methylprostaglandin $F_{2\alpha}$ can be administered intramuscularly and repeated up to a total of four doses if necessary. In an abdominal delivery, the same dose may be administered directly into the myometrium. In patients with a history of asthma or glaucoma, 15-methylprostaglandin $F_{2\alpha}$ is contraindicated.

If atony persists, a gloved fist should be placed immediately in the vagina, pushing the uterus up and out of the pelvis, with the other hand providing counterpressure through the abdominal wall to anteflex the fundus over the vaginal fist. (At this point, the lower uterine segment should be palpated carefully to insure that a rupture was not overlooked at the initial examination.) If atony can be corrected by this maneuver, the uterus should be held in an elevated position for at least 5 min more.

When the above measures fail and the patient is jeopardized by continuing active hemorrhage, the lower abdominal aorta should be occluded by transabdominal compression against the sacral promontory while blood replacement and other measures are being prepared. At this point, a uterine pack can be considered. Infection and continuing hemorrhage behind the pack are the principal complications and, therefore, it is not commonly used at our institution. Hot intrauterine douches sometimes are recommended, but we have not been impressed with their effectiveness.

For intractable cases, operative intervention may be necessary. Before considering hysterectomy, bilateral ligation of the ascending uterine arteries should be attempted. This is easily and quickly accomplished by passing absorbable sutures through the angles of the lower uterine segment and around the vessels, taking care not to perforate the bladder. (If in doubt, a bladder flap should be mobilized.) Additional hemostasis can be obtained by placing second sutures around the ovarian branches of the ascending uterine arteries in the cornual areas. Experience with this procedure suggests that reproductive function is not jeopardized seriously by uterine artery ligation.

As an alternative, ligation of the hypogastric arteries can be considered, particularly when the cervical branches of the uterine arteries seem to be contributing to the hemorrhage. In practice, hypogastric ligation does not add much to uterine artery ligation, and certain additional risks are involved, particularly when the operator is unfamiliar with the procedure. Possible complications include inadvertent ligation of the external iliac artery and laceration of the underlying hypogastric vein. Both are potentially lethal.

One other approach for intractable cases involves angiography by way of the right common femoral artery, followed by the deposition of a material, such as Gelfoam particles, that induces clot formation in the bleeding vessel.

Hysterectomy may become necessary as a last resort. Total hysterectomy is performed most often, although a subtotal operation probably would be just as effective and much safer for a patient who has become a poor operative risk.

Finally, it should not be forgotten that uterine atony can be associated with a coagulation disorder. In that event, correction of the clotting deficiency becomes a vital step in the patient's management.

Uterine inversion

Puerperal uterine inversion is an uncommon obstetric emergency which must be considered in cases of postpartum hemorrhage and shock. When inversion occurs, immediate measures must be undertaken to prevent maternal morbidity and possible mortality.

Major risk factors for uterine inversion include primiparity, delivery of a macrosomic fetus, fundally implanted placenta, patients receiving oxytocin and mismanagement of third stage of labor due to excessive cord traction, Credé fundal pressure, or both. Hemorrhage, shock, and pain, either singly or in combination, are common complications of inversion. Shock disproportionate to blood loss has long been noted as a cardinal symptom, but this has not been a significant finding in more recent series.

Palpable "cupping" or an apparent absence of the fundus on abdominal examination suggests inversion, but indentation is overlooked easily and diagnosis ultimately depends upon demonstrating the mass in the vagina. Routine examination of the cervix postpartum will establish the diagnosis and may do so before the appearance of any symptoms. Although spontaneous inversion may occur, preventive measures should be directed toward careful management of the third stage of labor.

The usual measures to counteract shock should be undertaken, and whole blood should be made available immediately. Oxytocic agents should be withheld and an attempt made to reposition the uterus manually via the vagina. Removal of placenta before replacement carries some risk of excessive blood loss and shock. Therefore, manual replacement is attempted without removing the placenta. After repositioning the uterus the placenta usually is easily removed. Only if the uterus cannot be returned to its normal position can removal of the placenta be attempted. If there is a tendency toward cervical contraction, traditionally general anesthesia (halothane, a potent uterine relaxant) is recommended to produce uterine relaxation, but this also carries a risk of aspiration of the gastric contents, further aggravating hypotension. More recently, specific uterine relaxants like terbutaline and magnesium sulfate have been used successfully.

Terbutaline, given as a 0.25-mg iv bolus, will relax the contraction ring in about 80% of patients, thus avoiding the need for general anesthesia. Terbutaline should not be used in patients with significant hypotension and shock. With hypotension, terbutaline is contraindicated, and magnesium sulfate can be used as a 2-g iv bolus given over 10 min.

The portion of the uterus that inverted last should be replaced first to avoid multiple thicknesses of the myometrium in the cervical ring. Once the uterus has been replaced, the hand should be left in the endometrial cavity until there is firm contraction and intravenous oxytocics are being administered. Regardless of the method of vaginal replacement, careful manual exploration of the uterus afterward is essential to rule out the possibility of uterine rupture. Intramyometrial or intramuscular injections of 250 μg 15-methylprostaglandin $F_{2\alpha}$ may prove beneficial in intractable cases, as described earlier.

In those patients in whom immediate replacement is not successful, an operative approach may be indicated. This also is required in patients with subacute or chronic inversion where there is tight contraction of the cervical ring and some degree of involution of the uterus. The procedure

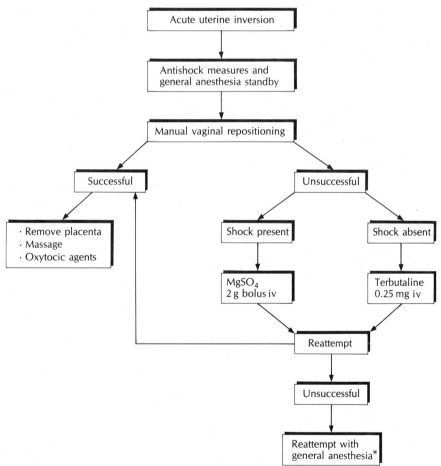

* This was only necessary in subacute and chronic cases

Fig. 36.1 Suggested management protocol for uterine inversion.

of Haultain involves incision of the cervical ring posteriorly through an abdominal approach. Spinelli described a vaginal procedure in which the bladder is dissected away from the cervix and lower uterine segment and then the cervical ring is divided anteriorly.

Based on our experience, the recommended management is shown in Fig. 36.1. A satisfactory postpartum course and successful outcome of all patients can be attributed primarily to immediate recognition and rapid manual replacement. The former is insured by a policy of routine examination of the cervix and vagina after delivery. A high index of suspicion should be maintained for the possibility of inversion of the uterus in all cases of postpartum hemorrhage. Manual replacement should be possible in nearly all cases. Abdominal or vaginal operative procedures rarely will be required for acute inversion, but they generally are effective if needed.

SUGGESTED READING

BASSAW B, ROOPNARINESINGH S. Post partum shock and uterine inversion. *West Indian Med J* 1990;39:178–179.

BRAR HS, GREENSPOON JS, PLATT LD, PAUL RH. Acute puerperal uterine inversion. New approaches to management. *J Reprod Med* 1989;34:173.

BROWN BJ, POULSON AM, MINEAU DE, MILLER JR FJ. Uncontrollable postpartum bleeding: new approach to hemostasis through angiographic arterial embolization. *Obstet Gynecol* 1979;54:361.

HAYASHI M, CASTILLO MS, NOAH ML. Management of severe postpartum hemorrhage due to uterine atony using an analogue of prostaglandin F_2. *Obstet Gynecol* 1981;58:426.

HSIEH TT, LEE JD. Sonographic findings in acute puerperal uterine inversion. *J Clin Ultrasound* 1991;19:306–309.

KITCHIN JD, THIAGARAJAH S, MAY HV, *et al.* Puerperal inversion of the uterus. *Am J Obstet Gynecol* 1975;123:51.

MOIR DD, AMOA AB. Ergometrine or oxytocin? Blood loss and side-effects at spontaneous vertex delivery. *Br J Anaesth* 1979;51:113.

MOMANI AW, HASSAN A. Treatment of puerperal uterine inversion by the hydrostatic method; reports of five cases. *Eur J Obstet Gynecol Reprod Biol* 1989;32:281–285.

PLATT LD, DRUZIN, ML. Acute puerperal inversion of the uterus. *Am J Obstet Gynecol* 1981;141:187.

ROMO MS, GRIMES DA, STRASSLE PO. Infarction of the uterus from subacute incomplete inversion. *Am J Obstet Gynecol* 1992;166:878–879.

THIERY M, DELBEKE L. Acute puerperal uterine inversion: two step management with a β-mimetic and a prostaglandin. *Am J Obstet Gynecol* 1985;153:891.

TOPPOZADA M, EL-BOSSATY M, EL-RAHMAN HA, EL-DIN AHS. Control of intractable atonic postpatum hemorrhage by 15-methyl prostaglandin F_2. *Obstet Gynecol* 1981;58:327.

WATSON P, BESCH N, BOWES Jr WA. Management of acute and subacute puerperal inversion of the uterus. *Obstet Gynecol* 1980;55:12.

WEEKES LR, GANDHI S. Five year study of postpartum hemorrhage: Queen of Angels Hospital, 1973–1977. *J Natl Med Assoc* 1979;71:829.

WIEDSWANG G, MOEN MH. Non-puerperal inversion of the uterus. *Acta Obstet Gynecol Scand* 1989;68:559–560.

ZAHN CM, YEOMANS ER. Postpartum hemorrhage: placenta accreta, uterine inversion, and puerperal hematomas. *Clin Obstet Gynecol* 1990;33:422–431.

37

Macrosomia

KIM R. LIPSCOMB

Definition

Macrosomia is arbitrarily defined as a birth weight above the 90th percentile for gestational age or >4000–4500 g at term. The overall incidence for infants weighing >4000 g is 5–10%, and 1–2% for infants weighing >4500 g. Macrosomic infants and their mothers are at increased risk for maternal and perinatal morbidity and mortality, therefore the identification and management of macrosomia are of ongoing importance in obstetrics.

Risk factors

Less than 40% of macrosomic infants are born to patients with identifiable risk factors. The majority are infants of diabetic mothers. The incidence of macrosomia increases as the degree of glucose intolerance increases. The incidence of fetal weight exceeding 4000 g is 12% with one abnormal glucose value on the 3-h glucose tolerance test and almost 50% with gestational or pregestational diabetes.

The pathophysiology of excessive fetal growth in the infant of the diabetic mother is complex; however, the most widely accepted hypothesis is that maternal hyperglycemia stimulates fetal hyperinsulinemia as a result of elevated fetal glucose levels. This, in turn, mediates accelerated fuel utilization and growth. The features of this growth abnormality include abnormal adipose deposition and distribution, visceral organomegaly, and acceleration of muscle and skeletal growth. Skeletal growth is less sensitive to insulin influence compared to soft tissue, thus the head circumference remains in the normal range. The infant becomes asymmetrically large with an increased abdominal-to-head circumference or weight-to-length ratio.

The remaining risk factors are maternal obesity (>70–90 kg), excessive maternal weight gain (>20 kg), history of large maternal birth weight, previous delivery of a large infant, and postdatism. As many as 30% of postdate pregnancies deliver macrosomic infants. This problem has resulted from expectant management schemes that permit the continued growth of normal infants, whereas compromised slowly growing fetuses are identified by surveillance techniques and delivered. Postdate morbidity now is often related to the big neonate while the postmaturity problem has been eliminated.

Predictability

The prenatal diagnosis of the macrosomic infant would be of value in determining timing and route of delivery and in reducing maternal and perinatal risks. Unfortunately, the clinician's ability to diagnose accurately macrosomia through palpation and fundal height measurements is poor. Even with the introduction of real-time ultrasonography and standard measured parameters to estimate fetal weight, we are left with limited capabilities.

Multiple formulas using measurements of fetal biparietal diameter (BPD), femur length (FL), head circumference (HC), abdominal circumference (AC), and FL:AC ratio have been studied. Repeated reports corroborate that the formulas using FL and AC to estimate fetal weight are superior in predicting birth weight in the macrosomic population. BPD and AC formulas are probably less predictive due to the slow growth, position, and molding of the fetal head. Even with the best formulas, progressively greater underestimation occurs with increasing birth weights. This results in mean errors and standard deviations of 10–15%, which obviously decrease the clinical usefulness of these estimations. Studies have suggested, however, that an AC greater than the 90th percentile or an FL:AC ratio less than the 10th percentile may identify the asymmetric fetus at risk for becoming macrosomic and more careful monitoring of growth may be performed.

Complications

The risks that the macrosomic infant and mother encounter are associated with the delivery process itself. Complications cited in the literature include: increased cesarean section rate, increased operative vaginal deliveries, postpartum hemorrhage, maternal vaginal lacerations, shoulder dystocia-associated injuries, and birth asphyxia.

The main indication for cesarean section is usually cephalopelvic disproportion as compared to repeat cesarean section for the normal-weight population. The rate of delivery with the vacuum extractor and, less commonly now, mid-forceps is higher. As will be discussed in Chapter 38, the association of mid pelvic operative procedures and subsequent shoulder dystocia is well known. Shoulder dystocia occurs in 8–30% of macrosomic deliveries, resulting in lower Apgar scores, potential asphyxia, and fetal trauma. Because of the concerns for birth complications, there has been an increase in the cesarean section rate when macrosomia is suspected. In spite of this rise in abdominal deliveries, perinatal outcome associated with the macrosomic infant has not improved.

Evacuation of the overdistended uterus and the passage of the large infant through the birth canal lead to a higher rate of postpartum hemorrhage due to uterine atony and lacerations. Routine use of oxytocin following delivery probably decreases the need for transfusions in these cases.

Management

Prevention of macrosomia and thoughtful intrapartum management must be the focus, as there is no accurate method to diagnose macrosomia, and no justification for elective cesarean section for macrosomia since most women deliver these infants vaginally. One should always individualize care and fully discuss the options with the patient. There are no strict rules; however, it is the author's opinion that the following guidelines are reasonable:

1 perform a baseline ultrasound to establish accurate dating on all patients with risk factors for macrosomia:
  (a) diabetes;
  (b) maternal obesity (>90 kg);
  (c) excessive weight gain (>20 kg);
  (d) history of large maternal birth weight;
  (e) birth of a previous macrosomic infant;

2 perform ultrasound in the third trimester on any patient who develops risk factors or exhibits a size greater than date discrepancy;

3 liberally use ultrasound at term in patients with risk factors for macrosomia or patients with postdate pregnancy;

4 consider serial ultrasound examinations on infants with AC greater than the 90th percentile or a FL:AC ratio less than the 10th percentile to detect macrosomia;

5 consider induction of labor at term, given good dates, when there is evidence of macrosomia to avoid further growth;

6 aim for excellent glucose control in the diabetic patient to prevent accelerated fetal growth;

7 consider performing intrapartum ultrasound on all patients with risk factors for macrosomia if no prior data exist;

8 consider that there may be an error of 10–15% in the estimate of fetal weight;

9 consider elective cesarean section for infants with weights of ⩾4500 g or a history of shoulder dystocia;

10 consider elective cesarean section for infants with weights of ⩾4250 g in the diabetic patient;

11 avoid a prolonged second stage of labor and mid pelvic operative vaginal delivery;

12 have skilled physicians available who are prepared to manage a shoulder dystocia, as well as anesthesia and blood products.

In conclusion, macrosomia is strongly associated with diabetes, maternal obesity, excessive weight gain, history of large maternal birth weight, and birth of a previous macrosomia infant. In recent years, postdate pregnancy has become a major contributing factor to the macrosomic newborn population. These infants and their mothers are at increased risk for morbidity and mortality due to increased cesarean rate, operative vaginal deliveries, hemorrhage, and shoulder dystocia. With less than optimal ways to identify macrosomia and predict which infants will experience shoulder dystocia, we must focus on prevention and careful intrapartum management to prevent complications.

SUGGESTED READING

CHERVENAK JL, DIVON MY, HIRSCH J. Macrosomia in the postdate pregnancy: is routine ultrasonographic screening indicated? *Am J Obstet Gynecol* 1989;161: 753–756.

HADLOCK FP, HARRIST RB, FEARNEYHOUGH TC, et al. USE of femur length/abdominal circumference ratio in detecting the macrosomic fetus. *Radiology* 1985;154:503–505.

HERGET ED, EBERHARD M. Pregnancy outcome following ultrasound diagnosis of macrosomia. *Obstet Gynecol* 1991;78:340–343.

HIRATA GI, MEDEARIS AL, HORENSTEIN J, et al. Ultrasonographic estimation of fetal weight in the clinically macrosomic infant. *Obstet Gynecol* 1990;162:238–242.

KLEBANHOFF MA, MILLS JL, BERENDES HW. Mother's birth weight as a predictor of macrosomia. *Am J Obstet Gynecol* 1985;153:253–257.

LAZER S, BIALE Y, MAZOR M, et al. Complications associated with the macrosomic fetus. *J Reprod Med* 1986;31:501–505.

LEIKIN EL, JAMES JH, GERRI A, et al. Abnormal glucose screening tests in pregnancy: a risk factor for fetal macrosomia. *Obstet Gynecol* 1987;69:570–573.

MILLER JM, KORNDORFFER FA, GABERT HA. Fetal weight estimates in late pregnancy with emphasis on macrosomia. *J Clin Ultrasound* 1986;14:437–442.

MILLER JM, BROWN HL, KHAWLI OF, *et al*. Ultrasonographic identification of the macrosomic infant. *Am J Obstet Gynecol* 1988;159:1110–1114.

SPELLACY WN, MILLER S, WINEGAR A, *et al*. Macrosomia – maternal characteristics and infant complications. *Obstet Gynecol* 1985;66:158–161.

38

Shoulder dystocia

KIM R. LIPSCOMB

Definition

Shoulder dystocia is encountered after the delivery of the fetal head, when further delivery of the infant is prevented by the impaction of the fetal shoulder behind the maternal symphysis, requiring specific maneuvers to effect delivery.

Incidence

Shoulder dystocia occurs infrequently, with an incidence of 0.15–1.7% of all vaginal deliveries. This wide range is due to inherent subjectivity of the definition of dystocia by clinicians, the degree of reporting, and differences in defining the study population.

Risk factors

Shoulder dystocia is strongly correlated with macrosomia. Repeated studies have shown that infants weighing >4000 g are at statistically increased risk for shoulder dystocia when compared to those weighing <4000 g. An infant weighing between 4000 and 4500 g has an 8–10% chance, whereas an infant weighing ≥4500 g has a 20–30% chance of shoulder dystocia. As mentioned in Chapter 37, the macrosomic infant has a trunk or chest circumference that is larger than the head circumference. This dimension and the large arms contribute to the greater dimensions of the upper body. This bulk may block the fetal shoulder rotation from the anteroposterior position to a more desirable oblique position for delivery. Although macrosomia is clearly a risk factor for shoulder dystocia, it must be remembered that 50–60% of shoulder dystocias occur in infants weighing <4000 g.

The majority of macrosomic infants occur in pregnancies complicated by diabetes mellitus. Infants of diabetic mothers have been shown to experience a significantly higher shoulder dystocia rate than infants of nondiabetics of a similar birth weight, with a incidence range of 13–31%. This rate is even higher in infants weighing >4500 g. To date there has been no comparison in the incidence of shoulder dystocia in insulin- versus noninsulin-dependent diabetics.

Other clinical factors associated with shoulder dystocia include: post-datism, male fetus, maternal obesity, previous history of a macrosomic infant, previous history of shoulder dystocia and, more importantly, second-stage labor disorders, and operative vaginal delivery. Benedetti and Gabbe, as well as others, have shown an association between prolonged second stage of labor, mid pelvic delivery and shoulder dystocia. They reported an almost 28-fold increase in dystocia when a mid pelvic procedure was performed after a prolonged second stage. Furthermore, in this study, clavicular and humeral fractures and nerve palsies were more frequent with assisted macrosomic deliveries. Acker *et al.* found that in infants weighing between 3500 and 4000 g with any abnormality of labor and instrumental delivery, the incidence of shoulder dystocia doubled.

Complications

All investigators have reported an increased perinatal morbidity and mortality in association with shoulder dystocia. Perinatal mortality varies from 21 to 290:1000 deliveries complicated by shoulder dystocia and immediate neonatal morbidity has been reported in 20% of cases. Brachial plexus injury occurs in 15–22% of cases and fractures occur in 14–18% of cases. Almost 95% of brachial plexus injuries are of the Erbs–Duchenne type. This results in C5–6 nerve involvement with 85% of infants recovering totally. Klumpe's-type nerve injury, involving C8–T1 nerves, has a recovery rate of 40% in the first year. Humeral as well as clavicular fractures occur and usually resolve uneventfully. Severe fetal asphyxia is rare, occurring in 143:1000 deliveries complicated by shoulder dystocia as compared with 14:1000 deliveries overall. Fetal morbidity can be delayed and McCall found that 28% of infants born with a shoulder dystocia demonstrated neuropsychiatric dysfunction at a 5–10-year follow-up.

The true risk of permanent injury in shoulder dystocia has been reported as only 0.3%. It appears that many prophylactic cesarean sections would need to be performed in order to avoid one permanent injury in a group at high risk for shoulder dystocia.

Predictability

Efforts to diagnose accurately macrosomia prenatally or predict shoulder dystocia have been poor. The diagnosis of macrosomia can be made in only 30% of these cases. When performed, ultrasound estimation of fetal weight is accompanied by a 10–15% error. This is a result of maternal obesity, fetal body composition, and fetal head position. The predictability becomes more dismal, with 50% of shoulder dystocias occurring with birth weights <4000 g, when the physician is less suspicious. Until better ultrasonic parameters and/or ratios have been standardized, we are left with a high index of suspicion and readiness for management as our best tools.

Management

Although the optimum management of shoulder dystocia is debatable, all would agree that the first step is anticipation. Every effort should be made to identify the mother and fetus at risk and prepare a clear plan of management of labor and the delivery process.

The patient should be completely informed of the risks and benefits of a trial of vaginal delivery. Prophylactic cesarean section may be strongly considered when the estimated fetal weight is >4500 g, or >4000–4250 g in the diabetic, or with a prior history of shoulder dystocia. This decision should be made in consideration of the experience of the physician and attendant personnel and with the patient's wishes in mind.

Physicians should systematically review the presentation and management of shoulder dystocia prior to the time of delivery, including the worst-case scenario. Anesthesia should be readily available, as should blood products. Delivery should be performed in the delivery room, not the labor room. Ideally three persons will need to be present, as well as the pediatrician.

Mid pelvic operative procedures should be avoided in the setting of macrosomia and/or abnormal labor pattern.

It is crucial to recognize the signs of shoulder dystocia. As the shoulders descend in response to maternal efforts, the anterior shoulder moves from the oblique position under one of the pubic rami. If the anterior shoulder descends in the anteroposterior diameter of the outlet, an impaction behind the symphysis may occur and further descent is blocked. Rapid delivery of the head, vacuum extraction, and overzealous external rotation of the head can cause shoulder dystocia.

Shoulder dystocia is usually heralded by the classic turtle sign. After the fetal head delivers it retracts back on to the maternal perineum. As maternal efforts to expel the fetal body continue, the fetal shoulder become impacted behind the symphysis.

Having recognized a shoulder dystocia, if alone, call for assistance. Do not attempt to suction or relieve a tight nuchal cord since prematurely cutting off blood supply may be deleterious for the fetus. The mother is instructed to stop pushing. All attendants should refrain from applying fundal pressure which can only make the impaction worse.

The normal term fetus can endure up to 10 min of asphyxia before permanent neurologic injury is likely to occur. A previously compromised fetus will probably have less time. During the first 5 min the major harm to the neonate is most likely to be an iatrogenic injury. Pulling and twisting the head and neck will only increase the chances of a neurologic injury.

The first attempt to effect delivery is by gentle posterior and inferior traction of the fetal head, thus disimpacting the anterior shoulder while the posterior shoulder fills the sacrum. Often simultaneous suprapubic pressure slightly away from behind the bone or to one side will displace the impacted anterior shoulder into the oblique diameter and allow delivery.

If this is not successful, attempt the McRobert's maneuver, which is hyperflexion of the maternal legs on to her abdomen. This brings both the pelvic inlet and outlet into a more ventral position, facilitating delivery of the fetal shoulders. As shoulder dystocia is thought to be a bony dystocia, cutting a proctoepisiotomy may not be necessary. If the McRobert's maneuver fails, enlarging the episiotomy, however, may allow more room for the next proposed maneuvers.

Next, by gently placing the physician's hand into the vagina, the anterior shoulder may be rotated to the oblique lie, thus effecting delivery. Alternatively, the posterior shoulder may be rotated 180° and passed under the pubic rami. This is defined as the Woods or corkscrew maneuver. As the posterior shoulder rotates anteriorly, it will often deliver. These maneuvers are often unsuccessful in severe dystocia, and excessive time should be avoided.

Should the above maneuvers fail, the physician's hand can be passed into the vagina following the posterior arm to the elbow. The arm is flexed and then swept out over the infant's chest and delivered over the posterior perineum. Rotation of the trunk bringing the posterior arm anteriorly may be required. This appears to be the most expeditious means of delivery.

Fracture of the clavicle may be attempted by applying direct pressure away from the fetal lung. This will hopefully diminish the size of the shoulder girdle and effect delivery. This fracture occurs spontaneously most often but in reality it is difficult to achieve in the management of a shoulder dystocia.

The knee–chest position has been described and advocated by nurse midwives, again to place the pelvic girdle more ventral. This probably effects a similiar benefit as the McRobert's maneuver and the latter is easier to achieve. This appears awkward and may expend needed time. Squatting also has been advocated and reportedly increases pelvic capacity by 30%.

If all else fails and there is still a reasonable chance for safe delivery and a good fetal outcome, a symphysiotomy or the Zavanelli procedure may be performed. For a symphysiotomy the patient is placed under anesthesia. After displacing the urethra, the symphysis is separated by sharp dissection in hopes of disimpacting the anterior shoulder and achieving a vaginal delivery. The final resort is the Zavanelli maneuver, where the fetal head is replaced in the vagina in the flexed position and a cesarean section is performed.

In conclusion, shoulder dystocia is a very frightening, potentially catastrophic, and often unexpected experience. It is associated with macrosomia, diabetes, postdatism, maternal obesity, previous history of macrosomia and shoulder dystocia, as well as second-stage labor abnormalities, and operative vaginal deliveries. Birth trauma accompanying a shoulder dystocia carries an increased risk of perinatal morbidity and mortality as well as maternal morbidity. Even in the hands of the best clinicians, the predictability of shoulder dystocia is not very good. As a result, physicians must have a high index of suspicion for infants in the above risk groups. Hopefully, with adequate anticipation and preparation for shoulder dystocia, adverse sequelae may be avoided in order to insure a good outcome for the mother and her baby.

SUGGESTED READING

ACKER DB, SACHS BP, FRIEDMAN EA. Risk factors for shoulder dystocia. *Obstet Gynecol* 1985;66:762–768.

ACKER DB, SACHS BP, FRIEDMAN EA. Risk factors for shoulder dystocia in the average-weight infant. *Obstet Gynecol* 1986;67:614–617.

BENEDETTI TJ, GABBE SG. Shoulder dystocia, a complication of fetal macrosomia and prolonged second stage of labor with mid-pelvic delivery. *Obstet Gynecol* 1978;52:526–529.

BOYD ME, USHER RH, MCLEAN FH. Fetal macrosomia: predication, risks, proposed management. *Obstet Gynecol* 1983;61:715–722.

EL MADANY AA, JALLAD KB, RADI FA, *et al.* Shoulder dystocia: anticipation and outcome. *Int J Gynecol Obstet* 1990;34:7–12.

GROSS TL, SOKOL RJ, WILLIAMS T, *et al.* Shoulder dystocia: a fetal–physician risk. *Am J Obstet Gynecol* 1987;156:1408–1418.

GROSS SJ, SHIME J, FARINE D. Shoulder dystocia: predictors and outcome. *Am J Obstet Gynecol* 1987;156:334–336.

KELLER JD, LOPEZ-ZENO JA, DOOLEY SL, *et al.* Shoulder dystocia and birth trauma in gestational diabetes: a five year experience. *Am J Obstet Gynecol* 1991; 165:928–930.

KOROKAWA J, ZILKASKI M. Adapting hospital obstetrics to birth in the squatting position. *Birth* 1985;12:87–90.

LANGER O, BERKUS MD, HUFF RW, *et al.* Shoulder dystocia: should the fetus weighing ≥4000 grams be delivered by cesarean section? *Am J Obstet Gynecol* 1991;165:831–837.

LEVINE MG, HOLROYDE J, WOODS JR, *et al.* Birth trauma: incidence and predisposing factors. *Obstet Gynecol* 1984;63:792–795.

MCCALL JR JO. Shoulder dystocia: a study of aftereffects. *Am J Obstet Gynecol* 1962;83:1486–1490.

O'LEARY JA, LEONETTI HB. Shoulder dystocia: prevention and treatment. *Am J Obstet Gynecol* 1990;162:5–9.

SANDBERG EC. The Zavanelli maneuver extended: progression of a revolutionary technique. *Am J Obstet Gynecol* 1988;158:1347–1353.

SEEDS JW. Malpresentations. In: Gabbe SG, Niebyl JR, Simpson JL, eds. *Obstetrics Normal and Problem Pregnancies*. 2nd edn. New York: Churchill Livingstone, 1991:539–572.

39

Suppression of postpartum lactation

DANIEL R. MISHELL, JR

Clinicians should encourage breast-feeding as infant morbidity from respiratory and gastrointestinal diseases as well as overall morbidity and mortality are significantly less among infants who have breast-fed than those who have received artificial milk. Nevertheless, in certain instances mothers may elect not to nurse their babies, such as following a preterm birth or neonatal illness. For women who do not desire to nurse their infants, suppression of postpartum breast engorgement and lactation may be accomplished by either mechanical compression of the breasts with or without fluid restriction or by administration of hormones. Either bromocriptine mesylate (Parlodel), a peptide ergot alkaloid, or various estrogens with or without androgens have been utilized to suppress postpartum lactation. These two types of hormones have different actions. While bromocriptine is a dopamine agonist and thus inhibits prolactin release directly, the estrogenic formulations inhibit the action of prolactin upon the breasts by blocking the receptors in the target tissue.

The benefits derived from the use of either of these hormonal preparations have to be weighed against their potential risks and compared with the benefits and risks of mechanical compression alone. Postpartum breast engorgement and lactation normally begin 40–72 h after delivery and persist for at least 1 week in the absence of nursing. During this period the symptoms may be treated by such measures as breast-binders, ice bags, and analgesics. Although restriction of oral fluid intake and the use of diuretics have been advocated to enhance relief of breast discomfort, Kochenour reported that these measures do not provide additional symptomatic relief. The degree to which hormonal preparations are superior to breast compression or placebos varies in different studies depending on the study population, experimental design, and the specific drugs being evaluated.

Estrogens

The conclusion of most prospective studies has been that long-acting intramuscular estrogen preparations effectively prevent symptoms, without rebound engorgement, in about 80% of patients. This rate is significantly better than that obtained with placebos. Treatment needs to be initiated as soon after delivery as possible to be effective.

Morris *et al.* in a randomized, double-blind study compared a testosterone enanthate–estradiol valerate combination (Deladumone) with a placebo. When evaluated on the third, fourth, and fifth postpartum days, the hormonal preparation was significantly more effective than the placebo in preventing lactation, engorgement, and discomfort. Similar results were obtained by questionnaire at 14 days postpartum. At the 6-week examination, the placebo- and drug-treated groups were indistinguishable in regard to breast and uterine involution, lochia, and resumption of menses. In another randomized, double-blind study, Varga *et al.* found that oral stilbestrol suppressed postpartum lactation to a significantly greater extent than placebo.

A problem with nearly all randomized drug–placebo studies dealing with inhibition of lactation is the lack of use of breast-binders in the placebo group. But in a double-blind, placebo-controlled study performed by Schwartz *et al.*, all patients were fitted with tight bras soon after delivery. On the third and fourth postpartum days, patients treated with any of the three estrogens used in the trial – chlorotrianisene (TACE), diethylstilbestrol, and Deladumone – had significantly less breast tenderness and lactation than the placebo group. However, about half of all patients had continued or rebound breast engorgement after leaving the hospital, and the differences between the four groups were not significant at 5 weeks postpartum.

The results of this study indicate that estrogen therapy is superior to the use of breast-binding alone in suppressing postpartum breast tenderness and lactation during the first few postpartum days. But this improvement is not sustained during the next few weeks.

The benefits of estrogenic drugs must be weighed against their risks and side-effects. The most important of these is their reported association with venous thrombosis and thromboembolism. There is normally a hypercoagulable state postpartum, and the addition of high-dose estrogen increases production of clotting factors and thus could increase the risk of venous thrombosis. Retrospective studies have suggested such

a relationship, but the incidence of thrombosis in estrogen-treated puerperal is unknown. Estrogen should not be administered to patients with
a history of thrombosis or thromboembolism. Other individuals at increased risk for postpartum thrombosis are those over age 35 and those
who have had an operative delivery. Such individuals should not receive
estrogenic steroids to suppress lactation. Breast carcinoma and active
hepatic disease are also contraindications. Uterine subinvolution and
endometrial hyperstimulation have been reported to occur more frequently with estrogen therapy, but the addition of an androgen to the
estrogenic agent appears to prevent these effects.

In summary, long-acting estrogen–androgen preparations are effective in preventing puerperal breast engorgement, lactation, and discomfort in about 80% of patients. Their use carries very low risk in most
cases.

Bromocriptine

When bromocriptine is given in the recommended dose of 2.5 mg b.i.d.
with meals for 15 days, it is very effective in preventing breast secretion,
engorgement, and congestion.

Several randomized studies have compared bromocriptine with estrogen (either diethylstilbestrol or chlorotrianisene). In these studies
bromocriptine was found to be as, or slightly more, effective than estrogen for inhibition of lactation and breast engorgement as well as relief of
breast pain. No comparison of bromocriptine and Deladumone has been
reported, but Shapiro and Thomas reported that bromocriptine reduced
the symptoms of breast pain and engorgement secretion significantly
better than the use of breast-binders and analgesics.

About one-fourth of women receiving bromocriptine report adverse
symptoms. Most common are headache, dizziness, nausea, vomiting,
and skin rash, necessitating discontinuation of therapy in as many as 10%
of patients. Bromocriptine also produces hypotension in about one-third
of patients; therefore, treatment should not be initiated until at least 4 h
after delivery, after vital signs have been stabilized and while the patient
is in a recumbent position. Blood pressure should be monitored during
the first few hours of treatment. Although there have been a few case
reports of development of myocardial infarction and cerebrovascular
accident in the postpartum period among patients who received bromocriptine, there is no epidemiologic evidence of a causal relation between use of this drug, which causes vasal dilatation, and an increased
incidence of either myocardial infarction or stroke.

As many as 40% of women experience some degree of rebound lactation after the medication is discontinued, but these symptoms are usually

mild and can be relieved by an additional 7 days of treatment with one 2.5 mg tablet daily. After lactation has been initiated, bromocriptine, unlike estrogen, is still able to suppress lactation because of of its effect in lowering prolactin. Treatment with estrogens will not inhibit lactation once it has been initiated. Thus bromocriptine is the agent of choice for the inhibition of lactation in women who must discontinue nursing for any reason.

A long-acting, microencapsulated form of bromocriptine has been developed but it is not currently available in the USA. A single long-acting injection suppresses prolactin for 60 days. Several European studies indicate that a single injection of 50 mg of this long-acting preparation given within 3 h of delivery is extremely effective (>95%) for prevention of breast engorgement and milk secretion and has a very low incidence of side-effects without rebound lactation. Thus the initial studies of this agent are encouraging.

SUGGESTED READING

Crosignanni PG, Lombrosco GC, Caccamo A. Suppression of puerperal lactation by metergoline. *Obstet Gynecol* 1978;51:113.

Delitala G, Masala A, Alatgna S, *et al*. Metergoline in the inhibition of puerperal lactation. *Br Med J* 1977;1:744.

Kochenour NK. Lactation suppression. *Clin Obstet Gynecol* 1980;23:1045–1059.

Kremer JAM, Thomas CMG, Rolland R, Lancranjan I, van der Heijden PFM. Return of gonadotropic function in postpartum women during bromocriptine treatment. *Fertil Steril* 1989;51:622.

Kremer JAM, Rolland R, van der Heijden PFM, Schellekens LA, Vosmar MBJG, Lancranjan I. Lactation inhibition by a single injection of a new depot-bromocriptine. *Br J Obstet Gynaecol* 1990;97:527–532.

Morris JA, Creasy RK, Hohe PT. Inhibition of puerperal lactation. Double-blind comparison of chlorotrianisene, testosterone enanthate with estradiol valerate and placebo. *Obstet Gynecol* 1970;36:107–114.

Pepperell RJ. Suppression of lactation. *Med J Aust* 1986;144:37.

Peters F, Del Pozo E, Conti A, Breckwoldt M. Inhibition of lactation by a long-acting bromocriptine. *Obstet Gynecol* 1986;67:82.

Schwartz DL, Evans PC, Garcia L-R, *et al*. A clinical study of lactation suppression. *Obstet Gynecol* 1973;42:599–606.

Varga L, Lutterbeck PM, Pryor JS, *et al*. Suppression of puerperal lactation with an ergot alkaloid: a double-blind study. *Br Med J* 1972;2:743–744.

40

Drugs in pregnancy

ROBERT HURD SETTLAGE

Americans use drugs—irrespective of sex, age, socioeconomic stratum, region of residence, or reproductive status. Inducements to use drugs flood our commercial media. Ungoverned peer pressure, particularly in adolescence, tips unprepared young people toward casual use for experiences.

Pregnancy confers no immunity to the urge to "take medicine," cited by Sir William Osler (1849–1919) as "perhaps, the greatest feature that distinguishes man from other animals." Yet in spite of widespread and increasing use of drugs since World War II—old, new and novel formulations—direct evidence fails to reveal a corresponding increase in birth defects attributable to drug use.

In this chapter, the following topics will be addressed, emphasizing strategies for the safe selection and use of prescription drugs:

1 extent of drug use by gravidas;
2 vulnerability of the embryo and fetus to drug injury;
3 pharmacologic considerations associated with pregnancy;
4 prescribing advice from the Food and Drug Administration (FDA);
5 examples of drugs by FDA category;
6 conclusions.

Extent of drug use by gravidas

Most pregnant women take medicine. In a 1991 study of 4186 New Haven gravidas, only 34% abstained from all drug use during the first trimester of their pregnancies. A 1987 survey of 492 women in New York State

237

revealed that 91% used prescribed or over-the-counter drugs during their last pregnancies. A 1978 prospective study of 168 women in Florida revealed that all 168 took at least two drugs prenatally, 93% took five or more, the mean number was 11, and the maximum was 32. During their intrapartum stay, patients who delivered vaginally received a mean of seven additional drugs. If delivery was by cesarean section, 15.2 drugs were used during labor, and another 2.5 drugs during the postpartum hospital stay. In a Texas population of 231 women, the mean number of drugs per patient was 9.6 before labor, 6.0 during labor, and 8.7 postpartum, for a total fetal/neonatal exposure of 18.7 drugs per neonate.

Finally, retrospective interview of 304 postpartum women in Florida identified 93 drugs used by or given to this group – 32% prescribed and 68% over-the-counter preparations. Most did not know what they received in labor. Although half knew the names of drugs they had taken prenatally, only 43% could relate the intended benefit; none could recall precautions, common side-effects, techniques for self-monitoring, drug–drug or drug–food interactions to avoid, or action to take if a dose were missed – all topics recommended for pharmacist counseling when prescriptions are filled.

Fetal vulnerability

Susceptibility of the fetus to the effects of maternal drug use varies with the stage of pregnancy. Obviously, complete information from human studies will never be available, because controlled trials cannot be conducted, but animal studies can provide some guidance.

In the preimplantation and presomite stages, from 0 to 18 days following conception in the human, drugs exert an "all-or-nothing" effect. The pregnancy is aborted or continues unscathed. Experimentally, ethanol has such an effect in canine species.

During the stage of organogenesis, from 19 to 80 days, the tissue or organ system that is developing most rapidly will suffer injury. Ethanol causes a distinctive fetal alcohol syndrome in a variety of species, including our own, exemplified by mid facial dysmorphia.

Finally, drugs can impair functional capacity in the absence of detectable physical change. Ethanol use after 80 days is strongly associated with mental retardation. In rats, maternal alcohol ingestion sharply reduces cerebral neuron arborization and complex connections.

Pharmacologic considerations in pregnancy

Between initial absorption and final excretion, a number of characteristics and processes influence drug effect. Pregnancy influences some but not all of them. For example, small, lipid-soluble molecules diffuse freely. Most drugs have low molecular weights, i.e., below 250. The human placenta allows bidirectional transfer of most molecules below molecular weights of 600. This explains why heparin, with a molecular weight well above 1000, is generally the preferred anticoagulant in pregnancy: it does not reach, and thus cannot harm, the fetus. Ethanol, at the other extreme, with its molecular weight of 26, diffuses so rapidly and extensively that kinetic studies remain nearly impossible despite modern analytic techniques. Other influences of pregnancy on drug effect include the following.

1 Pregnancy can alter the absorption of oral drugs. A gravida with hyperemesis might not retain a drug, whereas slowed gut peristalsis can increase exposure and absorption by delaying transit time.

2 Pregnancy can change the distribution of drugs through alteration in intravascular and extravascular volumes.

3 Pregnancy alters drug–receptor interactions because of the appearance and growth of new placental and fetal populations of drug receptors.

4 Pregnancy can alter excretion through increased renal plasma flow or hinder excretion through storage in added adipose tissue.

5 Generally not influenced by pregnancy are biotransformation, drug interactions, and pharmacokinetics.

Finally, although it is nearly as rich in drug-metabolizing enzymes as the maternal liver, placental tissue provides little protection to the fetus. Effectively, there is no "placental barrier" except to large proteins. The fetus lacks a full repertoire of drug-handling capacity and therefore relies on access to the maternal circulation for detoxification and excretion. Fetal handling capacity is particularly poor before term.

Guidance from the FDA

Prior to 1980, virtually all drugs came with the disclaimer, "Use in pregnancy has not been approved." This changed in 1980 with the publication by the FDA of the five "pregnancy categories," summarized as follows.

A *Controlled studies show no risk.* Adequate, well-controlled studies in pregnant women have failed to demonstrate risk to the fetus.

B *No evidence of risk in humans.* Either animal findings show risk, but human findings do not; or, if no adequate human studies have been done, animal findings are negative.

C *Risk cannot be ruled out.* Human studies are lacking, and animal studies are either positive for fetal risk, or lacking as well. However, potential benefits may justify the potential risk.

D *Positive evidence of risk.* Investigational or postmarketing data show risk to the fetus. Nevertheless, potential benefits may outweigh the potential risk.

X *Contraindicated in pregnancy.* Studies in animals or humans, or investigational or postmarketing reports, have shown fetal risk which clearly outweighs any possible benefit to the patient.

Briggs *et al.* have assembled useful data on more than 500 commonly used drugs, employing the FDA pregnancy categories. Drugs from the current Los Angeles County + University of Southern California Drug Formulary (July 1991) appear in Tables 40.1–40.5. Note that some drugs have split designations (e.g., B/D), intended to alert prescribers to possible problems if they are used just prior to delivery. For example, opiates can induce respiratory depression in the neonate; sulfonamides can

Table 40.1 Category A drugs

Potassium chloride, citrate, and gluconate
Thyroid preparations: levothyroxine, liothyronine, thyroglobulin, and thyroid
Vitamins: at dosages that do not exceed the recommended dietary allowances

Table 40.2 Category B drugs

Antihistamines
Chlorpheniramine, cimetidine, cyproheptadine, dimenhydrinate, meclizine, ranitidine

Antiinfectives
Antifungals: amphotericin B, clotrimazole, miconazole, nystatin
Cephalosporins (check specific drug)
Penicillins (check specific drug)
Other antiinfectives: clindamycin, erythromycin, polymyxin B, spectinomycin
Antituberculosis: ethambutol
Sulfonamides: sulfasalazine (B/D), sulfonamides (B/D)
Trichomonacides: metronidazole
Urinary germicide: nitrofurantoin

Autonomics
Parasympatholytics (anticholinergic): glycopyrrolate
Sympathomimetics (adrenergic): ritodrine, terbutaline
Sympatholytics: acebutolol, metoprolol, pindolol

Coagulants/anticoagulants
Thrombolytics: urokinase

Cardiovascular drugs
Acebutolol, pindolol

Continued

Table 40.2 *Continued*

Central nervous system drugs
Acetaminophen, butorphanol (B/D), fentanyl (B/D), hydromorphone (B/D), ibuprofen, indomethacin (B/D), magnesium sulfate, maprotiline, meperidine (B/D), methadone (B/D), morphine (B/D), nalbuphine (B/D), naloxone, naproxen, oxycodone (B/D), oxymorphone (B/D), pentazocine (B/D), sulindac (B/D)

Diagnostic agents
Indigo carmine

Diuretics
Amiloride

Antidiarrheals
Loperamide, paregoric (B/D)

Gastrointestinal agents
Dimenhydrinate, meclizine

Hormones
Adrenal: prednisolone, prednisone
Antidiabetic agents: insulin
Pituitary: desmopressin, vasopressin
Thyroid: calcitonin

Serums, toxoids, and vaccines
Immune globulin, hepatitis B, rabies, tetanus

Miscellaneous
Phenazopyridine, probenecid

Table 40.3 Category C drugs

Aminophylline	Furosemide
Aspirin	Gentamicin
Betamethasone	Guaifenesin
Chloral hydrate	Heparin
Chloramphenicol	Isoniazid
Chlorpromazine	Methyldopa
Codeine (D if use is sustained or at term)	Phenylephrine
	Prochlorperazine
Dexamethasone	Propoxyphene (D if use is sustained)
Dextroamphetamine	Pseudoephedrine
Diphenhydramine	Rifampin
Disulfiram	Theophylline
Docusate calcium/potassium/sodium	Trimethoprim
Ephedrine	

Table 40.4 Category D drugs

Azathioprine	Medroxyprogesterone
Chlorambucil	Meprobamate
Chlordiazepoxide	Methotrexate
Chlorpropamide	Pentobarbital
Cortisone	Phenobarbital
Coumarin derivatives	Phenytoin
Cyclophosphamide	Quinine
Diazepam	Reserpine
Ethanol (X if in large	Streptomycin
amounts or if sustained)	Tetracycline
Kanamycin	Tolbutamide
Lithium	

Table 40.5 Category X drugs

Aminopterin
Estrogens (all categories, including clomiphene)
Ethanol
Iodinated glycerol
Isotretinoin
Menadione (late)
Live vaccines (measles, mumps, rubella, smallpox)
Oral contraceptives
Phencyclidine
Ritodrine (before 20 weeks' gestation)
Sodium iodide radionuclides

displace bilirubin from neonatal albumin-binding sites (although frank kernicterus apparently has not been reported from this usage in pregnancy).

Current formularies and drug insert information for drugs should always be checked and appropriate caution used in recommending and prescribing all drugs, but especially those in categories C and D.

Conclusions

Cohlan, reviewing several decades of his career as a research teratologist, has made the following comment:

Despite the fact that there has been an exponential explosion all over the world during the past 50 years in the use of drugs and chemicals and in the exposure to a myraid of environmental pollutants, the overall incidence of congenital malformation has remained fairly constant.

Nevertheless, the most prudent course when considering drug use in pregnancy remains clear, simple, and straightforward:

1   have clear and specific indications for drug use;

2   choose the safest effective drug;

3   teach your patients to respect drugs;

4   model, through your behavior, the precept that "life is not a drug-deficiency state."

SUGGESTED READING

BRIGGS GG, FREEMAN RK, YAFFFEE SJ. *Drugs in Pregnancy and Lactation – A Reference Guide to Fetal and Neonatal Risk*. 3rd edn. Baltimore: Williams & Wilkins, 1993.

BUITENDIJK S, BRACKEN MB. Medication in early pregnancy: prevalence of use and relationship to maternal characteristics. *Am J Obstet Gynecol* 1991;165:33.

CHASNOFF IJ. Drug use in pregnancy: parameters of risk. *Pediatr Clin North Am* 1988;35:1403.

COHLAN SQ. Drugs and pregnancy. In: Young B, ed. *Perinatal Medicine Today*. New York: Alan R Liss, 1980:92.

COSTAS K, DAVIS R, KIM N, *et al*. Use of supplements containing high-dose vitamin A, New York State, 1983–1984. *MMWR* 1987;36:80.

DOERING PL, STEWART RB. The extent and character of drug consumption during pregnancy. *JAMA* 1987;239:843.

HARJULEHTO T, ARO T, SAXEN L. Long-term changes in medication during pregnancy. *Teratology* 1988;37:145.

HILL RM, CRAIG JP, CHANEY MD, *et al*. Drug utilization during the perinatal period. *Pediatr Res* 1977;11:417.

MEDICAL ECONOMICS DATA. *Physician's Desk Reference*. 46th edn. Montvale, NJ: Medical Economics, 1992.

SLOVITER R. *Pharmacology*. Washington, DC: Council on Resident Education in Obstetrics and Gynecology, 1984.

41

Exposure to teratogens

BRUCE W. KOVACS

Principles of teratology

Teratogens are exogenous agents or factors which have the potential to cause fetal wastage, malformations, or central nervous system dysfunction when exposure occurs during gestation. In general, teratogens can be divided into three broad categories: drugs or chemicals, infectious agents, and physical agents.

Teratogens affect embryologic development by interfering with cellular growth, differentiation, interaction, and migration, all of which are critical processes in embryogenesis. In most cases teratogenic agents affect more than one tissue or organ system because the insult occurs in many cell types. Thus, dysfunctions in the tissues of the developing embryo occurring as a result of teratogenic agents can produce hypoplasia or hyperplasia of developing structures, incomplete differentiation of organs, or disruption of the normal morphologic patterns.

Considering the vast number of potential teratogens to which the human embryo may be exposed, relatively few are known to cause serious malformations in exposed individuals. The efficacy of a particular teratogen is, in part, dependent on the genetic make-up of both mother and fetus, as well as on a number of factors related to the maternal–fetal environment. Most importantly, however, the timing of the exposure during gestation is the primary factor which determines whether or not a teratogenic effect will be seen and which organ system or systems are affected. In humans, the most vulnerable period is between 3 and 8 weeks after the last menstrual period, during the period of organogenesis. Unfortunately, most women do not realize they are pregnant until this critical period of development is well underway and will not have taken precautions to avoid exposure to known teratogenic agents.

Lastly, many congenital anomalies caused by teratogenic agents such as oral clefts, congenital heart disease, and neural tube defects also occur in fetuses not exposed to teratogens. These types of birth defects are thought to be due to a combination of several inherited susceptibility factors and exposure to environmental insults. In this regard there are probably a number of agents which, given a unique set of circumstances (metabolic status of the mother, a susceptible fetus, an embryologically vulnerable period, and a large teratogenic dose) are capable of producing teratogenic effects. Thus, a number of abnormalities which are described as multifactorial in etiology may have a teratologic component to their pathogenesis.

Clinical teratology

Teratology as a clinical discipline began after the teratogenic effects of intrauterine rubella infection were demonstrated in 1941. In the succeeding decades, greater consideration has been given to exogenous environmental factors and their potential for deleterious effects on the fetus. In 1960, when thalidomide was shown to cause phocomelia and other malformations in the children of mothers who had been given the drug during pregnancy, additional concern was raised about the use of prescription drugs in pregnancy. Thus in 1962, drug law amendments were enacted that led to regulations requiring that new drugs not be administered to pregnant women until preliminary studies indicated reasonable evidence of the drug's safety and effectiveness in animals, and later humans. Subsequently the Food and Drug Administration has devised a system for classifying therapeutic drugs for use in pregnancy based on the degree to which risk to the fetus has been ruled out (Table 41.1). In most cases, animal studies have been used extensively to determine the possible teratogenic effects of drugs. Although such studies may be helpful, their results do not always reliably predict the response in humans. For example, in rats and mice, thalidomide was shown not to cause malformations that were later seen in human fetuses. Conversely, corticosteroids can produce cleft palate in mice, but there is not a proven risk in human studies.

Because of these uncertainties in extrapolations from animal studies to humans, the critical value of case reports and human teratogen registries in identifying the teratogenic potential of drugs is obvious. Importantly, however, when studies of birth defects in humans are evaluated, the statistics presented should be reviewed with caution. Retrospective and

Table 41.1 Drugs in pregnancy: FDA categories

Category A applies to drugs for which controlled studies in women fail to demonstrate a risk to the fetus

Category B indicates that either: (a) animal studies have not demonstrated a fetal risk, but no adequate studies have been done in humans; or (b) animal studies have uncovered some risk that has not been confirmed in controlled studies in humans

Category C also has two meanings: (a) animal studies have revealed adverse fetal effects, but no adequate controlled studies have been done in humans; or (b) studies in humans and animals are not available

Category D applies to drugs associated with birth defects in humans, but with potential benefits that may outweigh their known risks

Category X indicates drugs for which abnormalities have been demonstrated in animal or human studies. The potential risks of the drugs in this category clearly outweigh their potential benefits. Such drugs are contraindicated in pregnancy

uncontrolled studies, as well as individual case reports, may be misleading about the risk of exposure to specific drugs during pregnancy, especially those that are commonly used during gestation. Because there is an empiric background risk that offspring in any large population of women using any drug during pregnancy will be born with birth defects, large and carefully conducted studies are required to prove an agent is a teratogen. Failure to take these concepts into account may lead to spurious claims of a causal relationship. Thus, it is important to remind patients that reports in lay literature often ignore these factors.

Counseling in exposed patients

Most commonly, it is exposure to drugs and chemicals that leads to concern. It has been estimated that as many as 32% of pregnant women are exposed to common pharmacologic agents such as analgesics, antimicrobials, sedatives, tranquilizers, and antidepressants. Importantly, this figure does not take into account exposure to substances such as tobacco, alcohol, cocaine, and others abused by women in our society. In addition, pregnancies complicated by maternal illnesses or trauma may also result in exposures to various other drugs or radiation. Environmental exposure to noxious solvents and chemicals in the workplace and home is also relatively common in pregnancy.

Counseling regarding an exposure to a potential teratogen should be performed in a sympathetic manner so that the patient is not unduly alarmed or burdened by guilt. Most often patient inquiries are related to substances or agents with relatively low-level risk for teratogenicity. These situations should be managed by careful explanation, reassurance, and further counseling in order to minimize the risk for the remainder of the pregnancy. Certain patients, however, have been exposed to agents that are known to be associated with significant increased risk for fetal malformation and/or mental retardation. In these circumstances a referral of such a patient to a health professional with special education or experience in teratology and birth defects is most appropriate. Importantly, in these patients additional studies usually consisting of detailed and serial ultrasound evaluations of fetal morphology are warranted. However, genetic amniocentesis for chromosomal studies is not usually of value, in that gross chromosomal abnormalities are not present in fetal cells even when defects have been produced by a teratogen. In addition, reassurance may also be obtained by maternal α-fetoprotein screening, although its efficacy for this purpose is unproven. More recently, the prenatal diagnosis of fetal infections which may cause teratogenesis has become available to evaluate potential risk and is advisable for documented exposures.

Lastly, it is important to be aware that, despite our ability to evaluate fetal morphology, in cases of known exposure we are still severely limited in our ability to predict neurodevelopmental outcome. There is an increasing awareness that some teratogenic agents primarily manifest their adverse effects in the central nervous system. Such neurobehavioral teratogens do not produce infants with profound structural anomalies but rather cause subtle damage in the central nervous system which only becomes apparent as the child develops. Therefore, patients must also be made aware of the diagnostic limitations and not be given inflated predictions, based only on anatomic integrity. Thus, even when objective data do not suggest malformations, some patients may request pregnancy termination. In these cases and in those with identified fetal malformations, psychologic support for the patient's decision should be provided along with follow-up counseling after the termination.

In cases where prenatal diagnosis has established that there is a morphologic anomaly present and termination in a previable period has not been accomplished it is important to maximize the potential for neonatal well-being. A neonatalogist should be advised and present at the delivery in that multispecialty support for the liveborn but damaged infant is often essential. In discussing the absolute recurrence risk for a similar abnormality in subsequent pregnancies with the patient it is important to emphasize that it is small. However, in view of the fact that some anomalies may reflect a component of polygenic susceptibility, the relative risk may be increased compared with the risk in the overall population. Preconception counseling and care are advised to minimize recurrence risk. In addition, psychologic counseling is advised to help the patient cope with the delivery of an affected child.

Teratogenic agents

Drugs and chemicals

Alcohol

Ethanol is one of the most commonly abused substances in the USA. The incidence of the *fetal alcohol syndrome* (FAS) runs as high as 0.2%, and an additional 0.4% of newborns show less severe features of the disorder. The range and severity of anomalies caused by the prenatal ingestion of ethanol appear to be dose-related. Risk due to ingestion of one or two drinks per day (1–2 oz) is not well defined but may cause a small reduction in average birth weight. Fetuses of women who drink six drinks per day (6 oz) are at 40% risk to show some features of FAS. The most consistent findings in babies with this disorder include: (1) prenatal growth deficiency for weight, height, and head circumference; (2) distinct craniofacial features; and (3) mild to moderate mental retardation. The average IQ among FAS individuals is 65, but may range from 16 to 105. Hypotonia is a frequent finding, along with poor motor coordination. Because even moderate exposure has been related to FAS, the best advice is to avoid alcohol consumption during pregnancy.

Antibiotics

Studies on the teratogenicity of the majority of antibiotics have failed to reveal an increased risk to the human fetus. A few, however, appear to pose a potential for damage. Tetracycline exposure beyond the fourth month of pregnancy has been shown to result in deciduous teeth that appear yellow with hypoplasia of the enamel. Streptomycin and related compounds will produce eighth nerve damage with subsequent hearing loss in about 10–15% of fetuses exposed.

Antihypertensive agents

Over the years a number of these agents from various classes have been suspected of causing birth defects. However, until recently no distinct association has been established for any agent despite rather widespread use of many antihypertensives. In the past few years, a new class of antihypertensive agents, angiotensin-converting enzyme inhibitors, has been shown to be associated with oligohydramnios and neonatal anuria. No specific malformation pattern has yet been reported in human case reports. Nonetheless, these medications are contraindicated in pregnancy.

Antineoplastic agents

Amniopterin and methotrexate, both of which are folic acid antagonists, are proven teratogens. Exposure in the first 6 weeks of gestation is usually lethal to the embryo; later exposure during the first trimester produces fetal effects which include intrauterine growth retardation, craniofacial anomalies, abnormal positioning of extremities, and mental retardation.

Some alkylating agents have been associated with severe intrauterine growth retardation, and fetal anomalies such as cleft palate, microphthalmia, limb reductions, digit anomalies, and poorly developed external genitalia. The first trimester is a particularly dangerous time for use of these drugs; however, a number of patients so treated have produced normal offspring. Cyclophosphamide also has teratogenic potential but the exact risk is unclear in that a number of normal offspring have been born after first-trimester exposure. Other agents used for cancer chemotherapy appear to have less risk for teratogenic effects in humans.

Anticoagulants

The use of coumarin derivatives (warfarin, coumadin) during the first trimester is associated with an increased risk of spontaneous abortion, intrauterine growth retardation, central nervous system defects, stillbirth, and a characteristic syndrome of craniofacial features known as the fetal warfarin syndrome. Embryologically, the most vulnerable time appears to be between 8 and 11 weeks after the last menstrual period. Because of this teratogenic risk, heparin has major advantages over coumarin anticoagulants during pregnancy because it does not cross the placenta. Thus, it is the drug of choice for anticoagulation during the first trimester and after 36 weeks' gestation. Patients using coumarin drugs for prophylaxis should be changed to heparin prior to conception.

Anticonvulsants

The incidence of epilepsy in pregnant women in the USA is about 1:200, and these women have an increased risk for significant fetal abnormalities. It is not clear whether the major proportion of this risk is due to anticonvulsant therapy or to a potential teratogenic effect of the underlying convulsive disorder. However, specific patterns of fetal malformations have been associated with different anticonvulsant agents. Diphenyl-hydantoin (Dilantin) can produce a specific pattern of malformations known as the fetal hydantoin syndrome, the clinical features of which include craniofacial abnormalities, limb reduction defects, prenatal-onset growth deficiency, mental retardation, and cardiovascular anomalies. Overall, approximately 10% of exposed fetuses have the syndrome, and an additional 30% may have only isolated features.

Valproic acid (Depakene) is a relatively new anticonvulsant, which produces congenital malformations similar to those found in the fetal hydantoin syndrome. Although normal births associated with prenatal valproic acid exposure have been reported, this drug should be avoided during pregnancy.

Carbamazepine (Tegretol) also appears to have a potential for teratogenesis, perhaps as a result of its metabolic breakdown. The malformations reported include minor craniofacial defects, nail hypoplasia, and neurodevelopmental delays. However, the incidence of the defects is less than that associated with Dilantin.

Trimethadione (Tridione) and paramethadione (Paradione), used to treat *petit mal* epilepsy, have been associated with a characteristic pattern of malformations. The features include craniofacial abnormalities, intrauterine growth retardation, mental retardation, and cardiovascular abnormalities. In addition, exposure to these agents has been associated with an increased risk for fetal loss. Taken together, women using trimethadione or paramethadione face an 85% risk for pregnancy loss or major congenital anomalies. In light of the relatively minor nature of *petit mal* seizures, these anticonvulsants should not be used during pregnancy.

Cocaine

The prevalence of cocaine use in pregnancy is unknown but is likely to be >10% in many areas. Cocaine use in the perinatal period is associated with an increased incidence of prematurity, intrauterine growth retardation, microcephaly, and fetal death. In addition there is evidence of teratogenic effects on central nervous system (CNS) structure, and cocaine use has the potential to cause cerebral infarcts in the fetal brain. However, although the long-term neurologic outcome of infants exposed to cocaine *in utero* is not yet known, it is prudent to consider it a neurobehavioral teratogen.

Heavy metals

The nonessential metallic elements, mercury, lead, and cadmium, are reproductive and developmental toxicants; however, only mercury and lead have proven teratogenic potential. Mercury, especially compounds like methylmercury, produce CNS damage and dysfunction with microcephaly in fetuses exposed during gestation, leading to cerebral palsy. Most exposures occur as a result of the ingestion of foods contaminated with industrial waste or mercury-containing antifungals. Similarly, lead and lead-containing compounds are neurodevelopmental teratogens. Since both substances are abundant in industrial society, clinicians need to question patients about potential exposures to these agents in the home or at work.

Organic solvents and compounds

This group of chemicals are as diverse as they are widely used in the USA. In general, exposure occurs as a result of inhalation of vapors or as absorption through the skin. Fortunately, although there are other adverse effects associated with exposures to these substances, few have any teratogenic effects in humans. However, polychlorinated biphenyls (PCBs) are a notable exception to this situation. Ingestion of these chemicals due to contamination of cooking oil has been reported and has caused darkened skin pigmentation and growth retardation. No pattern of structural malformations was noted; however, there was an increase in the incidence of several common malformations reported.

Psychotropic agents

This group of drugs is of special interest because it contains major tranquilizers and antianxiety agents, which are some of the most commonly prescribed drugs in the USA. However, the data regarding their teratogenicity are conflicting and, in general, no specific pattern of teratogenesis is apparent. Exceptions include lithium salts, diazepam (Valium), meprobamate, and impramine, all of which cross the placenta and have been associated with birth defects. However, of these, only lithium is a proven teratogen.

Steroid hormones

Exposures to progestins and estrogen–progestin combinations in the first trimester occur fairly commonly due to their use in the management of threatened abortion or because women continue taking birth-control pills, unaware that they are pregnant. The most consistent abnormality associated with the use of progestins during pregnancy is masculinization of the external genitalia in female fetuses. The magnitude of this risk appears to be between 1 and 2%.

The teratogenicity of estrogen and progestin combinations is more difficult to assess. Potential problems include congenital heart defects, nervous system defects, limb reduction malformations, and modified development of sexual organs. However, except for the latter category, no firm evidence for a causal relationship exists and inadvertent use of low-dose birth-control pills in the first trimester has not been associated with teratogenic effects.

Tobacco smoke

Maternal tobacco smoking reduces the chance for a normal pregnancy outcome, but is not teratogenic. The effects on pregnancy include decreased birth weight, birth length, and head circumference, as well as an increased risk for spontaneous abortions, intrauterine fetal death, neonatal death, and prematurity. Because of this and its other adverse effects, pregnant women should be counseled to reduce smoking as much as possible.

Vitamins

Lack of adequate folate is associated with increased incidence of neural tube defects and deficiencies of other vitamins and trace elements. It appears to result in increases in pregnancy loss, growth retardation, and malformed fetuses. However, in certain cases large doses of vitamins or their derivatives can be teratogenic.

Vitamin A and analogs such as isotretinoin (Accutane) used for treatment of severe acne appear to be teratogenic. Affected infants demonstrate craniofacial malformations, psychomotor retardation, congenital heart defects, and CNS malformations. Thus, physicians have an important responsibility to discuss the risks with all female patients before beginning treatment. The exact risk for serious defects following exposure during the first trimester has not yet been established, but it appears to be substantial.

Vitamin D may also have teratogenic potential when given in very high doses; however, more data are needed to substantiate the validity of this reported association.

Infectious agents

Various species of bacteria, parasites, and viruses can have teratogenic effects and produce congenital anomalies and neurodevelopmental abnormalities. The best known are the TORCHES agents (toxoplasmosis, rubella, cytomegalovirus, herpes, and syphilis) which are proven teratogens and produce a characteristic pattern of abnormalities.

Toxoplasmosis infection must occur as a primary infection in gestation to have teratogenic effects. Primary infection in the first trimester produces fetal infection in about 15% of cases. However, these infections result in the most severe fetal effects. The majority of the adverse effects are in the CNS and include microcephaly, intracranial calcifications, seizures, hydrocephalus, mental retardation, and chorioretinitis. Toxoplasmosis infections which occur later in gestation more often result in fetal infections (about a 60% rate in the third trimester) which usually are mild. Treatment of maternal disease with Spiramycin and fetal disease with pyrimethamine and sulfonamide has been advocated by some; however, this only decreases the risk of fetal infection. Measures to prevent this infection, such as avoiding cat litter, handwashing after handling cats, and eating only well-cooked meats, should be emphasized to patients at risk.

Rubella infections result in fetal infections with associated anomalies in about 20% of cases acquired in pregnancy. First-trimester infections are the highest risk both for transplacental passage and subsequent congenital effects. Anomalies produced include cataracts, deafness, patent ductus arteriosus, mental retardation, and growth retardation. Rubella vaccine should not be given during pregnancy; however, when inadvertent vaccination has occurred, it has not been reported to produce anomalies.

Cytomegalovirus infection occurs relatively commonly during pregnancy yet much about its teratogenicity is uncertain. About 40% of infants born to mothers with either primary or recurrent cytomegalovirus infections during gestation will have evidence of congenital infection. Thus, it is the most common cause of intrauterine infection. However, only about 10% of these infants will demonstrate clinical signs of the infection at birth. The CNS is usually involved in those infants with the most severe manifestations of this disease, most often resulting in microcephaly, mental retardation, spastic diplegia, optic atrophy, blindness, deafness, and seizures. The long-term follow-up of the 90% of infants who are asymptomatic at birth reveals a high incidence of hearing loss, neurodevelopmental delay, and below-average IQ and behavioral problems.

Herpes simplex (types I and II) infection in the first trimester can result in malformations only when they are primary maternal infections. The anomalies produced include microcephaly, chorioretinitis, hydroencephalus, and patent ductus. However, the transmission rate to embryo and fetus is low and most often congenital herpes occurs during the perinatal period.

Syphilis is one of the best-known teratogens and its effects have been understood for about 500 years. Transplacental infection is rare before the fourth month of gestation, thus the primary effects relate to organ dysfunction rather than malformations. Early congenital syphilis presents in the first 2 years of life manifested by hepatosplenomegaly, lyphadenitis, mucocutaneous rashes or eruptions, osteitis, nephrosis, meningitis, CNS lesions, hydrocephalus, palsies, chorioretinitis, uveitis, and optic atrophy. Late congenital syphilis has widespread manifestations but most diagnostic are interstitial keratitis, sensorineural deafness, notched incisors (Hutchinson teeth), mulberry molars, saddle-nose deformity, Clutton joints, and mental retardation. Prompt treatment of syphilis during pregnancy can prevent congenital sequelae.

Varicella-zoster virus causes chicken pox and shingles and is an established teratogen. However, there is uncertainty as to the magnitude of the risk to the fetus with first- and second-trimester exposures. The characteristic pattern of anomalies produced by congenital infections consists of cortical atrophy, chorioretinitis, limb and/or digit hypoplasia, and cicatricial (scar-like) skin lesions. Infants born after *in utero* exposure to the varicella-zoster virus have growth deficiency, mental retardation, hearing loss, and seizures. Varicella-zoster immune globulin, if given to exposed pregnant patients immediately after a known exposure, may prevent fetal sequelae.

Physical agents

Radiation can be divided into two broad categories; ionizing radiations and nonionizing radiations. Exposure to ionizing radiation in pregnancy occurs relatively frequently as a result of diagnostic medical or dental procedures and less frequently as therapy. The forms of ionizing radiation consist of high-energy external radiation like γ- or X-rays and lower-energy radiation like α and β particles emitted from radioisotopes. The biologic effects of these ionizing radiations are dose-, rate-, and source-dependent and include teratogenesis, mutagenesis, and carcinogenesis.

The amount of energy absorbed from an external ionizing radiation source has traditionally been measured in radiation-absorbed dose (rad) and for X-rays 1 rad is absorbed from 1 röntgen (R). More recently, the term gray (Gy) has come into common usage and is equivalent to 100 rad. α and β particles derived from radioisotopes yield higher rates of energy transferred to tissue and the term radiation-equivalent measurement (REM) reflects the difference in efficacy of these sources to produce damage. One REM is based on 1 rad of absorbed X-ray and a sievert (Sv) is equivalent to 100 REM.

Medical diagnostic radiation with exposure to <10 rad has little or no teratogenic effect and at doses <5 rad poses to risk to the developing embryo. Much higher doses (>50 rad) are required to produce fetal malformations in animals, including humans. The developing CNS appears to be the most vulnerable organ and microcephaly, microphthalmia, cataracts, retinal pigment changes, and mental retardation are the fetal anomalies which have been attributed to these very high doses of γ- or X-rays. Other organs and structures appear to be relatively insensitive to γ- or X-rays, perhaps due to the regenerative capacity in these tissues. In light of this, it is estimated, but not established, that a radiation dose of 10–25 rad to the fetus during the first 6 weeks post-conception increases the risk of an anomaly by an additional 0.5% over the background rate of 3–5% in nonexposed gestations. Prior to implantation, mammalian embryos are minimally sensitive to the teratogenic and growth-reducing effects of high-dose radiation exposure: if any effect at all occurs, it is increased early pregnancy loss. After about the 16th week postconception the only reported effect of ionizing radiation on the fetus has been related to the potential for leukemia in exposed individuals. In general, doses <10 rad increase the chance of leukemia from a background rate of 1:3000 to 1:2000.

Most diagnostic radiation studies deliver ≤5 rad to the mother and only a small fraction of any dose is delivered to the developing embryo or fetus. If the abdomen is shielded, the dose may be negligible. For example, an upper and lower gastrointestinal series, an intravenous pyelography, and a lower pelvic study would together deliver a total of <3 rad to the fetus. Thus, in most cases, women exposed to diagnostic radiation can be counseled that the risk is extremely small. Therefore, under ordinary circumstances, it is only therapeutic levels of radiation which present a significant risk to the fetus. In these cases counseling must be more precise and take into account the source of radiation, the dose rate, and the specific time of gestation during which therapy was being administered.

Nonionizing radiation exposures occur from a large variety of sources including ultrasound equipment, video display terminals, microwave devices, magnetic resonance imagers, and electric power lines. While there remains some debate as to whether or not some of these types of exposures have detrimental health consequences with long-term exposures in adults, there is no evidence that they have any teratogenic effects in humans. Patients who have concerns regarding such exposures should receive sympathetic and thoughtful counseling to assuage their fears.

High levels of thermal energy (heat) during embryogenesis have been suggested as having a teratogenic effect in humans. However, no conclusive evidence has yet been presented to support this contention. While there have been defects produced in animals by elevations of core temperature, in humans no consistent pattern of anomalies has yet been established. Moreover, in many case reports the maternal hyperthermia was due to infections of unknown etiology, confounding causality. A recent study which relied on self-reporting of hot-tubs or sauna use, or fevers and neural tube defects, suggested that the relative risk for neural tube defects was doubled when there was a history of these heat exposures. However, the level of hyperthermia and the duration of exposure were not quantitated, which complicates accurate counseling. Unfortunately, the lay press has heightened maternal anxiety by popularizing the notion that hot-tubs, saunas, and even electric blankets are now established teratogens. Patients who present with concern due to possible hyperthermic episodes in the first trimester should receive assurance that the absolute risk is low and they should be offered maternal serum α-fetoprotein testing with ultrasonographic evaluation for fetal malformations in the second trimester.

SUGGESTED READING

BRENT RL. Radiation teratogenesis. *Teratology* 1980;21:281.

BRUNELL PA. Fetal and neonatal varicella-zoster infections. *Semin Perinatol* 1983; 7:47.

HANSON JL. Teratogenetic agents. In: Emery AE, Rimoin DL, eds. *Principles and Practice of Medical Genetics*. 2nd edn. Edinburgh: Churchill Livingstone, 1990;183.

HEINONEN OP, STONE D, SHAPIRO S. *Birth Defects and Drugs in Pregnancy*. Littleton, CO: Publishing Sciences Group, 1977.

JONES KL, SMITH DW, ULLELAND N, *et al*. Pattern of malformation in offspring of chronic alcoholic mothers. *Lancet* 1973;1:1267.

MILUNSKY A, ULCICKAS M, ROTHMAN KJ, *et al*. Maternal heat exposure and neural tube defects. *JAMA* 1992;268:882.

42

Gestational age assessment

CHARLES J. MACRI & JEFFREY S. GREENSPOON

Knowledge of the correct gestational age is essential for the proper management of pregnancy. Some antenatal tests require accurate pregnancy dating for the correct interpretation, e.g., maternal serum α-fetoprotein. Other tests are performed at specific times during the antepartum period, e.g., amniocentesis for fetal karyotype or glucose screening for gestational diabetes. Accurate dating of pregnancy by early or mid-trimester ultrasound revealed that 80% of pregnancies that were postterm by menstrual dating actually had inaccurate dating and, therefore, did not require antepartum surveillance for postdates. Especially if postterm pregnancy is managed with induction of labor, then it is critical to date pregnancy correctly.

Human gestation lasts 280 days from the first day of the last menstrual period, assuming a 28-day menstrual cycle, or 266 days from ovulation. The gestational age can be determined from the first day of the last menstrual period when a woman has regular menses and has not used oral contraceptives (which can delay ovulation) in the preceding 2 months. Naegele's rule predicts that the estimated date of confinement (EDC) is equal to the first day of the last menstrual period plus 7 days minus 3 months. This method subtracts a time interval of 85 days from the length of a year in days in order to determine when the gestation will be 280 days in length. If ovulation is timed or a woman undergoes assisted transfer of zygotes or embryo transfer, these events may be used to predict the EDC reliably.

If a woman does not have regular ovulatory cycles or if she was using oral contraceptives during the 2 months prior to her last menstrual per-

Table 42.1 Criteria for fetal maturity prior to repeat elective delivery. Adapted from the American College of Obstetricians and Gynecologists

---

In a pregnancy that is at least 39 weeks' duration from the last menstrual period with normal menstrual cycles and no immediate antecedent use of oral contraceptives, fetal maturity can be assumed if one of the following clinical criteria for estimating gestational age is supported by at least one of the following laboratory determinations. If criteria are not met, amniotic fluid analysis for fetal lung maturity should be performed prior to elective induction or cesarean delivery.

Clinical criteria
1 Fetal heart tones have been documented for at least 20 weeks by nonelectronic fetoscope (DeLee) or at least 30 weeks by Doppler
2 Uterine size has been established by pelvic examination prior to 16 weeks of gestation

Laboratory determinations
1 Thirty-six weeks have elapsed since a positive serum or urine human chorionic gonadotropin pregnancy test
2 Ultrasound:
   (a) Measurement based on the crown–rump length obtained between 6 and 12 weeks of gestation
   (b) Other ultrasound confirmation of gestational age obtained before 24 weeks of gestation

---

iod, ovulation might have been delayed, and her menstrual dates might be incorrect. The gestational age of her pregnancy must be established using other criteria.

A pregnancy with excellent obstetric dates meets the criteria that have been proposed by the American College of Obstetricians and Gynecologists (Table 42.1). A patient who does not meet these criteria has "poor" dates.

Uterine size estimated by an experienced examiner correlates well with gestational age during the first 16 weeks of pregnancy. This can be taught as described by Fox.

Fetal heart tones (FHTs) can be heard by Doppler technique as early as 8–10 weeks. Hertz *et al.* reported first hearing FHTs by nonelectronic (DeLee) stethoscope at a median of 21 weeks; the mean gestational age was 22 weeks because the data were skewed by some excessively delayed recordings of FHTs. Andersen *et al.* reported first hearing with the DeLee stethoscope FHTs at a mean gestational age of 20.5 weeks, whereas Jimenez *et al.* reported first hearing FHTs at a mean gestational age of 17.1 weeks.

Some other clinical parameters have been used in the past to determine gestational age, although they are not reliable enough to be used to establish fetal maturity.

Table 42.2 Gestational age as estimated from the crown–rump length. From MacGregor *et al.*

Crown–rump length (cm)	Gestational age (weeks + days)		
	MacGregor *et al.*	Robinson & Fleming	Drumm *et al.*
1.0	7 + 5	7 + 0	6 + 6
1.1	7 + 6	7 + 1	7 + 1
1.2	8 + 0	7 + 3	7 + 2
1.3	8 + 1	7 + 4	7 + 3
1.4	8 + 1	7 + 5	7 + 4
1.5	8 + 2	7 + 6	7 + 5
1.6	8 + 3	8 + 0	7 + 6
1.7	8 + 4	8 + 1	8 + 0
1.8	8 + 5	8 + 2	8 + 1
1.9	8 + 5	8 + 3	8 + 2
2.0	8 + 6	8 + 4	8 + 3
2.1	9 + 0	8 + 5	8 + 4
2.2	9 + 1	8 + 6	8 + 5
2.3	9 + 1	8 + 6	8 + 6
2.4	9 + 2	9 + 0	9 + 0
2.5	9 + 3	9 + 1	9 + 1
2.6	9 + 4	9 + 2	9 + 2
2.7	9 + 4	9 + 3	9 + 3
2.8	9 + 5	9 + 3	9 + 3
2.9	9 + 6	9 + 4	9 + 4
3.0	9 + 6	9 + 5	9 + 5
3.1	10 + 0	9 + 6	9 + 6
3.2	10 + 1	9 + 6	10 + 0
3.3	10 + 2	10 + 0	10 + 0
3.4	10 + 2	10 + 1	10 + 1
3.5	10 + 3	10 + 1	10 + 2
3.6	10 + 4	10 + 2	10 + 3
3.7	10 + 4	10 + 3	10 + 3
3.8	10 + 5	10 + 3	10 + 4
3.9	10 + 6	10 + 4	10 + 5
4.0	10 + 6	10 + 5	10 + 5
4.1	11 + 0	10 + 5	10 + 6
4.2	11 + 1	10 + 6	11 + 0
4.3	11 + 1	11 + 0	11 + 0
4.4	11 + 2	11 + 0	11 + 1
4.5	11 + 3	11 + 1	11 + 2
4.6	11 + 3	11 + 1	11 + 2
4.7	11 + 4	11 + 2	11 + 3
4.8	11 + 5	11 + 3	11 + 4
4.9	11 + 5	11 + 3	11 + 4
5.0	11 + 6	11 + 4	11 + 5
5.1	12 + 0	11 + 4	11 + 5

Continued on p. 260.

Table 42.2 *Continued*

Crown–rump length (cm)	Gestational age (weeks + days)		
	MacGregor *et al.*	Robinson & Fleming	Drumm *et al.*
5.2	12 + 0	11 + 5	11 + 6
5.3	12 + 1	11 + 5	12 + 0
5.4	12 + 1	11 + 6	12 + 0
5.5	12 + 2	11 + 6	12 + 1
5.6	12 + 3	12 + 0	12 + 2
5.7	12 + 3	12 + 1	12 + 2
5.8	12 + 4	12 + 1	12 + 3
5.9	12 + 4	12 + 2	12 + 3
6.0	12 + 5	12 + 2	12 + 4
6.1	12 + 6	12 + 3	12 + 5
6.2	12 + 6	12 + 3	12 + 5
6.3	13 + 0	12 + 4	12 + 6
6.4	13 + 0	12 + 4	12 + 6
6.5	13 + 1	12 + 5	13 + 0
6.6	13 + 2	12 + 5	13 + 0

Hertz *et al.* demonstrated that fetal movement (quickening) was first perceived by nulliparas at a mean of 18.6 weeks, and in multiparas at a mean of 18.4 weeks. Andersen *et al.* noted that multiparas perceived quickening at a mean of 17 weeks and nulliparas perceived it 1–2 weeks later. The patient may recall quickening because it is an emotionally important event during her pregnancy.

Fundal height corresponds to the menstrual age between 18 and 30 weeks in most patients. It is measured in centimeters by a tape measure from the symphysis pubis to the top of the fundus. Andersen *et al.* found that the fundus reached the umbilicus at a mean gestational age of 19.9 weeks (± a standard deviation of 14.9 days). Jimenez and colleagues performed a longitudinal study and reported that the fundus reached the umbilicus at a mean gestational age of 16.6 weeks (± a standard deviation of 6 days).

Ultrasound is the most reliable method to determine gestational age. When the gestational age is determined by crown–rump length measurement, the estimated gestational age has a 95% confidence interval that is ±5 days (Table 42.2). Later in pregnancy, the 95% confidence interval is wider. By obtaining the arithmetic average of the four commonly measured parameters biparietal diameter, head circumference, abdominal circumference, and femur length, one can estimate gestational age more accurately than by using single parameters (Table 42.3). If a

Table 42.3 Estimated fetal age based on biparietal diameter, head circumference, abdominal circumference, and femur length. From Hadlock *et al.*

Menstrual age (weeks)	Biparietal diameter (cm)*	Head circumference (cm)†	Abdominal circumference (cm)‡	Femur length (cm)§
12.0	1.7	6.8	4.6	0.7
12.5	1.9	7.5	5.3	0.9
13.0	2.1	8.2	6.0	1.1
13.5	2.3	8.9	6.7	1.2
14.0	2.5	9.7	7.3	1.4
14.5	2.7	10.4	8.0	1.6
15.0	2.9	11.0	8.6	1.7
15.5	3.1	11.7	9.3	1.9
16.0	3.2	12.4	9.9	2.0
16.5	3.4	13.1	10.6	2.2
17.0	3.6	13.8	11.2	2.4
17.5	3.8	14.4	11.9	2.5
18.0	3.9	15.1	12.5	2.7
18.5	4.1	15.8	13.1	2.8
19.0	4.3	16.4	13.7	3.0
19.5	4.5	17.0	14.4	3.1
20.0	4.6	17.7	15.0	3.3
20.5	4.8	18.3	15.6	3.4
21.0	5.0	18.9	16.2	3.5
21.5	5.1	19.5	16.8	3.7
22.0	5.3	20.1	17.4	3.8
22.5	5.5	20.7	17.9	4.0
23.0	5.6	21.3	18.5	4.1
23.5	5.8	21.9	19.1	4.2
24.0	5.9	22.4	19.7	4.4
24.5	6.1	23.0	20.2	4.5
25.0	6.2	23.5	20.8	4.6
25.5	6.4	24.1	21.3	4.7
26.0	6.5	24.6	21.9	4.9
26.5	6.7	25.1	22.4	5.0
27.0	6.8	25.6	23.0	5.1
27.5	6.9	26.1	23.5	5.2
28.0	7.1	26.6	24.0	5.4
28.5	7.2	27.1	24.6	5.5
29.0	7.3	27.5	25.1	5.6
29.5	7.5	28.0	25.6	5.7
30.0	7.6	28.4	26.1	5.8
30.5	7.7	28.8	26.6	5.9
31.0	7.8	29.3	27.1	6.0
31.5	7.9	29.7	27.6	6.1

Continued on p. 262.

Table 42.3 *Continued*

Menstrual age (weeks)	Biparietal diameter (cm)*	Head circumference (cm)†	Abdominal circumference (cm)‡	Femur length (cm)§
32.0	8.1	30.1	28.1	6.2
32.5	8.2	30.4	28.6	6.3
33.0	8.3	30.8	29.1	6.4
33.5	8.4	31.2	29.5	6.5
34.0	8.5	31.5	30.0	6.6
34.5	8.6	31.8	30.5	6.7
35.0	8.7	32.2	30.9	6.8
35.5	8.8	32.5	31.4	6.9
36.0	8.9	32.8	31.8	7.0
36.5	8.9	33.0	32.3	7.1
37.0	9.0	33.3	32.7	7.2
37.5	9.1	33.5	33.2	7.3
38.0	9.2	33.8	33.6	7.4
38.5	9.2	34.0	34.0	7.4
39.0	9.3	34.2	34.4	7.5
39.5	9.4	34.4	34.8	7.6
40.0	9.4	34.6	35.3	7.7

*BPD = $-3.08 + 0.41$ (MA) $- 0.000061$ MA^3; $r^2 = 97.6\%$; 1 SD = 3 mm.
†HC = $-11.48 + 1.56$ (MA) $- 0.0002548$ MA^3; $r^2 = 98.1\%$; 1 SD = 1 cm.
‡AC = $-13.3 + 1.61$ (MA) $- 0.00998$ MA^2; $r^2 = 97.2\%$; 1 SD = 1.34 cm.
§FL = $-3.91 + 0.427$ (MA) $- 0.0034$ MA^2; $r^2 = 97.5\%$; 1 SD = 3 mm.
BPD, Biparietal diameter; MA, menstrual age; HC, head circumference; AC, abdominal circumference; FL, femur length.

parameter is known to be affected by a fetal condition, e.g., abdominal circumference in a poorly controlled diabetic patient, the parameter should not be included with those used to determine gestational age.

Figure 42.1 shows the gestational age as estimated from the presence of fetal structures on transvaginal ultrasound examination. Table 42.2 shows the gestational age as estimated from the crown–rump length. Table 42.3 shows the gestational age as estimated from fetal structures.

When the menstrual dates are within the variation of the ultrasound examination, it is appropriate to accept the menstrual dates (Fig. 42.1).

SUGGESTED READING

AMERICAN COLLEGE OF OBSTETRICIANS AND GYNECOLOGISTS. *Committee Opinion.* Number 77. Washington DC: ACOG, 1990.
ANDERSEN HF, JOHNSON TR Jr, BARCLAY ML, FLORA JD Jr. Gestational age

Weeks of gestation	4	5	6	7	8	9	10	11	12
Gestational sac only	100								
Yolk sac	0	91	100						
Fetal pole with heart motion	0	0	86	100					
Single ventricle	0	0	6	82	70	25	0	0	0
Falx	0	0	0	0	30	75	100	100	100
Midgut herniation	0	0	0	0	100	100	100	50	0
Total cases	6	11	15	17	10	13	15	11	6

Percentage of Embryonic Structures Present or Absent

☐ Structure present ▢ Structure absent

Fig. 42.1 Summary of detection of six embryonic structures in the first trimester of pregnancy. **Bold line** differentiates weeks of gestation in which the majority of embryos/fetuses displayed change in ultrasonographic appearance. From Warren *et al.*

assessment. I. Analysis of individual clinical observations. *Am J Obstet Gynecol* 1981;139:173–177.

ANDERSEN HF, JOHNSON TR Jr, FLORA JD Jr, BARCLAY ML. Gestational age assessment. II. Prediction from combined clinical observations. *Am J Obstet Gynecol* 1981;140:770–774.

FOX GN. Teaching first trimester uterine sizing. *J Fam Pract* 1885;21:400–401.

HADLOCK FP, DETER RL, HARRIST RB, PARK SK. Estimating fetal age; computer-assisted analysis of multiple fetal growth parameters. *Radiology* 1984;152:497–501.

HADLOCK FP, HARRIST RB, SHAH YP, KING DE, PARK SK, SHARMAN RS. Estimating fetal age using multiple parameters: a prospective evaluation in a racially mixed population. *Am J Obstet Gynecol* 1987;156:955–957.

HANNAH ME, HANNAH WJ, HELLMANN J, HEWSON S, MILNER R, WILLIAN A, AND THE CANADIAN MULTICENTER POST-TERM PREGNANCY TRIAL GROUP. Induction of labor as compared with serial antenatal monitoring in post-term pregnancy: a randomized controlled trial. *N Engl J Med* 1992;326:1587–1592.

HERTZ RH, SOKOL RJ, KNOKE JD, ROSEN MG, CHIK L, HIRSCH VJ. Clinical estimation of gestational age: rules for avoiding preterm delivery. *Am J Obstet Gynecol* 1978;131:395–402.

JIMENEZ JM, TYSON JE, REISCH JS. Clinical measures of gestational age in normal pregnancies. *Obstet Gynecol* 1983;61:438–443.

KRAMER MS, MCLEAN FH, BOYD ME, USHER RH. The validity of gestational age estimation by menstrual dating in term, preterm, and postterm gestations. *JAMA* 1988;260:3306–3308.

MacGregor SN, Tamura RK, Sabbagha RE, Minogue JP, Gibson ME, Hoffman DI. Underestimation of gestational age by conventional crown–rump length dating curves. *Obstet Gynecol* 1987;70:344–348.

Warren WB, Timor-Tritsch I, Peisner DB, Raju S, Rosen MG. Dating the early pregnancy by sequential appearance of embryonic structures. *Am J Obstet Gynecol* 1989;161:747–753.

43

Wound infections

ALAN FISHMAN

Operative wound infections have been a continuous complication of clinical practice since the very first surgical procedures were performed, and are clearly documented in medical literature dating back to the 16th century. While the frequency, prognosis, and pathogenesis of surgical wound infections have been significantly altered by antibiotics and modern surgical technique, lowering the incidence of wound infections provides an ongoing challenge for the practitioner. Abdominal wound infections following cesarean delivery or gynecologic surgery account for significant increases in the length and cost of hospitalization, and in overall patient morbidity. The total cost of an infected wound has been estimated to be as high as $30 000/case. The increased cost of wound infections is mostly due to prolonged hospital stay, but other costs, including antibiotics, supplies, additional surgical procedures, and prolonged disability from work, all contribute.

Cesarean delivery is one of the most common operations in the USA and carries a higher rate of wound infections than most abdominal surgical procedures. Reviews of abdominal surgery in general have revealed wound infection rates in the 5–7% range. Hysterectomy, the most common major gynecologic procedure, has a 6% infection rate, while reports for cesarean delivery reveal an average wound infection rate of 10%. Part of the difficulty in discussing the incidence of wound infections is that different investigators have differing opinions as to what constitutes a wound infection. Some authors rely on bacteriologic results; however, many wound infections may not yield positive cultures due to antibiotic therapy or inadequate culture technique. Conversely, many wounds are colonized with bacteria, so a positive culture is not necessarily pathologic. For the purposes of this discussion wound infection is defined as any collection of serous fluid, purulent material, or blood that requires drainage or drains spontaneously. This definition is more clinically oriented since it accounts for all of the conditions that will result in an open wound after surgery, even if there is no bacteriologic evidence of wound infection.

Surgical wounds can be divided into categories based on the type of procedure, and the likelihood of subsequent infection. The wound classification scheme adopted by the American College of Surgeons is as follows.

Clean wound (1.7% infection rate): gastrointestinal, genitourinary, or respiratory tracts are not entered, no inflammation is encountered, and there is no break in aseptic technique.

Clean contaminated wound (10% infection rate): uninfected gastrointestinal, genitourinary, or respiratory tracts are entered without spillage. Included are procedures that enter into the vagina. Cesarean delivery with ruptured membranes is included in this group.

Contaminated wound (20% infection rate): acute inflammation is encountered, or a major break in aseptic technique occurs, or gross spillage from the gastrointestinal tract occurs. Incisions into an infected genitourinary tract or a cesarean delivery with chorioamnionitis would be included in this category.

Dirty wound (30% infection rate): presence of pus, perforated viscus, or wounds caused by traumatic injury are classified as dirty wounds. The main dirty wounds that obstetrician/gynecologists encounter are ruptured appendix or ruptured tuboovarian abscess.

Risk factors and prevention

Risk factors for the development of wound infection have been well defined in the surgical literature. Cruse and Foord looked prospectively at more than 23 000 patients over a 5-year period. They identified eight major risk factors, including age, obesity, bacterial contamination of the wound, operating time, use of drains, duration of preoperative hospitalization, break in the surgeon's gloves, and shaving the hair at the surgical site. Other investigators have looked at specific risk factors for infection after cesarean delivery. These have been shown to include duration of labor, interval from rupture of the membranes to delivery, number of vaginal exams, and duration of internal monitoring. It is no coincidence that these risk factors are also associated with chorioamnionitis.

The two major determinants for the development of a wound infection are the size of the bacterial inoculum, and the resistance of the patient. In obstetrics and gynecology the primary endogenous sources of bacteria are the abdominal skin and the vagina. The importance of these endogenous contamination sources is apparent when we look at the progression from a 2% infection rate in clean cases to a 30% rate in dirty cases. Since there are large amounts of normal flora in the vagina and on the skin it is especially important for adequate surgical preparation for any procedure. Specific steps in the preparation of the patient for surgery that can minimize the risk of infection include:

1   all bacterial infections, excluding ones for which the surgery is being performed, should be eradicated before the procedure if possible;

2   hair removal should only be done if the hair directly interferes with the surgical procedures, and should be done with atraumatic clippers, depilatory agents, or scissors, and not by a razor;

3   the extended operative field should be scrubbed and covered (painted) with an antiseptic solution;

4   the vagina must be prepped for any procedure that will likely enter the vagina;

5   nonpermeable, disposable drapes which expose only the operative field should be used.

Specific surgical techniques and principles that can reduce the incidence of wound infections include:

1   gentle handling of the tissue;

2   meticulous hemostasis;

3   minimizing the presence of foreign body, i.e., suture material;

4   elimination of dead space;

5   Scarpa's fascia may be reapproximated but, in general, suture material should be kept to a minimum in closing the subcutaneous tissues or in securing hemostasis;

6   the old surgical axiom, "approximation not strangulation," retains its validity, especially with regard to fascial closure;

7   electrocautery should be used with care, and the surgeon must keep in mind that reduced operative time and blood loss need to be balanced against increased tissue devitalization and increased potential for infection;

8   closed suction drains, through their own separate incisions, may be used to reduce the accumulation of serosanguineous fluids.

The condition of the wound greatly influences local resistance to infection. It takes a minimum of 10^5 bacteria/ml to produce infection in otherwise healthy tissues but the presence of foreign bodies or hematomas reduces the minimum inoculum size required to produce infection by a factor of 10 000.

Clinical presentation

Wound infections can be divided into early-onset and late-onset subsets. The vast majority of wound infections become apparent between post-operative days 4 and 7. These so-called late-onset infections usually present with swollen, erythematous, and draining wounds, with or without fever. The early-onset wounds present during the first 48 h postoperatively. An English study by Moir-Bussy that looked at post-cesarean wounds reported that approximately 20% of infections in this series were early wound infections and the remainder were late infections.

Early wound infections usually present with fever, and a margin of discoloration around the incision. This margin may be a spreading cellulitis or, rarely, a margin of necrosis representing necrotizing fasciitis. Early-onset wound infections are frequently the result of a single organism, most commonly group A or B *Streptococcus*, *Staphylococcus*, or *Clostridium perfringens*. Culture of the wound either by biopsy of the wound edge or by aspiration is important for these aggressive infections. Treatment of these infections consists of thorough debridement of all nonviable tissue, and parenteral antibiotic therapy. If a superficial cellulitis is present, antibiotic therapy should consist of a penicillinase-resistant penicillin such as oxacillin or dicloxacillin. If a clostridial infection is present the cellulitis is usually accompanied by a watery discharge. These symptoms may or may not be associated with the classical findings of bronze-colored skin, and crepitus.

Late-onset wound infections usually present with swelling, erythema, and drainage from the incision. Treatment for such wounds basically consists of incision and drainage. Even in the presence of fever, antibiotics are not usually required unless there are signs of superficial cellulitis present around the wound margins. Once the wound is opened and thoroughly debrided, the patient's symptoms of pain and fever should rapidly abate within a 24-h period. If the patient remains febrile after this time, broad-spectrum antibiotic therapy aimed at mixed flora should be instituted. Unlike the case with early-onset wound infections, which are usually single-organism infections, late-onset infections are often mixed bacteria, and aerobes and anaerobes must be covered if antibiotics become necessary.

Management of open wounds

Incisional wounds that are classified as contaminated or dirty should not be closed primarily. These wounds can either be closed by delayed primary closure or left open to granulate secondarily. Delayed primary closure is preferable since secondary closure takes an average of 8 weeks to heal completely, with poorer cosmetic results. If the wound is to be left open postoperatively, a fine-mesh gauze such as burn gauze is packed into the open wound and covered with a sterile dressing in the operating room. This dressing can be left in place until the wound is to be evaluated for delayed primary closure on postoperative day 4 or 5, unless it becomes saturated with exudate, in which case the wound must be irrigated and repacked. Closure of such wounds should not be attempted prior to the fourth postoperative day due to higher risk of infection. When the incision is evaluated for closure the sides of the incision should look clean and viable. If there are any signs of inflammation or necrotic tissue, wound closure should be delayed. Delayed primary closure can be performed with sterile tape strips alone or with supportive monofilament vertical mattress sutures if necessary to accomplish good approximation of the wound edges.

Late-onset wound infections will usually present with copious serosanguineous or purulent drainage. Prior to opening, these wounds must be probed with a sterile cotton bud to ensure that the fascia is intact. If a defect in the fascia is noted, further opening and debridement should be carried out in the operating room, due to the possibility of evisceration, which represents a true surgical emergency. If the fascia is intact, the wound is opened and debridement of necrotic tissue should be performed under adequate anesthesia. Usually a short-acting sedative or narcotic and local anesthesia are adequate for wound care. Irrigation may be performed with either sterile saline alone or with a 1:1 solution of sterile saline and Dakin's solution. We favor the Dakin's solution initially as this helps keep the wound edges clean and free of necrotic tissue, and minimizes the amount of subsequent sharp debridement. After 1–2 weeks when healthy granulation tissue can be seen the Dakin's is replaced with plain sterile saline. Irrigation should be under pressure to aid in mechanical debridement. Adequate pressure can be developed by using an 18 G angiocath over a 60 ml syringe. Large-volume irrigation with a catheter-tip syringe is ineffective and therefore not recommended. After adequate debridement and irrigation, the wound should be packed with Kerlex, or Nu-gauze. The packing adjacent to the wound should be moistened while the remainder of the packing should be dry, and this packing should be changed 2–3 times/day. These open wounds may also be considered for secondary wound closure after they are granulating well (2–3 weeks). Secondary wound closure is performed using the same procedures described above for delayed primary closure. This procedure has been used with significant reduction in healing time when compared to traditional healing by secondary intention, but carries with it a 15–20% failure rate.

Various compounds have been evaluated for their potential to increase wound healing. An Egyptian medical document dated to 1700 BC describes how a variety of severe wounds were treated with a poultice of butter and honey. This combination became known as the balms of Gilead and has been in use for thousands of years by peoples around the world. At least two groups have studied granulated sugar or honey as a wound balm in the 1980s, and have found improved wound healing with these agents. Another ancient remedy has recently been studied for its potential to affect wound healing. Aloe vera dermal wound gel was applied to open wounds, and compared with standard open wound treatment. Schmidt and Greenspoon found that the use of Aloe vera was associated with a significant delay in wound healing. Other enzyme compounds or membranes that have been used for decubitus ulcers have been suggested, and are currently under investigation. Any agent that can be shown to increase wound healing will have broad clinical applications.

Parenteral antibiotic prophylaxis should be used with any operations that are associated with a high risk of infection, or are associated with life-threatening consequences if infection occurs, i.e., in immunocompromised patients. Except in cesarean deliveries where the antibiotic can be given after cord clamping, parenteral antibiotic prophylaxis should be started prior to surgery, preferably within the hour before the operation. Ideally a single preoperative dose of an antibiotic should be administered. Antibiotics administered to patients whose incisions are considered dirty or contaminated should be considered as therapeutic rather than prophylactic. Topical antibiotics should not be used at the time of primary closure of the operative incision; however, they may be considered for delayed primary closure since parenteral antibiotics do not achieve appreciable levels in granulation tissue.

Necrotizing fasciitis

Necrotizing fasciitis is a rare and life-threatening wound infection that requires prompt recognition and treatment for a good outcome. Early clinical signs are nonspecific, and may have subtle cutaneous findings. The infection is polymicrobial in origin and spreads very rapidly along the relatively ischemic fascial planes. There is extensive thrombosis of the penetrating vessels which causes the skin to become devascularized. The diagnosis should be suspected when the patient appears critically ill in the presence of a dusky or necrotic-looking wound margin. The extent of fascial necrosis is usually much greater than the skin appearance indicates. Definitive early diagnosis can be confirmed by frozen biopsy of the wound, obtained under local anesthesia; however, the diagnosis is not usually discovered until it becomes apparent that the patient needs extensive surgical debridement. The histologic findings necessary to make the diagnosis include necrosis of the superficial fascia, fibrinous thrombi of the blood vessels penetrating the fascia, infiltration of the deep dermis and fascia by polymorphonuclear leukocytes, and an absence of muscle involvement.

Treatment of necrotizing fasciitis is by aggressive excision of all affected tissue, parenteral antibiotic therapy, and supportive therapy. Prognosis is dependent on when in the disease process the diagnosis is made. Most series report a mortality rate in the 50% range.

SUGGESTED READING

CRUSE PJ, FOORD R. A five year prospective study of 23 649 wounds. *Arch Surg* 1973;107:206.

CRUSE PJ, FOORD R. A 10 year prospective study of 62 930 wounds. *Surg Clin North Am* 1980;60:27.

GIBBS RS, SWEET RL. *Infectious Diseases of the Female Genital Tract.* 2nd edn. Baltimore, MD: Williams & Wilkins, 1990:374.

GILSTRAP LC, CUNNINGHAM FG. The bacterial pathogenesis of infection following cesarean section. *Obstet Gynecol* 1979;53:1979.

LAC + USC WOMEN'S HOSPITAL PERI-OPERATIVE INCISION MANAGEMENT PROTOCOL. *J Perinat Neonatal Nurs* 1990;4:25.

LYKEGAARD-NIELSEN M, MOESGAARD F, LARSEN PN, HJORTRUP A. Early reclosure vs. conventional secondary intention of incisional abscesses. *Scand J Infect Dis* (Suppl) 1984;43:67.

SCHMIDT JM, GREENSPOON JS. Aloe vera dermal wound gel is associated with a delay in wound healing. *Obstet Gynecol* 1991;78:115.

STAMENKOVIC I, LEW PD. Early recognition of potentially fatal necrotizing fasciitis. The use of frozen section biopsy. *N Engl J Med* 1984;310:1737.

SWEET RL, LEDGER WJ. Puerperal infections: a two year review. *Am J Obstet Gynecol* 1973;117:1093.

PART 2

Perinatal Medicine

44

Pregnancy monitoring with α-fetoprotein

ARNOLD L. MEDEARIS

α-Fetoprotein (AFP) is the major circulating protein of the early fetus. Synthesis in the early fetus occurs mainly in the yolk sac. Later, most fetal AFP is produced from the fetal liver with smaller amounts produced in the gastrointestinal tract and placenta. Its physiologic function has best been described as immunoregulatory.

Normal concentrations of AFP

The concentration of AFP in the fetal tissue varies. In fetal blood it peaks at 2–3 mg/ml between the 13th and 15th weeks of gestation, after which the level decreases as pregnancy progresses. In the amniotic fluid AFP is present in microgram levels. Like fetal serum, the amniotic fluid levels reach a peak early in pregnancy and decline gradually during the second trimester. The major source of AFP in the amniotic fluid is likely fetal urine.

In other fetal tissues, the concentration of AFP reaches a peak between the 22nd and 32nd weeks of gestation and parallels circulating maternal levels. Maternal serum AFP (MSAFP) levels occur in nanogram amounts. In the mother, circulating AFP normally rises at the 7th week of gestation and reaches a peak around the 32nd week of pregnancy (range 27–36 weeks) and then declines toward term. The range of values around the mean is very wide, particularly in the last weeks of pregnancy. The normal nonpregnant adult basal level of AFP is approximately 25 ng/ml with a half-life of 1–6 days.

Measurement of AFP

Since AFP has no biologic activity, measurement depends on immunologic methods. Many techniques are used, including immunodiffusion, immunoelectrophoresis, hemagglutinin inhibition, enzyme-linked immunosorbent assay and, most commonly, by radioimmunoassay (RIA). A sensitive technique is required for detecting the nanogram amounts of AFP in pregnancy and RIA is the assay that provides the greatest degree of sensitivity. Because of the limited availability of highly purified protein for iodination and standardization, there are different ranges of normal in different laboratories, and this must be borne in mind when interpreting results. Measurement of MSAFP is calculated in multiples of the median (MOM). This method allows for comparison among laboratory standards.

Medical conditions other than pregnancy can cause changes in serum AFP. Primary carcinoma of the liver (hepatoma) and some germ cell tumors in women lead to elevation of blood AFP. The increase presumably reflects the tendency of dedifferentiated cells to return biochemically to the embryonic state. Elevation of AFP levels may be found in some nonneoplastic conditions of the liver. Although rare, the possibility of an extrauterine source of AFP production should always be considered in the differential diagnosis of increased levels of AFP during pregnancy, particularly when no fetal abnormality is identified.

Abnormally high MSAFP

The detection of neural-tube defects by measuring abnormally high values of AFP in maternal serum was initially the primary use of this screening test. Later, it was shown that when the maternal serum AFP values are low there is an increased incidence of fetal aneuploidy. Pregnancy screening with AFP for high (neural-tube defects) and low levels of serum AFP (fetal trisomy) will be discussed.

To minimize the incidence of results that are either false-positive (high levels with a normal fetus) or false-negative (normal levels with an affected fetus) in the determination of serum AFP levels, the selection of the normal range is critical. Setting a high level reduces false-positive rates in the detection of neural-tube defects but also reduces the number of cases detected. Setting a lower level improves the detection rate at the expense of an increasing false-positive ratio.

False-negative results arise from the fact that the range of normal values in affected cases overlaps the normal range. Technical errors can also occur. Up to 20% of all mothers whose fetuses have open neural-tube defects may have a normal serum AFP value. Failure of detection will not lead to termination of a normal pregnancy, but false-positive results may. Therefore, the reasons for false-positive results are important to remember. They are: (1) overlap of the upper end of the normal range with the lower end of the abnormal range; (2) technical errors in estimation; (3) multiple pregnancy; (4) concurrent maternal liver disease or neoplastic process secreting AFP; (5) collection of blood samples after amniocentesis, which can cause fetal maternal bleeding and consequently elevates MSAFP; and (6) inaccurate gestational age assessment.

Careful histories must be obtained from each patient as MSAFP is affected by a variety of factors. For example, diabetic patients have been shown to have a lower threshold level of AFP for the detection of neural-tube defects. Maternal weight and race also affect thresholds. These factors must be considered when evaluating the raw level of AFP.

Careful attention to physical examination and the use of diagnostic ultrasound eliminates many of the reasons for false-positive results. An extremely important point, which cannot be overemphasized in evaluating both high and low AFP levels, is the accurate dating of the gestation. A careful history combined with a physical exam and, if indicated, an ultrasound examination should be used to obtain an accurate estimate of gestational age. The optimal time for sampling of MSAFP is at 15–20 weeks' gestation. AFP is increasing during this time and false-positive results may occur if the pregnancy is >2 weeks from the initial assessment.

Elevated MSAFP levels in the second trimester lead to the detection of >80% of neural tube defects. In closed spina bifida, AFP levels are usually normal or only slightly increased. Because serum measurements of AFP are only a screen for neural tube defects and other malformations, obtaining an abnormal value in pregnancy dictates the use of ultrasound and possibly amniocentesis to evaluate further the findings. If a high MSAFP (>2.5 MOM for singleton pregnancy) or a very high MSAFP (>3.5 MOM for singleton pregnancy) is obtained, a detailed ultrasound examination must be carried out to confirm the gestational age. Often patients are uncertain as to the date of their last menstrual period and high values may simply be reflecting the patient being further along in pregnancy. In addition, multiple pregnancies have higher normal mean values of MSAFP (twins, high AFP >4.5 MOM and very high >5.5 MOM). Elevated levels of MSAFP in the second trimester screening can identify pregnancies with anencephaly with >95% accuracy, open spina bifida with >85% accuracy, and other structural fetal anomalies can be detected with varying degrees of accuracy.

The source of increased amniotic fluid AFP is presumably leakage of the fetal cerebrospinal fluid or transudation from fetal capillaries directly exposed to the amniotic fluid. The source of the elevated maternal serum levels of AFP is presumably amniotic fluid absorbed through the fetal membranes. Amniotic fluid analysis for AFP levels is important in cases at increased risk for neural-tube defects, patients who have a neural-tube defect, or who have had a previous pregnancy with a neural-tube defect. The risk of a neural-tube defect is 3–5 times higher in this group than among normal women.

Follow-up for abnormally high MSAFP

Ultrasound for a high MSAFP should diagnose anencephaly with 100% accuracy, eliminating the need for amniocentesis. Remaining neural-tube defects are identified with approximately 95% accuracy. Maternal size, fetal size, fetal position, location, type, and size of the defect affect the diagnostic accuracy of ultrasound in clinical cases.

Amniocentesis for the measurement of amniotic fluid AFP and a detailed ultrasound examination by an experienced ultrasonographer should be performed as the confirmatory steps in detection of a neural-tube defect. In addition, obtaining a fetal karyotype is important in delineating syndromes associated with neural-tube defects.

Elevated levels of amniotic fluid AFP have been observed in encephalocele, hydrocephalus, esophageal atresia, tetralogy of Fallot, congenital nephrosis, Turner syndrome (45,X monosomy), cystic hygromas, omphalocele, gastroschisis, and ventral wall defects. In particular, the detection of defects of the fetal abdominal wall has been a major benefit of MSAFP screening.

The identification of a small neural-tube defect is difficult. The ultrasound signs suggesting a neural-tube defect, however, have been helpful. These signs include the "lemon" sign – irregular shape of the fetal head – and the "banana" sign, suggesting a herniation of the cerebellum with an open neural-tube defect. When there is a raised AFP level in the amniotic fluid with or without an obvious neural-tube defect, other tests can be carried out to help explain the raised value. The most commonly used ancillary test is acetylcholinesterase in amniotic fluid as assessed by gel electrophoresis technique. Acetylcholinesterase is a neurotransmitter identified in amniotic fluid. A specific band of acetylcholinesterase is found in the presence of a neural-tube defect. A patient with raised AFP values and positive acetylcholinesterase and no ultrasound evidence of neural-tube defect should be evaluated by centers with special competence in the detection of neural-tube defects.

MSAFP levels may be increased in association with fetal death occurring between 20 and 36 weeks' gestation. It has not been determined whether there is a consistent rise in AFP just before fetal death. The cause is probably a disturbance of the placenta site.

High levels of AFP in patients with no evidence of congenital abnormalities have been associated with increased pregnancy loss in the late second and early third trimester. These patients are at increased perinatal risk for premature delivery and/or possible growth retardation. The etiology of these findings is unclear, but may be associated with bleeding, vaginal or intraamniotic, or a higher incidence of maternal medical complications in these patients. Further studies are being undertaken to delineate preventable causes of the adverse outcome in patients with high AFP and otherwise normal fetal findings.

Abnormally low MSAFP

In 1984 Merkatz *et al.* described the association between low MSAFP and fetal aneuploidy. Many subsequent publications confirmed this observation. AFP screening programs now evaluate patients in whom the level of MSAFP is significantly below the median. In the initial study, patients with an MSAFP of 0.4 MOM or lower had a much higher risk of having a baby with trisomy 21. This approach has been modified to an adjusted cut-off value based on the maternal age. In patients in whom, for example, the MOM MSAFP value is 0.7, but their age is 34, their risk for having a Down's syndrome baby is adjusted to that of a woman aged 35. Clearly, while the risk of having a Down's syndrome baby is greater over age 35, most aneuploidies are born to women less than age 35. Twenty percent of fetal aneuploidy can be detected with this approach. Similar to screening for elevated MSAFP, it is best to use the same gestational age range, 15–20 weeks.

More recently, it has been determined that by utilization of β subunit human chorionic gonadotropin (hCG) and unconjugated estriol in combination with MSAFP, the detection of women carrying fetuses with trisomy 21 can be increased to approximately 60%. A complex algorithm of the biochemical values is used to identify patients at risk for Down's syndrome. In these patients, the MSAFP and unconjugated estriol are low, while the β subunit hCG shows approximately a twofold rise. Utilization of this screening technique also may be helpful in identifying patients carrying trisomy 18 fetuses where all values measured are very low.

This "triple screen" will provide a more sensitive method of detection of fetal chromosomal abnormalities than has been previously available with just the AFP. The use of combination biochemical testing is now standard clinical practice. A diagram for the assessment of the patient with an abnormal triple screen is seen in Fig. 44.1. The cut-off for evaluation in a screening program (1/190 in Fig. 44.1) can be altered to increase or decrease the risk of Down's syndrome. Increases in the ratio (e.g., 1/270) will result in a decrease in the number of cases diagnosed and a

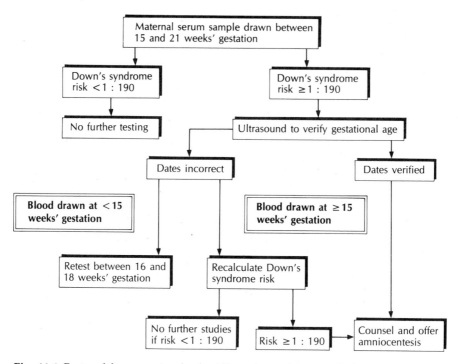

Fig. 44.1 Protocol for screening for fetal Down's syndrome with the use of measurements of α-fetoprotein, unconjugated estriol, and chorionic gonadotropin in maternal serum. From Haddow *et al.*

decrease in the number of aminocenteses performed. Optimal curves for balancing the number of procedures and the number of cases diagnosed must be determined for each screening program.

The utilization of maternal age (35 years) for screening for patients with chromosomal abnormalities detects only 20% of Down syndrome, with the remaining infants being born to women under 35. From a public health management viewpoint, it may be of greater benefit to screen all women with triple screen, including those 35 or over, and only offer amniocentesis to those who show a positive marker. Identified patients at increased risk should receive genetic counseling before proceeding to amniocentesis. As with assessment of increased AFP, an accurate estimation of gestational age is extremely important in the interpretation of results.

Summary

The use of MSAFP as a screen for both neural-tube defects and fetal aneuploidy is now standard clinical practice. The importance of this surveillance is not only the identification of neural-tube defects, but also the detection of other major congenital anomalies, including defects of the fetal abdominal wall.

When MSAFP is elevated, ultrasound examination must be performed to rule out erroneous dating, fetal death, multiple pregnancy, or congenital malformations associated with these elevations. If these cannot be detected, amniocentesis should be carried out under ultrasound guidance to measure levels of amniotic fluid AFP. When findings are normal, assurance can be given to the patient that her fetus is at a very low risk to have a detectable anomaly. When the amniotic AFP is elevated, the chance that the fetus will be abnormal is increased. Both ultrasound and ancillary biochemical testing, such as amniotic fluid acetylcholinesterase measurement, should be completed to confirm the diagnosis. With the combined use of amniotic fluid AFP, acetylcholinesterase, and ultrasound, the rate of detection of open spina bifida in the second trimester of pregnancy should approach 100% in patients at increased risk for neural-tube defects because of an abnormal MSAFP screen or a history of previous neural-tube defect. The relationship between abnormal MSAFP levels and high-risk pregnancy conditions is just beginning to be defined. In addition, the ability to screen women for fetal aneuploidy using MSAFP in conjunction with β-hCG with or without estriol (multiple marker screen) increases the rate of detection of Down's syndrome babies to 55–60% in patients undergoing subsequent aminocentesis.

SUGGESTED READING

BURTON BK, PRINS GS, VERP MS. A prospective trial of prenatal screening for Down syndrome by means of maternal serum α-fetoprotein, human chorionic gonadotrophin, and unconjugated estriol. *Am J Obstet Gynecol* 1993;169:526–530.

CRANDALL BR. The identification of development defects: the AFP model. In: Crandall BF, Brazier MAB, Eds. *Prevention of Neural Tube Defects: The Role of Alpha-Fetoprotein.* New York: Academic Press, 1978.

FERGUSON-SMITH MA, GIBSON AM, WHITFIELD CR, *et al.* Amniocentesis and the alpha fetoprotein screening programme. *Lancet* 1979;1:39.

HADDOW JE, PALOMAKI GE, KNIGHT GJ, *et al.* Prenatal screening for Down's syndrome with use of maternal serum markers. *N Engl J Med* 1992;327:588.

KJESSLER B, JOHANSSON SGO, LIOBJORK G, *et al.* Alpha fetoprotein levels in maternal serum in relation to pregnancy outcome in 7158 pregnant women prospectively investigated during their 14th–20th week post last menstrual period. *Acta Obstet Gynecol Scand* 1977;69:25.

MACRI JN, WEISS RR. Prenatal serum alpha fetoprotein screening for neural tube defects. *Obstet Gynecol* 1982;59:633.

MERKATZ IR, NITOWSKY HM, MACRI JN, JOHNSON WE. An association between low maternal serum alpha-fetoprotein (AFP) and fetal chromosomal abnormalities. *Am J Obstet Gynecol* 1984;148:886.

MILUNSKY A, ALPERT E, WEFF RK, FRIGOLETTO F. Prenatal diagnosis of neural tube defects. IV. Maternal serum alpha fetoprotein screening. *Obstet Gynecol* 1980;55:60.

PHILLIPS OP, ELIAS S, SHULMAN LP, ANDERSEN RN, MORGAN CD, SIMPSON JL. Maternal serum screening for fetal Down's syndrome in women less than 35 years of age using alpha-fetoprotein, hCG, and unconjugated estriol: a prospective 2-year study. *Obstet Gynecol* 1992;80:353.

WALD NJ, KENNARD A, DENSEM JW, CUCKLE HS, CHARD T, BUTLER L. Antenatal maternal serum screening for Down's syndrome: results of a demonstration project. *Br Med J* 1992;305:391.

WHYLEY GA, WARD H, HARDY NR. Alpha-fetoprotein levels in amniotic fluid in pregnancies complicated by Rhesus iso-immunization. *J Obstet Gynaecol Br Commonw* 1974;81:459.

45

Antepartum fetal evaluation

ARNOLD L. MEDEARIS

The purpose of this chapter is to familiarize the obstetrician with the current testing approach used at Los Angeles County–University of Southern California Medical Center. The primary goal of antepartum fetal surveillance is to identify the fetus at risk of death *in utero* and, secondarily, to identify the fetus at risk for fetal distress and abnormal neonatal outcome. Historically, the initial focus was on fetal heart rate (FHR) alteration during uterine contractions (contraction stress test). Later, uterine contractions were not required for evaluation of the fetal status, which led to the development of the nonstress test (NST). In the 1980s, real-time ultrasonography enabled the physician to assess additional factors in the evaluation of the intrauterine condition of the fetus, including fetal breathing, fetal movement, fetal tone, and amniotic fluid volume. These observations of fetal status were added into antepartum fetal surveillance schemes. This approach, know as the fetal biophysical profile (BPP), combines the NST with real-time ultrasound parameters. Recently, clinical attention has focused on the NST and amniotic fluid volume as indicators of fetal status before the onset of labor in the term and postterm pregnancy. Current fetal surveillance techniques should include some form of amniotic fluid volume assessment to predict reliably the fetus at risk of intrauterine death. Our primary fetal surveillance protocol is the NST in combination with a four-quadrant technique for amniotic fluid volume assessment, the amniotic fluid index (AFI). The complete BPP is used when the NST is nonreactive secondary to fetal immaturity.

Indications for fetal surveillance

The current indications for antepartum fetal surveillance, the gestational ages for starting testing, and the frequency of testing are illustrated in Table 45.1. Fetal surveillance begins customarily at or around 34 weeks' gestation. Depending on the clinical circumstances, fetal assessment may

Table 45.1 Current indications for antepartum fetal surveillance, the gestational age when testing is begun, and the frequency of testing

Indication	Gestational age	Frequency of testing
Medical problems		
Diabetes mellitus		
DMA1 (uncomplicated)	40 weeks (280 days)	Twice a week
DMA1 (complicated)	34 weeks (238 days)	Twice a week
DMA2-R	34 weeks (238 days)	Twice a week
Collagen vascular disease	34 weeks (238 days)	Twice a week
Cardiac disease	34 weeks (238 days)	Once a week
Chronic hypertension	34 weeks (238 days)	Twice a week
Renal disease	34 weeks (238 days)	Once a week
Thyroid disease	34 weeks (238 days)	Once a week
Sickle cell disease	34 weeks (238 days)	Once a week
Obstetric problems		
Abnormal fetal heart tones, arrhythmia, abnormal nonstress test	When diagnosed	One test at time of diagnosis. If normal, refer to clinic
Amniotic fluid		
Increased ≥24 cm	When diagnosed	Once a week
Decreased ≤5 cm	When diagnosed	Admit
Meconium-stained	When diagnosed	One test at time of diagnosis
Cholestasis of pregnancy	36 weeks (252 days)	Once a week
Pregnancy induced hypertension	When diagnosed	Twice a week
Intrauterine growth retardation – probable	When diagnosed	Twice a week
Intrauterine growth retardation – possible	When diagnosed	Once a week
Postdates	287–293 days	Once a week
	294 days	Twice a week
Previous stillborn	One week before previous loss or 34 weeks (238 days)	Once a week
Spontaneous premature rupture of membranes	When diagnosed	Daily

Continued

Table 45.1 *Continued*

Indication	Gestational age	Frequency of testing
Discordant twins: ≥20% difference in estimated fetal weight	When diagnosed	Twice a week
Rh disease	Individualize	Once a week

Additional criteria

1 The earliest that antepartum fetal surveillance will be initiated is an estimated fetal weight of ≥650 g or 25 weeks' gestational age
2 Whenever the condition for which antepartum testing was initiated is resolved or ruled out, testing will be cancelled
3 There are certain other conditions that may significantly increase the risk for the fetus. These include, but are not limited to: systemic lupus erythematosus, chronic hypertension, and complicated cases of diabetes mellitus. These cases will be individualized and antepartum testing may begin earlier

be initiated earlier, if the clinical situation warrants earlier testing, it is not begun until the fetus is potentially viable. Our institutional criteria are a gestational age of 25 weeks or greater or a sonographic estimated fetal weight of 750 g. In pregnancies complicated by post dates, diabetes mellitus, and intrauterine growth retardation, testing is done twice a week. All other patients undergo testing once a week unless clinical circumstances dictate more frequent testing.

Fetal surveillance criteria

A reactive FHR pattern is diagnosed when there are two or more FHR accelerations of at least 15 bpm lasting 15 s from the time the FHR leaves baseline until it returns during a 10 min moving window. A reactive NST within 7 days of delivery is recognized as a sign of fetal well being and carries a low probability of fetal demise or distress. Moreover, reactivity, whether spontaneous or evoked by acoustic or physical stimulation is associated with a favorable outcome. If an acceptable fetal heart acceleration is not observed during a 40 min observation period, the test is considered nonreactive. Fetuses who exhibit a nonreactive FHR pattern are at a greater risk of meconium stained amniotic fluid, cesarean delivery, cesarean delivery for fetal distress, and perinatal mortality than patients with a reactive test. The risk of perinatal mortality is 7–10 times higher among these fetuses.

Frequently, FHR decelerations will be observed during the performance of an NST. For management purposes, these FHR decelerations have been defined as decline in FHR of 30 bpm or more and lasting 30 s from the time the deceleration leaves the baseline until it returns. If a deceleration occurs immediately after an acceptable FHR acceleration (15 bpm by 15 s), it is not considered abnormal. The presence of prolonged FHR decelerations during an NST may suggest cord compression. The most common reasons for these decelerations are oligohydramnios, abnormal cord positions, or fetal anemia. Their presence represents a sign of potential fetal jeopardy and is associated with a greater risk of harm than a reactive NST without FHR decelerations. The possibility of aorto-caval supine hypotension must be ruled out when decelerations are seen. Late decelerations by spontaneous contractions are a possible indication of fetal compromise and must be evaluated if observed during antepartum testing.

Besides FHR assessment, our current protocol uses the AFI to assess the amniotic fluid volume. There are two techniques for the assessment of amniotic fluid. They include a single measurement of the largest vertical pocket of amniotic fluid or the summation of the largest vertical pockets from four quadrants of the uterus measured during real-time ultrasound examination. We use the four-quadrant technique in our testing pro-tocols. The uterus is divided in quadrants. The linea nigra divides the uterus into right and left halves and the umbilicus divides it into upper and lower halves. The ultrasound transducer is placed along the longitu-dinal axis of the mother perpendicular to the floor. The vertical diameter of the largest pocket in each quadrant is identified and measured. The total of all four quadrants is summed and the total represents the AFI. In a low-risk population the average AFI is 16.2 ± 5.3 cm. The amniotic fluid is considered decreased (oligohydramnios) whenever a patient has an AFI of ≤5.0 cm. Amniotic fluid is considered increased if the AFI ≥24.0 cm.

When the results of the AFI and the NST are compared, an inverse relationship between the AFI and the incidence of nonreactive NST and FHR decelerations is found. In the presence of a reactive NST, fetuses with sonographic evidence of oligohydramnios (AFI ≤5.0 cm) have a greater risk of perinatal morbidity. Patients with decreased AFI are more likely to develop fetal distress in labor than patients with a nonreactive NST.

The most common cause of nonreactive NST is fetal immaturity, and additional ultrasound observations that have been correlated with well-being are valuable in assessing the status of the fetus. The fetal BPP is used to supplement the NST whenever a nonreactive test is encountered. The components of the profile include breathing, movement, tone, am-niotic fluid volume, and the NST. For each component that is present, the fetus receives two points. A score of 8 or 10 is considered normal. A profile score of 6 is considered suspicious and warrants repeat testing within 24 h. A fetal BPP score of 4 or less is associated with a substantial risk of adverse outcome and patients are considered for delivery.

Current testing and management protocol

All patients who present for antepartum fetal surveillance are evaluated with NST and AFI. The management of these patients is based not only on the results of testing but also on the clinical findings in the patient at the time of testing. Once the monitor is applied, a baseline FHR is established for approximately 10 min. If no FHR accelerations are apparent, fetal acoustic stimulation is applied using the external auditory larynx. The use of acoustic stimulation has increased the incidence of reactive tests and shortened testing time, while providing an outcome comparable to that of fetuses with spontaneous FHR accelerations. Those patients who exhibit a reactive test and a normal AFI (>5.0 cm) are tested either once or twice a week depending on their indication of testing (Table 45.1) Those patients with a nonreactive NST are evaluated with the remaining components of the fetal BPP. By using this approach, our total testing time is reduced. Moreover, this testing approach can be applied uniformly to a high-risk population regardless of gestational age and the indication for testing.

The criteria for consideration of delivery are listed in Table 45.2. These intervention criteria apply to term, postterm, or fetuses with evidence of fetal lung maturity. In the preterm fetus, management is individualized depending on the status of fetal lung maturity and the circumstances of the case. Nonetheless, the preterm fetus who manifests these findings is at a greater risk of harm. Continuous electronic fetal monitoring should be considered, if delivery is not feasible. In the term fetus, the indications for intervention include the presence of oligohydramnios (AFI ≤5.0 cm), a FHR bradycardia or a fetal BPP score ≤4. For term fetuses who exhibit a FHR deceleration during their NST and have a normal AFI (>5.0 cm), repeat testing in 3–4 days is recommended. If at the time of repeat testing in the term fetus the FHR deceleration pattern persists, consideration should be given to delivery by a trial of labor. In postdate pregnancy, however, the fetus who exhibits a FHR deceleration is at a significant risk of meconium-stained amniotic fluid, fetal distress, and perinatal death.

Table 45.2 Delivery is considered under these circumstances

Amniotic fluid index ≤5.0 cm
Prolonged fetal heart rate bradycardia
Biophysical profile score ≤4
Postdate pregnancy with fetal heart rate deceleration

Under these circumstances, induction for labor with oxytocin and continuous fetal surveillance during labor have reduced the fetal morbidity associated with this FHR pattern in postdate pregnancy.

Results

By combining the NST with the AFI as the primary form of fetal surveillance, the risk of fetal death has been reduced in our patient population. Over the last 5 years our antepartum fetal stillbirth rate in patients tested within 4 days of delivery has been less than 2:1000.

SUGGESTED READING

BOCHNER CJ, MEDEARIS AL, OAKES GK, et al. Antepartum predictors of fetal distress in postterm pregnancy. *Am J Obstet Gynecol* 1987;157:353–358.

MANNING FA, MORRISON I, LANGE IR, et al. Fetal assessment based on fetal biophysical profile scoring: experience in 12 620 referred high-risk pregnancies – I. Perinatal mortality by frequency and etiology. *Am J Obstet Gynecol* 1985;151: 343.

MEDEARIS AL. Detection and management of intrauterine growth retardation: an American approach. In: Chervanck FA, Isaacson GC, Campbell S, eds. *Texbook of Ultrasound in Obstetrics and Gynecology*, vol 2. Boston/Toronto/London: Little, Brown & Company, 1993:1437–1440.

PLATT LD, PAUL RH, PHELAN J, et al. Fifteen years of experience with antepartum fetal testing. *Am J Obstet Gynecol* 1987;156:1509–1515.

RUTHERFORD SE, PHELAN JP, SMITH CV, et al. The four-quadrant assessment of amniotic fluid volume: an adjunct to antepartum fetal heart rate testing. *Obstet Gynecol* 1987;70:353–356.

SMITH CV, PHELAN JP, PLATT LD, et al. Fetal acoustic stimulation testing. (The FAS-TEST.) II. A randomized clinical comparison with the nonstress test. *Am J Obstet Gynecol* 1986;155:131.

46

Fetal lung maturity

SIRI L. KJOS

Fetal lung development occurs on three levels: anatomic, biochemical, and physiologic. Each level has its own time-course of maturation. Understanding these interrelationships provides the basis for antenatal evaluation of fetal lung maturity.

Anatomic development

1 *Pseudoglandular stage* (conception through 16 weeks' gestation): beginning as a budding of the foregut into the mesoderm, the pulmonary tree forms by dichotomous division to form a mature bronchial tree by the 16th week of gestation.

2 *Canalicular stage* (17 through 24 weeks): the primitive airways begin to canalize, and the glandular-appearing cells of the second stage become cuboidal. Paralleling the airway branching is the pulmonary vascular branching.

3 *Alveolar stage* (24 weeks' gestation to term): further division continues, forming respiratory bronchioles that form saccules in which alveoli appear. Alveolar development continues into the second year of life.

A parallel branching and growth of the pulmonary vasculature occurs in step with the respiratory tree. At the end of the canalicular stage, arterial branching is complete. Rapid proliferation of capillaries also develops around the alveolar ducts. Thus, by 24–25 weeks' gestation, anatomic development is complete for effective gas exchange.

Biochemical development

At approximately 24 weeks' gestation, type 2 pneumocytes containing lamellar bodies appear. These lamellar bodies contain surfactant and are secreted directly into the alveolar space. Surfactant acts as a detergent, that spreads over the alveolar surface, creates an interface with the air that lowers alveolar surface tension, and prevents the alveoli from collapsing during expiration. This follows from the law of LaPlace: $P = 2T/r$ (where P = the retractive force, T = surface tension and r = the radius of the alveolus). During expiration, as the radius of the alveolus decreases, increased force is required to prevent atelectasis. Surfactant counteracts this process by lowering the surface tension.

Surfactant is a collective term for a group of compounds produced by the type 2 pneumocytes. These compounds are composed primarily of phospholipids. At term, the major phospholipids are composed of phosphatidylcholine (lecithin), 70–80%; phosphatidylglycerol (PG), 10–15%; and phosphatidylinositol (PI), 5–10%. Phospholipids are composed of a glycerol backbone with two fatty-acid chains and a third molecule that specifically identifies each phospholipid. In lecithin, this is phosphatidylcholine; PG contains glycerol, and PI contains myoinositol. Furthermore, the most active of the lecithins is dipalmitoylphosphatidylcholine (DPPC), in which both fatty-acid chains are saturated palmitic acids. The various phospholipids follow a sequential but variable time-course in appearance, which permits measurement of a lung profile to evaluate maturity.

Physiologic development

Fetal breathing movements are visible during the last half of gestation. This activity most likely corresponds to a maturing of the central nervous system and is associated with low-voltage, high-frequency electrocortical activity. By about 34 weeks' gestation, the healthy fetus spends over half of its time "breathing" at a rate of 30–60 "breaths" per minute. Fetal breathing movements also may play a role in the generation of fetal lung fluid. The fetus produces an ultrafiltrate lung fluid that differs from amniotic fluid and plasma and that changes in electrolyte composition with advancing gestational age. This most likely reflects the increased alveolar secretion of surfactant.

Methods to determine lung maturity

Indirect evaluation of fetal maturity

Many different fetal parameters have been studied in an attempt to ascertain fetal lung maturity (Table 46.1). These can be grouped into indirect

Table 46.1 Methods to determine fetal lung maturity

Test	Maturity value	Requirements	Comments
Ultrasound	BPD >9.2 cm and/or grade III placenta and/or FL >7.3 cm	Negative diabetes screen	Used to evaluate term fetus with poor dating criteria
Shake test (Luminex foam stability index)	Stable ring 1:2 dilution (>47% FSI)	Uncontaminated specimen	Rapid, inexpensive, simple FSI: semiqualitative
Microviscosimetry (FELMA)	$P <0.320$	Uncontaminated specimen	Use with caution in premature gestations
Optical density (OD_{650})	>0.150	Uncontaminated specimen	Rapid, inexpensive, simple, semiqualitative: transitional values (0.100–0.149)
Rapid slide agglutination PG (Amnistat-FLM/AFLM)	+PG (+4 or +2)	Not affected by blood or meconium	Rapid, simple. May be contaminated by bacterial PG from vaginal secretions
Lung profile 2-D thin-layer chromatography			Time- and labor-intensive, expensive
L:S ratio	>2.0 (in most laboratories)	Uncontaminated	Use with caution in diabetic patients. May use 1-D TLC
% DPPC (lecithin)	>50%	Affected by blood	Reaches maturity at 35–36 weeks. Major surface active phospholipid
% PI	Variable	Affected by blood	Rises from 30 weeks to 25%, then decreases

Continued on p. 292.

Table 46.1 *Continued*

Test	Maturity value	Requirements	Comments
% PG	>2%	Not affected by blood, meconium, or vaginal secretions	Represents final maturation stage in surfactant. Presence assures protection from RDS in diabetes

BPD, Biparietal diameter; FL, femur length; FSI, foam stability index; PG, phosphatidylglycerol; 2-D, two-dimensional; L:S, lecithin:sphingomyelin; 1-D, one-dimensional; TLC, thin-layer chromatography; DPPC, dipalmitoylphosphatidylcholine; PI, phosphatidylinositol; RDS, respiratory distress syndrome.

determinants of fetal age (either biochemical or biophysical) and direct determinants which measure pulmonary surfactant. Indirect biochemical parameters measured from amniotic fluid (creatinine, cortisol, prolactin, amniotic fluid osmolarity, and bilirubin) have been correlated with fetal maturity but have unacceptably high false-positive and false-negative rates that limit their utility.

The most useful indirect assessment of fetal maturity is ultrasound determination of fetal weight and gestational age. It is most effectively used to establish correct gestational age when performed prior to 24 weeks' gestational age. Frigoletto reported that a pregnancy that reaches 38 weeks' gestation, as determined by early clinical markers or early ultrasound, has virtually no risk of respiratory distress syndrome (RDS). Neither amniocentesis nor a repeat ultrasound is necessary. Often, however, a patient presents late for her prenatal care and requires assessment of fetal maturity.

Several investigators have used cephalometry and/or placental grading to evaluate the term fetus when considering elective induction of labor or repeat cesarean section. They found that when either a biparietal diameter (BPD) was ≥9.3 cm or there was a grade III placenta present, no cases of RDS were found.

We employ the schema prospectively studied by Golde for timing elective cesarean sections. First, all women are screened for diabetes using a random 1-h postglucose blood sugar level of <140 mg%. For levels <140 mg%, diabetes is excluded. Patients then receive ultrasound assessment of maturity. A BPD >9.2 cm and/or the presence of a grade III placenta indicates fetal maturity. If these requirements are met, no amniocentesis is performed, and the patient is delivered using these criteria. At this institution, 247 nondiabetic patients met the ultrasound screening criteria for maturity. Only one case of mild RDS occurred. Recently, we evaluated the use of femur length ≥ 7.3 cm as additional evidence of maturity and found this method also to be highly predictive. In summary, ultrasound measurements can be used successfully to evaluate term nondiabetic gestations for elective delivery.

Direct evaluation of pulmonary surfactant

All screening and semiquantitative methods for surfactant evaluation are based on an understanding of the anatomic and biochemical maturational process of the fetal lung.

Lecithin:sphingomyelin ratio

In a method first developed by Gluck, lipids in the amniotic fluid are separated by one-dimensional, thin-layer chromatography (TLC) into lecithin and sphingomyelin. Lecithin or phosphatidylcholine is the primary surface active phospholipid. Concentrations of lecithin and sphingomyelin can be measured by densitometry or planiometry and are reported as a ratio (L:S). The concentrations of lecithin gradually increase until term, with sphingomyelin remaining constant. This results in a gradual increase in the L:S ratio until term. At approximately 34–36 weeks of gestation the L:S ratio equals or exceeds 2.0, indicating fetal lung maturation. With a ratio of ≥ 2.0, only a 2.0–7.4% incidence of RDS has been reported. The higher false-positive rate has been reported in earlier gestational ages and in pregnancies complicated by diabetes. Contamination by blood, meconium, and vaginal secretions can alter results unpredictably.

Lung profile

Essentially a modification of the L:S ratio, the lung profile employs two-dimensional chromatography to separate the components of phospholipids. In addition to the L:S ratio, the lung profile measures the percentage of DPPC, PI, and PG. Although there are several modifications in technique (acetone precipitation, lamellar body fraction analysis), the lung profile has become the "gold standard" for assessment of fetal lung maturity. It can be performed on contaminated samples and allows a more accurate prediction of "transitional" profiles, where the L:S ratio is 1.5–1.9 and no PG is present. Infants with these ratios have approximately a 15–20% risk of RDS, which is usually mild in its presentation.

The most active and largest component of surfactant, DPPC, gradually increases with gestational age, generally achieving a maturity value of 50% and higher after 34 weeks. PI follows a variable time-course, rising until approximately 35–36 weeks' gestation to a 25% value and then decreasing until term, but it has no maturity value. PG appears at approximately 35 weeks and continues to rise to term. Its presence (>2%) indicates the final stage of biochemical maturity and is associated with a L:S ratio greater than 2.0. For this reason, the presence of PG is also a predictor of fetal lung maturity. The drawback to the lung profile is the time and laboratory sophistication required. It is usually only available in referral centers and during weekday work hours.

Screening test

Shake test (foam stability index)

Based on the ability of surfactant to form highly stable surface films able to support foam in the presence of ethanol, a simple 15-min test for lung maturity was developed. This test uses gross visualization. A mature test is defined as a stable ring of foam in a 1:2 dilution with ethanol. The false-positive rate is only about 1.0%, but this test is associated with a high false-negative rate and must be performed on uncontaminated specimens. A commercial modification and simplification of this technique is the Luminex foam stability index consisting of six premeasured wells that contain different amounts of ethanol. This test allows a semi-quantification of maturity, with a value of 47 or greater considered mature and not associated with RDS. Values <45 are strongly predictive of RDS.

Optical density at 650 nm (OD_{650})

The absorbance of amniotic fluid at 650 nm is due primarily to the phospholipid turbidity and minimally to biologic pigments such as meconium, blood, and bilirubin. Investigators have demonstrated an optical density measurement ≥0.150 to be predictive of fetal lung maturity in healthy as well as in premature and diabetic pregnancies. Further work by Sbarra *et al.* has shown that OD_{650} reflects the actual concentration of lecithin, not simply the ratio. The drawback of this simple, rapid and inexpensive test is that the results are affected by fluid grossly contaminated with blood and meconium. Recently, Sbarra *et al.* demonstrated the validity of the OD_{650} using free-flowing, vaginally obtained amniotic fluid. Care must be taken to centrifuge the fluid at 2000 g for 10 min, as the rate and length of centrifugation affect absorbance values.

Microviscosimetry (FELMA)

Shinitzky *et al.* quantified the relationship between lipid microviscosity and surface tension using a fluorescent hydrocarbon probe, defined as the *P* value. The *P* value decreases with gestational age, and the fetus is considered mature when the *P* value is <0.320. A linear relationship between the decreasing *P* values and L:S ratios between 0.5 and 2.5 has been established. In term gestations, a *P* value <0.320 is highly predictive of lung maturity (93.8–100%), but a negative test has a low predictive value of maturity. The technique is rapid and simple, but it requires expensive equipment and uncontaminated specimens.

Rapid slide agglutination of PG (Amniostat FLM/AFLM)

An immunologic slide agglutination test for PG has been developed that requires only 0.1 ml of amniotic fluid and 15 min to perform. It is not affected by blood or meconium and correlates well with two-dimensional, TLC PG. A strongly positive PG by slide agglutination is predictive of the absence of RDS. PG is detected in only 50% of fetuses after 36 weeks' gestation and, therefore, accounts for the poor ability to predict RDS (15–35%). This test is suited for use in the patient with premature rupture of the membranes where accelerated fetal lung maturity often is reported to be present and the fluid is contaminated. It is also well suited for diabetic patients in whom the presence of PG indicates that RDS is not present.

Summary

In conclusion, most of the tests for fetal lung maturity have a very high predictive value for absence of RDS if the test indicates maturity (98–100%), but all share a lower predictive value for presence of RDS with a test that indicates immaturity (13–64%). Thus, they are used as screening tests. When screening tests are positive, there is usually no need for further testing.

It is critical, however, when developing a testing protocol to understand the limits of each test as well as the individual patient's situation, which demands knowledge of fetal lung maturity. With the exception of PG determination either by two-dimensional TLC or by rapid slide agglutination, all tests, including the L:S ratio, are altered by blood and meconium contamination. Vaginally obtained fluid has not been shown to alter testing if it is not grossly contaminated. Fluid extracted from peripads can be used to obtain amniotic fluid from patients with premature rupture of the membrane and has been demonstrated to yield valid L:S ratios and lung profiles. Although the rapid slide agglutination test for PG can be performed easily on all specimens, it should be remembered that PG is present in only 50% of samples by 37 weeks' gestation. In prematurity, the OD_{650} is extremely reliable (90%). Similar reliability of the foam stability index has been reported in preterm and growth-retarded fetuses. All screening laboratory tests should be performed in the hospital laboratory to insure quality control. One or more screening tests should be available on a 24-h basis.

At Los Angles County–University of Southern California Women's Hospital, nondiabetic patients who are candidates for elective delivery with poor dating criteria undergo an ultrasound evaluation for maturity. If the BPD is 9.2 cm or greater, if there is a grade III placenta, of if the femur length is 7.3 cm or greater, delivery is undertaken without amniocentesis. Patients without ultrasound criteria for maturity undergo amniocentesis. Maturity can be documented with a screening test such as an OD_{650}, Amniostat FLM/AFLM, or shake test. Immature test results require a lung profile. Pregnancies complicated by diabetes undergo amniocentesis when there is either poor dating criteria or poor glycemic control prior to elective delivery. RDS in infants of diabetic mothers as currently managed, with euglycemia controlled and early ultrasound dating, is an increasingly rare event.

On our labor floor, two screening tests are employed in assessing high-risk pregnancies on a 24-h basis. The OD_{650} is used with great reliability on uncontaminated specimens. The Amniostat FLM/AFLM is used primarily in cases of contaminated specimens and vaginally collected specimens. Clinical management decisions are based on the initial screening tests. Immature screening results are always followed up with a complete lung profile, which is only performed during weekday work hours. All specimens are evaluated by the pathology laboratory.

SUGGESTED READING

KJOS SL, WALTHER FJ, MONTORO M, PAUL RH, DIAZ F, STABLER M. Prevalence and etiology of respiratory distress in infants of diabetic mothers: predictive value of fetal maturation tests. *Am J Obstet Gynecol* 1990;163:898–903.

LIPSHITZ MB, WHYBREW WD, ANDERSON GD. Comparisons of the lumadex-foam stability index test, lecithin:sphingomyelin ratio and simple shake test for fetal lung maturity. *Obstet Gynecol* 1984;63:349.

SBARRA AJ, MICHLEWITZ H, SELVARAJ RJ, *et al.* Relation between optical density at 650 nm and L/S ratios. *Obstet Gynecol* 1977;50:723.

SBARRA AJ, CETRULO CL, SELVARAJ RJ, *et al.* Surfactants, L/S ratio, amniotic fluid optical density and fetal pulmonary maturity. *J Reprod Med* 1982;27:34.

SHINITZKY M, GOLDFISHER A, BRUCK A, *et al*. A new method for assessment of fetal lung maturity. *Br J Obstet Gynaecol* 1976;83:838.

TURNER RJ, READ JA. Practical use and efficiency of amniotic fluid OD650 as a predictor of fetal pulmonary maturity. *Obstet Gynecol* 1983;61:551.

47

Management of infants at risk of neonatal respiratory distress syndrome: the use of antenatal corticosteroids and neonatal surfactant therapy

SIRI L. KJOS

Premature birth prior to fetal lung maturity frequently results in hyaline membrane disease (HMD), a cause of neonatal respiratory distress syndrome (RDS) secondary to deficient surfactant production. Early symptoms of grunting, intercostal retractions, nasal flaring, and cyanosis are produced by the collapse of the alveoli during expiration, secondary to deficient surfactant. In severe cases, fatigue, hypoxia, acidosis, and eventual death may result. HMD accounts for 20% of all neonatal mortality. Its course is swift, with 92% of deaths due to HMD occurring within the first 4 days of life.

Investigation has been directed toward understanding the mechanism of lung maturity and the use of pharmacologic agents to induce surfactant production in premature fetuses. Current studies are examining the possible role of antenatal thyroid hormones, β-sympathomimetics, prolactin, and glucocorticoids in accelerating surfactant production. Postnatally the administration of exogenous surfactant has remarkably reduced the morbidity of RDS.

Mechanism of action of glucocorticoids

Mounting evidence suggests that glucocorticoids are involved in surfactant production and regulation. Fetal lung tissue contains 2–5 times the number of glucocorticoid receptor sites compared with fetal heart, liver, brain, muscle, and kidney tissue. Glucocorticoid receptors are present in lung tissue from the 12th gestational week. It is proposed that glucocorticoids bind to the type II alveolar cells to induce or increase surfactant production via the choline incorporation pathway system.

A qualitative difference in the fatty acid composition of phosphatidyl-choline is present in infants with hyaline membrane disease compared with infants free of disease. These fatty acids in phosphatidylcholine undergo a sequential maturational process, changing to the final, mature saturated palmitic acid (DPPC). Which controlling enzyme(s) could be induced or sequentially induced in lung maturation by glucocorticoids is not known, but many are thought to be affected. In rabbit fetuses injected with steroids compared with those injected with normal saline, the lung tissue of the cortisol-injected fetuses showed a higher lecithin and cholino-phosphotransferase content. This was probably secondary to *de novo* induction of an enzyme. Others have demonstrated an increase in lung compliance in monkeys after betamethasone administration, but no increase in lecithin concentration was shown. The steroid benefit was secondary to structural changes in connective tissue.

Clinical trials of corticosteroids

In 1972, the first double-blind clinical trial was performed by Liggins & Howie. They reported that the betamethasone-treated group had a decrease in RDS to 9.0%, compared with the control group rate of 25.8%. Furthermore, this difference was confined largely to gestations of 32 weeks or less, in which delivery had occurred 24 h or longer after the administration of betamethasone. No advantage of steroid therapy was found 7 days after injection or after 34 weeks' gestation. These findings were confirmed in a large retrospective study in which a significant reduction in RDS occurred only in infants weighing 751–1250 g, who were delivered more than 48 h after receiving steroids. Several other studies have addressed this question with conflicting results. Caution must be used in data analysis, as gestational age, maternal and fetal diagnosis, adequate population size in each subgroup, and timing of delivery all affect outcome.

The National Institutes of Health (NIH) sponsored Collaborative Group on Antenatal Steroid Therapy addressed this question in a blinded, randomized trial of 696 pregnant women at risk for preterm delivery. A reduction in RDS was seen in infants born after 24 h of steroid therapy (12.8 versus 18.0%). In further analysis of subgroups, the significant protective benefit was limited to female infants, nonlaboring patients, and singleton gestations. No benefit was seen for male infants, pregnancy-induced hypertension, multiple gestations, laboring patients or those with premature ruptured membranes (PROM). No increase in postpartum or neonatal complications was noted in mothers receiving steroids or in their infants. Interestingly, the occurrence of RDS in both the steroid and placebo groups in this study was significantly less than the incidence predicted by earlier studies (25–80%). More recently, meta-analysis of 12 controlled trials involving over 3000 pregnancies found a 70% reduction in the development of neonatal RDS after corticosteroid administration among babies born between 24 h and 7 days after therapy. Additional secondary benefits of corticosteroid therapy were decreased risk of periventricular hemorrhage, necrotizing enterocolitis, and neurologic abnormalities.

The safety and efficacy of steroid administration in patients with preterm premature rupture of membranes (PPROM) has been addressed by several studies. Some reported a significantly increased rate of neonatal infection, septicemia, with no decrease in RDS. In contrast, other studies showed a reduction in RDS in patients with PROM who received steroids. A metaanalysis of five randomized controlled trials did demonstrate a decrease in RDS in infants born at 28–34 weeks of gestation to mothers with PROM. However, the authors clearly qualified the inference of their study by stating the significance is based on one of the five studies, which was of poor study design. When the problematic study was excluded, no benefit to steroid therapy could be demonstrated. The authors also found a significant increase in risk of maternal endometritis and a trend toward increased neonatal infections. Their summary, along with the conflicting literature, concludes that the safety and efficacy of corticosteroid therapy in PPROM patients has not been established.

Administration of steroids

Glucocorticoids have numerous and diversified physiologic effects. They have potent antiinflammatory and immunosuppressant effects as well as being diabetogenic and having a sodium retention capacity. Both dexamethasone and betamethasone are used preferentially over other glucocorticoids because of their equally low maternal:fetal gradients of 3:1, which allows lower maternal doses to be given to achieve sufficient fetal levels.

Ballard *et al.* studied fetal betamethasone levels (expressed in cortisol equivalents) following the usual 12 mg dose given twice, 24 h apart. Reassuringly, levels were comparable with those of physiologic stress in infants (i.e., with PROM and RDS), and they never exceeded three times that of normal levels. The half-life of betamethasone in the fetus is 14 h. By the third day after therapy, the fetus cortisol level returned to normal.

Betamethasone is administered as two 12 mg im doses given, 24 h apart. Dexamethasone is administered as four 5 mg im doses given every 12 h.

Long-term effect of corticosteroids

Glucocorticoid therapy for induction of lung maturity first began in the 1970s. A follow-up of 406 of the 696 patients enrolled in the NIH Collaborative Antenatal Steroid Study showed no differences in cognitive, motor, or neurologic function between the steroid and placebo group at 3 years of age. In a 5-year follow-up study of extremely-low-birth-weight infants (500–999 g) an increased survival was found in those receiving antenatal steroid therapy, with no increased risk of chronic illness or impaired neurodevelopment.

Caution should be noted based on several animal studies which have shown multisystemic adverse effects that include: (1) decreased organ weight and DNA content of brain, heart, lung, liver, pancreas, and adrenals; (2) decreased total cell number; (3) decreased central nervous system DNA synthesis and increased gliosis; (4) impaired myelination; (5) impaired immune response; and (6) increased thymic involution. Studies on rhesus monkeys given 2 mg im betamethasone from day 120 to day 133 of gestation and delivered 1 month later showed persistent steroid effects, as indicated by decreased organ weight. These effects are consistent with long-standing adrenal insufficiency. Although these are animal studies using different dosing regimens, they present serious questions regarding long-term use and effects of glucocorticoid in pregnancy.

Surfactant replacement therapy

In 1980, Fujiwara *et al.* first reported that the use of modified bovine surfactant markedly improved gas exchange in neonates with severe RDS. Subsequent large randomized clinical trials have demonstrated a reduction in oxygen requirements and mean airway pressures in infants treated prophylactically or symptomatically (requiring mechanical ventilation). Improved oxygenation with surfactant therapy resulted in decreased mortality, decreased RDS, and less chronic lung disease. These studies used preparations of either natural (from human amniotic fluid or cow, calf, or bovine lung) or synthetic surfactant. Currently two preparations are commercially available in the USA; Exosurf, an artificial surfactant, and Survanta, obtained from bovine lung.

Both preparations are administered via an endotracheal tube and can be given either prophylactically at birth, before the development of signs and symptoms of RDS, or after symptoms have developed. Their onset of action occurs immediately after administration, with the neonate requiring lower oxygen concentrations and lower ventilatory pressure. Repeated doses may be required as the effect may be transient.

The use of surfactant therapy in the neonate has been a major contribution to the increased survival in preterm infants. The most dramatic improvement is in the very preterm infant, 24–25 weeks' gestational age, in which current survival rates of 50–70% are not uncommon in tertiary neonatal centers. It is critical for the delivery of these infants to occur at hospitals offering surfactant therapy and experienced in neonatal intensive care.

Summary

The use of glucocorticoids should be restricted to patient groups shown to have maximal benefits: (1) fetuses at <34 weeks' gestation or weight of 900–1500 g; (2) fetuses with immature surfactant levels; and (3) patients in whom a delay in delivery of >24 h can be achieved. Steroid administration has no demonstrable benefit in infants delivered 7 days after steroid administration. Even though the NIH study found that the reduction in RDS appeared to be limited to female infants, singleton gestations, and nonlaboring patients, it is premature to add these as strict criteria necessary for steroid administration. Each case must be assessed individually. A review addressing this issue found that only 10.7% of threatened preterm deliveries were candidates for treatment with steroids. If steroids are administered to patients with preeclampsia or PPROM, extreme caution and close surveillance are mandatory. Glucocorticoids are contraindicated in diabetic patients.

At Los Angeles County–University of Southern California Women's Hospital, patients with threatened preterm deliveries undergo ultrasound evaluations to estimate gestational age and weight. Amniocentesis under ultrasound guidance is performed if possible, not only to document pulmonary status but to rule out occult amnionitis. Lung maturity and infection are obvious contraindications to steroid administration, as is a medical need for immediate delivery. Barring contraindications, corticosteroid therapy is given in selected patients at risk for preterm delivery and neonatal RDS (i.e., <34 weeks or absence of pulmonary maturity, delayed delivery >24 h, and no signs of infection). Tocolytics are instituted as needed. Close fetal surveillance is achieved by continuous external fetal heart rate monitoring and tocodynamometry. Consultation with the neonatologist is obtained antenatally to coordinate and optimize delivery and fetal care. Finally, traumatic or stressful labor and delivery are to be avoided in these fragile infants.

SUGGESTED READING

AVERY ME, AYLWARD G, CREASY R, *et al*. Update on prenatal steroid for prevention of respiratory distress: report of a conference, September 26–28, 1985. *Am J Obstet Gynecol* 1986;155:2.

BALLARD PL, GRANBERG P, BALLARD RA. Glucocorticoid levels in maternal and cord serum after prenatal betamethasone therapy to prevent respiratory distress syndrome. *J Clin Invest* 1975;56:1548.

BALLARD RA, CALLARD PL. Prenatal administration of betamethasone for prevention of respiratory distress syndrome. *J Pediatr* 1979;94:97.

BECK JC, JOHNSON JWC. Maternal administration of glucocorticoids. *Clin Obstet Gynecol* 1980;23:93.

COLLABORATIVE GROUP ON ANTENATAL STEROID THERAPY. Effects of antenatal dexamethasone administration in the infant: long-term follow-up. *J Pediatr* 1984;104:259–267.

CORBET A, BUCCIARELLI R, GOLDMAN S, *et al*. Decreased mortality rate among small premature infants treated at birth with a single dose of synthetic surfactant: a multicenter controlled trial. American Exosurf Pediatriac Study Group I. *J Pediatr* 1991;118:277.

CROWLEY P, CHALMERS I, KEIRSE MJ. The effects of corticosteroid administration before preterm delivery: an overview of the evidence from controlled trials. *Br J Obstet Gynaecol* 1990;97:11.

DOYLE LW, KITCHEN WH, FORD GW, *et al*. Antenatal steroid therapy and 5-year outcome of extremely low birth weight infants. *Obstet Gynecol* 1989;73:743.

EPSTEIN ME, FARREL PM, SPARKS JW, *et al*. Maternal betamethasone and fetal growth and development in the monkey. *Am J Obstet Gynecol* 1977;127:261.

FARRELL PM, WOOD RE. Epidemiology of hyaline membrane disease in the United States: analysis of national mortality statistics. *Pediatrics* 1976;58:167.

FARRELL PM, ZACHMAN RD. Induction of choline phosphotransferase and lecithin synthesis in the fetal lung by corticosteriods. *Science* 1973;179:279.

FUJIWARA T, MEATA H, CHIDA S, *et al*. Artificial surfactant therapy in hyaline membrane disease. *Lancet* 1980;1:55.

GARITE TJ, FREEMAN RK, LINZEY EM, *et al*. Prospective randomized study of corticosteroids in the management of premature rupture of the membranes and the mature gestation. *Am J Obstet Gynecol* 1981;141:598.

JOHNSON JWC, MITZNER W, LONDON WT, *et al*. Betamethasone and the rhesus fetus: multisystemic effects. *Am J Obstet Gynecol* 1979;133:677.

JOHNSON JWC, MITZNER W, BECK JC, *et al*. Long-term effects of betasone on fetal development. *Am J Obstet Gynecol* 1981;141:1053.

KENDIG JW, NOTTER RH, COX C, *et al*. A comparison of surfactant as immediate prophylaxis and as rescue therapy in newborns of less than 30 weeks gestation. *N Engl J Med* 1991;324:865.

LIGGINS GC, HOWIE RN. A controlled trial of antepartum glucocorticoid treatment for prevention of the respiratory distress syndrome in premature infants. *Pediatrics* 1972;50:515.

MERRITT TA, HALLMAN M, BERRY C, *et al*. Randomized, placebo-controlled trial of human surfactant given at birth versus rescue administration in very low birth weight infants with lung immaturity. *J Pediatr* 1991;118:581.

OHLSSON A. Treatments of preterm premature rupture of the membranes: a meta-analysis. *Am J Obstet Gynecol* 1989;160:890.

PHIBBS RH, BALLARD RA, CLEMENTS JA, *et al*. Initial clinical trial of EXOSURF, a protein-free synthetic surfactant, for the prophylaxis and early treatment of hyaline membrane disease. *Pediatrics* 1991;88:1.

SHELLEY SA, KOVACEVIC M, PACIGA JE, *et al*. Sequential changes of surfactant phosphatidylcholine in hyaline-membrane disease of the newborn. *N Engl J Med* 1979;300:112.

SIMPSON GF, HARBER GM. Use of β-methasone in management of preterm gestation with premature rupture of membranes. *Obstet Gynecol* 1985;66:168.

48

Fetal heart rate and uterine activity monitoring: what every practitioner must know about the equipment

RICHARD H. PAUL

Electronic fetal heart rate (FHR) monitoring has become an integral part of current obstetric practice. The basis and development of monitoring found its origins in the pioneer work of Hon who undertook the continuous intrapartum plotting of instantaneous FHR from the fetal electrocardiogram (FEKG). The assessment of fetal well-being, during both the antepartum and intrapartum period, relies almost exclusively on continuous FHR evaluation. In the antepartum period, primarily during the third trimester, the utilization of concepts developed from intrapartum observations led to the initial widespread use of contraction stress testing. Subsequently, observations in the nonstressed fetal state, in which the association between FHR acceleration and fetal movements was established, have proven to be a most valuable prognostic evaluator of the well fetus. Widespread use of intrapartum monitoring has resulted in a virtual disappearance of intrapartum fetal death and a probable decline in the occurrence of severe fetal asphyxia with its potential deleterious consequences. When used improperly, FHR monitoring is commonly blamed for the dramatic increase in cesarean births, often felt unnecessary. The initial concern regarding maternal febrile morbidity associated with direct intrapartum monitoring has not materialized. Only rare isolated instances of fetal trauma and sepsis have been reported as a result of scalp electrode applications. It would seem to many careproviders that the advantages of properly utilized fetal monitoring far outweigh the relative disadvantages.

The cardiotachometer

The basis of FHR determination lies in the instantaneous evaluation of cardiac cycles, whose length is inversely proportional to the FHR. Thus, a derived FHR is equal to 60 000 divided by the cycle interval in milliseconds. If the initial interval is 600 ms in the first cycle, the instantaneous rate would be displayed as 100 bpm; if the subsequent interval is 400 ms, the instantaneous rate would be 150 bpm and a subsequent 300 ms interval would be displayed as a 200 bpm rate. The FHR monitor calculates intervals between successive cardiac cycles and converts them into proportional voltage outputs which are displayed as specific FHRs on the strip chart recorder. In the simplest terms, the primary advantage that an electronic fetal monitor provides is that it can instantaneously calculate successive intervals and display a rate which otherwise must be averaged by the human ear. The electric and mechanical activities of the heart provide markers which serve to calculate cycle intervals. These successive intervals and the derived rate form the basis for display of continuous FHR patterns.

The direct (internal) system

The direct (internal) system involves the attachment of a small stainless steel spiral electrode, whose penetration depth is limited to 2 mm, into the presenting part of the fetus. This method of direct monitoring must necessarily occur with a cervical dilatation of at least 1–2 cm, following rupture of membranes, and only after the proposed application site on the presenting part is clearly identified. Caution is warranted when application is made in any unusual presentations such as breech, face, etc. Likewise, electrode application with known maternal infections, such as group B *Streptococcus*, HIV, and herpes, are contraindications to direct monitoring. Such patients can almost always be clinically monitored by external or indirect methods, as will be described.

The fetal electrode is bipolar with the penetrating spiral portion serving as one element and a secondary reference electrode which comes in contact with the maternal vaginal secretions. The two leads from the spiral electrode are connected to a ground plate which is usually attached to the mother's thigh. The bipolar electrode senses differential voltages between the two electrodes and, as a result, obtains the FEKG as well as other electric signals conducted to the application site.

Usually, the directly derived FEKG signal amplitude far exceeds the maternal EKG and is efficiently amplified and counted by the monitor. In the process of obtaining the fetal signal, an automatic gain-control amplifier is used in order to amplify the FEKG signal complex sufficiently to trigger the cardiotachometer. At times, when a fetus has died, this same automatic gain-control feature may amplify the maternal EKG and lead to the erroneous assumption that the heart rate displayed is that of the fetus. Unfortunately, this misinterpretation has led to inappropriate intervention due to erroneous diagnosis of fetal distress. The most precise FHR that may be calculated is derived from successive R waves of the FEKG which serve to trigger the cardiotachometer. This reference FHR is the "gold standard" against which all other heart rate methods must be judged. The evaluation of FHR variability of the heart rate is most precisely determined, both in a long-term and a short-term sense, from the directly derived FEKG and heart rate display.

Troubleshooting the direct system

Evaluation of the noisy or uninterpretable record

As noted above, the monitor derives the heart rate by measuring the interval between two successive signal triggers and converting it to an instantaneous rate. When the system is properly attached, the R wave of the FEKG serves as the repetitive trigger for the cardiotachometer. An improperly applied spiral electrode or loose ground plate may result in a low signal-to-noise ratio. When a low-amplitude FEKG and electric noise are simultaneously present, these signals will often lead to miscalculation of intervals, and widely fluctuating erroneous rates, or "noisy tracings" are recorded. In order to evaluate this problem, the first step is to auscultate the fetal heart tones and rule out a fetal arrhythmia. If an irregular rhythm is heard on auscultation, the diagnosis of fetal arrhythmia is established. If the fetal rhythm is regular, one is dealing with a system problem. If the system is suspect, one should check the electrode placement and ground plate application and reattach these if necessary. A defective electrode or malfunctioning monitor is rarely the problem. The problem is nearly always a loose connection or poor electrode application. Rapid intermittent changes in heart rate every three to five beats may represent a true fetal arrhythmia. The most commonly observed FHR arrhythmia is a premature ventricular contraction (PVC); this may be confirmed by evaluating the direct FEKG signal which may be obtained from an output in the rear of the monitor. Additionally, ultrasonic evaluation or echocardiography may be used to establish the origin and characteristics of the arrhythmia.

Evaluation of persistent bradycardia

The fetal monitor can measure only the time interval between successive triggers and cannot selectively discriminate between maternal and fetal R waves. If the spiral electrode is applied to the cervix or the vaginal mucosa, the monitor may display a maternal heart rate. In the case of the dead fetus mentioned above, maternal EKG complexes may be transmitted to the spiral electrode and the resultant recording of the maternal heart rate may be interpreted as fetal bradycardia and diagnosed as fetal distress. Legitimate causes of fetal bradycardia are rare and are most often related to a congenital heart block and at times structural defects. When a heart rate in the bradycardic range is encountered, it is wise to determine that it is indeed of fetal origin. This may be accomplished by simultaneous auscultation or recording of the maternal heart rate. Synchrony of audible signals would confirm that both are of maternal origin. Currently, the ready availability of real-time ultrasonic imaging of the fetal heart activity will unequivocally define the origin of a bradycardic heart rate.

The indirect (external) system

There are three common methods of indirect or external recording of the fetal heart rate. Two of these systems, Doppler ultrasound and phonocardiography, derive the heart rate from the mechanical activity of the heart. The Doppler system sends out ultrasonic energy and detects frequency shifts in the returning reflected waves from the moving heart structures, such as the ventricular wall, septum, or valves. The Doppler system is a very reliable means of obtaining a FHR signal; a coupling gel must be applied to the maternal abdomen to which the transducer is applied. The phonocardiogram detects the mechanical sound produced by the fetal heart and converts the intervals into a rate. This system is passive and does not require any preparation or coupling to the maternal skin on the abdomen. This technique is largely impractical due to its sensitivity to movements and interference produced by extraneous noise. With either system, the mechanical motion and sounds that provide the trigger signal may vary somewhat from one contractile cycle to the next. For example, valve motion may provide one trigger and the septum motion a slightly different trigger source. Thus, neither system provides absolute precision relating to beat-to-beat FHR variability on a short-term basis. A change in the relationship of either the Doppler or phonocardiogram transducer to the fetal heart, caused by either maternal or fetal movement, can result in signal loss. Because these movement events occur, most external systems must utilize some form of signal conditioning logic, or editing in the determination and presentation of rate. The essential function of fetal heart signal-processing is to enhance appearance while maintaining a reasonable representation of the actual or true FHR. The specific characteristics of editing logic will vary from one instrument to another and it is important that the users be particularly aware of the specific type of signal-processing used in their given machine. The currently used and reasonably reliable ultrasonic signal utilizes a process termed autocorrelation. This type of ultrasound signal-processing attempts to extract any recurring signal source from a background of relative signal noise. The process, given five or six successive signals, develops a template signal stored within the machine processor. Incoming signals are then compared to the existing template. If no incoming template-like signal is encountered within 1–2 s, the machine usually discontinues recording the FHR and the process starts again. With autocorrelation any consistently reflected signal can be counted. Thus, a transducer focused on the maternal aorta may reflect signals of maternal origin and present a heart rate (maternal) which could be erroneously confused as fetal. Here again, definition of the presence of fetal heart activity must be certain.

An additional potential pitfall that one may encounter with external systems is the confusion that may occur as a result of complex signal characteristics. In particular, it is possible through the editing and logic systems to display one-half of the actual rate or, in other cases, doubling of a low rate. FHRs below 100 bpm may result in double-counting, whereas rates above 180 bpm may be halved. In order to confirm the true rate, one may auscultate the fetal heart or undertake ultrasonic imaging to define the FHR. The tip-off that halving or doubling is occurring lies in observation of abrupt and rapid changes in the heart rate recording, which are not physiologic and should lead one to suspect machine-produced artifact.

The final method of external FHR recording utilizes the FEKG signal which is conducted to the surface of the maternal abdomen. The magnitude of this signal on the maternal abdomen is related to gestational age as well as fetal position. Electrodes are placed on the maternal abdomen and systematically moved until the largest FEKG complex is detected. This fetal signal is generally of much lower amplitude than the maternal EKG and thus a mixture of both EKG signals is derived by an abdominal EKG system. In order to produce the FHR, extensive logic and conditioning must be utilized. Cancellation of the maternal signal and various approaches have failed to make this approach practical. The theoretic advantage of such a system would be that one could accurately ascertain FHR beat-to-beat variability. Most monitors provide switches of defeating logic applications with external systems.

Troubleshooting the indirect system

The most frequent cause of an unsatisfactory external FHR record is the improper positioning of the transducer. This problem is usually easily corrected by merely moving the transducer to a position from which it can obtain an improved signal. Subsequently, the transducer may be fixed in this position and readjusted should the FHR tracing become unsatisfactory. Occasionally, one will have to hand-hold and frequently readjust the transducer angle in order to obtain a countable signal, particularly when the patient is very obese or when the fetus is actively moving. It should be reemphasized that in some circumstances, using autocorrelation techniques, it is possible to count various recurrent signals. Thus, rates such as maternal heart rate may be derived from maternal arterial vessels and/or consecutive repetitive movements of the abdominal wall, leading to an erroneous conclusion of fetal status. When faced with questions regarding the FHR, a definitive evaluation of the fetus utilizing either auscultation or ultrasonic imaging is mandatory.

Methods of recording uterine activity

The direct or indirect system

The direct or indirect system commonly involves the placement of a fluid-filled plastic catheter through the vagina and cervix into the intrauterine cavity and the connection of this to a pressure-sensitive transducer. The pressure transducer will sense changes in hydrostatic pressure in the fluid-filled catheter and provide an accurate measurement of intrauterine pressure. The transducer should be placed at the estimated position of the catheter tip. Thus the transducer is generally placed at the position of the xiphisternum. In addition, the pressure transducer system must be properly zeroed at atmospheric pressure, filled with fluid, free of air bubbles, and electronically calibrated to guarantee system reliability. When properly calibrated, the direct system precisely measures the relative intrauterine resting tone and the amplitude of uterine contractions. The resting tone may be helpful in evaluating states of altered uterine activity associated with abruptio placentae or the occurrence of uterine hyperstimulation.

A falsely elevated resting tone occurs when the pressure transducer is improperly positioned below the tip of the intrauterine catheter. Similarly, true resting tone may be falsely low when the pressure transducer is elevated above the catheter tip. A rough guide in evaluating tone is that a 30 cm column of water will raise the apparent tone by 20 mmHg.

Perforation of the lower uterine segment by the rigid catheter guide has been reported. Care must be taken not to pass the guide past the tip of the examining fingers during the cathether insertion. It is unlikely that the flexible catheter itself causes uterine perforation. With current information, there is essentially no direct evidence linking the insertion of intrauterine catheters with an increased intrauterine or postpartum incidence of maternal febrile morbidity. Previous observations regarding the occurrence of infection were more likely related to the length of labor, the duration of ruptured membranes, and the number of vaginal examinations. Recently, self-contained, disposable, microchip pressure transducer devices have been used. Their reliability is comparable to the fluid-filled systems. The advantages of such systems are the ease of use and elimination of flushing, and effects of positional change. These systems are more expensive.

The indirect system

The indirect system of uterine recording involves the placement of a pressure-sensitive tocodynamometer on the maternal abdomen, usually in the region of the uterine fundus. The tocodynamometer detects forward motion and rotation of the uterus with a uterine contraction and is reflected on the uterine activity recording channel. This system provides reasonably accurate information regarding the duration and frequency of contractions, but does not accurately reflect intensity. Likewise, tone as it appears is a relative product of the belt tension. Belts are commonly used to attach the toco device to the abdomen. The use of external systems for measuring uterine activity is purely passive and is not associated with any known maternal or fetal complication. Current evidence suggests that indirect systems provide adequate information regarding uterine activity for clinical management. The main disadvantages are the need for repositioning and patient discomfort from the belt-attached systems.

SUGGESTED READING

DIVON M, TORRES FP, YEH S-Y, PAUL RH. Autocorrelation techniques in fetal monitoring. *Am J Obstet Gynecol* 1985;151:61–64.

FREEMAN RK, GARITE TJ (eds). *Fetal Heart Rate Monitoring*. Baltimore, MD: Williams & Wilkins, 1981.

HON EH. Intrapartum fetal electrocardiography. In: Crosigani PG, Pardi G, eds. *Fetal Evaluation During Pregnancy and Labor*. New York: Academic Press, 1971: 240.

PARER JT (ed). *Handbook of Fetal Heart Rate Monitoring*. Philadelphia, PA: WB Saunders, 1983.

PAUL RH, HON EH. A clinical fetal monitor. *Obstet Gynecol* 1970;35:161.

PAUL RH, PETRIE RH. *Fetal Intensive Care*. North Haven, CT: William Mack, 1979.

STRONG TH, PAUL RH. Intrapartum uterine activity: evaluation of an intrauterine pressure transducer. *Obstet Gynecol* 1989;73:432–434.

49

Interpretation of fetal heart rate records: baseline heart rate and variability

RICHARD H. PAUL

Proper interpretation and assessment of fetal heart rate (FHR) patterns presume that there is an intact central nervous system as well as a fetal heart that has become functionally responsive to neural input. In addition, for the proper control of this integrated system, both the heart and central nervous system must be properly oxygenated in order to be responsive.

Control of the FHR

The regulation of heart rate is a complex function invoking both intrinsic and extrinsic mechanisms. Numerous sites within the fetal heart may serve as inherent pacemakers. Most commonly, spontaneous discharge from the sinoatrial (SA) node is the predominant driving force for cardiac function. In the near-term fetus its heart responds predictively to many neural and humeral influences that may modify or alter the pacing action of the SA node. Drugs such as atropine and epinephrine usually provoke a rise in rate, while agents such as propranolol induce a fall. In addition, a number of physiologic or pathophysiologic mechanisms such as cord compression or direct pressure applied to the fetus may lead to a slowing of the FHR. The individual fetal response to given stimuli or drugs is highly variable and tends to be more exuberant as gestational age advances.

In addition to the above-mentioned mechanisms involving heart rate function, the maturing fetus develops cyclic episodes of sleep and wakefulness similar to those seen in the newborn. During periods of fetal activity, such as fetal movement, there are alterations in rate both of acceleratory and deceleratory nature as well as increases in the FHR variability related to fetal state changes. During active state, the baseline FHR is often more difficult to define at a specific level. Fetuses that are subjected to external stimuli such as acoustic stimulation may have their intrinsic state pattern altered and respond by observable changes in the FHR pattern. The usual response is that of a startle with associated fetal movement and a reactive FHR pattern. When neural and humeral influences affecting the pacemaker function are diminished, such as in the premature infant or during asphyxia, variations around the basal intrinsic rate often diminish. Thus, the controlling mechanisms which regulate cardiac function on a moment-by-moment basis appear to reflect fetal status more definitively than the mere FHR level, either high- or low-rate. It is no longer reasonable to accept isolated episodes of FHR bradycardia or tachycardia (<120 or >160 bpm) as a singular definitive observation regarding fetal distress. Aberrations in FHR provide early information about the development of fetal hypoxemia and acidemia, as well as the integrated function of both the neurologic and fetal cardio-vascular systems.

Effects of uterine contractions

The historical perspective relating to initial evaluation of FHR patterns related intrapartum events in which the FHR changes in response to uterine contractions were noted. Uterine contractions represented a repetitive stimulus and stress to the fetus. These uterine contractions historically have been associated either with rises in FHR, termed accelerations, or by falls in rate associated with contractions, termed deceleration patterns. In addition, the possible effects of uterine contractions include direct pressure on the fetus, including the presenting part, with intrinsic increases in intracranial pressure as well as potential entrapment of the umbilical cord.

The most obvious and consistent effect of uterine contractions relates to the diminished uterine blood flow that is inversely related to the amplitude and duration of contractions. During contractions the fetus is functionally isolated from the maternal source of nutrient and gas exchange. Under usual circumstances the intact fetus can tolerate this transitory decrease in the availability of oxygen and exhibits few or no accumulative effects as a result of this tolerable intermittent stress. In the compromised fetus, contractions judged clinically "normal" may provoke signs of stress, as reflected in the FHR. When contractions are excessive in amplitude or frequency, even the normal fetus may experience a fall in oxygen content, becoming hypoxemic, and may exhibit the typical FHR pattern – late deceleration, indicative of this stress response. In this sense, the diagnosis and etiology of fetal stress and distress are more certain than when one observes unusual or abnormal FHR patterns in the absence of uterine activity. Thus, labor presents an opportunity which repetitively stresses the fetus and the evoked responses may be interpreted and related to outcome measures that are temporally proximate.

Terminology of FHR monitoring

As exposure and experience were gained with FHR interpretation, a necessary step became the definition of terms which would standardize communication regarding FHR observations. *Baseline heart rate* refers to those features of FHR that occur between uterine contractions, whereas *periodic FHR changes* are those which are related to uterine contractions. By convention, the terms *bradycardia*, *tachycardia*, and *variability* refer to baseline heart rate changes, whereas *acceleration*, *deceleration*, and *FHR irregularity* are descriptive terms that are contraction-related.

Baseline FHR

The so-called baseline FHR is usually equated with the observations made between uterine contractions. The exception to this general rule is when a contraction provokes a FHR response which extends beyond the termination point of the uterine contraction. The pattern most commonly exhibiting this characteristic is late deceleration. The average or normal baseline FHR at term is approximately 140 bpm, with the normal range being 120–160 bpm. Maturation of the fetus is associated with apparent increases in vagal tone and a progressive decrease in rate with advancing gestational age. By convention, a baseline heart rate determination requires a minimum of 10 min observation before establishing a baseline rate.

A baseline FHR of less than 120 bpm is termed bradycardia, whereas a rate which exceeds 160 bpm is labeled tachycardia.

The observation of bradycardia in the range of 100–120 bpm may occasionally be encountered as a normal variant for a given fetus. This is usually associated with normal outcome when associated with FHR variability characteristics which are average or normal. However, bradycardia may also be a sign of fetal problems, such as persistent umbilical cord compression, severe fetal hypoxic events, or an intrinsic arrhythmia. Commonly, during sustained bradycardia at levels of 60–70 bpm, the FHR exhibits absent variability which is usually the result of a nodal rhythm. In general, a marked bradycardia (100 bpm and less) is clinically equated with probable severe fetal asphyxia, although, in retrospect, it is apparent that this FHR response was merely a protective reflex to stress.

Fetal heart block may be a cause of sustained fetal bradycardia and this disorder is currently best evaluated and diagnosed by fetal echocardiography and ultrasonic imaging. It is important to recognize the association of FHR bradycardia and structural abnormalities of the fetal heart. Thus, the sonographic examination should fully evaluate structure as well as functional parameters. As noted in Chapter 48, care must be taken to determine properly the source of an apparent bradycardic heart rate in that many electronic fetal monitors may display rates other than the FHR, leading to misinterpretation and inappropriate intervention. Fetal tachycardia, as defined above, is most commonly associated with maternal fever. Fetal sepsis is also a recognized cause of fetal tachycardia; however, this diagnosis is difficult to establish with certainty prior to the delivery. The evolution, over time, of tachycardia in conjunction with late or variable decelerations may portend an ominous outcome. This trend is particularly significant when the preexistent observations have demonstrated a reactive pattern with a normal baseline level. Tachycardia alone probably reflects two additional pathologic states: the first are the fetal anemias due to a twin–twin transfusion, fetomaternal bleed, isoimmune disorders, or congenital infection. Fetal anemia should be suspected if one encounters a sinusoidal pattern. Second is probable relatively subacute or chronic hypoxemia, with or without acidemia. Recent observations have associated an elevated fixed FHR and the occurrence of intrauterine injury which has presumably impaired normal central nervous system control functions. Such FHR patterns may additionally exhibit decreased variability and atypical decelerations or minimal responses to uterine contractions. During labor most tachycardia that is unassociated with ongoing deceleration patterns is caused by mechanisms other than hypoxia. Infrequent provokers of tachycardic events during labor can relate to the maternal administration of β-mimetic drugs or atropine-like substances which readily cross the placenta. Thus, the observation of tachycardia should lead to an appraisal of the maternal status, including infection, hyperthyroid state, as well as recent medications that the mother has received. Finally, other causes of fetal tachycardia include cardiac arrhythmias such as supraventricular atrial tachycardia. These arrhythmias can be defined and diagnosed using ultrasonic techniques.

FHR variability

The term beat-to-beat FHR variability (FHRV) represents the continuous and subtle interaction of the sympathetic and parasympathetic nervous system and their impact which produce alterations in cardiac rate. Reflex neural inputs such as those related to chest wall movement or sinus arrhythmia are associated with variations in R-R intervals. It would appear that the impulses from higher cortical centers within the fetal brain have an impact on the FHRV, as reflected in alterations during acoustic stimulation and/or alterations in the fetal state such as sleep and wakefulness.

In normal circumstances, the FHR is modulated by a balance between the parasympathetic vagal system and the sympathetic cardiac nerves. These counterbalancing influences tend to slow and increase the rate and produce somewhat irregular alterations in the heart rate pattern, termed variability. By convention, variability has been divided into both long- and short-term components. Abrupt short-lived changes in the beat-to-beat interval are termed *short-term variability*, whereas the more gentle oscillations of 2–5 cycles/min with an amplitude of 5–15 bpm are termed *long-term variability*. While short-term variability is difficult to quantitate, its presence probably reflects an intact, well-oxygenated, functioning autonomic system and is an important predictor of the fetus that is responsive, nonacidemic, and probably well at that moment.

In general, the presence of average short-term variability, even in the face of other FHR abnormalities, portends a good outcome. Appraisal of both long- and short-term variability clinically occurs simultaneously and most classifications of FHR variability endorse this approach in making clinical assessments.

FHR variability is best assessed in the stable baseline heart rate period preceding contractions. Decreased variability <5 bpm may reflect fetal hypoxemia or an acidemic state. Clearly compromised infants usually demonstrate absent or markedly diminished variability, often accompanied by or preceded by deceleration patterns. On occasion, diminished variability may be associated with drug administration such as narcotics and tranquilizers. Such occurrences of decreased variability can be logically ascribed to the pharmacologic agent rather than to probable asphyxial origins.

Decreased variability occurrences during the labor process may also reflect fetal sleep or relative fetal inactivity. During fetal rest or inactivity, movements and FHR accelerations as well as variability are diminished. The baseline FHR is stable, lower, and more easily defined. In contrast, during fetal activity, accelerations are frequently present, FHR variability increased, and the baseline more unstable. Thus, the alternating or cyclic fetal sleep/wake states may be appreciated during labor as well as during antepartum evaluation, which is more thoroughly understood.

The clinical significance of increases in FHR variability of >15 bpm is poorly understood. In most circumstances, these episodes of increased variability or so-called saltatory patterns are associated with normal outcome. In general, increases and rapid fluctuations of rate denote an intact and functional cardiovascular reaction to central nervous system input. The heart rate composed of only long-term variability, which boringly oscillates, has been termed a sinusoidal pattern. It has most commonly been associated with the anemic fetus, as mentioned above. Instances of *sinusoidal-like pattern* may also be associated with the administration of certain narcotics such as alphaprodine during labor. When a so-called sinusoidal pattern is observed, a potential cause should be sought. When appropriate, fetal blood sampling may be undertaken to evaluate the possibility of anemia or the potential of a fetal maternal bleed, which may be evaluated by inspecting the mother's circulation for fetal blood cells.

SUGGESTED READING

FREEMAN RK, GARITE TJ (eds). *Fetal Heart Rate Monitoring*. Baltimore, MD: Williams & Wilkins, 1981.

MILLER FC, PAUL RH. Intrapartum fetal heart rate monitoring. In: Makowski EL, ed. *Clinical Obstetrics and Gynecology*, vol 21. Hagerstown: Harper & Row, 1978: 561–577.

PARER JT (ed). *Handbook of Fetal Heart Rate Monitoring*. Philadelphia, PA: WB Saunders, 1983.

PAUL RH, PETRIE RH. *Fetal Intensive Care*. North Haven, CT: William Mack, 1979.

PAUL RH, KHAZAIN SA, SUIDAN A, YEH S-Y, SCHIFRIN BS, HON EH. Clinical fetal monitoring. VII. The evaluation and significance of intrapartum baseline FHR variability. *Am J Obstet Gynecol* 1975;123:206–210.

PAUL RH, YONEKURA ML, CANTRELL CJ, TURKEL S, PAVLOVA Z, SIPOS L. Fetal injury prior to labor: does it happen? *Am J Obstet Gynecol* 1986;154:1187–1193.

SHIELDS JR, SCHIFRIN BS. Perinatal antecedents of cerebral palsy. *Obstet Gynecol* 1988;71:899–905.

SMITH CV, PHELAN JP, PLATT LD, BROUSSARD P, PAUL RH. Fetal acoustic stimulation testing (the "FAS-TEST"). II. A randomized clinical comparison with the nonstress test. *Am J Obstet Gynecol* 1986;155:131–134.

50

Periodic changes in fetal heart rate

RICHARD H. PAUL

By convention, periodic changes of the fetal heart rate (FHR) are those alterations related to uterine contractions (UCs) which are referred to as accelerations and decelerations.

Acceleration

Acceleration of the FHR is often associated with the occurrence of uterine contractions or with fetal movements. During the antepartum period, the appearance of FHR accelerations of 15 bpm or more forms the basis for nonstress testing. This observation, associated with fetal movement or UCs, is the best prognosticator of fetal well-being. The presence of acceleration patterns, even when fetal movement or UCs are not observed, still portends the well fetus. Historically, it has been observed that accelerations of rate are commonly encountered in early labor and in nonvertex or breech presentations. Recent evaluations during the intrapartum period have demonstrated that the accelerations which are provoked in response to tactile or acoustic stimulation are associated with a nonacidotic fetus.

It is uncertain what provokes or evokes periodic accelerations, but this FHR response may represent early selective occlusion of the umbilical vein while arterial circulation remains open. In this circumstance, the venous return to the right heart is decreased and the fetus may compensate by developing an increased heart rate. Such periodic accelerations may later be associated with the occurrence of variable decelerations. Accelerations which immediately precede and follow variable decelerations are the so-called shoulders, which embrace this pattern. Thus, brief sporadic accelerations accompanying variable decelerations are probably a positive sign of fetal well-being, particularly when coupled with normal or average variability.

The observation of a uniform acceleration or "overshoot" following variable deceleration patterns should be viewed with suspicion and ominous prognosis. In this circumstance, FHR irregularity within the periodic pattern is often absent and the deceleration pattern frequently has no preceding acceleratory component. The presence of this combination of decelerations with a uniform acceleratory overshoot suggests fetal compromise.

Deceleration

There are three classically recognized periodic FHR deceleration patterns which have been extensively evaluated and defined. The deceleration patterns are named by their relationship to the onset of a uterine contraction as well as their waveform and shape. The patterns which are recognized are early deceleration, variable deceleration, and late deceleration. In addition, combinations or mixtures of these patterns are commonly encountered and it is convenient to have a category in which one may place unusual or combined patterns.

Early deceleration

Early decelerations are benign and rarely associated with a depressed newborn or fetal acidosis. The onset of early deceleration begins simultaneously with the onset of a UC with the nadir corresponding to the peak and recovery to baseline by the end of the contraction. The waveform is uniform and appears as a mirror reflection of the underlying uterine contraction. In a usual sequence, the amplitude and duration of the deceleration are proportional to the amplitude and duration of the UC. Early decelerations rarely exhibit a fall below 100 bpm or exceed a 30 bpm fall from the baseline.

Early decelerations are of reflex origin, being a vagal response to apparent increases in intracranial pressure. This pattern may be reproduced in the fetus or newborn by manual compression of the head and is blocked by the administration of atropine. Early decelerations may be encountered throughout labor, but are most commonly seen when the vertex is descending into the pelvis with the cervix being 5–6 cm dilated. Early deceleration patterns are infrequently seen in breech presentation and are thought to require no specific therapy in view of their association with a good outcome.

Variable deceleration

Variable decelerations are the most common pattern observed during labor. They often occur without warning at any time during the process of labor and delivery. Variable decelerations can be experimentally produced by varying degrees of umbilical cord compression and are presumptively related to mechanical alterations which cause impingement upon the umbilical circulation. These patterns occur more often in patients with decreased amniotic fluid volume.

Occlusion of the umbilical vein and arteries alters the fetal blood pressure and, through baroreceptor mechanisms, evokes a reflex vagal slowing of the FHR. Variable decelerations are so named since they possess a variable waveform and bear an irregular or variable relationship to the onset of uterine contractions. Additional features which may be associated with variable decelerations are the presence of a precedent irregular acceleration immediately prior to and following the deceleration pattern. In addition, the fall in rate is abrupt and changes of 30 beats or more between cardiac cycles can be recognized by careful inspection of the FHR pattern. Recovery is most often equally rapid and these rapid FHR adaptations probably denote neurogenic integrity in the compensating fetus. Variable decelerations may mimic or be mistaken for early or late decelerations, but their waveform and intermittent nature should lead to the proper recognition of variable decelerations.

Variable decelerations may be produced by mechanical impingement upon the cord through abdominal palpation. Likewise, such patterns may be eliminated by alterations in maternal position and probable relief of pressure on the umbilical cord. Intrapartum restoration of amniotic fluid volume has been shown to be efficacious in reducing the occurrence of variable and prolonged FHR decelerations. Subsequently, intrapartum fetal distress with resultant operative interventions are effectively decreased. An evaluation of the accumulative effect of repetitive fetal stress, as suggested by variable deceleration, is usually made by evaluation of the baseline heart rate. The baseline heart rate level, as well as the presence or absence of FHR variability (FHRV), in association with the repetitive deceleration pattern, forms the basis on which judgments regarding asphyxial stress are made. If FHRV and baseline rates remain normal, babies are generally born nonasphyxiated and in a responsive state, irrespective of the deceleration magnitude. On the other hand, a rising baseline rate and decreasing variability apparently reflect an increasing stress state and the impending development of asphyxial distress. Severe variable decelerations may be occasionally accompanied by brief episodes of cardiac asystole or standstill. These episodes represent an exuberant vagal response and are usually encountered in the otherwise healthy fetus. They are invariably associated with an average or increased baseline variability after the deceleration, and fetal outcome has been generally good. Commonly, severe variable decelerations are associated with a heart rate level of 60 bpm or less. During this low rate a nodal rhythm develops and irregularity is usually absent. During such repetitive events, as stated above, it is not infrequent that asystole occurs and this should not cause major alarm, but should be treated similarly to severe variable decelerations. The ultimate significance of the severity of the deceleration patterns will lie in the evaluation of baseline heart rate characteristics, coupled with the clinical status of the patient as clinical decisions are made.

Late deceleration

Late deceleration has a uniform waveform which is late in onset related to the onset of the UC. The nadir of the deceleration follows the peak of the contraction and the return to baseline extends beyond the end of the UC. Late decelerations are the exception to contraction-related periodic responses as they extend into what otherwise would be called the baseline heart rate interval. In general, the degree of FHR fall of the late deceleration is related to the degree of fetal stress. Thus, smaller falls, although implying hypoxemia, do not bear the same connotation as larger falls in rate. In general, the degree of late deceleration will be proportional to the intensity and duration of UCs. The hallmark of late decelerations is that they are repetitive and not isolated.

Late decelerations are the result of a fall in the fetal P_{O_2}, which is most commonly caused by interruption of or insufficient intervillous space blood flow. The degree of fetal hypoxemia depends upon the duration and the amplitude of the uterine contraction. The late deceleration reflects the uterine activity as well as the intrinsic fetal reserve or tolerance to this stress. Decreased intervillous perfusion may result from placental separation, excessive uterine activity, or hypotensive perfusion pressures, which can provoke this pathologic FHR pattern in the otherwise totally normal fetus. Conversely, in the marginally compensated or compromised fetus, late decelerations may be provoked even with minimal uterine contractions and minor falls in the P_{O_2}, which the normal fetus would easily tolerate.

The mechanism whereby fetal hypoxemia provokes late deceleration is not fully understood. There are two mechanisms which are recognized as capable of producing late deceleration. The most common is a vagally mediated reflex response to hypoxemia wherein the aortic chemoreceptors detect a low fetal P_{O_2}. Each fetus apparently has an individual P_{O_2} level below which a vagally induced discharge and reflex slowing of the heart rate will occur. The reflex late deceleration is initially characterized by increased irregularity during the deceleration pattern. Reflex late decelerations imply an operative fetal central nervous system and in the early evolutionary stages of late decelerations it is unlikely that the fetus is acidotic or severely depressed. Nevertheless, even with the presence of irregularity within the late deceleration pattern, immediate correction is desirable. Steps taken to alleviate late deceleration are alterations in maternal position, diminishment of uterine activity, if feasible, and the administration of maternal oxygen. The second recognized cause of late deceleration is that of direct myocardial depression. In the terminal stages of fetal distress and asphyxia the myocardial cells are probably directly injured and a slowing of rate will be seen as myocardial dysfunction progresses. This direct late effect is not blocked by the maternal administration of atropine and is usually associated with other ominous FHR pattern findings, such as absent FHRV and compensatory tachycardia. As death approaches, the FHR declines, passing through bradycardic levels to final cessation of cardiac function. Thus, the presence of recurrent or repetitive late deceleration patterns in association with absent variability and tachycardia demands immediate clarification. Attempts should be promptly undertaken to relieve potential stress factors and further define the fetal condition. Mechanisms for the evaluation of fetal status in view of these findings include fetal stimulation via acoustic or tactile measures in an attempt to provoke FHR accelerations. If FHR accelerations, with variable characteristics, are provoked, it is most unlikely that fetal acidemia is present. Some would feel that fetal scalp pH provides a useful commentary.

The appearance and identification of late deceleration, no matter how subtle, must be considered a sign of fetal stress and hypoxemia. The occurrence of repetitive late deceleration over periods of time measured in hours under experimental conditions may bear a relationship to the subsequent brain injury. Thus, the recognition and alleviation of late deceleration, which implies fetal hypoxemia, are desirable. The observation of this periodic pattern demands prompt identification and appropriate corrective interventions.

SUGGESTED READING

CLARK SL, PAUL RH. Intrapartum fetal surveillance: the role of fetal scalp blood sampling. *Am J Obstet Gynecol* 1985;153:717–720.

FREEMAN RK, GARITE TJ (eds). *Fetal Heart Rate Monitoring*. Baltimore, MD: Williams & Wilkins, 1981.

MILLER FC, PAUL RH. Intrapartum fetal heart rate monitoring. In: Makowski EL, ed. *Clinical Obstetrics and Gynecology*, vol 21. Hagerstown: Harper & Row, 1978: 561–577.

MILLER FC, PEASE KE, PAUL RH. Fetal heart rate pattern recognition by the method of auscultation. *Obstet Gynecol* 1984;64:332–336.

PARER JT (ed). *Handbook of Fetal Heart Rate Monitoring.* Philadelphia, PA: WB Saunders, 1983.

PAUL RH, PETRIE RH. *Fetal Intensive Care.* North Haven, CT: William Mack, 1979.

PAUL RH, KHAZAIN SA, SUIDAN A, YEH S-Y, SCHIFRIN BS, HON EH. Clinical fetal monitoring. VII. The evaluation and significance of intrapartum baseline FHR variability. *Am J Obstet Gynecol* 1975;123:206–210.

SMITH CV, NGUYEN HN, PHELAN JP, PAUL RH. Intrapartum assessment of fetal well-being: a comparison of fetal acoustic stimulation with acid base determinations. *Am J Obstet Gynecol* 1986;155:726–728.

51

Fetal acid-base assessment

RICHARD H. PAUL

Since the introduction of fetal blood sampling (FBS) by Saling in 1962, the assessment of fetal scalp blood pH has provided adjunctive data regarding fetal status during labor. At present, the two most commonly used methods to assess intrapartum fetal status are continuous electronic fetal monitoring (EFM) and intermittent assessment of fetal capillary pH (FBS). The theory behind acid-base assessment of the fetus is an attempt to discriminate normal and abnormal tracings with a pH measurement, thus reflecting hypoxia and acidosis. As demonstrated by Saling & Schneider, fetuses with a pH <7.20 were more likely to be delivered depressed. Conversely, a normal fetal outcome was associated with a fetal pH ≥7.20.

Scalp FBS, however, has never achieved widespread acceptance, in contrast to continuous EFM. FBS suffers from clinical and practical problems; for instance, the lack of trained personnel, accessible equipment for pH analysis, and the questionable reliability of laboratory results when such analysis is available. In addition, there are frequently clinical circumstances, such as a nondilated cervix or intact membranes, which make the procedure technically impossible. Other factors, such as the time delay in obtaining results, misinterpretation of pH data, and the cumbersome procedure, are drawbacks. Finally, the intermittent nature of FBS and the need for repetitive sampling during labor limits usage.

Historically, in our institution, which serves a large high-risk population, approximately 2% of women in labor undergo scalp FBS. More recently, alternative noninvasive methods, to assess fetal condition and draw relationships with acid-base status during labor, have been investigated and found to be reliable. The purpose of this chapter is to familiarize the clinician with the use of various techniques to establish fetal well-being and to provide a management scheme in the event that a laboring patient has an abnormal FHR tracing.

Indications for fetal acid-base assessment

Current acceptable criteria for considering pH assessment during labor are illustrated in Table 51.1. The usual and customary indications for acid-base assessment are repetitive late decelerations, diminished fetal heart rate (FHR) variability (≤5bpm), repetitive severe variable decelerations, sinusoidal FHR pattern and the clinically confusing FHR tracing. In addition to these, atypical variable decelerations (Table 51.2), as described by Krebs *et al.*, represent a different approach to the interpretation of variable FHR decelerations. These investigators found that when atypical variable decelerations were present during labor, there was a greater likelihood of fetal acidosis and a higher probability of an adverse fetal outcome. A persistent, nonreactive FHR pattern for more than 80min is also associated with a significant increase in perinatal mortality and fetal acidosis. Thus, if a fetus fails to exhibit accelerations, either spontaneous or evoked, during labor, FBS may be considered.

Table 51.1 Indications for fetal acid-base assessment

Repetitive late decelerations
Diminished fetal heart rate variability
Repetitive severe variable decelerations
Atypical variable decelerations
Sinusoidal patterns
Persistent nonreactive fetal heart rate pattern
A clinically confusing fetal heart rate pattern

Table 51.2 Characteristics of atypical variable fetal heart rate (FHR) decelerations

Loss of initial FHR acceleration
Delayed return of FHR to baseline
Loss of secondary FHR acceleration
Prolonged acceleration after the deceleration
A biphasic deceleration
Decreased FHR variability within the deceleration
Continuation of the baseline rate at a level lower than that preceding the deceleration

Establishing the diagnosis of fetal acidosis

If a fetus manifests one of the FHR patterns in Table 51.1, fetal pH assessment may be considered before undertaking delivery. As previously demonstrated by Kubli, infants with a pH <7.20 are more likely to be depressed at delivery, whereas those infants with a normal fetal outcome were associated with a lack of acidosis or pH ≥7.20. However, when fetal scalp pH is correlated with the Apgar score, Bowe *et al.* reported an incidence of false-normal pH and false-abnormal pH of 10.4 and 7.5%, respectively. Possible explanations for the relatively high incidence of pH–Apgar score discrepancies are listed in Tables 51.3 and 51.4. In the false-normal pH group the most common error in interpretation is the failure to consider the effects of maternal hyperventilation. Thus, whenever FBS is performed, a maternal venous pH evaluation is desirable. A maternal venous–fetal pH difference of less than 0.15 is considered within the normal range. In the case of maternal hyperventilation, the fetal pH may become falsely elevated secondary to maternal respiratory alkalosis. As demonstrated in Table 51.4 the most common reason for a false-low pH is that the FBS is done in close proximity to or during a uterine contraction, in association with a FHR deceleration. Under these circumstances, the fetal scalp pH, secondary to increased carbon dioxide, is more likely to be lower than between uterine contractions.

Despite theoretic benefits, there is only limited use of FBS by clinicians today. Clark & Paul demonstrated an average use in 3% of patients. As a

Table 51.3 Clinical situations associated with false-normal scalp blood pH

Maternal hyperventilation
Drugs
Neonatal airway obstruction
Congenital anomalies
Infection
Premature fetus
Acidosis between sampling and delivery

Table 51.4 Clinical conditions associated with false-low pH

Anesthesia/analgesia
Maternal acidosis
Stage of labor
Delay of analysis
Timing of sampling in relation to uterine
  contraction or fetal heart rate deceleration

result, alternative methods to assess fetal well-being, as judged by acid-base pH status, have been investigated. One method, the continuous pH electrode, has been tested and has not been found to be sufficiently reliable to be used clinically. More recently, attention has been directed at the presence of spontaneous or evoked FHR accelerations and their relationship to fetal acid-base status. The presence of FHR accelerations of 15 bpm for 15 s from the time the FHR leaves baseline until it returns is associated with a nonacidotic fetus. This has led to the exploration of noninvasive techniques to assess fetal well-being.

Initially, Clark *et al.* reviewed the FHR tracings of 200 fetuses who had undergone FBS. Of these, 169 had a FHR acceleration in response to scalp incision during FBS. All of these had a pH ≥7.20. In the 31 fetuses who failed to exhibit an acceleration, 50% were acidotic. Subsequently, Clark *et al.* prospectively investigated the scalp stimulation test which used digital scalp palpation or a pinch using an Allis clamp to evoke or produce a FHR acceleration. In the 100 fetuses exhibiting abnormal FHR tracings suggestive of fetal compromise, the scalp stimulation test provoked an acceleration in 51 fetuses. Of these, a single fetus (2%) demonstrated a pH <7.20. In that fetus with a pH <7.20, the scalp samples were pH 7.19, 7.20, and 7.19. This fetus had Apgar scores of 6 and 8 at 1 and 5 min, respectively. Of those fetuses who failed to exhibit a FHR acceleration in response to scalp stimulation, acidosis (pH <7.20) was identified in about 40%.

Subsequently, Smith and associates studied a less invasive technique, acoustic stimulation, as a provocative stimulus to assess fetal status. In a series of 64 fetuses with abnormal FHR tracings, these investigators evaluated the fetal response to externally applied acoustic stimulation, from an electrolarynx, and the presence of acidosis. Of the 64 fetuses studied, 30 fetuses exhibited a reactive FHR pattern in response to acoustic stimulation. All had a pH ≥7.25. Of the 34 nonresponding fetuses, 53% were considered to be acidotic. Thus, the finding of spontaneous or evoked FHR accelerations (15 bpm × 15 s) is associated with a normal fetal scalp pH.

Management of suspected fetal stress/distress and FHR abnormalities

The management of a patient with an abnormal FHR pattern should be accomplished in a stepwise manner. Initially, the patient should be repositioned on her left side, administered with oxygen, and intravenous fluids. If oxytocin is being infused, it should be discontinued. If the pattern becomes normal within a reasonable period of time, continued observation of the patient is reasonable. However, if the FHR pattern persists despite these initial attempts to remedy the FHR abnormality, fetal scalp stimulation or acoustic stimulation should be undertaken. If a reactive (15 bpm × 15 s) pattern is observed, a nonacidotic fetus is reasonably assured. If the fetus fails to manifest an acceptable FHR acceleration with either scalp or acoustic stimulation, FBS can be considered or delivery should be undertaken. Generally, if the scalp blood sampling is used, a pH <7.20 calls for a repeat confirmation of the low pH and expeditious delivery. If the pH is between 7.20 and 7.25, repeat FBS is arranged at frequent intervals every 30–60 min. A fetal scalp pH ≥7.25 warrants continued observation and repeat sampling as indicated. The need to repeat FBS is a major limitation of FBS, particularly if a labor is anticipated to require hours of observation. A major advantage of acoustic stimulation is the ease of repeated application, its inexpensive cost, and immediate result. Using this approach over a period of 5 years has virtually eliminated FBS in our institution. During this time, cesarean delivery for fetal distress has decreased and the occurrence of low Apgar scores and perinatal asphyxia has been stable.

SUGGESTED READING

BOWE ET, BEARD RW, FINSTER M, *et al.* Reliability of fetal blood sampling. *Am J Obstet Gynecol* 1970;107:279.

CLARK SL, PAUL RH. Intrapartum fetal surveillance: the role of fetal scalp sampling. *Am J Obstet Gynecol* 1985;153:717.

CLARK SL, GIMOVSKY ML, MILLER FC. Fetal heart rate response to scalp blood sampling. *Am J Obstet Gynecol* 1982;144:706.

CLARK SL, GIMOVSKY ML, MILLER FC. The scalp stimulation test: a clinical alternative to fetal scalp blood sampling. *Am J Obstet Gynecol* 1984;148:274.

EDERSHEIM TG, HUTSON M, DRUZIN ML, KOGUT EA. Fetal heart rate response to vibratory acoustic stimulation predicts fetal pH in labor. *Am J Obstet Gynecol* 1987;157:1557–1560.

KREBS HB, PETRES RE, DUN LH. Intrapartum fetal heart rate monitoring. VII. Atypical variable decelerations. *Am J Obstet Gynecol* 1983;145:297.

KUBLI FW, HON EH, KHAZIN AF, *et al.* Observations in heart rate and pH in the human fetus during labor. *Am J Obstet Gynecol* 1969;104:1190.

POLZIN GB, BLAKEMORE KJ, PETRIE RH, AMON A. Fetal vibroacoustic stimulation: magnitude and duration of fetal heart rate accelerations as a marker of fetal health. *Obstet Gynecol* 1988;72:621–626.

ROWE ET, BEARD RW, FINSTER M, *et al.* Reliability of fetal blood sampling. *Am J Obstet Gynecol* 1970;107:279.

SALING E, SCHNEIDER D. Biochemical supervision of the fetus during labor. *J Obstet Gynecol Br Commonw* 1967;74:799.

SMITH CV, NGUYEN HN, PHELAN JP, *et al.* Intrapartum assessment of fetal well-being: a comparison of fetal acoustic stimulation with acid-base determinations. *Am J Obstet Gynecol* 1986;155:726.

THEARD FC, PENNEY LL, OTTERSON WH. Sinusoidal fetal heart rate: ominous or benign? *J Reprod Med* 1984;29:265.

52

Effects of drugs on fetal heart rate

RICHARD H. PAUL

The fetal heart rate (FHR) forms the primary basis of fetal evaluation during both the antepartum and intrapartum periods of pregnancy. Use of clinical FHR monitoring has become widespread over the last 20 years and is employed in two-thirds of births in the USA. With widespread application many procedures, including drug administration, have been shown to demonstrate effects which are identified by changes in FHR. At best, the FHR is merely an indirect reflection of fetal status. However, careful observation of FHR changes, coupled with our present under-standing of the pathophysiology of FHR response, permits us to draw some conclusions regarding the effects of various drugs used in clinical care of pregnant patients. FHR responses to drugs may be evoked by multiple mechanisms. Three primary factors must be considered indi-vidually and collectively in dealing with maternal drug administration and its potential effects on the fetus. One must ask: Are the observed FHR responses a direct drug effect on the fetus subsequent to maternal transfer of this agent? Are the changes in FHR an indirect result of alterations in uterine activity or alterations in the maternal cardiovascular system? Individually, each of these mechanisms may significantly affect the FHR response and, at times, it seems that a combined effect, likely involving all of these separate mechanisms, is responsible. In general, most drugs and anesthetic gases promptly cross the placenta with one notable exception, heparin. Although succinylcholine, which is com-monly administered during cesarean birth, crosses the placenta, it does so only at a slow rate.

Antepartum period

With the exception of propranolol and phenobarbital, little is known about the FHR effects of most drugs used clinically during the antepartum period. Propranolol, a sympathetic blocking agent, may cause fetal bradycardia, which, if unrecognized as being drug-induced, may lead to unnecessary intervention. Phenobarbital, as used in the treatment of gestational hypertension, including preeclampsia, has been associated with a higher incidence of abnormal antepartum FHR testing patterns. There is little doubt that other drugs probably have an effect on FHR characteristics. However, our identification and definitive understanding of such agents and their effects remain grossly deficient. As an example, the utilization of agents such as the β-sympathomimetic drugs which appear to have an initial effect of increasing the baseline FHR subsequently disappear with chronic use. Administration of agents to correct maternal arrhythmias, such as adenosine, seemingly has little identifiable effect on FHR characteristics. Finally, even though an unusual or suspect FHR observation is made, the subsequent clinical significance and management implications are difficult to define.

Intrapartum period

One must assume that drugs commonly administered to the mother, with the notable exception of heparin, will rapidly cross the placenta and enter the fetal circulation. Agents such as antibiotics, vitamins, and anesthetic gases clearly enter the fetal compartment but scanty information exists regarding their effects on the FHR. Compared with the antepartum period, intrapartum observation regarding the effects of various drugs on the FHR forms a larger area of understanding including the following major categories: narcotic analgesics, local anesthetic agents, labor-inhibiting agents, anticonvulsant sedatives, oxytocic agents, and agents affecting the autonomic nervous system. It must be reemphasized that these agents may evoke their effects through various mechanisms. For instance, local anesthetic agents may directly affect the fetal myocardium, uterine activity, and the maternal cardiovascular system.

The principal observed effect of narcotic analgesics is a propensity to decrease FHR variability. This is thought to reflect a depressant effect on the fetal central nervous system after rapid transplacental passage. Quantitative evaluation of data regarding these effects is currently minimal but worthy of future investigation. The clinical significance of such observations remains unknown but a conscious recognition of this effect is important since FHR variability evaluation is important in judging clinical condition of the fetus. More subtle FHR effects emerge as narcotic agents are evaluated relative to their potential effects on uterine activity. Narcotic-associated increases in uterine activity may be due to direct myometrial stimulation or indirectly related to relief of pain and alterations in maternal catecholamine release. The infrequent narcotic-provoked maternal respiratory arrest and resultant maternal hypoxia will dramatically affect the FHR, usually being evidenced by a prolonged deceleration. This complication is largely avoidable with careful patient observation, appropriate drug dosage, and proper administration. A final peculiar observation relating to narcotic agents is that some fetuses, following administration of these agents, will demonstrate what is described as a sinusoidal FHR pattern. The mechanism that provokes this associated pattern and its clinical significance remain unclear. The primary benefit of understanding this particular relationship lies in the fact that this type of sinusoidal pattern frequently disappears. Thus, this observation needn't imply fetal distress or raise a suspicion of potential fetal anemia or compromise.

Local anesthetic agents may produce FHR changes by two major mechanisms. First, their oxytocic potential may interfere with uteroplacental exchange and/or cause umbilical cord compression. More commonly, FHR changes are due to alterations in the maternal cardiovascular system. The most commonly encountered FHR changes involved with local anesthetic agents relate to their use in conduction anesthesia. Thus, the use of saddle block or epidural anesthesia, by blocking sympathetic tone, and resultant maternal hypotension will frequently evoke a FHR response. The fetus most often responds to these temporary stress factors by exhibiting hypoxemically induced late deceleration patterns. An uncommon form of FHR response, seen in the past, would be that seen secondary to paracervical block (PCB) anesthesia. This technique has largely fallen out of favor in current practice but when used may result in a local vasoconstrictive effect on the uterine arteries, thus reducing uterine blood flow, producing fetal stress and a bradycardic event. The clinical term used to describe this event is postparacervical block bradycardia. The onset is often 7–8 min after administration and recovery usually occurs in the same time-frame. When this occurs, subsequent use of PCB anesthesia is contraindicated.

Studies relating to administration of labor-inhibiting agents, such as the β-sympathomimetics or magnesium sulfate, generally relate to occurrences and treatment of presumed preterm labor. Consequently, FHR measurement has generally been limited to applications of external monitoring techniques which impose limitations regarding the quantitative parameters of FHR evaluation. Thus, little information exists regarding the specific FHR effects of drugs such as ritodrine, terbutaline, and indomethacin. Intrapartum experience with the administration of the β-sympathomimetic drugs is also limited, even though these drugs may be given over periods of hours. The most commonly encountered alteration is the rise in baseline FHR which occasionally reaches tachycardiac levels. These tachycardiac levels are not infrequently associated with a concomitant diminishment of the baseline FHR variability. As stated previously, the chronic administration of oral tocolytic agents, although producing an initial rise in FHR, seems to disappear as a result of tachyphylaxis or as the fetus matures.

Anticonvulsive sedative agents may be used at times for treatment of gestational hypertension. Intrapartum parenteral administration of magnesium sulfate, extending over many hours, has been associated with diminished FHR variability, in contrast to an apparent increase of FHR variability during initial intravenous bolus administration. Administration of other anticonvulsant agents, such as diazepam, barbiturates, and hydroxyzine, is commonly associated with diminished FHR variability.

The ability of oxytocin, in a worst-case scenario, to induce uterine tetany will provoke dramatic FHR decelerations and bradycardia. The resultant cessation of intervillous blood flow and fetal hypoxemia cause profound FHR changes. Carefully controlled oxytocin administration is thus mandatory and usually is associated with little or no apparent FHR effect. A commonly accepted and reasonable interval for increasing oxytocin dosage is 30–60 min. It is questionable whether direct transfer of oxytocin impacts the fetus or whether it may have an identifiable effect.

Drugs that affect the maternal autonomic nervous system also pass to the fetus and result in an identifiable FHR response. As noted previously, propranolol may be associated with fetal bradycardia, whereas atropine or scopolamine may eliminate or modify the vagal component of FHR control. Atropine is thus associated with a fetal tachycardia and concomitant loss of FHR variability. Such agents, often used preoperatively, may confound interpretation of FHR patterns. Additionally, even though they may dramatically alter abnormal FHR patterns, the fetal condition is *not* improved.

Numerous additional drugs no doubt have effects that are likely reflected in the FHR. The mechanism of their action must be individually considered. For example, an antihypertensive agent such as hydralazine would probably cause FHR changes by reducing maternal blood pressure and decreasing intervillous perfusion pressure and blood flow. The potential physiologic effect of antepartum and intrapartum administration of drugs and their associated FHR changes deserves careful critical attention.

SUGGESTED READING

Freeman RK, Garite TJ (eds). *Fetal Heart Rate Monitoring*. Baltimore, MD: Williams & Wilkins, 1981.

Keegan KA, Paul RH, Broussard PM, McCart D, Smith MA. Antepartum fetal heart rate testing. III. The effect of phenobarbital on the nonstress test. *Am J Obstet Gynecol* 1979;133:579.

Mason BA, Goodman JR, Koos BJ. Adenosine in the treatment of maternal paroxysmal supraventricular tachycardia. *Obstet Gynecol* 1992;80:3.

Parer JT (ed). *Handbook of Fetal Heart Rate Monitoring*. Philadelphia, PA: WB Saunders, 1983.

Paul RH, Petrie RH. *Fetal Intensive Care*. North Haven, CT: William Mack, 1979.

Petrie RH, Yeh SY, Murata Y, et al. The effect of drugs on fetal heart rate variability. *Am J Obstet Gynecol* 1978;130:294.

Yeh S-Y, Paul RH, Cordero L, Hon EH. A study of diazepam during labor. *Obstet Gynecol* 1974;43:363.

53

Abnormal fetal heart rate patterns: diagnosis and management

RICHARD H. PAUL

Definitions

Fetal heart rate (FHR) monitoring is widely used to evaluate fetal status with a goal of detecting fetal distress in labor. Fetal distress is the term generally equated with fetal hypoxia, with the potential risk of fetal and subsequent infant injury. Historically, certain patterns of FHR have been associated with fetal acidosis, depressed newborns, and, rarely, intrapartum death. Thus, the diagnosis of fetal distress is clinically imprecise when applied. In practice, fetal distress is the clinical diagnosis made when the practitioner feels that the fetus cannot safely remain *in utero* without risk of compromise or injury.

Classically, FHR patterns have been used to screen for fetal distress. It may be helpful to divide these FHR patterns into three groups, as follows: (1) unstressed; (2) stressed with compensation; and (3) decompensated (Table 53.1). It should be emphasized that these groups are based primarily on *interpretation* of the FHR patterns. The definitive diagnosis of fetal distress remains fetal hypoxia and acidosis, which many times must be necessarily retrospectively determined at birth. Often times the prospectively assigned diagnosis fetal distress is contradicted and proved incorrect, as judged by a normal newborn.

Fetal distress is often discussed as though its acute occurrence is limited to labor. It has become increasingly clear that fetal hypoxia and probable injury occur as a result of acute or chronic processes that precede labor. Furthermore, a chronically stressed fetus probably responds differently to the acute stresses of labor than a normal fetus. The FHR

Table 53.1 Classification of fetal heart rate (FHR) patterns in labor

| Pattern class | Characteristics | |
	Baseline	Periodic
Unstressed	120–160 bpm	Accelerations present Normal variability No late decelerations May have early or small variable decelerations
Stressed	Normal–decreased Usually normal range, trend for level to have risen over time of observation	Accelerations present Decreased variability May have more severe variable decelerations
Distressed	Elevated or decreased >160 or <120 bpm	Accelerations absent Decreased/absent variability May have severe periodic decelerations or atypical deceleration pattern The preterminal baseline FHR will become bradycardiac, unstable and "wandering"

characteristics of acute and chronic stress and distress are somewhat different, as is the treatment.

Diagnosis

FHR records are interpreted by reviewing two facets: the baseline, and any periodic changes. Either or both of these aspects may be abnormal.

Baseline

Normal baseline FHR is defined as a rate between 120 and 160 bpm. In fact, a baseline greater than 140–145 bpm is quite unusual in a term fetus. Conversely, a baseline as low as 100 bpm may also be quite normal, and even lower baseline rates may be seen without hypoxia or fetal compromise with congenital heart block. A higher baseline heart rate may reflect a fetal tachyarrhythmia or maternal fever or medication effect. FHR variability is an important indicator of fetal health or stress and its quantitation in an absolute sense is impractical. Variability of 5–15 bpm is classified as normal and is thought to be induced by a constant interplay of fetal sympathetic and parasympathetic influences. Nonstress-related factors which influence baseline variability include gestational maturation, movements, the fetal sleep/wake state, and maternal drug ingestion.

Baseline findings are used in an attempt to define fetal stress and distress. In general, subacute or chronic fetal stress will cause a flattening of the baseline (loss of variability), and is often associated with an elevation of the baseline heart rate.

Acute fetal distress (such as that caused by a cord prolapse) is accompanied by a sudden profound decrease in the baseline heart rate. This may be referred to by some authors as a bradycardia but is more appropriately termed a prolonged deceleration.

Periodic changes

Periodic FHR changes include accelerations and three types of decelerations (Fig. 53.1). Accelerations are universally reassuring signs which indicate an intact neurologic system with appropriate cardiac response.

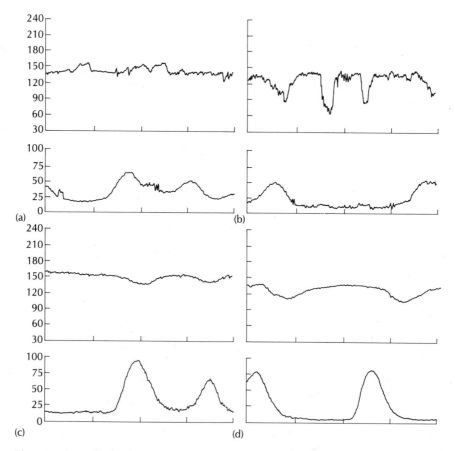

Fig. 53.1 Periodic fetal heart rate changes: (a) acceleration; (b) variable deceleration; (c) early deceleration; and (d) late deceleration.

The presence of FHR accelerations (15 bpm × 15 s) virtually precludes significant fetal acidosis. Variable decelerations are thought to be associated with cord compression. Previously, small variable decelerations associated with normal baseline findings were thought to be of minor clinical importance. It has now become apparent that even these subtle decelerations may indicate fetal vulnerability in certain instances such as antepartum testing or prolonged pregnancy. It is now clear that these findings are commonly associated with decreased amniotic fluid volume. During labor such variable decelerations may progress to a fetal stress pattern with decreasing variability and a rising baseline heart rate. With repetitive occurrence over sufficient time of cord occlusion, fetal distress with failure to recover to baseline between decelerations may occur. This pathologic progression may be ameliorated by use of intrapartum amnioinfusion.

Other types of decelerations include early decelerations, thought to be related to fetal head compression, and late decelerations, which are due to reduction in the uteroplacental blood flow. Early decelerations do not herald fetal compromise, but may be confused with late decelerations. Late decelerations may, early in their evolution, be associated with normal baseline findings, in which case they constitute a fetal stress pattern. With repetitive occurrence of late deceleration, there will be progression to a pathologic baseline FHR in a full-blown picture of fetal distress. The latter is evidenced by a rising flat baseline, often to tachycardiac levels, and a loss of reactivity or absent accelerations.

Management

FHR monitoring is a screening tool for fetal well-being. As such, it is a much more accurate indicator of fetal normality than of fetal stress/distress. When FHR monitoring was first introduced, this principle was not clearly understood, and operative delivery rates climbed as infants were delivered as an emergency procedure for abnormal FHR findings. This chapter discusses interpretation of the abnormal FHR with the aid of other tests, and management of the fetus with an abnormal FHR.

Interpretation

Many events in labor may lead to a FHR recording typical of fetal stress, and on some occasions with fetal distress. The classic method for resolving these observations was to measure fetal capillary pH directly. Fetal pH determinations have never been widely used outside of academic centers due to the quality control and other problems. Recent data have shown that a FHR acceleration associated with fetal stimulation was associated with a normal pH ($\geq$7.20) in nearly all instances. The methods of fetal stimulation used have included palpation of or pinching the fetal scalp with an Allis clamp, incising the scalp for pH evaluation, and sound stimulation with an artificial larynx. Sound and scalp stimulation are simpler, better tolerated, and more practical than fetal pH determinations. Fetal pH may be reserved for those cases not resolved by these means, but in our institutional practice has decreased in use to <1:1000 births.

Other methods, such as the biophysical profile, are occasionally used intrapartum, especially in the evaluation of the very preterm fetus whose FHR findings may be confusing. The biophysical profile and amniotic fluid index (a measure of amniotic fluid pockets in four quadrants) are much more useful in antepartum patient surveillance. Even so, application of these techniques provides useful guidance or screening for patients in early labor. Patients exhibiting a normal admission or screening profile have less intrapartum morbidity.

Finally, several groups have attempted to develop continuous fetal pH, $P\text{CO}_2$ and oximetry monitors. These devices have not been of significant clinical value to the present time due to various technical problems.

Delivery

The first principle of management of the abnormal FHR is to correct the abnormality. This is most commonly achieved by altering the maternal position with a presumed benefit of restoring blood flow through the umbilical cord and/or intervillous space. Even in the patient who has obvious fetal distress demanding a prompt operative delivery, 15–30 min commonly elapse between diagnosis and delivery. This time can be used to promote fetal recovery *in utero* if certain steps are taken.

1 Maternal drug administration should be evaluated and excluded as the provocative factor eliciting the FHR abnormality.

2 Oxytocin infusions should be stopped. On occasion, when excessive uterine activity is the inciting factor judged to be causing fetal distress, such activity can be decreased by using a tocolytic agent.

3 Maternal fever should be treated with antipyretics and, if necessary, a cooling blanket.

4 Maternal hypotension should be corrected, and placental blood flow optimized by proper positioning. Volume restoration and even the use of pressor agents may be necessary in the case of hypotension due to regional anesthesia.

5 For a pattern suggestive of cord compromise, maternal reposition from back to sides to knee–chest position may be helpful. One should obviously have ruled out cord prolapse.

6 Amnioinfusion may be utilized to restore a decreased amniotic fluid volume. This will often reduce or eliminate variable deceleration patterns.
7 Oxygen may be administered to the mother by mask.

The basis for the correction of FHR abnormalities, evoking the diagnosis of fetal distress, is restoration of blood flow. Two circulations are thus considered: mother–intervillous blood flow and fetal–umbilical blood flow.

Most of these maneuvers can be instituted by nursing personnel while awaiting physician response. The more specific and complicated decision involves the route and urgency of delivery in the patient with an abnormal FHR pattern. In general, immediate delivery is advised for the fetus with a new onset of bradycardia of<90 bpm which does not recover and exceeds 3–5 min. Operative delivery should also be considered for the patient who has a FHR pattern suggestive of distress with no response to digital palpation or sound stimulation.

Conclusion

FHR remains the first-line screen for fetal well-being. Abnormal FHR should be interpreted with the adjunctive help of other techniques, such as fetal stimulation. As the goal of this surveillance is the birth of a healthy, normal infant, it should not be a surprise or a disappointment that many infants delivered after a suspicious or abnormal FHR tracings are normal. It is, however, important to use all the available tools to minimize nonindicated surgical interventions as well as fetal harm. With such an approach the rate of intervention, by cesarean, for this diagnosis in our hospital is approximately 2%.

SUGGESTED READING

CLARK SL, GIMOVSKY ML, MILLER FC. The scalp stimulation test: a clinical alternative to fetal scalp blood sampling. *Am J Obstet Gynecol* 1984;148:274.

MACRI CJ, SCHRIMMER DB, LEUNG A, GREENSPOON JS, PAUL RH. Prophylactic amnioinfusion improves the outcome of pregnancy complicated by thick meconium and oligohydramnios. *Am J Obstet Gynecol* 1992;167:117–121.

PAUL RH, KHAZAN SA, SUIDAN A, YEH S-Y, SCHIFRIN BS, HON EH. Clinical fetal monitoring. VII. The evaluation and significance of intrapartum baseline FHR variability. *Am J Obstet Gynecol* 1975;123:206.

PAUL RH, PETRIE RH, RABELLO YA, MUELLER EA. *Fetal Intensive Care.* New Haven, CT: William Mack, 1979.

SARNO AP JR, MYOUNG OA, PHELAN JP, PAUL RH. Fetal acoustic stimulation in the early intrapartum period as a predictor of subsequent fetal condition. *Am J Obstet Gynecol* 1990;162:762–767.

SHAW KJ, PAUL RH. Fetal responses to external stimuli. *Obstet Gynecol Clin North Am* 1990;17:235–240.

SMITH CV, PHELAN JP, PAUL RH, BROUSSARD P. Fetal acoustic stimulation testing: a retrospective experience with the fetal acoustic stimulation test. *Am J Obstet Gynecol* 1985;153:567.

STRONG TH, HETZLER G, SARNO AP, PAUL RH. Prophylactic intrapartum amnio-infusion: a randomized prospective clinical trial. *Am J Obstet Gynecol* 1990;162: 1370–1375.

ZANINI B, PAUL RH, HUEY JR. Intrapartum fetal heart rate: the correlation with scalp pH in the preterm fetus. *Am J Obstet Gynecol* 1980;136:43.

54

Genetic counseling and the obstetric patient

DENA TOWNER

Reproduction is intimately tied to congenital and genetic defects and as such every pregnancy should be screened for risk factors. There is a 3–4% risk that any pregnancy will result with an infant found to have a congenital birth defect noted in the first month of life. By puberty 10–15% of children will be diagnosed with a congenital or genetic condition. By assessing for risk factors during the pregnancy, the obstetrician can identify some of these women. Unfortunately, most birth defects occur in pregnancies without risk factors. As a result, screening tests are being developed to identify affected fetuses in women at low risk. This screening has increased the detection rate for many common birth defects. Parental carrier testing is available for many common genetic diseases.

Risk assessment

Initial genetic risk screening by the obstetrician should begin with a family history for birth defects, diseases that run in the family, mental retardation, stillbirths, multiple pregnancy losses, and family ethnicity. Prior pregnancy outcome should be reviewed, with special attention to recurrent pregnancy losses of two or more spontaneous abortions, a prior anomalous infant, or known genetic disease in a prior infant. If an abnormal outcome occurred in a prior pregnancy, was there a genetic evaluation performed, and are the records available for review? It is nearly impossible to counsel a patient adequately for recurrence risk if an evaluation was not performed and the child is not alive to be examined. Many times the patient had counseling about recurrence risk, but she doesn't remember what she was told and needs to be counseled again.

Ethnic background holds important clues for certain diseases as some disorders have an increased frequency in certain populations. Tay–Sachs disease in Ashkenazi Jews, sickle cell disease in American blacks, α-thalassemia in Asians, and β-thalassemia in Greeks and others of Mediterranean descent are classic examples. Carrier status can be tested for these diseases.

Pedigree analysis of the extended family may identify a fetus at risk. In most cases the fetus is found not to be at risk, which eases the parents' minds. Most isolated defects are sporadic events and thought to be multifactorial in etiology. As a result, only first-degree relatives are at increased risk. For example, there is a cousin with cleft lip, so there is concern for the fetus. Recurrence risk is generally 5% when either a parent or a sibling has the defect. When a more distantly related family member has the defect, the risk is <1% and approaches that of the general population. When asking about birth defects it is prudent to name a few examples as many people may not consider that the uncle who had an extra finger or the cousin who had open heart surgery at 2 months had birth defects, if there was no long-term problem and mental function was normal. Patterns of inheritance should be identified if there are multiple affected family members.

Mental retardation has many known and unknown etiologies, with two of the three most common forms amenable to prenatal diagnoses — trisomy 21 and fragile X. The third most common cause of mental retardation is alcohol abuse. Specific attention should be paid to mental retardation and learning disorders that affect predominantly males in a family. This may represent the X-linked form of mental retardation called fragile X, which is the most common form of inherited mental retardation and can be tested for with DNA analysis. Trisomy 21 is the other common cause and will be discussed later.

Parental ages and maternal medical problems should be assessed. Maternal age is associated with increasing risk for chromosomal abnormalities, particularly trisomy 21. Age 35 at the time of delivery is the generally accepted age to offer genetic amniocentesis, as the incidence of a chromosomally abnormal fetus is equivalent to the historical loss rate due to amniocentesis of 1:200. Advanced paternal age (over 45 years) is associated with increasing chances for new spontaneous dominant mutations, such as achondroplasia, neurofibromatosis, osteogenesis imperfecta, etc.

Maternal medical diseases can have an impact on fetal development. Insulin-requiring diabetes is associated with an increased spontaneous abortion rate and up to a 20-fold increase in fetal anomalies if euglycemia is not maintained at the time of conception and during organogenesis. These anomalies include major structural defects such as neural tube defects, caudal regression syndrome, and heart anomalies, specifically transposition of the great arteries and ventral septal defect. Women with systemic lupus erythematosus are at risk to have a fetus with complete heart block if anti-Ro antibodies are present. This is due to the autoimmune destruction of the fetal cardiac conduction system.

A review of early pregnancy exposure to potential teratogens is mandatory. This includes asking about fevers, rashes, or viral syndromes. Toxoplasmosis, cytomegalovirus, rubella, and varicella are all well documented to be associated with fetal malformation. High persistent fever and exposure to prolonged hot-tub or sauna use are associated with an increased risk for neural-tube defects (and possibly other defects) due to cell death and abnormal tissue migration.

Ingested substances can also be teratogenic. The most common and preventable cause of mental retardation and learning disabilities is alcohol abuse. No level is considered safe, but up to three "binges" in the first trimester has not been associated with fetal alcohol syndrome. Cocaine use has been associated with genitourinary abnormalities and vascular disruption sequences such as gastroschisis, transverse limb defects, etc. Review of medications (prescription and nonprescription) taken should be explored. Generally no medication has been taken or only products considered safe in pregnancy have been ingested. In this case reassurance can be given. In some cases, pregnancy is unplanned and a known or suspected teratogen was ingested. This would include retinoic acid, lithium, chemotherapeutic agents, coumarin, and anticonvulsants.

Radiation exposure is also important to inquire about. The level set as being unsafe is >10 rad, 2–10 rad is of uncertain risk, and <2 rad is with minimal risk. Preimplantation exposure is either lethal or no risk to the embryo. For exposure later in pregnancy the risk is for microcephaly, growth retardation, and a possible twofold increased risk for childhood leukemia and other cancers. For a reference point, a barium enema results in a 0.5 rad dose to the skin. The fetal dose is much lower as the radiation dose decreases with the square of the distance traveled through tissue.

Referral for genetic counseling should be made if any of the above risk factors are found. Genetic counselors can be of great assistance in more precisely determining the genetic and teratogenetic risks to the fetus.

Prenatal testing

Maternal serum α-fetoprotein (MSAFP) testing is offered to women between 15 and 20 weeks' gestation. Initially this test was used to identify fetuses with neural tube defects. However, it became apparent that fetuses with other defects also had elevated levels. Most frequently this included abdominal wall defects. As experience accumulated it was noted that low MSAFP was associated with Down's syndrome and other chromosomal abnormalities. MSAFP testing will correctly identify 80% of spina bifida and 95% of anencephaly. Thirty percent of infants with Down's syndrome will have low MSAFP levels.

Other maternal serum markers have been identified that further enhance the detection of chromosomally abnormal fetuses. Estriol and human chorionic gonadotropin in conjunction with AFP are able to identify up to 75% of fetuses with Down's syndrome. Trisomy 18 and triploidy likewise have a characteristic pattern. The use of these three tests is termed triple screen.

Amniocentesis and chorionic villus sampling are the standard means by which fetal tissue is obtained for prenatal diagnosis. Women who will deliver at or after 35 years of age should be routinely offered either procedure, as the risk for a chromosomally abnormal fetus increases each year (Table 54.1). The maternal serum triple screen will also identify younger women at increased risk who would then be offered amniocentesis. Karyotypic analysis only identifies chromosomal structural and numerical abnormalities. It does not identify single-gene disorders or microdeletions.

Families at risk for a known inherited disease may be able to have prenatal testing. Many metabolic disorders, hematologic disorders, and X-linked diseases can be tested for in the fetus by DNA analysis of cells obtained by amniocentesis or chorionic vilus sampling or examination of the amniotic fluid for abnormal metabolites (Table 54.2). As the current human genome mapping project for mapping and sequencing the entire human genome continues, more genetic diseases will become candidates

Table 54.1 Chromosomal abnormalities with advancing maternal age

Maternal age (years)	Risk of Down's syndrome	Risk of all chromosomal abnormalities
20	1:1667	1:526
25	1:1250	1:476
30	1:952	1:384
35	1:385	1:204
37	1:227	1:130
40	1:106	1:65
42	1:64	1:40
45	1:39	1:20
48	1:14	1:10

Table 54.2 Common genetic diseases for which prenantal diagnosis is available

Disease	Inheritance	Diagnosis: DNA or enzyme
Sickle cell	Autosomal recessive	DNA
Hemophilia A	X-linked recessive	DNA
α-Thalassemia	Autosomal recessive	DNA
Tay–Sachs	Autosomal recessive	Enzyme
Duchenne muscular dystrophy	X-linked recessive	DNA
Phenylketonuria	Autosomal recessive	DNA
Maple syrup urine disease	Autosomal recessive	Enzyme
Cystic fibrosis	Autosomal recessive	DNA
Adult polycystic kidney disease	Autosomal dominant	DNA
Fragile X	X-linked	DNA
Myotonic dystrophy	Autosomal dominant	DNA

for prenatal diagnosis. However there needs to be a family history of an affected individual, otherwise there would be too many diseases to test for indiscriminately. Alternatively, diseases with a high carrier frequency in a population that have poor prognosis should be screened for. This has been successful for Tay–Sachs disease in Ashkenazi Jews.

Targeted ultrasound between 18 and 20 weeks' gestation performed by a person trained in fetal anatomy, and in particular cardiac anatomy, is utilized by many centers to screen for major congenital anomalies. If one major structural abnormality is noted there is roughly a 10% chance that there is a chromosomal abnormality present. This depends on the anomaly, as some are more specific than others. For example, there is a 50% chance of Turner syndrome with a cystic hygroma, 30% chance of Down's syndrome when there is duodenal atresia, but <5% chance of a chromosomal lesion with a neural-tube defect. If there is more than one structural abnormality the risk for a chromosomal abnormality increases. A major structural anomaly is an indication for chromosomal analysis.

SUGGESTED READING

BRIGGS GG, FREEMAN RK, YAFFE SJ. *Drugs in Pregnancy and Lactation.* Baltimore, MD: Williams & Wilkins, 1986.

THOMPSON JS, THOMPSON MW. *Genetics in Medicine.* Philadelphia: WB Saunders, 1991.

VOGEL F, MOTOLSKY AG. *Human Genetics: Problems and Approaches.* Berlin: Springer-Verlag, 1986.

55

Genetic implications of pregnancy loss

DENA TOWNER

Pregnancy loss is one of the most emotionally devastating situations faced by many couples. There is frequently blame placed on oneself. If one carefully looks at the myriad of processes involved in achieving a successful pregnancy, it is understandable why there are frequent losses. It has been proposed that of 100 conceptions, only 30–35 pregnancies reach term. Once conception has occurred, cell division and blastocele formation must progress normally such that implantation can occur while the uterus is hospitable. Implantation, embryologic development and differentiation then must proceed normally. There are many factors that impinge on normal pregnancy maintenance, with genetic factors being prominent, especially in the early phases. This chapter deals with these genetic factors. Other etiologies for pregnancy loss will be addressed in Chapter 113.

Early pregnancy loss

Chromosomal abnormalities are known to contribute significantly to first-trimester losses. The earlier in gestation the loss, the greater is the likelihood that it is due to a karyotypic abnormality. Cytogenetic studies on abortuses have found that 50–60% will have karyotypic abnormalities. Autosomal trisomies (2n+1 or 47 chromosomes) collectively constitute the largest proportion of the abnormal karyotypes – approximately 50%. Trisomy of all chromosomes except number 1 have been found and trisomy 16 is the most common. Twenty-five percent of abortuses with abnormal karyotypes will have monosomy X (Turner syndrome, 45,X), 20% will be triploid (3n or 69 chromosomes), 5% tetraploid (4n or 92 chromosomes), and 3–5% various other structural abnormalities (deletions, duplications, translocations, etc). Autosomal monosomies (2n−1 or 45 chromosomes) are almost never identified. Karyotypic analysis of spermatozoa and fertilized ova at the pronuclear stage has identified equal numbers of cells missing a chromosome or having an extra one. From this one can conclude that autosomal monosomies are lost prior to the pregnancy being clinically evident.

Trisomy generally results from nondisjunction during meiosis during gametogenesis. Utilizing molecular DNA analysis in families with Down's syndrome it has been established that 95% of the time the parent of origin is the mother and 5% of the time the father. Maternal nondisjunction events occur at meiosis I 75% of the time and meiosis II 25%. In contrast the opposite is true for paternal nondisjunction with 25% meiosis I errors and 75% meiosis II errors. The distribution of maternal age was the same in both types of errors. Nondisjunction is clearly increased with advancing maternal age and the smaller chromosomes are affected more often. Rarely a mitotic error in one of the early cell divisions will result in a trisomic fetus due to anaphase lag. In this case the fetus may be mosaic for the trisomic and normal cell lines.

Sex chromosome abnormalities have an interesting pattern. Monosomy X (45,X) is frequently seen in abortuses and in fact is the most common single chromosomal abnormality. Alternatively, sex chromosome trisomies (47,XXY, 47,XXX, and 47,XYY) are rarely seen in abortuses. Parental age has no effect on incidence of sex chromosome aneuploidy. Monosomy X more commonly results from the loss of the paternal X or Y chromosome than a maternal X.

Triploidy usually results from dispermic fertilization but can result from failure to extrude the polar body at the time of fertilization. Triploid conceptions may occur more often when there is delayed fertilization. It is estimated that 1.5% of all conceptions are triploid. In *in vitro* programs 5–10% of fertilized ova contain three pronuclei, implying that those would develop into triploid embryos. Tetraploidy results from failure of cell division after the first mitosis, leading to a cell with 92 chromosomes.

Unbalanced chromosomal complements (deletions, duplications, rearrangements, etc.) can result *de novo* during gametogenesis or be the result of unbalanced segregation of a parental balanced translocation.

It is intuitively easy to understand why a chromosomal abnormality can lead to loss and easy for the parents to comprehend. But what about the other 50% of abortuses that are chromosomally normal? Single-gene mutations can influence the development of the embryo. Extensive research in the mouse and other animals has identified numerous genes called homeobox genes. These genes have a very important role early in development and differentiation as they regulate normal body axis formation and organ induction. Genes are also involved with the organization of the early blastocyst and morula. If the inner cell mass, which is the precursor to the embryo proper, does not form properly, the pregnancy will be lost. Many of the gross early malformations lead to an anembryonic pregnancy and are termed blighted ovum. In one study of 1000 abortuses, nearly 50% were anembryonic. In another study of abortuses with a crown–rump length <30 mm, 70% were morphologically abnormal. From work with *in vitro* fertilization, if a heart beat is seen with ultrasound at 4 embryonic weeks there is a >95% chance of a term pregnancy. However, if the heart beat is not seen until 5 weeks, there is a 50% chance of embryonic loss. This implies that abnormal development from a very early stage leads to pregnancy loss.

Evidence for lethal single-gene mutations comes from X-linked diseases. There is increased loss of male fetuses with incontinentia pigmenti and oral facial digital type I. Retts syndrome is seen only in females and is thus assumed to be lethal in male fetuses. In research species, such as *Drosophila*, there are many known recessive lethal genes. It can be assumed that these genes also exist in humans. Candidates for lethal recessive genes would be those involved with biosynthesis of amino acids, mucopolysaccharides, fatty acids, etc. There are no known inborn errors of metabolism for biosynthesis of organic molecules, only diseases related to errors in degradation of these compounds.

Women who have had an abortion with a normal karyotype are more likely to have karyotypically normal abortions subsequently. The converse, however, is not true: a karyotypically abnormal abortion does not increase the likelihood of a later abortion being karyotypically abnormal. Studies from the 1970s suggested there was an increased risk (76%) that an abortion following a known trisomic abortus would also be trisomic. Remember that the risk of any abortus being karyotypically abnormal is 50–60% and a subsequent abortus would be at a more advanced maternal age, also known to be associated with increased trisomic risk. A recent large study of 273 women with two karyotyped spontaneous abortions, controlled for maternal age, has shown that there is no increased risk. This information implies that chromosomal abnormalities are a random event leading to pregnancy loss. This is in contrast to a liveborn with a trisomy, where there is a 1% recurrence risk for another trisomy. This may relate to a parent having gonadal mosaicism or maternal factors preventing abortion of the less lethal trisomies and not a predisposition to aneuploid conceptions. Conversely, repetitive euploid pregnancy loss suggests a recurrent process that may not be due to the genetic make-up of the embryo.

Late pregnancy loss

As gestation progresses the proportion of losses due to genetic factors declines and those due to maternal or other environmental factors increases. As mentioned above, in losses in the first trimester there is a chromosomal abnormality 50–60% of the time. In the second trimester, 10–15% are due to chromosomal abnormalities. In the third trimester, 5% of stillbirths have chromosomal abnormalities. This is still higher than the 0.6% seen in liveborn infants. The type of chromosomal abnormalities seen in third-trimester stillbirths is similar to those seen in liveborns, predominantly trisomy 13, 18, and 21, monosomy X, and structural rearrangements. Why some of these fetuses are lost early, others stillborn, and yet others liveborn is a question that nobody has been able to answer. Single-gene disorders can also lead to stillbirth, for example Neu–Loxova syndrome, lethal multiple pterygium syndrome, Meckel–Gruber syndrome, and several skeletal dysplasias.

When there is a stillborn infant without an obvious cause, such as a complete placental abruption, a genetic etiology should be sought after, as the family will want to know what was the reason for the stillbirth and the chance it could happen again. The obstetrician should perform a thorough exam (include checking for anal patency, iris, pupils, and palate) and document physical findings with a clear note and photographs. The physical exam may be extremely limited as the fetus may be quite macerated or very premature. Photographs of the face, hands, feet, and ears are the most helpful if a dysmorphologist is to look at them later. Ideally if there is any suggestion of malformations a clinical geneticist should examine the fetus. An autopsy should be requested to aid in the search for malformations and/or to make a diagnosis. X-rays should also be obtained as this may make a diagnosis or differentiate between dominant and recessive forms of diseases, such as osteogenesis imperfecta. The view most beneficial is the whole-body anteroposterior with head slightly extended, arms straight with hands supinated and fingers extended. Lateral views may help if a vertebral body defect is suspected.

Karyotype analysis should be done, especially if a malformation is present, as 25–35% will have a chromosomal abnormality. Overall, 5% of stillbirths will have a chromosomal abnormality and some of these fetuses will not have a malformation. A variety of tissue sources can be utilized for the chromosomal analysis. Unclotted blood obtained from cardiac puncture is excellent if the demise was recent. Other tissues used have included liver, spleen, thymus, and pericardial sac. One must also consider doing an amniocentesis prior to the delivery, especially if the patient is not in labor and wants to await spontaneous labor. Another excellent source that is frequently overlooked is the fetal membranes. After delivery, using aseptic techniques, the chorion and amnion are carefully separated and pieces of chorion are snipped away. This is easiest done over the fetal vessels. If the demise has been long-standing, fibroblasts from connective tissue are the best bet for a successful culture. The easiest source to obtain is the fascia lata from the lateral thigh. Tissue should be obtained with aseptic technique and ideally it is placed in culture media, but normal saline temporarily would be a fine substitute. If a structural chromosomal anomaly is found, parental karyotypes should be done to determine if either is a carrier for a balanced translocation. In most cases the rearrangement is spontaneous.

To complete the evaluation, a full family history needs to be obtained. Emphasis should be on other pregnancy losses in the parents and grandparents, neonatal deaths, congenital malformations, and mental retardation. Once there is a stillborn, especially if it is malformed, much hidden family history comes to light. After all of the information is collected and it appears that the loss potentially was due to a genetic abnormality, the family should be referred for genetic counseling. This is best done as soon as possible but also at a reasonable time – usually 1–2 months – after the delivery so that the parents have had time to grieve and are ready to understand the information given to them.

SUGGESTED READING

ANTONARAKIS SE, AND THE DOWN SYNDROME COLLABORATIVE GROUP. Parental origin of the extra chromosome in trisomy 21 as indicated by analysis of DNA polymorphisms. *N Engl J Med* 1991;324:872–876.

EDWARDS R. Causes of early embryonic loss in human pregnancy. *Hum Reprod* 1986;1:185–198.

THOMPSON JS, THOMPSON MW. *Genetics in Medicine.* Philadelphia: WB Saunders, 1991.

VOGEL F, MOTOLSKY AG. *Human Genetics: Problems and Approaches.* Berlin: Springer-Verlag, 1986.

WARBURTON D, KLINE JK, STEIN Z, HUTZLER M, CHIN A, HASSOLD T. Does the karyotype of a spontaneous abortion predict the karyotype of a subsequent abortion? Evidence from 273 women with two karyotyped spontaneous abortions. *Am J Hum Genet* 1987;41:465–483.

56

Autoimmune disorders during pregnancy

T. MURPHY GOODWIN & JEFFREY S. GREENSPOON

Although several autoimmune disorders may affect reproductive-age women, this chapter will discuss only systemic lupus erythematosus (SLE), immune thrombocytopenic purpura (ITP), myasthenia gravis (MG), and rheumatoid arthritis (RA). The first three disorders can affect the fetus and neonate also, through the passive transfer of maternal antibody mediating the disease process. Therefore, women suffering from these disorders should be managed by a team that includes an obstetrician, an internist, and a pediatrician. In addition, peer support groups can provide emotional support and improve self-esteem.

There is no evidence that the glucocorticoid medications, which frequently are used to treat these disorders, increase malformations above the general rate of 27.5:1000 births. However, their use may result in adrenal suppression. Patients at risk for adrenal suppression should receive hydrocortisone 100 mg iv every 6–8 h during periods of stress, including the peripartum and any perioperative period. Patients receiving glucocorticoids should be screened for:
1 evidence of tuberculosis, which may be reactive during therapy;
2 steroid-induced glucose intolerance before and during pregnancy. Prior to conception, the patient should consult a physician to determine if any medications should be changed to avoid teratogenesis.

Systemic lupus erythematosus

SLE is a chronic inflammatory autoimmune disease that affects many different organ systems. One woman in 700 has SLE, and about one pregnancy in 1660 is complicated by SLE. SLE is important to the obstetrician because it predominantly affects reproductive-age women. The sex ratio is 9:1 female:male.

Maternal complications

A diagnosis of SLE can be made with certainty when the patient fulfills four of the criteria listed in Table 56.1. These strict criteria were established to facilitate the clinical study of SLE. Therefore, the diagnosis may be appropriate even when strict criteria for SLE are not met. Fertility is not impaired in women with SLE unless they are so ill as to be anovulatory or they have received cytotoxic therapy that has damaged the

Table 56.1 Criteria for the diagnosis of systemic lupus erythematosus (SLE)

A patient with any four of the following criteria, either serially or simultaneously, may be classified as having SLE:

Malar rash (fixed erythematous rash over the malar eminences, sparing the nasolabial folds)
Discoid rash (erythematous raised patch with keratotic scaling and follicular plugging; older lesions may be atrophic)
Photosensitivity
Oral ulcers (usually painless)
Arthritis (nonerosive arthritis involving two or more peripheral joints)
Serositis
    (1) Pleuritis or pleural effusion or
    (2) Pericarditis or pericardial effusion
Renal disorder
    (1) Proteinuria of 0.5 g/day
    (2) Cellular casts
Neurologic disorder
    (1) Seizures in the absence of other causes or
    (2) Psychosis in the absence of other causes
Hematologic disorder
    (1) Hemolytic anemia with reticulocytosis or
    (2) Leukopenia $<4000 \, mm^3$ on at least two occasions or
    (3) Lymphopenia $<1500 \, mm^3$ or
    (4) Thrombocytopenia $<100\,000 \, mm^3$
Immunologic disorder
    (1) Positive LE cell preparation
    (2) Anti-DNA antibody to native DNA
    (3) Anti-Sm antibody or
    (4) False-positive serologic test for syphilis for at least 6 months
Antinuclear antibody

ovary. There is a higher rate of spontaneous abortion and fetal demise. Intrauterine fetal growth retardation, fetal distress, preeclampsia, and preterm delivery are more frequent in these patients.

Approach to SLE in pregnancy

There are five major areas to evaluate when considering the risks of pregnancy in a patient with SLE: (1) disease activity; (2) end-organ damage (especially renal impairment); (3) medications required to maintain remission; (4) presence or absence of the antiphospholipid antibody syndrome; (5) presence of anti-SS-A because of its association with the neonatal lupus syndrome.

Disease activity is important for anticipating SLE exacerbation and superimposed pregnancy-induced hypertension. The estimated risk of exacerbation of disease during pregnancy varies widely, from 30 to 77%. Patients in remission for 6 months or longer before pregnancy have a 35% risk of exacerbation during pregnancy, but these patients have a better than 90% chance of having a viable pregnancy outcome. Patients not in remission for 6 months prior to pregnancy have approximately a 48% chance of exacerbation and generally have a poorer pregnancy outcome than the group in remission for 6 months or more. Patients with active disease at the onset of pregnancy have lower fetal survival rates of 50–75%. However, only 10% of those having an exacerbation suffered permanent deterioration of function, usually renal. Recent case-controlled studies showed that postpartum exacerbation occurred no more frequently in women with SLE than in control nonpregnant SLE patients when both groups were followed the same length of time.

Patients with active renal disease (or, less commonly, cardiac disease) have a poor prognosis. A total of 40–60% develop superimposed preeclampsia, which may be difficult to distinguish from an SLE exacerbation. An active urinary sediment and low levels of serum complement may be helpful in making the distinction. Preeclampsia is usually associated with an increased serum complement level.

The goal of medical therapy is to reduce medication to the least number of safe medications. If the patient can tolerate it, change nonsteroidal antiinflammatory drugs and hydroxychloroquine to prednisone, because of prednisone's better safety record with regard to fetal effects. Maternal complications of glucocorticoids include glucose intolerance, gastric ulceration, truncal obesity, cutaneous atrophy, poor wound healing, glaucoma, cataracts, osteoporosis and, less commonly, steroid myopathy, aseptic necrosis of the femoral head, and transient fetal adrenal suppression.

Fetal complications

There is an increased incidence of intrauterine growth retardation in the fetuses of women with SLE. This may be a multifactorial process to which systemic vasculitis contributes, as do renal disease, chronic hypertension, and superimposed preeclampsia. Furthermore, maternal indications, such as worsening preeclampsia or the development of fetal distress, may lead to preterm delivery. At present, all fetuses undergo antepartum fetal surveillance because of concern for increased fetal loss even in the absence of acute disease.

The neonatal lupus syndrome consists of complete congenital heart block and/or a typical skin rash. The presence of the maternal antibody anti-SS-A/Ro in a patient with SLE is associated with development of the neonatal syndrome in 3.3% of newborns. The presence of anti-SS-A/Ro is associated with a 2–10% risk of neonatal lupus rash. Recently, the maternal antibody anti-[1]RNP (anti-nRNP) also has been associated with the neonatal lupus syndrome.

Management guidelines

Our basic management of the pregnant patient with SLE is shown in Table 56.2. A baseline set of serologic tests is obtained, including those studies shown in Table 56.2. Blood pressure and fetal growth are monitored carefully.

Delivery is often provoked by fetal or maternal indications. However, in the patient who is stable and has a healthy fetus, labor at term can be expected. Cesarean section is done only for the usual obstetric indications. If SLE is complicated by immune thrombocytopenia, the route of delivery is determined as described below. Postpartum exacerbation is managed expectantly with a satisfactory outcome anticipated.

Antiphospholipid antibody syndrome

Antiphospholipid antibody syndrome (APS), an important cause of maternal and fetal morbidity in pregnancy, is diagnosed when clinical events such as arterial or venous thrombosis, thrombocytopenia, or recurrent fetal loss occur in association with a positive laboratory test for antiphospholipid antibodies (e.g., anticardiolipin antibodies or the lupus anticoagulant; Table 56.2). The syndrome may occur alone (primary APS) or in conjunction with SLE or other rheumatologic diseases.

The lupus anticoagulant (LAC) is an antibody that was (mis)named due to: (1) its original identification with SLE, although it has since been identified in persons without SLE; and (2) the *in vitro* phenomenon of

Table 56.2 Approach to the pregnant patient with systemic lupus erythematosus (SLE)

Serial ultrasound for fetal growth
Modified biophysical profile twice a week from 25 weeks
Umbilical artery Doppler if IUGR suspected
1-h glucola at 20, 28, 32 weeks if the patient is on steroids
Special consideration if the patient is at high risk for APS, CCHB (see text)

Rheumatologic studies which may be ordered by the consultant

Antibody	Frequency in SLE (%)	Clinical significance associations
Antinuclear antibody	>90	
Anti-ds DNA	>80	Correlates with disease activity, specific for SLE
Anti Sm	30	Specific for SLE
aCL	40 ⎫	Correlates with fetal loss and
LAC	20 ⎬	thrombotic events
RPR	⎭	
Anti-SSA (Ro)	25	Both associated with
Anti-SSB (la)	20	NLE/CCHB and with Sjögren's syndrome
Anti-RNP	25	SLE, NLE
Every 1–3 months		
aCL*	⎫	
Anti-ds DNA	⎬	Useful for following disease
Platelets	⎬	activity
Renal function studies	⎭	

* If positive initially.
aCL, Anticardiolipin antibody; APS, antiphospholipid antibody syndrome; CCHB, congenital complete heart block; IUGR, intrauterine growth retardation; LAC, lupus anticoagulant; NLE, neonatal lupus erythematosus; RPR, rapid plasma reagin.

prolonging phospholipid-dependent coagulation tests such as the activated partial thromboplastin time. It does not cause a bleeding defect; in fact, it is associated with both venous and arterial thrombosis. LAC is associated with recurrent abortion, intrauterine growth retardation, and severe preeclampsia. APS may explain some of the increase in fetal wastage associated with SLE.

The rate of fetal loss may exceed 90% in patients with APS. Therapy for recurrent pregnancy loss associated with APS is still evolving. A 75% success rate was described by Cowchock *et al.* using a protocol including aspirin 80 mg daily, and subcutaneous heparin every 12 h in a dose that did not prolong the activated partial thromboplastin time. Heparin therapy was initiated after fetal viability was confirmed by ultrasound. No benefit was noted when prednisone was included in the regimen. Formal prospective evaluation of this regimen against aspirin alone or heparin alone has not been repeated. The use of immunoglobulin infusion is under investigation for patients who fail to achieve a successful pregnancy with conventional aspirin and heparin therapy.

The antibody to cardiolipin appears to have a specific association with fetal demise or fetal distress in patients with SLE. Patients with SLE and this antibody deserve intense antepartum surveillance. Preliminary information suggests that the development of variable decelerations or oligohydramnios is ominous and probably requires continuous monitoring until delivery.

Immune thrombyocytopenic purpura

ITP should be distinguished from the new entity incidental thrombocytopenia of pregnancy. Incidental thrombocytopenia is described below.

The prevalence of ITP is approximately 7.5:100 000 persons. Approximately 5% of those afflicted die, usually of central nervous system hemorrhage. ITP is diagnosed by exclusion. The criteria for diagnosis include a platelet count below normal ($<150 000/mm^3$), no other cause for thrombocytopenia (including drugs or systemic disease), and no evidence of a coagulopathy. A bone marrow biopsy should reveal normal or increased numbers of megakaryocytes, which is consistent with a peripheral destructive process. Platelet antibodies have little value in the management or diagnosis of the disease.

The pregnant patient should be evaluated for other causes of thrombocytopenia. The peripheral smear should be inspected to insure that the thrombocytopenia is not a laboratory artifact from platelet clumping caused by the anticoagulant that was used to collect blood. The patient should be examined for preeclampsia, hyperthyroidism, syphilis, malaria, infection with the human immunodeficiency virus, liver disease with portal hypertension, and splenomegaly or lymphoma. Pancytopenia suggests a primary bone marrow disorder (such as vitamin B_{12}, folate, or iron deficiency) or infiltration of the marrow with a neoplastic or granulomatous process. Common drugs associated with thrombocytopenia include quinine and quinidine, carbamazepine, alcohol, and heroin. ITP associated with SLE is managed as ITP; however, the other manifestations of SLE must be followed as well. There are two clinical presentations of ITP. In children, the acute form is more frequent following a viral infection and usually resolves completely. The chronic form predominantly affects women of child-bearing age and may cause recurrent episodes throughout life. About 75% of patients with the chronic form of ITP achieve remission with splenectomy.

Therapy

A patient with ITP is treated to maintain a platelet count $>50\,000/mm^3$. The initial dose of prednisone is $1.0–1.5\,mg/kg$ per day. A response occurs within 21 days. The dose is tapered to maintain a count $>50\,000/mm^3$. The patient should not receive aspirin or other nonsteroidal anti-inflammatory drugs because they interfere with platelet function. Patients who are refractory to glucocorticoids may be candidates for splenectomy during the early second trimester. As pregnancy proceeds and the uterus enlarges, a splenectomy becomes more difficult. Occasionally, splenectomy is performed at the time of cesarean section.

Intravenous immunoglobulin, usually given in a dose of $400\,mg/kg$ per day for a 5-day course, has been effective in raising platelet counts in refractory patients. A response usually occurs in 4–5 days. Immunoglobulin is expensive and the effect is transient, but a patient may be able to undergo splenectomy or delivery during the remission. The mechanism of action is thought to be blockage of the macrophage Fc receptor of the reticuloendothelial system. Some physicians have used immunoglobulin infusions rather than glucocorticoids to maintain an adequate maternal platelet count, although this approach is very expensive. Another potential advantage of immunoglobulin therapy during pregnancy is that it may increase the platelet count in a thrombocytopenic fetus whereas glucocorticoids do not consistently increase fetal platelet counts.

Route of delivery

Unfortunately, no laboratory test on maternal blood has been completely reliable in predicting fetal thrombocytopenia. Women with low maternal platelet counts may have normal infants; conversely, women in remission, or years after a splenectomy, may have a thrombocytopenic fetus. The usefulness of platelet-associated immunoglobulin G (PAIgG) is limited because it is not specific, i.e., it is frequently falsely positive for the prediction of a thrombocytopenic fetus. Many women with ITP who have PAIgG deliver infants without thrombocytopenia.

A review of 474 infants born to mothers with ITP noted that 10% of infants had moderate thrombocytopenia (platelets $51\,000–100\,000/mm^3$), and 15% had severe thrombocytopenia ($<50\,000/mm^3$). The risk of intracranial hemorrhage was 3% among infants with moderate or severe thrombocytopenia and was not statistically associated with the vaginal route of delivery.

If percutaneous blood sampling or intrapartum scalp sample for platelet estimate is undertaken, cesarean delivery is performed when the fetal platelet count is <50 000 mm^3, although the benefits of cesarean delivery have not been demonstrated prospectively. The patient should be informed that the risks associated with percutaneous umbilical blood sampling and cesarean delivery may exceed the benefits of identifying a thrombocytopenic fetus.

Doppler ultrasound, rather than a scalp electrode, should be used to monitor the fetal heart rate. The mother can have an epidural anesthetic if she has a normal platelet count or normal bleeding time. A marked drop in the maternal platelet count in the peripartum period may be a sign of preeclampsia or sepsis. A difficult delivery with the use of forceps or the vacuum extractor should be avoided because the fetus may develop neonatal thrombocytopenia.

Platelets should be available at the time of cesarean or vaginal delivery if the maternal platelet count is approximately 50 000/mm^3, but the platelets should not be transfused unless clinical bleeding is encountered, which is unlikely.

There are no exact guidelines regarding when platelets should be transfused. It is generally agreed that there is a risk of spontaneous bleeding with counts <20 000/mm^3; however, patients with ITP frequently tolerate lower counts without difficulty if they are not subjected to surgical or accidental trauma. If thrombocytopenia is the only clotting abnormality, it is unlikely that bleeding will occur with counts of 50 000/mm^3 or more. Each unit of platelets will increase the platelet count by 8000 to 10 000/mm^3. Transfused platelets do not persist for a long duration in the recipient because they are destroyed by the same immune-mediated process that is causing the thrombocytopenia.

Fetal and neonatal thrombocytopenia

The neonatal platelet count reaches a nadir 2–6 days after delivery. Platelet counts should be measured, although the thrombocytopenic neonate usually has petechiae. The platelet count usually returns to normal within 2 months after birth. There is a theoretic, but unlikely, risk that breast-feeding may transfer maternal antibody to the neonate.

Incidental thrombocytopenia of pregnancy

The widespread use of automated platelet counting during pregnancy has led to the identification of a previously unrecognized condition called incidental thrombocytopenia of pregnancy or pregnancy-associated thrombocytopenia. Approximately 6% of healthy, asymptomatic pregnant women may develop mild to moderate thrombocytopenia (70 000–150 000/mm^3). These patients do not have a history of thrombocytopenia or a bleeding diathesis and are otherwise healthy. The rate of thrombocytopenia (platelet counts <150 000/mm^3) in their newborn infants is 4%, which is not different from those observed in women without the condition. None of the newborns in prospective series has platelet counts <50 000/mm^3. Neither mother nor infant has had bleeding complications in association with this disorder. Many gravidas have received epidural anesthesia during labor and delivery without complication. The incidental thrombocytopenia usually resolves spontaneously by 6 weeks postpartum, although it may recur in subsequent pregnancies. No special management is required for patients with incidental thrombocytopenia of pregnancy.

Myasthenia gravis

MG is caused by an antibody directed against the postsynaptic membrane acetylcholine receptor. Clinical weakness occurs, which may be limited to ocular muscles, affect other muscle groups, such as the facial and pharyngeal and limb girdle, or cause generalized weakness. The major maternal risk involves respiratory failure or aspiration of oropharyngeal secretions. A total of 1:20 000–40 000 persons is affected by MG; and there is a predilection toward young women. In one series, thymoma was present in 10% of patients.

Plauche has summarized the outcome of 292 pregnancies in 202 women. The antepartum course was associated with remission in 30% of cases, exacerbation in 45%, and no change in 35%. A postpartum exacerbation occurred in 31%. Some patients experienced both an exacerbation and a remission in different trimesters of the same pregnancy. Maternal death occurred in 4% of patients, nearly always due to myasthenic crisis. Women who have undergone thymectomy have fewer exacerbations during pregnancy.

Women with MG have more frequent episodes of preterm labor and preterm delivery than normal pregnant women. The incidence of pre-eclampsia is increased. Magnesium sulfate should not be given to MG patients because it is a neuromuscular blocking agent. Phenytoin may be used to prevent eclamptic seizures.

After the diagnosis of MG, the patient is treated with cholinesterase inhibitors, such as pyridostigmine. Glucocorticoid treatment (prednisone 60–80 mg daily) is begun. Some 80–90% of patients will improve markedly or enter remission and be able to discontinue or decrease the cholinesterase inhibitor. These patients can be maintained on lower-dose, alternate-day glucocorticoid therapy.

The edrophonium (Tensilon) test may be used to confirm the diagnosis of MG or to differentiate exacerbation of MG from a cholinergic crisis (due to excessive cholinesterase inhibition). The weakness of MG is improved by edrophonium; cholinergic crisis is worsened by edrophonium. Edrophonium (1 mg) is injected intravenously, and then the effects on muscle weakness are observed for 2 min; an additional 3 mg is injected and observation continues for 2 min longer. If no effect is apparent, 6 mg is injected intravenously and observation continues.

Cholinesterase inhibitor drugs should be continued parenterally during labor because gastrointestinal absorption may be unreliable. Equivalent doses are approximately 0.5 mg iv neostigmine = 1.5 mg im neostigmine = 15 mg oral neostigmine = 60 mg oral pyridostigmine = 2.0 mg im pyridostigmine = 3.0–4.0 mg iv pyridostigmine. Neostigmine is given every 2–4 h; pyridostigmine is given every 3–6 h.

Analgesia during labor may be provided by an epidural anesthetic. Amide-type local anesthetics, such as lidocaine, should be used because they are metabolized normally. Ester-type local anesthetics should be avoided because the normal metabolism of these drugs by the cholinesterase system is inhibited. The second stage of labor may be shortened by a mid pelvic delivery to decrease maternal fatigue associated with labor. Because many medications exacerbate weakness, caution should be exercised. Increased weakness may be due to an exacerbation of MG, cholinergic crisis (due to excessive cholinesterase inhibition), a new medication increasing neuromuscular blockage (for example, an aminoglycoside), hypokalemia, coincident hyperthyroidism, or fatigue. The need to intubate the patient to support ventilation can be assessed by serial bedside measurements of vital capacity and peak flow. Congenital MG may cause decreased fetal movement, breathing movements, and contractures, which can be identified sonographically.

Neonatal MG occurs in 12–20% of neonates born to women with MG. Symptoms appear within 24 h of birth, occasionally as late as the third day after delivery. Neonatal symptoms resolve by 3 months, coincident with the fall of the passively acquired maternal antibody. Long-term follow-up of 31 children born to women with MG indicates that MG does not cause neuromuscular disease in the offspring. Modern techniques to support respiration and maintain nutrition during exacerbations as well as the availability of plasmapheresis in selected severe cases to shorten the length of crises make the outcome of pregnancy associated with MG better than older series would suggest.

Rheumatoid arthritis

RA is a chronic systemic disease that causes inflammation of the peripheral synovial joints in a symmetric distribution. Seventy percent of cases occur in the third to seventh decades of life; peak onset is in the fourth decade. Women are affected three times as frequently as men, and the incidence ranges from 0.5 to 3.8% of women.

RA improves during pregnancy in about 75% of patients. The remainder tend to undergo no change. About 90% will have a recurrence of symptoms within 2 months of delivery. The improvement seems to be due to increases in the levels of pregnancy-associated α_2-macroglobulin, a glycoprotein with known immunosuppressive activity. Patients with RA do not present many specific problems during pregnancy; the main issue is drug therapy.

Prospective studies of aspirin use in pregnancy did not find that it increased malformations in human beings. However, long-term aspirin use increased the frequency of anemia, antepartum and postpartum hemorrhage, and preeclampsia in women with RA. Aspirin also has been associated with prolonged lengths of gestation. Aspirin can cause hemostatic abnormalities in the fetus. It increases the incidence of intracranial hemorrhage and persistent pulmonary hypertension, and it carries the theoretic risk of premature closure of the ductus ateriosus. For these reasons, it is prudent to use the lowest possible dose of glucocorticoid instead of aspirin to treat arthralgia during pregnancy. The safest drug is acetaminophen, which should be used if it is effective.

Juvenile RA is seen infrequently by the obstetrician. There are three subgroups: primary systemic symptoms, polyarticular disease, and pauciarticular disease (involving only a few joints). The patient may have a small pelvis due to the effects on growth of chronic illness and treatment with glucocorticoids. A small pelvis may result in cephalopelvic disproportion and thus increase the need for cesarean section. Hip replacements may dislocate when the thighs are abducted. The anesthesiologist should be aware of the risk of atlantoaxial subluxation and micrognathia in these patients.

SUGGESTED READING

Autoimmune diseases and pregnancy

BYRON MA. Prescribing in pregnancy: treatment of rheumatic diseases. *Br Med J* 1987;294:236.

MOR-YOSEF S, NAVOT D, RABINOWITZ R, SCHENKER JG. Collagen diseases in pregnancy. *Obstet Gynecol Surv* 1984;39:67.

Incidental thrombocytopenia of pregnancy

BURROWS RF, KELTON JG. Incidentally detected thrombocytopenia in healthy mothers and their infants. *N Engl J Med* 1988;319:142–145.

BURROWS RF, KELTON JG. Low fetal risks in pregnancies associated with idiopathic thrombocytopenic purpura. *Am J Obstet Gynecol* 1990;163:1147–1150.

BURROWS RF, KELTON JG. Thrombocytopenia at delivery: a prospective survey of 6715 deliveries. *Am J Obstet Gynecol* 1990;162:731–734.

CHRISTIAENS GCML, HELMERHORST FM. Validity of intrapartum diagnosis of fetal thrombocytopenia. *Am J Obstet Gynecol* 1987;157:684–685.

CINES D, DUSAK B, TOMASKI A, MENNUTI M, SCHREIBER AD. Immune thrombocytopenic purpura and pregnancy. *N Engl J Med* 1982;306:831–836.

CONSENSUS CONFERENCE. Platelet transfusion therapy. *JAMA* 1987;257:1777.

COOK RL, MILLER RC, KATZ VL, CEFALO RC. Immune thrombocytopenic purpura: a reappraisal of management. *Obstet Gynecol* 1991;78:578–583.

KARPATKIN M, PORGES RF, KARPATKIN S. Platelet counts in infants of women with autoimmune thrombocytopenia. Effect of steroid administration to the mother. *N Engl J Med* 1981;305:936–939.

LAVERY JP, KOONTZ WL, LIU YK, et al. Immunologic thrombocytopenia in pregnancy; use of antenatal immunoglobulin therapy: case report and review. *Obstet Gynecol* 1985;66:41S.

MARTIN JN, MORRISON JC, FILES JC. Autoimmune thrombocytopenic purpura: current concepts and recommended practices. *Am J Obstet Gynecol* 1984;150:86.

NATIONAL INSTITUTES OF HEALTH CONSENSUS CONFERENCE. Intravenous immunoglobulin. Prevention and treatment of disease. *JAMA* 1990;264:3189–3193. [Usual course is 400 mg/kg daily for 5 days.]

PATRIARCO M, YEH S-Y. Immunological thrombocytopenia in pregnancy. *Obstet Gynecol Surv* 1986;41:661.

SAMUELS P, BUSSEL JB, BRAITMAN LE, et al. Estimation of the risk of thrombocytopenia in the offspring of pregnant women with presumed immune thrombocytopenic purpura. *N Engl J Med* 1990;323:229–235.

Antiphospholipid antibody syndrome

BRANCH DW, SILVER RM, BLACKWELL JL, READING JC, SCOTT JR. Outcome of treated pregnancies in women with antiphospholipid syndrome: an update of the Utah experience. *Obstet Gynecol* 1992;80:614–620.

COWCHOCK FS, REECE EA, BALABAN D, BRANCH DW, PLOUFFE L. Repeated fetal losses associated with antiphospholipid antibodies: a collaborative randomized trial comparing prednisone with low-dose heparin treatment. *Am J Obstet Gynecol* 1992;166:1318–1323.

LUBBE WF, LIGGINS GC. Lupus anticoagulant and pregnancy. *Am J Obstet Gynecol* 1985;153:322.

PEACEMAN AM, REHNBERG KA. The immunoglobulin G fraction from plasma containing antiphospholipid antibodies causes increased placental thromboxane production. *Am J Obstet Gynecol* 1992;167:1543–1547.

REECE EA, GABRIELLI S, CULLEN MT, ZHENG X-Z, HOBBINS JC, HARRIS EN. Recurrent adverse pregnancy outcome and antiphospholipid antibodies. *Am J Obstet Gynecol* 1990;163:162–169.

TRIPLETT DA, BRANDT JT, MAAS RL. The laboratory heterogeneity of lupus anticoagulants. *Arch Pathol Lab Med* 1985;109:946.

TRIPLETT DA, BRANDT JT, MUSGRAVE KA, et al. The relationship between lupus anticoagulants and antibodies to phospholipid. *JAMA* 1988;259:550.

WAPNER RJ, COWCHOCK FS, SHAPIRO SS. Successful treatment in two women with antiphospholipid antibodies and refractory pregnancy losses with intravenous immunoglobulin infusions. *Am J Obstet Gynecol* 1989;161:1271–1272.

Systemic lupus erythematosus

DRUZIN ML, LOCKSHIN M, EDERSHEIM TG, *et al*. Second trimester fetal monitoring and preterm delivery in pregnancies with systemic lupus erythematosus and/or circulating anticoagulant. *Am J Obstet Gynecol* 1987;157:1503.

GIMOVSKY ML, MONTORO M, PAUL RH. Pregnancy outcome in women with systemic lupus erythematosus. *Obstet Gynecol* 1984;63:686.

LOCKSHIN MD, DRUZIN ML, GOEL S, *et al*. Antibody to cardiolipin as a predictor of fetal distress or death in pregnant patients with systemic lupus erythematosus. *N Engl J Med* 1985;313:152.

RAMSAY-GOLDMAN R, HOM D, DENG J-S *et al*. Anti-SS-A antibodies and fetal outcome in maternal systemic lupus erythematosus. *Arthritis Rheum* 1986;29:1269.

Myasthenia gravis

AHLSTEN G, LEFRERT AK, OSTERMAN PO, STALBERG E, SAFWENBERG J. Follow-up study of muscle function in children of mothers with myasthenia gravis during pregnancy. *J Child Neurol* 1992;7:264–269.

FENNELL DF, RINGEL SP. Myasthenia gravis and pregnancy. *Obstet Gynecol Surv* 1987;41:414.

PLAUCHE WC. Myasthenia gravis in pregnancy: an update. *Am J Obstet Gynecol* 1979;135:691.

ROLBIN SH, LEVINSON G, SHNIDER SM, *et al*. Anesthetic considerations for myasthenia gravis and pregnancy. *Anesth Analg* 1978;57:441.

PART 3

Gynecology

57

Vulvovaginitis

SUBIR ROY

Vulvovaginitis, the most common problem in gynecologic office practice, has many causes and is often transmitted by sexual contact. The cardinal symptom of vaginitis is an abnormal vaginal discharge. If the vulva is involved, the patient may also complain of pruritus, burning pain, dysuria, and dyspareunia. The cause of symptoms is usually one or more microorganisms. A vaginal discharge can also be physiologic when due to mucus secretion from the endocervix at midcycle or to desquamation of epithelial cells premenstrually. Sometimes chemical irritation, an allergen, or a foreign body will produce an inflammatory reaction. Other factors that contribute to vulvovaginitis are poorly cornified vaginal epithelium, as seen in prepubertal girls and postmenopausal women, fecal contamination from the anus, sexual intercourse, chronic cervicitis, pregnancy, excessive local heat and moisture, broad-spectrum antibiotic therapy sufficient to destroy the normal bacterial flora, and coexisting systemic disease, particularly diabetes.

The vagina is normally acidic (pH 3.5–4.5) because of the lactic acid produced by Döderlein's bacillus (*Lactobacillus acidophilus*). Cervical mucus, menstrual blood, overgrowth of other organisims of the vaginal flora, and progesterone all raise the vaginal pH and favor the growth of trichomonads and *Gardnerella vaginalis* (previously known as *Corynebacterium vaginale* or *Haemophilus vaginalis*).

The history should include accounts of any previous vaginal infections and their treatment, as well as hygienic, contraceptive, and sexual practices. Microscopic examination of a wet smear will help to differentiate among infections due to fungi, trichomonads, and bacteria.

Trichomonas

Trichomoniasis of the urogenital tract is caused by the flagellated protozoan *Trichomonas vaginalis*, a sexually transmitted microorganism found in adults of either sex. A moderate rise in vaginal pH favors its growth. Another factor encouraging trichomonal infection is local erosion resulting from chemical or mechanical trauma, neoplasms, or other forms of vaginal infection. Presumably there is no significant host immunity to *Trichomonas*.

Clinical picture

Asymptomatic carrier

Approximately 15% of women in the reproductive years of life harbor *T. vaginalis*, but only one-third of these women have symptoms and signs of local inflammation, probably because the organism is more virulent. Asymptomatic carriers are identified by wet mount preparations at the time of routine gynecologic examination. These women should be treated to prevent transmission of the disease and to minimize the possibility that an acute infection will eventually be established.

Active infection

Trichomoniasis usually produces a malodorous discharge that may be frothy, profuse, thick, or thin, and green, yellow, gray, or white. If the vulva is involved, there may be local pain, itching, dyspareunia, dysuria, or urinary frequency. Erythema and edema of the vulva and vagina and punctate subepithelial hemorrhages or strawberry marks on the vagina and cervix are sometimes observed.

Diagnosis

In 80% or more of cases, a wet smear prepared with warm saline and examined immediately will contain motile trichomonads. They are easily identified by their size, shape, and flagellate motion. Other cases may be identified by cytologic smear, although there is a considerable incidence of both false-positive and false-negative reports. Staining methods add little to diagnosis, and cultures are seldom needed.

Systemic treatment

The drug of choice is metronidazole (Flagyl). A single dose of 2 g orally should be the initial treatment. Alternatively, 500 mg every 12 h for 7 days can be tried. With failure to eradicate, 2 g orally daily for 3–5 days can be attempted. Since the teratogenic potential of metronidazole is unknown, it seems prudent to withhold this drug during pregnancy except for patients with severe symptoms in the first trimester, in whom 2 g orally in a single dose may be considered. The short-term cure rate with this regimen approaches 98% and the complication rate is 10%, consisting chiefly of gastrointestinal complaints. Long-term cure rates depend on whether trichomoniasis is also eradicated from patients' sexual partners. Since a disulfiram-like reaction (nausea and flushing) can be induced when alcohol and metronidazole are ingested, patients should be advised not to ingest alcohol.

Topical treatment

A number of topical preparations are available, including suppositories, creams, and douches. They are not particularly effective, but may be useful in controlling symptoms in patients with multiple sexual partners when the partners cannot be treated. Metronidazole vaginal gel in a concentration of 0.75% delivers 37.5 mg of metronidazole in a 5-g applicator; when administered twice daily for 5 days, it may be tried to eradicate *T. vaginale*.

Therapy for sexual partners

Ideally, male sexual partners should be examined and treated if indicated. The diagnosis of trichomonads in the male is made on a wet mount of a urethral discharge obtained spontaneously or after prostatic massage. As a compromise, a couple can be treated concurrently. The male should use a condom during therapy to reduce the risk of reinfection. An alternative for the male partner is to abstain from intercourse for a month (or use a condom) in hopes that the infection will clear spontaneously.

Resistant disease

Continuing or recurring symptoms may be due to a coexisting pathogen such as *Candida*, to recurrent infection from an untreated partner, to drug resistance or to poor drug absorption, or to local inactivation of the drug by vaginal bacteria. In the last case, oral metronidazole should be repeated at a dose of 500 mg t.i.d. for 10 days.

Candida

Vulvovaginitis due to *Candida* is usually caused by the species *C. albicans*, a dimorphic fungus that forms yeast-like buds, pseudohyphae, and hyphae. This ubiquitous organism is frequently found as a saprophyte on the skin and in the bowel, oropharynx, and vagina. When host defenses are impaired, it becomes a pathogen. *C. albicans* is currently the most common cause of vaginitis during the reproductive years.

Factors that presumably predispose to candidal vulvovaginitis include an excess of vaginal glucose, as occurs in pregnancy or diabetes, reduction in vaginal bacterial flora, as occurs with the use of broad-spectrum antibiotics, and an excess of local moisture, as occurs during hot, moist weather or with tightly fitting clothing.

Clinical picture

Vulvitis

A candidal infection usually involves both the vulva and the vagina. The major vulvar symptom is pruritus, which may be associated with dysuria, dyspareunia, and local pain. The skin is erythematous, slightly edematous, and often excoriated.

Vaginitis

A typical vaginal discharge is thick, whitish, and resembles cottage cheese. The vagina may be erythematous but often appears normal.

Diagnosis

Candidiasis that produces a typical cheesy discharge can be diagnosed on sight. Other cases can be diagnosed by microscopic examination of a wet smear prepared by mixing a sample of the discharge with a few milliliters of normal saline to which several drops of 10% potassium hydroxide have been added. *Candida* cells are oval or round and approximately the size of a red blood cell. Elongated buds and pseudomycelia may also be present. Still other cases will require a culture for confirmation. Either Sabouraud's or Nickerson's medium inoculated with cells from a cotton swab will show evidence of growth in 2 or 3 days.

Treatment

1 The vagina is first cleansed as thoroughly as possible to remove excess discharge before the start of treatment.
2 A topical antifungal agent is prescribed. These are the most effective:
(a) Miconazole nitrate vaginal suppository 200 mg, intravaginally at bedtime for 3 days;

(b) Clotrimazole vaginal tablets 200 mg, intravaginally at bedtime for 3 days;

(c) Butoconazole 2% cream, 5 g, intravaginally at bedtime for 3 days;

(d) Terconazole 80 mg suppository or 0.4% cream, intravaginally at bedtime for 3 days.

3   Although messy and somewhat irritating, gentian violet solution (1% aqueous) is an effective adjuvant that can be applied at an office visit.

4   Coexisting vulvitis is best treated by local application of a corticosteroid cream plus an antifungal agent, e.g., Mycolog ointment, which has a higher pH than the vagina and therefore does not burn when applied to the vulva.

5   Clothing that increases local heat and moisture, such as nylon underwear and tightly fitting garments, should be avoided.

6   Intercourse should be avoided during the first few days of treatment or until it is no longer painful.

7   Broad-spectrum antibiotics (such as tetracycline for the treatment of acne) should be discontinued until the vulvovaginitis is eradicated.

Treatment failure

1   Reexamine the patient carefully to be certain that symptoms are not due to the emergence of a coexisting pathogen such as *Trichomonas*.

2   Evaluate the possibility of reinfection from a candidal infection of the patient's sexual partner's penile skin.

3   Retreat the patient with a combined topical and oral medication (one nystatin tablet 4 times a day) and consider such combined therapy for the partner as well or alternate vaginal preparations with 1% aqueous gentian violet painted on the vagina on 5 consecutive days.

4   Evaluate the possibility that the patient may have undiagnosed diabetes.

Bacteria

When vulvovaginitis is due to neither *Trichomonas* nor *Candida*, the diagnosis is usually labeled nonspecific vaginitis (NSV) or bacterial vaginosis (BV), especially if the pH >4.5, there is a positive potassium hydroxide whiff-test and clue cells are present. The term BV has been proposed for this condition since bacteria are involved but without leukocytes. In the majority of these cases, however, the infection is due to a specific, though unidentified, bacterium.

The microbiologic picture of NSV or BV consists of the presence of gram-variable coccobacilli, consistent with *Gardnerella vaginalis*, together with numerous anaerobic organisms. The latter are thought to be responsible for the production of aromatic amines with names such as putrescine and cadavarine, which are volatilized by the addition of 10% potassium hydroxide, resulting in the characteristic fishy odor associated with this disorder. Clue cells may be visualized (stratified squamous cells with a granular appearance due to a coating of organisms) when saline is mixed with vaginal fluids in this condition; however, it is not pathognomonic for this condition.

Local treatment with triple sulfa or nitrofuranzone (Furacin) cream for 10–14 days is sometimes ameliorative but usually not successful. Ampicillin 500 mg 4 times a day for 5 days may eradicate *Gardnerella*, but since it also kills *Lactobacillus*, it raises the vaginal pH, apparently facilitating reinfection. The cure rates with these therapies is only 14–60%. Metronidazole 500 mg twice daily for 7 days is the treatment of choice resulting in a cure rate of 75–80% 1 month later. A new therapy for this condition is metronidazole vaginal gel in a concentration of 0.75% which delivers 37.5 mg of metronidazole in a 5-g applicator and, when administered twice daily for 5 days, has been shown efficacious in treating BV with cure rates at 1 month of 85–97%. If reinfection occurs, the patient's sexual partner should also be treated with metronidazole on the supposition that he is harboring the organism. Another new therapy is clindamycin vaginal cream 2%, 5 g daily for 7 days (100 mg clindamycin), which has shown efficacy in this condition (with cure rates of 61–94% at 1 month). Both of these compounds eradicate *G. vaginalis* and other anaerobes while sparing the lactobacilli.

Neisseria gonorrhoeae

Gonococcal infection is discussed in Chapter 61.

Colon bacilli

A persisting vaginitis, particularly in children, can result from repeated contamination of the vulvar area by feces. Although any of the usual inhabitants of the lower bowel can be involved, *Escherichia coli* is most likely to be the offending organism. Teaching proper hygiene usually cures the infection. Acute vaginitis usually responds to a 4–5-day course of oral ampicillin.

Bacteroides species may be normally found in the vagina and may on occasion cause vaginitis that produces a malodorous discharge. A symptomatic infection from which *B. fragilis* has been cultured can be treated with oral metronidazole 250 mg t.i.d. or clindamycin (Cleocin) 300 mg q.i.d. for 10 days.

Miscellaneous bacteria

Many other bacteria are capable of causing vaginitis. Examples are streptococci, which produce a thin, watery discharge, and staphylococci, which can occur in hospital personnel.

Viruses

Herpes simplex virus

The most common venereal disease in women in many parts of the country is herpetic infection of the vagina and vulva. This topic is covered in Chapter 60.

Condyloma acuminatum

Condyloma acuminatum is a viral venereal infection that produces multiple small warts (caused by human papillomavirus) and is a sexually transmitted disease. These lesions are found most often on the vestibule but may also involve the labia, perianal skin, vagina, and cervix. Large lesions tend to coalesce and become secondarily infected.

Treatment is tedious and protracted. For small lesions, the best drug is podophyllin (20% in tincture of benzoin or a 25% ointment) applied directly to individual lesions. Fresh trichloroacetic acid 80% may be applied to resistant lesions. The surrounding skin should be protected against the irritating effects of these drugs by a coating of petrolatum, and the residual podophyllin or trichloroacetic acid should be washed away with soap and water 1–2 h later.

Therapy should be repeated at weekly intervals until all lesions are cleared. Any other coexisting infections, such as trichomoniasis or candidiasis, should be treated concurrently. Extensive lesions may require electrocautery, cryosurgery, laser therapy, or surgical excision under anesthesia.

Chemicals and allergens

Almost any agent that comes into contact with the vulva or vagina can cause erythema, irritation, ulceration, and/or discharge. The list includes soaps, douche materials, bubble bath, contraceptive preparations, powder, cloth dyes, perfumed or colored toilet paper, and local medications. Treatment begins with elimination of as many of these items as possible, including a change from nylon to cotton underwear.

Atrophic vaginitis

This topic is covered in Chapter 98 on hormone replacement therapy for menopausal symptoms.

Cervicitis

If the primary course of a vaginal discharge is extensive cervicitis, electrocautery, cryosurgery, or laser therapy may be necessary once neoplastic diseases or specific infective etiologies such as *N. gonorrhoeae*, *Chlamydia trachomatis*, herpes simplex virus or the human papillomavirus have been ruled out.

Pediculosis

An infestation with *Phthirus pubis* will cause chronic vulvar irritation but can easily be missed unless a careful examination is made for this tiny louse. Lindane (Kwell) lotion or shampoo is the treatment of choice. Clothing and linen should be changed frequently. Repeat treatment in 1 week is commonly required, as is treatment of sexual partners.

Pediatric vulvovaginitis

Infections in children are covered in Chapter 63.

Scabies

Scabies is due to the mite *Sarcoptes scabiei*, which produces small, itchy subcutaneous burrows, papules, and vesicles along the wrists, finger webs, and torso. Treatment is the same as for pediculosis.

SUGGESTED READING

BAKER DA, DOUGLAS JM, BUNTIN DM, *et al*. Topical podofilox for the treatment of condylomata acuminata in women. *Obstet Gynecol* 1990;76:656–659.

BELLINA JH. Use of carbon dioxide laser in management of condyloma acuminatum with 8-year follow-up. *Am J Obstet Gynecol* 1983;147:375–378.

CHEN KCS, FORSYTH PS, BUCHANAN TM, *et al*. Amine content of vaginal fluid from untreated and treated patients with nonspecific vaginitis. *J Clin Invest* 1979;63:828.

GARDNER HL. *Haemophilus vaginalis* vaginitis after twenty-five years. *Am J Obstet Gynecol* 1980;137:385.

HILLIER S, KROHN MA, WATTS DH, *et al*. Microbiologic efficacy of intravaginal clindamycin cream for the treatment of bacterial vaginosis. *Obstet Gynecol* 1990;76:407–413.

HOWETT MK, RAPP R. Basic biology of papillomavirus. *Contemp Ob/Gynecol* 1986; 28:110–123.

KAUFMAN RH. The origin and diagnosis of "nonspecific vaginitis". *N Engl J Med* 1980;303:637.

LUGO-MIRO VI, GREEN M, MAZUR L. Comparison of different metronidazole therapeutic regimens for bacterial vaginosis. *JAMA* 1992;268:92–95.

MCCORMICK WM, EVARD JR, LAUGHLIN CF, et al. Sexually transmitted conditions among women college students. *Am J Obstet Gynecol* 1980;139:130.

PHEIFER TA, FORSYTH PS, DURFEE MA, et al. Nonspecific vaginitis: role of *Haemophilus vaginalis* and treatment with metronidazole. *N Engl J Med* 1978;298:1429.

SCHMITT C, SOBEL JD, MERIWETHER C. Bacterial vaginosis: treatment with clindamycin cream versus oral metronidazole. *Obstet Gynecol* 1992;79:1020–1023.

SPIEGEL CA, AMSEL R, ESCHENBACH D, et al. Anaerobic bacteria in nonspecific vaginitis. *N Engl J Med* 1980;303:601.

US DEPARTMENT OF HEALTH AND HUMAN SERVICES, PUBLIC HEALTH SERVICE, DIVISION OF SEXUALLY TRANSMITTED DISEASES. Sexually transmitted diseases treatment guidelines. *Centers for Disease Control MMWR* 1989;38:1–41.

58

Sexually transmitted diseases

SUBIR ROY

Venereal diseases may be caused by a variety of agents. Bacterial diseases include syphilis, gonorrhea, chancroid, and granuloma inguinale. Lymphogranuloma venereum is caused by *Chlamydia*. Venereally transmitted *Mycoplasma* species include *M. hominis* and the T strain. Infections with herpes simplex type 1 and 2 and condyloma acuminatum are caused by viruses. Trichomonal vaginitis is caused by a protozoan while pediculosis pubis is caused by a louse.

Syphilis

The primary lesion of syphilis appears after 10–90 days of incubation (average 21 days) and consists of single or multiple painless chancres on the anus, vulva, vagina, cervix, nipples, or mouth. Regional lymph nodes will probably be enlarged. If a chancre is discovered, syphilis is best diagnosed by a dark-field examination to demonstrate the spirochete *Treponema pallidum*. To obtain a good specimen, the lesion is cleansed, abraded, and blotted free of blood, and a sample of oozing serum is placed on a slide and covered with a coverslip. The chancre heals in 3–6 weeks.

Serologic tests for syphilis become positive 4 or 5 weeks following an initial infection, or 1–2 weeks after a chancre appears. The nonspecific *Treponema* tests, such as flocculation tests (the Venereal Disease Research Laboratory (VDRL) and the rapid plasma reagin card (RPR) test) or complement fixation tests (Wassermann, Kolmer) are diagnostic if the titer is 1:32 or higher. Tests showing titers lower than 1:32 should be repeated.

Specific tests for treponemal antibodies (fluorescent treponemal antibody absorption test (FTS-ABS) and the *T. pallidum* hemagglutination assay (TPHA-TP) or microhemagglutination assay for antibody to *T. pallidum* (MHATP) test) should be performed because of the likelihood of obtaining a false-positive result with the complement fixation tests.

Secondary syphilis begins 2–8 weeks after eruption of the chancre and is manifested by cutaneous and mucous membrane lesions or by condylomas (condyloma latum) of the anogenital region. Because these lesions are teeming with spirochetes, either a dark-field examination or a biopsy can be used for diagnosis. Latent syphilis has no clinical manifestations and is diagnosed on the basis of positive serology after neurologic (negative cerebrospinal fluid) and cardiovascular involvement has been ruled out. It is also necessary to rule out other diseases that can produce a positive blood test: acute fevers, collagen disease, mononucleosis, malaria, leprosy, yaws, and lymphogranuloma.

If early and asymptomatic, syphilis that is primary, secondary, or latent and present for less than 1 year can be treated with benzathine penicillin G, 2.4 million units im or tetracycline 500 mg by mouth, 4 times a day for 14 days or erythromycin 500 mg by mouth, 4 times a day for 14 days. The latter therapies are effective for those patients who are penicillin-allergic. If the duration of the asymptomatic syphilis is unknown or has existed for more than 1 year (excepting neurosyphilis), then benzathine penicillin G 2.4 million units im once a week for 3 weeks (7.2 million units total) or tetracycline 500 mg by mouth, 4 times a day for 30 days or erythromycin 500 mg by mouth, 4 times a day for 30 days can be administered.

Neurosyphilis may be treated with 12–24 million units of penicillin G administered as 2–4 million units every 4 h iv for 10–14 days.

Gonorrhea

Gonorrhea is covered in Chapter 61.

Granuloma inguinale

Granuloma inguinale is due to a gram-negative bacterium, *Calymmatobacterium granulomatis*, that may be sexually transmitted, possibly by anal intercourse. The initial papular lesion is painless, ulcerates, and spreads via the lymphatics to regional lymph nodes with pseudobubo formation in the inguinal areas. With obstruction of lymphatics, elephantiasis may result. Suppuration and sinus formation are rare in female patients; when they do occur, the lesions may mimic carcinoma. The diagnosis is made by the observation of Donovan bodies (intracellular bacteria) in a biopsy specimen. It is not very contagious and is infrequently reported in the USA.

The treatment of choice is tetracycline 2 g daily for 14–21 days. Other antibiotics, such as erythromycin and gentamicin, are also effective. If the response is poor, treatment may be extended. Treatment of relapses is often necessary.

Chancroid (soft chancre)

Chancroid is a superficial infection caused by a small gram-negative rod, *Haemophilus ducreyi*. The typical lesion is a painful, shallow, circular vulvar ulcer with a necrotic erythematous border and yellow-to-gray base. Regional lymph nodes are often enlarged and may suppurate. Dark-field examination eliminates the diagnosis of a syphilitic chancre, and a gram stain of a smear usually demonstrates the bacilli arranged in a characteristic cluster.

The susceptibility of *H. ducreyi* to antimicrobial agents varies widely; therefore, response to therapy should be carefully monitored and adjustments to therapy should be instituted when necessary. Suggested therapies for cases and sex partners include erythromycin 500 mg by mouth 4 times daily for 7 days or ceftriaxone 250 mg im in a single dose or trimethoprim/sulfamethoxazole, one double-strength tablet by mouth twice daily for a minimum or 7 days or trimethoprim/sulfamethoxazole, four double-strength tablets by mouth in a single dose.

While ulcers generally show improvement within 7 days of instituting therapy, lymph nodes take longer. If lymph nodes are fluctuant, needle drainage through healthy skin may speed healing while incision and drainage of lymph nodes delays healing and is not advised. A follow-up test for syphilis is advisable.

Lymphogranuloma venereum

Lymphogranuloma venereum is produced by a bacterium, *Chlamydia trachomatis* (serotypes L_1, L_2, and L_3). The initial small erosion or painless ulcer presents 4–21 days after exposure. One to 4 weeks later, it progresses by lymphatic spread to the femoral and inguinal lymph nodes associated with systemic symptoms such as fever, headache, myalgia, and arthralgia. These nodes may separately enlarge, producing a "groove" along the inguinal ligament dividing the "saddle" nodes, two terms that have been used to characterize this lesion. Lymphatic buboes with ulceration and drainage are relatively uncommon in women. Lymphatic spread to the perirectal and pelvic nodes produces proctitis, followed by strictures and fistula formation. The urethra can also be involved. About

80% of patients will have a positive Frei test if injected intradermally with 0.1 ml of the antigen. A complement fixation test is more accurate in the earlier stages of the disease. Biopsies may be obscured by necrosis and infection and are not always diagnostic. Serologic tests for syphilis are apt to give a false-positive result.

Tetracycline 2 g daily for a minimum of 10–15 days, perhaps even for 3–4 weeks, may be necessary. Erythromycin 2 g daily or sulfamethoxazole 4 g daily each for 2–4 weeks are alternative therapies. A rectal stricture will require a colostomy.

Molluscum contagiosum

Molluscum contagiosum is caused by a DNA virus, is sexually and physically transmitted, and is usually asymptomatic, although irritation may lead to secondary infection and localized lymphadenopathy. The umbilicated papule typically appears 2–8 weeks after infection and characteristically contains yellow curd-like material; it can be expressed and stained with gram, Wright or Giemsa stain, revealing large intracytoplasmic molluscum bodies which are ovoid accumulations of maturing virons. Generally, no therapy is required. Although lesions can be sprayed with ethylchloride or frozen with liquid nitrogen, it is normally only necessary to express the contents with curettage of the base.

Mycoplasma

Mycoplasma hominis and T strains of this genus (unique bacteria that have no cell wall) frequently inhabit the vagina, are commonly associated with pelvic infections, and can be transmitted sexually.

While *Mycoplasma* has been implicated as a possible cause of abortion, chorioamnionitis, low-birth-weight infants, bartholinitis, salpingitis, tuboovarian abscess, urinary tract infection, and infertility, it appears to have a low rate of virulence. The antibiotic of choice is tetracycline 1 g daily for 7 days following a loading dose of 1–2 g.

Other diseases

Herpes simplex is discussed in Chapter 60, and condyloma acuminatum, trichomoniasis, pediculosis, and scabies are discussed in Chapter 57.

SUGGESTED READING

ABRAMS AJ. Lymphogranuloma venereum. *JAMA* 1968;205:59.
ALERGANT CB. Chancroid. *Practitioner* 1972;209:624.

PIOT P, PLUMMER FA. Genital ulcer adenopathy syndrome. In: Holmes KK, March P-A, Sparling PF, Wiesner PF, eds. *Sexually Transmitted Disease*. New York: McGraw Hill, 1990:771.

RUBIERO J. Granuloma inguinale. *Practitioner* 1972;209:628.

SPARLING PF. Diagnosis and treatment of syphilis. *N Engl J Med* 1971;284:642.

TAYLOR-ROBINSON D, MCCORMICK WM. The genital mycoplasmas. *N Engl J Med* 1980;302:1003.

US DEPARTMENT OF HEALTH AND HUMAN SERVICES, PUBLIC HEALTH SERVICE, DIVISION OF SEXUALLY TRANSMITTED DISEASES. Sexually transmitted diseases treatment guidelines. *Centers for Disease Control MMWR* 1985 (Suppl);34:1–35.

US DEPARTMENT OF HEALTH AND HUMAN SERVICES, PUBLIC HEALTH SERVICE, DIVISION OF SEXUALLY TRANSMITTED DISEASES. Sexually transmitted diseases treatment guidelines. *Centers for Disease Control MMWR* 1989;38:1–41.

59

Human immunodeficiency virus infection in women

DAVID A. GRIMES

Scope of the problem

The full fury of the worldwide epidemic of human immunodeficiency virus (HIV) infection has only begun to be felt. The majority of female acquired immune deficiency syndrome (AIDS) cases can be traced to intravenous drug use, although the second most common risk factor is heterosexual contact with a person at risk for AIDS. The proportion of AIDS cases in women attributed to heterosexual intercourse is growing rapidly (currently about one-third), suggesting that this may emerge as a major means of transmission, as is now the case in much of Africa. Since an estimated 1.5–2 million persons in the USA are currently infected with HIV, this will become an increasingly important problem in women's health in the years ahead.

Testing for HIV infection

The prevalence of infection varies widely in different populations within the USA. While rates of 0.01% have been found in voluntary blood donors, rates of 60% have been found in intravenous drug users in the metropolitan New York City area and 50% among women who are steady sexual partners of men with HIV infection. Voluntary testing, with appropriate informed consent and counseling, should be offered to women with a history of drug use themselves or drug use by a sexual partner. Women with multiple sexual partners, especially prostitutes, are appropriate candidates for testing. Sexual partners of hemophiliacs are also at increased risk. Women with a history of sexually transmitted diseases or who received blood products between 1980 and March of 1985 are at increased risk, as are women with a history of having a bisexual partner. Women who present with opportunistic infections or other constitutional signs and symptoms, such as persistent fever, diarrhea, lymphadenopathy, or lymphopenia, should be offered testing. Finally, women who have emigrated from countries where heterosexual transmission is thought to be prevalent (e.g., central and east Africa and Haiti) should be offered testing.

Current serologic tests for HIV infection are highly sensitive and specific. Within 2–3 months of infection, virtually all persons will develop circulating antibodies that can be detected by serologic tests. This "window phase" prior to antibody production may last as long as 6 months in some patients. Since HIV integrates into human genes, all antibody-positive persons should be considered potentially infectious.

The initial test used for HIV infection is usually an enzyme-linked immunosorbent assay (ELISA). If it is positive, the test is repeated using the same blood sample. If the repeat ELISA test is positive, a confirmatory test is usually done by the Western blot or immunofluorescence assay. Viral cultures of peripheral blood lymphocytes are expensive and not widely used for diagnosis.

Clinical course

Infection with HIV has a predilection for the T-cell lymphocytes (the primary orchestrator of the body's immune system) and for the central nervous system. Once infection occurs, the infection is presumed to persist for the duration of the patient's life. The initial infection can produce a febrile illness with rash and lymphadenopathy, or it may be entirely asymptomatic. The initial infection is followed by a symptom-free interval that may last from months to years. As time progresses, the infected person generally develops evidence of cellular immune dysfunction. Concomitantly, the patient manifests fever, weight loss, malaise, lethargy, central nervous system dysfunction, and opportunistic infections. Two classifications of HIV infections are used: that of the Centers for Disease Control is simpler than that of Walter Reed Hospital, which incorporates laboratory findings into the classification scheme.

Duration of infection appears to be the most important known risk factor. The most useful laboratory predictor of prognosis is the number of CD4-positive cells in the peripheral blood. Treatment with antiviral medications should be coordinated with an expert in infectious diseases. The longer the time since infection, the greater the risk of developing AIDS. In a group of male homosexuals, 75% had developed either AIDS or clinical illness within 8 years of infection.

Infection in pregnancy

HIV infection in pregnancy has important implications for both mother and fetus. Whether pregnancy may exacerbate the course of infection for the woman remains unclear. HIV infection can be transmitted vertically to the fetus. The precise mode of transmission is currently unknown, but there is ample evidence of *in utero* transmission as early as 13 weeks' gestation. Infection may be acquired during birth or after delivery, for example, through breast-feeding. Current estimates are that from 30 to 50% of infants born to HIV-infected women will acquire this infection. The clinical course of infants with HIV infection tends to be fulminant and devastating.

Prevention of infection

General recommendations

HIV infection is not easily acquired. It is much less infectious than hepatitis B, and casual contact will not lead to infection. Only three modes of infection are known: inoculation with body fluids, sexual contact, and perinatal transmission. The following recommendations are based on these modes of transmission.

Women can reduce their risk of acquiring HIV infection through changes in lifestyle and behavior. To minimize sexual transmission, abstinence is the only foolproof strategy. For sexually active women, a mutually monogamous relationship with an uninfected partner is strongly recommended. Laboratory studies have shown that condoms prevent transmission of HIV, and spermicides will inactivate the virus as well. Condoms used along with spermicides should provide the highest level of protection. Preliminary data from Africa suggest that condoms can help protect high-risk women from this infection.

Women who use intravenous drugs should be encouraged to stop. If unwilling or unable to do so, they should avoid sharing needles and other drug paraphernalia. If such supplies are shared, they should be disinfected with a dilute solution of household bleach between uses.

Prevention of infection in the workplace

The risk of health-care workers acquiring HIV infection in the workplace is small but not zero. The strategies used for preventing transmission of hepatitis B infection are appropriate for avoiding infection with HIV. Sharp items, such as needles and scalpel blades, should be considered potentially infectious and should be handled with great care. Sharp items should be disposed of appropriately, and needles should not be recapped or manipulated prior to disposal. When contamination with blood or other body fluids may occur, gloves alone or gloves supplemented by gowns, masks, and eye coverings may be appropriate. If contamination occurs with blood or body fluids, the health-care workers should wash the area immediately and thoroughly.

Prevention of infection during invasive procedures

Recommendations for preventing infection with hepatitis B are again appropriate. Persons who perform operative or obstetric procedures must wear gloves when touching mucous membranes or nonintact skin of patients. If aerosolization or splashes are likely to occur, masks, eye coverings, and gowns should be used. During obstetric procedures, appropriate barrier precautions should be used when handling the placenta or infant until blood and amniotic fluid have been removed from the infant's skin. Health-care workers with exudative lesions or weeping dermatitis should not be involved in invasive procedures or other direct patient-care activities.

Prevention of perinatal transmission

Women with HIV infection should be strongly encouraged not to become pregnant. Highly effective contraception or surgical sterilization should be used. If pregnancy occurs, patients should be informed of the risks of clinical deterioration associated with pregnancy as well as the projected rates of transmission to the fetus. All HIV-infected women should be advised of the availability of induced abortion as an option. Induced abortion will prevent perinatal transmission and may prevent aggravation of maternal illness as well.

SUGGESTED READING

FISCHL MA, DICKINSON GM, SCOTT GB, *et al.* Evaluation of heterosexual partners, children, and household contacts of adults with AIDS. *JAMA* 1987; 257:640.

GUINAN ME, HARDY A. Epidemiology of AIDS in women in the United States. *JAMA* 1987;257:2039.

HIRSCH MS. Clinical manifestations of HIV infection in adults in industrialized countries. In: Holmes KK, Mardh P-A, Sparling PF, Wiesner PJ, eds. *Sexually Transmitted Diseases.* 2nd edn. New York: McGraw-Hill, 1990:331–342.

HOLMBERG SD, CURRAN JW. The epidemiology of HIV infection in industrialized countries. In: Holmes KK, Mardh P-A, Sparling PF, Wiesner PJ, eds. *Sexually Transmitted Diseases.* 2nd edn. New York: McGraw-Hill, 1990:343–353.

Minkoff H, Nanda D, Menez R, Fikrig S. Pregnancies resulting in infants with acquired immunodeficiency syndrome or AIDS-related complex: follow-up of mothers, children, and subsequently born siblings. *Obstet Gynecol* 1987;69:288.

Rubinstein A. HIV infections in infants and children. In: Holmes KK, Mardh P-A, Sparling PF, Wiesner PJ, eds. *Sexually Transmitted Diseases*. 2nd edn. New York: McGraw-Hill, 1990:843–849.

60

Genital herpes

DAVID A. GRIMES

Genital herpes infection results from inoculation of the herpes virus on to a susceptible mucous membrane or through introduction into the skin by close contact with a carrier; the carrier may or may not have clinical signs of infection. Patients should be advised that nonsexual transmission by fomites, aerosol, hot-tubs, or swimming pools has not been documented. Most genital herpes infections are due to herpes simplex virus type 2 (HSV-2); the remainder, caused by HSV-1, can usually be traced to orogenital contact. The prevalence of antibodies to HSV-2 is influenced by age, sexual activity, and socioeconomic status. These antibodies increase with both age and sexual experience, and the prevalence is inversely related to socioeconomic status.

Although an epidemiologic association exists between HSV-2 and genital cancers, a causal link has not been established. Women with HSV-2 antibodies have a higher incidence of cervical dysplasia, carcinoma-*in-situ*, and invasive cancer than do women without these antibodies. Moreover, samples of tissue from cervical dysplasia, cervical carcinoma, and carcinoma-*in-situ* of the vulva have been found to contain HSV-2-specific DNA binding antigens. However, the association between squamous cancer and human papillomavirus infection appears stronger than that with HSV-2. Nevertheless, women with genital herpes infections should have a Pap smear at least annually.

Clinical presentation

The classification of herpes infections helps to determine management.

The initial genital infection with HSV can be symptomatic or asymptomatic. Among symptomatic infections, the infection may be primary or nonprimary. If the patient lacks antibodies to either type of HSV (more commonly HSV-1), the infection is considered to be primary, i.e., the patient has had no prior HSV infection. If the patient has HSV antibodies, the first genital infection is considered nonprimary, i.e., one that is caused by reactivation of latent virus. Recurrent infections are characterized by active lesions in a patient who has had previous ulcerations.

Primary infections tend to be longer and more severe than recurrent ones. With primary infections, multiple anatomic sites are often involved, and the patient may have signs and symptoms that are both local and systemic. The vesicular or ulcerated lesions can be very painful. In addition, genital herpes can lead to vaginal discharge from herpes cervicitis or urethral discharge from herpes urethritis. Tender inguinal adenopathy may be present.

With primary infections with HSV-2, constitutional symptoms, such as fever, malaise, and myalgias, occur in about 40% of men and 70% of women. The entire primary herpes episode lasts about a month, with symptoms occurring for approximately 2 weeks and healing over the next 1–2 weeks. In general, nonprimary first episodes of genital herpes are shorter and less painful than primary infections.

Several other complications of primary genital herpes can occur. In 4–8% of cases, viral meningitis is found; HSV encephalitis is even more rare. Involvement of the sacral autonomic plexus can lead to a hypotonic bladder, difficulty in voiding, and constipation. Herpes pharyngitis, from either HSV-1 or HSV-2, can be confused with streptococcal pharyngitis.

Recurrent genital herpes infections tend to be shorter and milder than primary infections. Most of these recurrences are caused by reactivation of latent virus rather than by reinfection. Often this occurs in a single nerve ganglion, which accounts for the unilateral distribution of most recurrent herpes. Some women experience itching, a tingling sensation, or neuralgia several hours or days before eruption of lesions. This often signals an impending recurrence. Recurrent genital herpes infections tend to occur 5–12 days before menses, and signs of infection disappear within about 10 days. The principal complication of recurrent herpes (other than neonatal transmission) is the psychologic burden of this chronic disease, especially its interference with sexual relationships. Fortunately, frequent recurrences happen in a minority of infected persons.

Infections in pregnancy

Pregnant women can have either localized genital infection or disseminated infection. In most women, the infection is limited to the oropharynx and genitals; when it spreads to the skin or viscera, the infection is associated with a maternal case-fatality rate of about 50%. Fetal losses are also very high.

Most neonatal herpes infections are caused by HSV-2 acquired during childbirth, although some are due to HSV-1. In addition, ascending infection and transplacental infection can occur.

The greatest risk to the fetus is caused by primary infections. When these occur in early pregnancy, the rates of spontaneous abortion and stillbirth are increased. Women with primary infection at the time of delivery have a higher risk of neonatal transmission than do women with recurrent lesions (50 versus 4%). Recurrent genital infection is much more common than primary infection in pregnancy.

Shedding of the herpes virus at the time of delivery is infrequent. Studies in unselected patient populations have found shedding to occur in only 0.1–0.4% of deliveries. Since the risk of neonatal infection is about 10-fold lower than these figures would suggest, some protective mechanism(s) must exist for the fetus.

After delivery, breast-feeding by infected mothers can be done, provided that care is taken to prevent transmission of the virus by direct contact. Infected family members should also observe similar techniques when handling newborn infants, since neonatal transmission from infected spouses has been reported. Likewise, hospital personnel with active lesions should not care for neonates, but the risk of transmission by this mode appears to be remote.

Although highly desirable, preventing neonatal infection is difficult to do. This is due to the fact that over 60% of women who give birth to infected infants have no signs or symptoms. Patients with recurrent herpes of the genitals should be asked to report to the hospital early in labor. The cervix and external genitals should be carefully examined, and culture of the cervix and/or vulva done. Women without evidence of lesions should be allowed to deliver vaginally. For women with active lesions or signs of asymptomatic infection in labor, cesarean delivery is the procedure of choice. Ideally, cesarean delivery should be carried out prior to or within 4–6 h of rupture of membranes, but some data suggest that cesarean delivery may be helpful in those with active infections regardless of the duration of ruptured membranes. Until a rapid and accurate diagnostic test that can be performed at the time of labor is widely available, the problem of neonatal herpes infections will persist.

Diagnosis

The clinical diagnosis of herpes infections can usually be made from the appearance of vesicles that progress to ulcers without scarring. If the patient gives a history of a prodrome and recurrence of such lesions, the clinical impression is further supported. However, because the diagnosis of genital herpes has such emotional impact – as well as lifelong consequences – a viral culture should be done for a definitive diagnosis. The sensitivity of the culture is greater in the vesicle or pustular stages (early lesions) than in the crusted stage (late lesion). The vesicle should be unroofed and the base swabbed, after which the swab is placed in a culture medium and sent to the nearest viral laboratory. Cytologic technics are faster but much less reliable. It should be remembered that neither a negative smear nor a negative culture excludes the disease. Serologic tests for herpes are not recommended for diagnosis.

Treatment

Although no cure exists for genital herpes infection, acyclovir can provide partial control of the signs and symptoms. However, the use of acyclovir does not influence the subsequent risk, frequency, or severity of recurrence after the drug is stopped.

First clinical episode

Before initiating therapy, one should determine that the patient's episode is a first episode of genital herpes. Treatment with acyclovir, 200 mg orally 5 times a day for 7–10 days (or until clinical resolution occurs), initiated within 6 days of the onset of symptoms, shortens the median duration of first-episode eruptions by 3–5 days. It may also reduce symptoms in primary episodes.

For those few patients who have symptoms or complications so severe as to require hospitalization, acyclovir can be given intravenously. The regimen is 5 mg/kg of body weight intravenously every 8 h for 5–7 days or until clinical resolution occurs. This treatment shortens the median course of first episodes by approximately 1 week.

Recurrent episodes

Treatment for recurrent episodes should be limited to those few patients who typically have severe symptoms and who are able to begin therapy at the onset of the prodrome or within 2 days of onset of lesions. Acyclovir, 200 mg orally 5 times daily for 5 days, or acyclovir 800 mg orally twice daily for 5 days initiated within 2 days of the onset of lesions shortens the mean clinical course by about a day. Neither intravenous nor topical acyclovir is indicated for recurrence.

Suppression of recurrences

Continuous treatment with acyclovir 200 mg orally 2–5 times daily or acyclovir 400 mg orally twice daily prevents recurrences in 65–85% of patients who experience frequent recurrences. The dose can and should be individualized for each patient. Once the acyclovir has been stopped, recurrences return at the same frequency. This regimen has been shown to be safe and effective up to 2 years, but the prolonged effects of acyclovir are not established. In addition, prolonged administration has the possibility of fostering the emergence of resistant strains. Hence, the cost, risks, and benefits should be carefully considered before embarking on this course. Women at risk of pregnancy should not use this suppressive regimen.

Counseling

Counseling is of pivotal importance in the management of herpes infections. Patients should be informed about the natural history of these infections, and they should be warned to avoid sexual contact when lesions are present. This advice holds also for patients using acyclovir. Transmission of HSV can occur during asymptomatic periods, but the risk of this is not well defined. Some experts advise that asymptomatic patients use condoms on a routine basis. When women become pregnant, they should advise their physicians if they or their sexual partner(s) have a history of genital herpes infections. Routine treatment of sexual partners is not indicated.

Genital herpes infections can be emotionally trying for the patient – as well as painful. Patients may benefit from individual or group counseling, and many communities have counseling services or support groups for such patients.

SUGGESTED READING

COREY L. The diagnosis and treatment of genital herpes. *JAMA* 1982;248:1041–1049.

COREY L. Genital herpes. In: Holmes KK, Mardh P-A, Sparling PF, Wiesner PF, eds. *Sexually Transmitted Diseases*. 2nd edn. New York: McGraw-Hill, 1990:391–413.

GUINAN ME. Oral acyclovir for treatment and suppression of genital herpes simplex virus infection. *JAMA* 1986;255:1747–1749.

SEXUALLY TRANSMITTED DISEASES TREATMENT GUIDELINES, SEPTEMBER, 1989. Atlanta, GA: US Department of Health and Human Services, 1989.

STAGNO S, WHITLEY RJ. Herpesvirus infections of pregnancy. Part II: herpes simplex virus and varicella-zoster virus infections. *N Engl J Med* 1985;313:1327–1330.

61

Pelvic infection

SUBIR ROY

Background

The vagina contains both aerobic and anaerobic organisms (anaerobes > aerobes). Pelvic infections may occur as a consequence of the introduction of pathogenic exogenous organisms (e.g., *Neisseria gonorrhoeae* (gonorrhea GC), *Chlamydia trachomatis* (CT), etc.) and/or by the presence of normal vaginal flora in an abnormal location (e.g., in the endometrium, oviducts, peritoneal cavity, etc.) in sufficient numbers to overwhelm the body's host defense system.

When an inoculation of mixed (aerobic and anaerobic) organisms derived from bowel flora is introduced into an abnormal location (e.g., peritoneal cavity), a biphasic infection pattern may ensue. Initially, peritonitis secondary to the effects of aerobic gram-negative organisms such as *Escherichia coli* precedes abscess formation composed largely of anaerobic organisms, predominantly of the *Bacteroides* group. Approximately 40% of laboratory animals infected in this manner but not treated with antibiotics have died of peritonitis while nearly 100% of surviving animals have developed abscesses.

Diagnosis

Historically, information suggestive of a sexually transmitted disease (STD) etiology is directly correlated with the following: relationship of onset of symptoms to onset of the last menstrual period (LMP), last sexual exposure, number of sexual partners (lifetime but, perhaps more importantly, over the last 2–3 months), history of previous STD (whether treated as outpatient or as inpatient), symptoms of sexual partner (complaint of urethral discharge or "drip") and contraceptive practices. A history of recent instrumentation may elucidate the mechanism by which endogenous flora may gain access to and produce disease of the upper genital tract and includes the following: dilatation and curettage (D&C) for diagnosis or elective termination of pregnancy, intrauterine contraceptive device insertion, or hysterosalpingography. Smoking predisposes the patient to more STDs, possibly because smokers are greater risk-takers and are more sexually active than nonsmokers and probably because smoking alters the host defense by reducing biologically active estrogens, impairing ciliary activity of oviductal cells, reducing leukocyte action, and putatively reducing immunoglobulin A activity in cervical mucus.

Many signs and symptoms may suggest infection of the pelvic structures. A patient may complain of fever, abdominal or pelvic pain, cervical or vaginal discharge, nausea, vomiting, right upper quadrant pain, etc. Upon examination, she may be found to have a normal temperature or temperature elevation; localized or generalized pain or tenderness with or without evidence of pelvic or abdominal peritonitis; discharge, the source, character and amount of which may be suggestive of the offending pathogen(s), etc. These may be characterized by the presence of "-ors," the classical findings associated with inflammation: color (heat), dolor (pain), rubor (redness), and tumor (mass). Additional findings may be characterized by utilizing the suffixes "-osis," the presence of pathogenic organisms without histologic changes induced in underlying tissues (e.g., nonspecific vaginosis); "-itis," the presence of pathogenic organisms with histologic changes induced in underlying tissues (e.g., vaginitis, endometritis, salpingitis); or abscess, a collection of pus and debris composed of desquamated or necrotic cells, tissues or organisms contained in a circumscribed location (e.g., appendiceal abscess, demarcated by loops of bowel), or by the destruction of organs or tissues (e.g., tuboovarian abscess).

Various simple tests may be performed in order to suggest the identity of the offending pathogenic organisms. A wet-mount smear with sodium chloride may aid in the diagnosis of nonspecific vaginosis, nonspecific vaginitis, or *Trichomonas vaginalis*, while one utilizing potassium hydroxide aids in the diagnosis of *Candida albicans*. Gram stains made of cervical discharge, vaginal discharge, wound infections, or from margins of abscesses permit identification of broad classes of organisms based on their morphologic appearance and gram-stain status. Empiric therapy may be selected, accordingly, while results of cultures are pending. These cultures should be obtained from portals or adjacent structures involved in sexual activities. These may include the oropharynx, urethra, cervix, vagina, and rectum. It may be necessary to obtain cultures for aerobic and anaerobic organisms, GC, genital mycoplasmas, as well as tissue cultures for CT.

Ultrasound of the female pelvis is frequently performed but it has not replaced the pelvic examination. If adnexal masses are visualized by ultrasound, suggesting inflammatory processes, the prudent physician does not aspirate them; instead, a trial of antibiotic therapy is instituted. A kidney, ureter, bladder X-ray of the pelvis may demonstrate gas in soft tissues; air under the diaphragm, suggestive of a perforated viscus; a mass lesion; ileus; etc. A computed tomography or magnetic resonance imaging scan may identify masses or blood-filled collections that are not discernible by other diagnostic studies. A barium enema (BE), upper gastrointestinal tract series (UGI) or intravenous pyelography may be useful in making or ruling out the diagnosis of gastrointestinal or genito-urinary conditions. Thus, standard diagnostic tests are useful in making the diagnosis of female pelvic soft tissue infections.

A white blood cell count, including erythrocyte sedimentation rate, by being elevated, may be helpful in making the diagnosis of genital tract infections; however, it is not mandatory that they be elevated in order to make this diagnosis.

Historically, the term febrile menses has connoted gonococcal salpingitis. This presumptive diagnosis is made when gram-negative intra-cellular diplococci organisms are seen on gram stain in an individual who has some or all of the following findings: lower abdominal pain, cervicovaginal discharge, cervical motion tenderness, bilateral adnexal tenderness, elevated white blood cell count, elevated sedimentation rate, and fever. While fever is commonly associated with the presence of GC, it is not essential in order to make the diagnosis. Nongonococcal salpingitis may be suggested with similar findings, except that it may occur at any time during the menstrual cycle (although it could occur with or soon after the onset of the LMP), may occur in the absence of fever, and is suggestive of CT if the gram stain demonstrates many polymorphonuclear neutrophils and few bacteria ("mucopus"). If the gram stain shows many polymorphonuclear neutrophils and bacteria, generally the patient has fever, and the presumptive diagnosis is based on the morphology of the predominant bacterial species identified.

Pain in the right upper quadrant in a woman with signs and symptoms of salpingitis suggests the Fitz-Hugh–Curtis syndrome in which the spread of pathogenic organisms (originally described with GC but now also reported for CT) along the colic gutters to the liver leads to adhesion formation.

If the patient does not fit the standard definition of salpingitis, and if she does not present with significant ileus or a large pelvic–abdominal mass, it may be possible to perform diagnostic laparoscopy to clarify the diagnosis. It has been reported that about 20% of such individuals will have normal-appearing pelvic structures, 3–4% each will be diagnosed as having ectopic pregnancy or appendicitis, and 2–4% will have a variety of other pelvic pathology (e.g., endometriosis, diverticulitis, etc.), while the remainder (about 65–70%) are found to have salpingitis.

Consequences

The consequences of infections of the female pelvic soft tissues include a three- to fourfold increase in pelvic pain, a seven- to 10-fold increase in ectopic gestation and a 15–60% increase in the incidence of infertility, proportional to the number of episodes of salpingitis that a patient has suffered.

Effects of birth control

With respect to patients using no method of birth control who are sexually active, barrier method users have half the risk (because of the barrier as well as use of nonoxinol-9-containing spermicidal jellies or creams which have been shown to impair the growth of GC or CT or kill the human immunodeficiency virus (HIV)), oral contraceptive users have a reduced risk (by virtue of the thick cervical mucus and, possibly, by the reduced menstrual flow that results from the progestagen component of the combination preparation). Intrauterine device (IUD) users have the same risk of developing salpingitis as controls, excepting those using the Dalkon Shield, or soon after IUD insertion when a small number of organisms are introduced into the endometrial cavity. The Dalkon Shield had a multifilament tail enclosed in a sheath which served as a wick, drawing bacterial organisms into the upper genital tract. Modern IUDs have a monofilament tail and their use is not associated with the problems generally associated with Dalkon Shield. Oral contraceptive users have been reported to harbor CT two- to threefold more frequently in their endocervix than nonoral contraceptive users. It has been suggested, although not proven, that oral contraceptive use alters or in some way makes the squamocolumnar junction tissues of the cervix more susceptible to inoculation by pathogenic organisms such as CT or the human papillomavirus.

Pathogenic organisms

Pelvic soft tissue infections are polymicrobial, with GC, CT, aerobic and anaerobic organisms and the genital mycoplasmas comprising the bulk of the community-acquired and endogenous flora responsible for these infections. Some investigators feel that the presence of the genital mycoplasmas is an indicator of sexual activity and that their presence is not necessarily associated with disease production. Usually, a combination of organisms is cultured from sites of infection, although occasionally, no pathogenic organisms are cultured; however, this need not mean that the patient is not infected since, typically, we only have access to the lower genital tract to obtain cultures (vagina, endocervix, or endometrium) while the disease may be occurring in the upper genital tract (oviducts or ovary), from which there may be no drainage to the lower genital tract or it may not be possible to obtain cultures.

CT is considered to be the most prevalent STD in the USA at this time with a prevalence of around 5 million annually. Cultures are time-consuming, expensive and have in many instances been replaced with more rapid but questionably accurate enzymatic or antibody tests. These tests may be responsible, because of their large false-positive rate when a low-prevalence population is screened, for the high rate of CT reported. It should be remembered, however, that the antibody titers to CT (immunoglobulin M and G) are higher in women who have an ectopic gestation (as compared to women with an intrauterine pregnancy of equal weeks' gestation) or in women who are infertile (as compared to fertile women). Thus, there is compelling reason to believe that CT has a pathophysiologic role in female genital tract tissues. GC, the classical STD, has been reported to have stabilized at approximately 2 million cases annually, equally divided by sex. In some settings (e.g., Los Angeles County –University of Southern Medical Center), GC is recovered from around 50% of the women hospitalized for the treatment of female pelvic soft tissue infections. In most reported series, GC is recovered from 40–60% and CT from 5–25% of such patients. Our CT recovery, based on endocervical culture, is around 5–10% from such patients. Both of these pathogens may be recovered simultaneously in high-risk patients.

In studies at Los Angeles County–University of Southern California Medical Center, *E. coli* was the most frequently recovered aerobic gram-negative pathogen, slightly more frequently than GC. Among the anaerobes, *Bacteroides bivius* and *B. disiens* were more frequently recovered than *B. fragilis* (only 5% of all anaerobes).

Both CT and GC are believed to injure the surface epithelium of the female genital tract in an ascending manner (via the endocervix to the oviducts). Subsequent infections with other offending pathogenic organisms may gain access to the underlying tissues (e.g., myometrium, parametrium) or to more remote locations (e.g., the ovary and the broad ligaments). These latter locations may be involved by direct extension or by seeding from hematogenous or lymphatic spread. As a consequence of genital tract tissue injury and because this tissue is generally incapable of complete restoration of structure and function, even after aggressive antibiotic therapy, the consequences of pelvic infection (pelvic pain, ectopic pregnancy, and infertility) are not surprising.

While HIV infection does not specifically lead to salpingitis, it is clearly another STD. HIV transmission among heterosexuals is increasing. Of those with HIV, 4% of males and 20% of females are reported to have acquired HIV heterosexually. The female-to-male ratio is still around 1:13, largely reflecting the high-risk groups (intravenous drug users, homosexuals, and prostitutes). However, in other parts of the world where intravenous drug use and homosexual practice, but not prostitution, are uncommon, there exists a 1:1 male-to-female ratio for HIV. HIV does not appear to affect fertility. Some 20–50% of mothers with HIV transmit the virus to the fetus, with manifestations of acquired immune deficiency syndrome appearing soon after birth, leading to death in the majority of cases, usually within 18 months. Many such mothers have chosen to undergo abortion. Condom use with nonoxinol-9 spermicidal jellies or creams appears to reduce the likelihood of HIV transmission by killing the organism.

Treatment

Ambulatory treatment for GC or CT requires therapy for the other pathogen as well. Commonly, a β-lactamase stable second- or third-generation cephalosporin is administered intramuscularly and a 7–10-day oral course of tetracycline, a synthetic tetracycline, or erythromycin is prescribed. Alternate new oral therapies are azithromycin 1 g (for CT) and cefixime 400 mg (for GC), one time only, or ofloxacin 200–400 mg b.i.d. for 10 days (for CT and GC).

Hospitalized therapy for female pelvic soft tissue infections follows a similar philosophy, although a greater concern to treat adequately the aerobic gram-negative and anaerobic organisms (both gram-negative and gram-positive) is required. Parenteral therapy with a β-lactamase stable cephalosporin with a synthetic tetracycline or erythromycin is generally recommended for salpingitis without a mass (on pelvic examination or ultrasound). If a mass is suspected on the basis of pelvic examination or ultrasound, then therapy directed against anaerobes is recommended. Clindamycin plus an aminoglycoside is frequently used. Clinidamycin may be able to eradicate CT. We generally recommend a repeat pelvic examination of the patient following 4–5 days of therapy (pelvic stress test), provided that there is significant clinical improvement (afebrile, if febrile on admission, reduction of abdominal and/or pelvic pain, return of gastrointestinal function, etc.) over the last 48 h of therapy. If the patient has significant resolution of tenderness upon examination and does not spike a fever following the examination, while continuing to receive the parenteral therapy during the ensuing 8–24 h, then she can be considered a candidate for discharge. Usually, a synthetic tetracycline or oral clindamycin is prescribed to complete a 10–14-day course of antibiotic therapy, although there are no firm data to conclude that oral therapy is beneficial following completion of parenteral therapy.

Approximately 30% of women hospitalized for antibiotic therapy for female pelvic upper genital tract infections will require surgical intervention with extirpation of some or all genital tract structures, either during or following the hospitalization, in order to be cured of their infection. There are reports, however, of patients with presumed or actual end-stage tubal disease (e.g., tuboovarian abscess on the basis of pelvic examination or pelvic ultrasound) who have responded to antibiotic therapy alone or with colpotomy drainage (drainage of a pelvic abscess via the posterior vaginal fornix, which is relatively safe to perform when the leading edge of the abscess extends to below the level of the external cervical os). These patients have had a resolution of the adnexal masses (the larger the mass, the longer the time required for its resolution) and some (generally between 10 and 15%) have conceived with no need for additional corrective surgery of their genital tract structures. It is not mandatory – although sometimes necessary – to remove the uterus when extirpative surgery is required. With the advances of *in vitro* fertilization or embryo transfer, if the uterus can be left *in situ*, then the patient has a chance for future fertility.

Patients who fail antibiotic therapy have successfully undergone ultrasound or computed tomography-guided aspiration of inflammatory masses, sparing them a laparotomy or extirpative surgery. It should be remembered that such aspirations cannot distinguish between an infected mass and an infected neoplasm. Aspiration of the latter could worsen the patient's prognosis.

SUGGESTED READING

AMIN-HANJANI S, NEELY T, CHATWANI A. Perihepatic adhesions: not necessarily pathognomonic of pelvic infection. *Am J Obstet Gynecol* 1992;167:115–116.

ARAL SO, MOSHER WD, CATES W. Self-reported pelvic inflammatory disease in the United States, 1988. *JAMA* 1991;266:2570–2575.

BOUVET E, SIMON F, SCHWARTZ D. Comparison of female to male and male to female transmission of HIV in 563 stable couples. *Br Med J* 1992;304:809–813.

CASOLA G, VANSONNENBERG E, AGOSTINO HB, et al. Percutaneous drainage of tubo-ovarian abscesses. *Radiology* 1992;182:399–402.

CHU SY, BUEHLER JW, BERKELMAN RL. Impact of the human immunodeficiency virus epidemic on mortality in women of reproductive age, United States. *JAMA* 1990;264:225–229.

CRAMER DW, GOLDMAN MB, SCHIFF I, *et al.* The relationship of tubal infertility to barrier method and oral contraceptive use. *JAMA* 1987;257:2446–2450.

EUROPEAN STUDY GROUP. Comparative evaluation of clindamycin/gentamicin and cefoxitin/doxycycline for treatment of pelvic inflammatory disease: a multi-center trial. *Acta Obstet Gynecol Scand* 1992;71:129–134.

GERSHMAN KA, ROLFS RT. Diverging gonorrhea and syphilis trends in the 1980s: are they real? *Am J Public Health* 1991;81:1263–1267.

GINSBURG DS, STERN JL, HAMOD KA, GENADRY R, SPENCE MR. Tubo-ovarian abscess: a retrospective review. *Am J Obstet Gynecol* 1980;138:1055.

HANDSFIELD HH, McCORMACK WM, HOOK E, *et al.* A comparison of single-dose cefixime with ceftriaxone as treatment for uncomplicated gonorrhea. *N Engl J Med* 1991;325:1337–1341.

HEMSELL DL, SANTOS-RAMOS R, CUNNINGHAM G, *et al.* Cefotaxime treatment for women with community-acquired pelvic abscess. *J Obstet Gynecol* 1985;151:771.

HENRY-SUCHET J, UTZMANN C, DE BRUX J, ARDOIN P, CATALAN F. Microbiologic study of chronic inflammation associated with tubal factor infertility: role of *Chlamydia trachomatis*. *Fertil Steril* 1987;47:274.

HILL GB. *Eubacterium nodatum* mimics *Actinomyces* in intrauterine device-associated infections and other settings within the female genital tract. *Obstet Gynecol* 1992;79:534–538.

HOFFMAN M, MOLPUS K, ROBERTS WS, LYMAN GH, CAVANAGH D. Tuboovarian abscess in postmenopausal women. *J Reprod Med* 1990;35:525–528.

HOLMES KK, ESCHENBACH DA, KNAPP JS. Salpingitis: overview of etiology and epidemiology. *Am J Obstet Gynecol* 1980;138:893.

JONES R, BARRY AL. Antimicrobial activity of ceftriaxone, cefotaxime, desacetyl-cefotaxime, and cefotaxime-desacetylcefotaxime in the presence of human serum. *Antimicrob Agents Chemother* 1987;31:818–820.

LANDERS DV, SWEET RL. Current trends in the diagnosis and treatment of tubo-ovarian abscess. *Am J Obstet Gynecol* 1985;151:1098–1110.

LAZZARIN A, SARACCO A, MUSICCO M, NICOLOSI A. Man-to-woman sexual transmission of the human immunodeficiency virus. *Arch Intern Med* 1991;151:2411–2416.

MARCHBANKS PA, LEE NC, PETERSON HB. Cigarette smoking as a risk factor for pelvic inflammatory disease. *Am J Obstet Gynecol* 1990;162:639–644.

PETERSON HB, GALAID EI, ZENILMAN JM. Pelvic inflammatory disease: review of treatment options. *Rev Infect Dis* 1990 (Suppl 6);12:S656–S664.

REES E. The treatment of pelvic inflammatory disease. *Am J Obstet Gynecol* 1980;138:1042.

REICH H, McGLYNN F. Laparoscopic treatment of tubo-ovarian and pelvic abscess. *J Reprod Med* 1987;32:747–752.

ROY S, WILKINS J. Cefotaxime in the treatment of female pelvic soft tissue infections. *Infection* 1985 (Suppl 1);13:56–61.

ROY S, WILKINS J, MARCH CM, *et al.* A comparison of the efficacy and safety of ceftizoxime with doxycycline vs. conventional CDC therapies in the treatment of upper genital tract infection with or without a mass. Clinical therapeutics. *Int J Drug Ther* 1990 (Suppl C);12:53–73.

SELLORS J, MAHONY J, GOLDSMITH C, *et al.* The accuracy of clinical findings and laparoscopy in pelvic inflammatory disease. *Am J Obstet Gynecol* 1991;164:113–120.

SENANAYAKE P, KRAMER DG. Contraception and the etiology of pelvic inflammatory disease: new perspectives. *Am J Obstet Gynecol* 1980;138:852.

US Department of Health and Human Services, Public Health Service, Division of Sexually Transmitted Diseases. Sexually transmitted diseases treatment guidelines. *Centers for Disease Control MMWR* 1985 (Suppl);34:45.

Shapiro CN, Schulz SL, Lee NC, Dondero TJ. Review of human immuno-deficiency virus infection in women in the United States. *Obstet Gynecol* 1989; 74:800.

Soper DE, Brockwell NJ, Dalton HP. Microbial etiology of urban emergency department acute salpingitis: treatment with ofloxacin. *Am J Obstet Gynecol* 1992; 167:653–660.

Sweet RL, Schacter J, Robbee MO. Failure of lactum antibiotics to eradicate *Chlamydia trachomatis* in the endometrium despite apparent clinical cure of acute salpingitis. *JAMA* 1983;250:2641.

Sweet RL, Blankfort-Doyle M, Robbie MO, Schacter J. The occurrence of chlamydial and gonococcal salpingitis during the menstrual cycle. *JAMA* 1986; 255:2062.

Teisala K, Heinonen PK, Punnonen R. Transvaginal ultrasound in the diagnosis and treatment of tubo-ovarian abscess. *Br J Obstet Gynaecol* 1990;97:178–180.

Tyrrel RT, Murphy FB, Bernardino ME. Tubo-ovarian abscesses: CT-guided percutaneous drainage. *Radiology* 1990;175:87–89.

Vancaillie T, Schmidt EH. Therapeutic laparoscopy: an update on the instrumentation. *J Reprod Med* 1987;32:891–894.

vanSonnenberg E, Agostino HB, Casola G, *et al.* US-guided transvaginal drainage of pelvic abscesses and fluid collections. *Radiology* 1991;181:53–56.

Walters MD, Gibbs RS. A randomized comparison of gentamicin-clindamycin and cefoxitin-doxycycline in the treatment of acute pelvic inflammatory disease. *Obstet Gynecol* 1990;75:867.

Washington AE, Gove S, Schachter J, Sweet RL. Oral contraceptives, *Chlamydia trachomatis* infection and pelvic inflammatory disease. A word of caution about protection. *JAMA* 1985;253:2246.

Westrom L. Incidence, prevalence and trends of acute pelvic inflammatory disease and its consequences in industrialized countries. *Am J Obstet Gynecol* 1980;138:880.

Wolner-Hanssen P. Oral contraceptive use modifies the manifestations of pelvic inflammatory disease. *Br J Obstet Gynaecol* 1986;93:619–624.

Wolner-Hanssen P, Svenson L, March P-A, Westrom L. Laparoscopic findings and contraceptive use in women with signs and symptoms suggestive of acute salpingitis. *Obstet Gynecol* 1985;66:233.

Wolner-Hanssen P, Eschenback DA, Paavonen J, *et al.* Decreased risk of symptomatic chlamydial pelvic inflammatory disease associated with oral contraceptive use. *JAMA* 1990;263:54–59.

62

Prevention of postoperative gynecologic infections

SUBIR ROY

Background

Contamination by endogenous bacteria may occur at the time of gynecologic operations despite vigorous preoperative vaginal cleansing. The combination of hemostatic sutures around crushed tissue, blood products, and bacterial contaminants from the vagina may lead to postoperative abdominal wound infections, pelvic (cuff) cellulitis or pelvic abscesses. Prolonged hospitalization with therapeutic antibiotic administration and a second operation may be necessary before the patient recovers.

Prevention

A variety of techniques may be used to reduce infection following gynecologic surgery. Foremost among these is the use of prophylactic antibiotics. Guidelines for the use of prophylactic antibiotics in gynecology are the following:

1 the operation should carry a significant risk of postoperative site infection;

2 the operation should cause significant bacterial contamination;

3 the antibiotic used for prophylaxis should have laboratory evidence of effectiveness against some of the contaminating microorganisms and demonstrate clinical effectiveness;

4 the antibiotic should be present in the wound in effective concentration at the time of incision;

5 a short-term, low-toxicity regimen of antibiotics should be used;

6 the benefits of prophylactic antibiotics must outweigh the dangers of antibiotic use.

In suitably chosen subjects, the use of prophylactic antibiotics has reduced operative site infection following vaginal hysterectomy from 40–70% to 5–20% and following abdominal hysterectomy from 20–30% to 5–10%. A study by Burke demonstrated that no benefit accrued to prophylactic antibiotics if they were administered more than 3 h after bacterial contamination occurred. Preoperative administration of an agent should precede any elective procedure requiring antibiotic prophylaxis. A short-term course not to exceed 24 h postoperatively is currently recommended. A variety of agents have been successfully utilized: ampicillin, doxycycline, metronidazole, and a variety of cephalosporins which, because of their broad bacterial spectrum and low toxicity, have been popular prophylactic agents: cephalothin, cephradine, cefazolin, cefoxitin, ceforanide, cefonicid, cefotetan, cefotaxime, ceftizoxime, and moxalactam provide a broader spectrum of bacterial coverage than the earlier agents and allow a shorter period of antibiotic administration. By contrast, metronidazole, which is considered effective only against obligate anaerobes, is also successful as a prophylactic agent.

Use of these newer agents for prophylaxis has raised concerns that resistant organisms may emerge; however, the short treatment course of these agents makes this unlikely. They should still not be utilized for prophylaxis unless their use is associated with a significant reduction of operative site infection following gynecologic surgery over that achieved with less potent agents. Studies to test this thesis are currently under way for many of these agents and have been completed successfully for cefotaxime and ceftizoxime. In a recently completed study at the University of Southern California, cultures from operative site infections recovered *Enterococcus* species from all patients; however, all such patients also had other pathogenic organisms recovered. Even though therapy was usually not directed toward this pathogen (*Enterococcus* species), the patients recovered. In day 3 regrowth of vaginal flora studies the recovery of *Enterococcus* species, *Escherichia coli*, and various bacteroides species was not predictive of infection and did not differ whether the patients were treated with a single preoperative dose of ceftizoxime or three doses of cefoxitin. Conversely, diphtheroids, *Peptostreptococcus* species and *Staphylococcus epidermidis* were more frequent after ceftizoxime, while *Enterobacter* species and *Pseudomonas aeruginosa* (organisms that are not part of the normal vaginal flora) were more frequent after cefoxitin. Hence, the drug/dose schedule may be important in altering the postoperative surgical field microbial milieu and the likelihood of development of operative site infection.

Hysterectomy is considered to be a clean contaminated procedure;

therefore, even with antibiotic therapy, Cruse has reported an expected operative site infection rate of approximately 7% for this class of surgery. In general, the use of prophylactic antibiotics at the time of vaginal hysterectomy regardless of menopausal status has been shown to reduce the occurrence of operative site infection. For abdominal hysterectomy cases, the data suggest that the use of prophylactic antibiotics reduces the incidence of postoperative urinary tract infections and also of wound infections if the rate of wound infections in the control group is high. Only two of 12 abdominal hysterectomy studies demonstrated a reduction of postoperative pelvic cellulitis. Discrepancies in the efficacy of abdominal hysterectomy prophylaxis studies are largely the result of varying therapeutic regimens and definitions of outcome. Some authors have compared standard febrile morbidity of all infection-related complications, while others have carefully defined and categorized outcome in terms of fever index, pelvic (vaginal cuff) cellulitis, vaginal cuff abscess, urinary tract infection, wound infection, need for therapeutic antibiotics (a sum of the four previous diagnoses), and duration of postoperative hospitalization. Only when the randomized groups are similar in terms of entry characteristics can the outcome of prophylaxis be meaningfully compared, as reported by Hemsell *et al*. Hemsell and co-workers have shown that prophylaxis with abdominal hysterectomy can lead to reduced operative site infections, whether compared to a randomly selected control group or whether a high-risk group is treated and compared to an untreated low-risk group.

Our experience also demonstrated the utility of prophylaxis at the time of abdominal hysterectomy, and indeed, the abdominal hysterectomy group had a higher postoperative infective morbidity at the operative site as compared to the vaginal hysterectomy group. Recently, patients with clue cells or with the diagnosis of nonspecific vaginosis or trichomoniasis have been reported to develop cuff cellulitis following abdominal hysterectomy without antibiotic prophylaxis at a greater rate (~30%) as compared to those without these diagnoses (8–10%). Since cuff cellulitis developed in about 10% of those without these diagnoses, studies using single-agent, single-dose antibiotic prophylaxis for abdominal hysterectomy should be performed to determine whether it would be cost-effective.

Examples of prophylactic regimens with recommendations are given in Tables 62.1 and 62.2. The initial dose of antibiotic is usually administered 30–60 min prior to incision in order to achieve satisfactory serum and tissue levels. Cefoxitin must be diluted with lidocaine prior to intramuscular injection to reduce pain at the injection site. A normal prothrombin time or 10 mg vitamin K administration is recommended prior to the use of drugs such as cefamandole, moxalactam or cefoperazone, which contain the N-methylthiotetrazole side chain, which may lead

Table 62.1 Hysterectomy prophylactic agents from the literature

Agents	Pre-op	+	Additional
Ampicillin	0.5 g	+	q 6 h × 4
Doxycycline	200 mg	+	q day × 2
Metronidazole	1 g	+	0.5 g or 1 g 6 h later
Cefazolin	1 g	+	0.5 g or 1 g intraoperatively + q 6 h × 4
Cefoxitin	2 g	or	
	2 g	+	2 g q 6 h × 2–4
Cefonicid*	1 g		
Cefotaxime*	1 g		
Moxalactam	2 g	or	
	1 g	+	1 g q 6 h × 2
Ceftizoxime*	1 g		
Cefotetan*	1 g		
Piperacillin	2 g	+	2 g q 6 h × 2

* Also may be used for cesarean section prophylaxis at cord clamping.

Table 62.2 Agents studied at the University of Southern California with good success for hysterectomy prophylaxis

Agents	Doses: pre-op + additional
Cefazolin	1 g + 1 g q 6 h × 4
Cefoxitin	2 g + 2 g q 6 h × 2–4
Cefotaxime	1 g
Moxalactam	2 g
Ceftizoxime	1 g
Cefmetazole	1 g or 2 g

to hypoprothrombinemia and/or platelet dysfunction with or without clinical bleeding.

Other factors, such as operative time, estimated blood loss, regrowth of vaginal flora, and associated procedures performed at the time of hysterectomy have been examined. Indications are that the subjects at higher risk for postoperative infection are those who have the greatest amount of surgery performed (e.g., vaginal hysterectomy with a Pereyra procedure or abdominal hysterectomy with a Burch procedure). These infections usually occur more than 72 h following surgery.

For those individuals who are allergic to antibiotics, Swartz and Tanaree have reduced infections following vaginal or abdominal hysterectomy by using a closed T-tube suction drainage in the space between the peritoneum and vaginal cuff for 36 h postoperatively. A vaginal pack coated with a sterile gel rather than an antibiotic cream can also reduce the amount of blood and blood products that accumulate between the peritoneum and vaginal cuff. Osborne *et al.* have reported that hot conization of the cervix, an area which harbors bacteria despite vaginal cleansing prior to hysterectomy, has also reduced postoperative infections. However, this requires additional surgery and may not be cost-effective in reducing infections.

It is best not to alter the normal flora of the vagina or abdominal skin prior to surgery. For vaginal hysterectomy patients a preoperative vaginal douche with an iodophor solution the night before surgery reduces the total number of organisms from about 10^8 to 10^6–10^7. However, a very thorough preoperative cleansing of the vagina renders the vagina essentially organism-free during the time required to perform a hysterectomy with associated anterior and posterior colporrhaphies. Therefore, vaginal douching the night before surgery is not recommended. For patients undergoing exploratory laparotomy or abdominal hysterectomy, it is necessary for them simply to bathe or shower normally the night prior to surgery. If they use an agent such as iodophor for many days prior to surgery, it could lead to an altered skin flora with predominance of gram-negative organisms, resulting in increased wound infections. It is preferable to have the patient simply remove debris from the skin surface. The skin preparation immediately prior to surgery will reduce the bacterial count sufficiently during the operative period.

Cruse has shown a reduced postoperative infection rate if the subjects are shaved just priorr to operation, if no electrocautery knives or adhesive plastic drapes are used, and if no drains are brought through the abdominal incision.

Fever in the postoperative period may have a natural (noninfective) basis with the release of endogenous pyrogens (such as interleukin 1 and 6, tumor necrosis factor, and prostaglandin E_2), which may act centrally to produce fever. Fever which persists beyond 4–6 h (excluding the first 24 h postoperatively), especially if it is associated with excessive tenderness in the perioperative tissues, or if cellulitis or purulent material exudes from the operative site, clinches the diagnosis of operative site infection and deserves antibiotic therapy. Patients may also have the clinical findings of operative site infection without having fever. Although the same antibiotic used for prophylaxis may be used to treat these infections, as usually the pathogenic organisms responsible for the infection may not be resistant, many authors have preferred to use alternative therapy (see Chapter 60).

If a practice is instituted to treat only those postoperative patients with findings of an operative site infection, with or without fever, especially excluding those who have febrile morbidity alone, then less antibiotic will be utilized, with a reduced chance of altering the microbial flora with resistant organisms. Additionally, the cost of hospitalization will be reduced.

There is no substitute for good operative technique with attention to hemostasis in reducing postoperative infections. No antibiotic or other aids will overcome poor operative technique in reducing postoperative infections. Indeed, simple steps such as irrigation of the abdomen and subcutaneous tissues prior to closure, and use of a Jackson–Pratt drain subcutaneously, which is brought out through a separate incision, may permit the primary closure of incisions associated with clean contaminated procedures in obese patients or those with chronic diseases which may impair their host defense systems, such as diabetes mellitus. Alternatively, or in contaminated cases, following irrigation of the abdomen and subcutaneous tissues, sutures can be placed in the incision but not tied and the incision may be packed with gauze with a covering bandage. After 4 days, the packing can be removed and, if the tissues appear uninfected, the sutures may be tied.

Patients undergoing contaminated procedures should be treated with therapeutic doses and durations of antibiotics and should not be considered for prophylactic antibiotic administration.

SUGGESTED READING

BURKE JF. The effective period of preventive antibiotic action in experimental incisions and dermal lesions. *Surgery* 1961;50:161.

CRUSE PJE. Some factors determining wound infection: a prospective study of 30 000 wounds. In: Pollle HC Jr, Stone HH, eds. *Hospital-Acquired Infections in Surgery*. Baltimore, MD: University Park Press, 1977:77–85.

DUFF P. Antibiotic prophylaxis for abdominal hysterectomy. *Obstet Gynecol* 1982; 60:25.

DUFF P, PARK RC. Antibiotic prophylaxis in vaginal hysterectomy. *Obstet Gynecol* 1980;55:1935.

DINARELLO CA. The endogenous pyrogens in host-defense interactions. *Hosp Pract* 1989;15:73–90.

DINARELLO CA, CANNON JG, WOLFF SM. New concepts on the pathogenesis of fever. *Rev Infect Dis* 1988;10:168.

HEMSELL DL, REISCH J, NOBLES B, *et al*. Prevention of major infection after elective abdominal hysterectomy: individual determination required. *Am J Obstet Gynecol* 1983;147:521.

LARSSON P, PLATZ-CHRISTENSES J, FORSUM U, PAHLSON C. Clue cells in predicting infections after abdominal hysterectomy. *Obstet Gynecol* 1991;77:450.

LEDGER WJ. Prevention, diagnosis and a treatment of postoperative infections. *Am J Obstet Gynecol* 1980;55:2035.

OSBORNE NG, WRIGHT RC, DUBAY M. Preoperative hot conization of the cervix. *Am J Obstet Gynecol* 1979;133:375.

ROY S, WILKINS J. Comparison of cefotaxime to cefazolin for prophylaxis of vaginal or abdominal hysterectomy. *Clin Ther* (Suppl A) 1982;5:74.

ROY S, WILKINS J. Single-dose cefotaxime versus 3 to 5 dose cefoxitin for prophylaxis of vaginal or abdominal hysterectomy. *J Antimicrob Chemother* (Suppl B) 1984;14:217–221.

ROY S, WILKINS J, HEMSELL DL, MARCH CM, SPIRTOS NM. Efficacy and safety of single-dose ceftizoxime vs. multiple-dose cefoxitin in preventing infection after vaginal hysterectomy. *J Repro Med* 1988;33:149–153.

ROY S, WILKINS J, GALAIF E, AZEN C. Comparative efficacy and safety of cefmetazole or cefoxitin in the prevention of postoperative infection following vaginal and abdominal hysterectomy. *J Br Soc Ant Chem* (Suppl D) 1989;23:109–117.

ROY S, WILKINS J, HEMSELL DL, MARCH CM, SPIRTOS NM. Efficacy and safety of single-dose ceftizoxime vs. multiple-dose cefoxitin in preventing infection after vaginal hysterectomy. *J Reprod Med* 1988;33:1.

ROY S, WILKINS J, MARCH CM, *et al*. Cefmetazole and cefonicid comparative efficacy and safety in preventing postoperative infections after vaginal and abdominal hysterectomy. *J Reprod Med* 1990;35:1082–1090.

SOPER DE, BUMP RC, HURT WG. Bacterial vaginosis and trichomoniasis vaginitis are risk factors for cuff cellulitis after abdominal hysterectomy. *Am J Obstet Gynecol* 1990;163:1016–1023.

SWARTZ WH, TANAREE P. Suction drainage as an alternative to prophylactic antibiotics for hysterectomy. *Obstet Gynecol* 1975;43:305.

63

Prepubertal vulvovaginitis

PAUL F. BRENNER

The most common gynecologic complaint of premenarchal patients is vaginal discharge. The risk of vaginal infections in young girls prior to puberty is increased by a thin vaginal mucosa, an exposed introitus, the close proximity of the vaginal opening and anal orifice, and poor perineal hygiene. The unestrogenized vaginal mucosa is very thin and easily susceptible to infection should bacteria gain access to the vagina. Failure of the labia minora to develop prior to puberty leaves the vaginal introitus relatively unprotected by labial fat pads and pubic hair. The anatomic proximity of the opening of the vaginal vault to the anus facilitates exposure to fecal bacteria. Most significant is the failure to instruct young girls in proper perineal hygiene. Girls who wipe the perineum from the anus towards the vagina after defecation and urination carry bacteria the short distance toward the exposed introitus and thin vaginal mucosa.

Differential diagnosis

A vaginal discharge in a premenarchal patient may be physiologic. Some estrogen of maternal origin remains in the newborn's circulation for the first 2 or 3 weeks of life. During this interval, under the influence of estrogen, the vaginal epithelium of the newborn is several layers thick, composed of glycogen-laden stratified squamous epithelial cells, and the vaginal pH is acidic. An increase in endogenous estrogen normally occurs early in puberty. The vaginal mucosa and cervix are quite sensitive to estrogen from any source. Small elevations of estrogen in the peripheral circulation increase the amount of cervical mucus present and the number

Table 63.1 Etiology of prepubertal vulvovaginitis

Physiologic
Postnatal
Premenarchal

Pathologic
Mixed enteric organisms
Sexually transmitted diseases
   Neisseria gonorrhoeae
   Chlamydia trachomatis
   Condylomata acuminata
   Herpes simplex
   Trichomonas
Foreign body
Contact irritant
Candidiasis
Enterobiasis
Shigellosis
Ear, nose, and throat pathogens
   Streptococcus
   Staphylococcus
Congenital anomaly
   Fistula
   Ectopic ureter
   Meningomyelocele
Skin disorders

---

of cells desquamated from the vaginal mucosa. Estrogen present in the first 2 or 3 weeks of life or in early puberty produces a physiologic leukorrhea which is characterized as milky-white or clear mucus discharge without an offensive odor or vulvar involvement.

There are several pathologic causes of vulvovaginitis in children (Table 63.1). Poor perineal hygiene may result in the transfer of mixed enteric organisms to the vagina. Sexually transmitted diseases (STDs) can occur in prepubertal girls of all ages. A foreign body placed in the vagina may lead to a vaginal discharge and contact irritants can cause vulvar–vaginal symptomatology. Candidiasis, enterobiasis, and shigellosis are infrequent specific causes of vaginal leukorrhea. Organisms responsible for ear, nose, and throat infections may be spread from their primary site to the vagina. Congenital anomalies of the urogenital system very rarely produce symptoms which may be interpreted as vaginal discharge.

Wiping the perineum in a direction from the anus to the vagina may allow a mixture of enteric organisms, including gram-negative coliform bacteria, enterococcus, and anaerobic bacteria to invade the vagina.

Mixed enteric organisms, also referred to as nonspecific vulvovaginitis, are the most common cause of leukorrhea in prepubescent girls.

Vaginal discharge may be a clinical manifestation of a STD, including *Neisseria gonorrhoeae*, *Chlamydia trachomatis*, condylomata acuminata, herpes simplex, and *Trichomonas*. STDs in prepubertal children have an association with sexual abuse. Other members of the immediate family or care-givers should be evaluated and cultured, as it is from one of them that the disease was acquired. When one STD is diagnosed it is entirely possible that the child may be coinfected with one or more other STDs and appropriate screening must be conducted. Some infants may acquire these vaginal infections through maternal colonization at the time of delivery. The incubation period for these infections may last up to 2 years. The most reliable diagnostic test for either gonorrhea or chlamydial vaginitis in a prepubertal girl is a culture. Condylomata acuminata (venereal warts) are dry warty lesions caused by the human papillomavirus, usually type 6 or 11 in children. Herpes simplex is characterized as small vesicular lesions on an erythematous base caused by the herpes simplex virus type 2. Examination under magnification of the scrapings taken from the herpetic lesions and prepared with Wright stain demonstrates multinucleated giant cells. *Trichomonas vaginalis* is expressed clinically as a frothy, watery yellow or green discharge. The motile flagellated parasites are identified in a saline wet-mount preparation. *Trichomonas* is very uncommon in prepubertal females.

A foreign body must always be included in the differential diagnosis of a pediatric patient who presents with a foul-smelling discharge admixt with blood. A small ball of toilet paper is the most common foreign body found in the vagina of a prepubertal child, but others include beads, marker tips, crayons, and pins. Most foreign bodies are not radiopaque and X-rays of the lower abdomen and pelvis are seldom helpful. A long list of contact irritants may inflame the vulvar tissue. Harsh soaps, detergents, disinfectants, bubble baths, powders, perfumes, feminine hygiene sprays, scented or colored toilet paper, cosmetics, chemicals, and topical medications are some of the agents which can act as contact irritants to vulvar tissue. Tight-fitting clothing, including leotards, tights, rubber pants, skin-tight jeans, nylon underclothing, and tight-fitting diapers are included in this category.

Vulvovaginal candidiasis is uncommon in the prepubescent female unless she has diabetes mellitus or has recently received antibiotic therapy. The child with vulvovaginitis due to *Candida albicans* has an inflamed, edematous, pruritic vulva and a thick, white, cheese-like vaginal discharge. A potassium hydroxide wet-mount preparation of the discharge demonstrates the characteristic spores and hyphae. *C. albicans* can be cultured on Nickerson, Sabouraud, or Biggy agar.

One-fifth of all prepubertal girls infected with *Enterobius vermicularis* — pinworms — develops vulvovaginitis. Pinworms inhabit the large intestine. Female pinworms emerge from the anus at night to deposit eggs on the perineum. With the aid of a flashlight these worms may be seen around the anus during the night. In the morning the eggs around the anus can be collected on the sticky side of Scotch tape and, following toluene treatment, can be seen with low-power microscopic magnification. Nocturnal perineal pruritus occurs as the pinworms contaminated with colonic bacteria egress from the anus and spread into the vagina. Prepubertal girls with pinworms often have other family members with these same parasites.

Colonization of the intestinal tract with *Shigella flexneri* or *S. sonnei* can cause symptoms of fever, malaise, diarrhea, and a mucopurulent vaginal discharge which sometimes contains blood. The diagnosis of shigellosis is confirmed by positive stool cultures.

Female children with otitis media, tonsillitis, or any upper respiratory tract infection due to *Streptococcus* or *Staphylococcus* species may have bacteria spread by manual transmission from the primary ear, nose, and throat location to the vulvovaginal area, resulting in a vaginal discharge. The diagnosis is confirmed when vaginal cultures are positive for the same organisms identified in the primary infection site.

Congenital anomalies in which a communication exists between the vagina and the rectum or bladder can be the cause of a vaginal discharge that has been present since birth. An ectopic ureter, particularly when the ureter drains directly into the vagina or introitus, has been the source of a continuous leakage of urine which is misinterpreted as a vaginal discharge. A meticulous search for the ectopic opening of the ureter is necessary and an intravenous pyelogram may be a useful diagnostic aid.

Lesions affecting the external genitalia of prepubescent girls may be a localized manifestation of a generalized skin disorder. Some skin disorders which affect the vulva include seborrheic dermatitis, psoriasis, atopic dermatitis, lichen sclerosis, vitiligo, eczema, erythema multiforme, and lichen planus. The treatment of the lesions found on the external genitalia is similar to that given for lesions from these skin disorders situated anywhere else on the body.

Vaginal discharge is the cardinal symptom of vaginitis. If the vulvar tissue is inflamed, it appears erythematous and edematous and associated symptoms of pruritus, dysuria, frequent urination, and enuresis may be present. The pertinent points in the history include the character of the discharge, the length of time the discharge has been present, the presence of odor, the presence of blood, the method of perineal hygiene, recent infections that might be streptococcal or staphylococcal in origin, recent venereal disease or parasites among immediate members of the family, nocturnal perianal pruritus, and the placement of a foreign body in the vagina.

Examination

The successful gynecologic examination of the prepubertal female is based on the examiner's ability to place the child at ease and to allow her to control the examination. Encouraging the child to participate in the history-taking process, a gentle but thorough physical examination, and the presence of a trusted family member all help to establish the appropriate level of rapport and confidence between the physician and young patient which is necessary. The inspection and subsequent vaginoscopy cannot be rushed. Attempts to hasten the procedure only result in an inadequate examination and a frightened patient. Selection of the position for the young patient during the gynecologic examination is based on the comfort of the patient and her ability to control the examination. The frog-leg position, the knee–chest position, and the dorsal lithotomy position have all been advocated for this exam. In my experience the dorsal lithotomy position is guaranteed to be uncomfortable and prevents the patient from exercising any control over the exam. I prefer the frog-leg position as it allows the patient the greatest degree of control. The patient may find it most comfortable to sit in her mother's lap during the exam. Inspection of the external genitalia and introitus may be accomplished by the examiner depressing the perineum on either side of the labia with both thumbs, by the examiner gently grasping each labia between thumb and index finger and separating the labia, or by the examiner placing the child's index fingers on the labia and separating them. A swab moistened with saline, a plastic eye-dropper, or a small plastic tube attached to the tip of an ordinary medicine dropper can be used to collect specimens for wet-mount preparations and cultures. The use of a dry cotton swab for this purpose should be avoided as a small child may find it painful. Xylocaine ointment applied to the vulva reduces the chance for discomfort.

An attempt should be made to examine the vagina of every child with prepubertal vulvovaginitis with the child awake. A variety of instruments are available for vaginoscopy of young patients, including fiberoptic vaginoscopes, the Killian nasal speculum, veterinary otoscopes, and urethroscopes. I find the Killian nasal speculum offers inadequate inspection of the upper vaginal vault and may be painful. A Welch–Allyn otoscope with veterinary otoscope attachments is both practical and inexpensive.

A rectal abdominal exam is an integral part of the gynecological exam. In addition to palpating a pelvic mass, a vaginal foreign body may be detected and discharge may be directed to the introitus. Any time the discharge is mixed with blood or the patient or her parents indicate that a foreign body has been placed in the vagina, adequate inspection of the vagina must be carried out. In such cases, if vaginoscopy cannot be completed successfully with the patient awake, she should be anesthetized. If the discharge does not contain blood, there is no history of a foreign body, and vaginoscopy is unsuccessful with the patient awake, vaginoscopy under anesthesia need not be performed.

Treatment

There are several nonspecific recommendations which will benefit any prepubertal girl with a vaginal discharge. The child should be instructed that following urination and defecation she should wipe away from the vulvovaginal area. Scented or colored toilet paper should not be used. A parent may have to supervise the child until it is certain she is practicing proper perineal hygiene. The child should switch from tight-fitting clothing and underwear made of wool or nylon to loose-fitting clothing, skirts, and white cotton underclothing. The underwear should be changed frequently. Sitz baths with warm water and preferably no soap or else very mild soap will provide symptomatic relief. When the child emerges from the tub, the vulvar tissue should be air-dried or, at most, dried very gently with a soft towel. Topical bland ointments or corticosteroid ointments (0.5 or 1.0% hydrocortisone) applied once or twice a day, at least once a day at bedtime, will relieve vulvar symptoms.

Specific treatment is available for prepubertal vulvovaginitis due to *Candida albicans* using topical antifungal creams: nystatin, miconazole, or clotrimazole for 7–14 days. Recurrent vaginal yeast infections may be treated with oral nystatin. Pinworms – enterobiasis – are treated with mebendazole (Vermox) one 100 mg chewable tablet and therapy is repeated in 2 weeks. Shigellosis is treated with trimethoprim–sulfamethoxazole 8–40 mg/kg per day orally for 7 days. Streptococcal and staphylococcal vaginitis is treated with the following oral antibiotics for 7–10 days: penicillin V potassium 125–250 mg q.i.d, cephalexin (Keflex) 25–50 mg/kg per day, dicloxacillin 25 mg/kg per day, and amoxicillin-clavulanate (Augmentin) 20–40 mg/kg per day.

STDs in a prepubertal female are treated with regimens appropriate for their body weight. Gonorrhea cultured from the vaginal discharge of a prepubescent female is treated with a single intramuscular injection with ceftriaxone 125 mg or spectinomycin 40 mg/kg for those children who cannot take ceftriaxone. A positive *Chlamydia* culture from the vaginal discharge is an indication for treatment with oral erythromycin 50 mg/kg per day for 10 days. Children approaching the age of puberty may receive oral doxycycline 100 mg b.i.d. for 1 week. *Trichomonas vaginalis* is treated with oral metronidazole (Flagyl) 15 mg/kg per day 3 times a day for 7–10 days. Herpetic lesions may be treated with 5% acyclovir ointment applied every 4–6 h as needed for relief of symptoms. Condylomata acuminata in very young children may be very difficult to treat. For those children with extensive lesions, laser ablation under general anesthesia has been quite successful.

Systemic antibiotics are used to treat a vaginal infection due to mixed enteric organisms in prepubertal girls. Amoxycillin 20–40 mg/kg per day, cephalexin 25–50 mg/kg per day, and ampicillin 50 mg/kg per day are available as liquid suspensions and are administered in divided doses 3 or 4 times a day for 7–10 days, the total dose corresponding to the patient's weight. A threefold regimen of improved perineal hygiene, systemic antibiotics, and topical corticosteroids resolves almost all vaginal infections due to mixed enteric organisms in premenarchal patients.

Contact irritants should be identified and removed from the perineal area. A foreign body requires removal from the vagina. Small foreign bodies may be flushed from the vagina using gentle irrigation with saline or water instilled through a small urethral catheter attached to a 25-ml syringe. Larger foreign bodies can be extracted from the vagina with bayonet forceps. The application of a local anesthetic ointment to the introitus may aid in the passage of any instrument into the vaginal vault of a prepubertal girl. Congenital anomalies found to be the cause of prepubertal vaginal discharge require surgical correction.

Persistent leukorrhea that fails to respond to therapy is an indication for vaginoscopy, even if it requires anesthesia. If a specific etiology is not found by vaginoscopy, persistent vulvovaginitis is treated with estrogen cream applied locally to the vulva for no more than 3 weeks. The estrogen thickens the vaginal mucosa, making it more resistant to infection.

SUGGESTED READING

PARADISE JE, CAMPOS JM, FRIEDMAN HM, FRISHMUTH G. Vulvovaginitis in premenarcheal girls: clinical features and diagnostic evaluation. *Pediatrics* 1982; 70:193–198.

ALTCHEK A. Pediatric vulvovaginitis. *J Reprod Med* 1984;29:359–375.

ARSENAULT PS, GERBIE AB. Vulvovaginitis in the preadolescent girl. *Pediatr Ann* 1986;15:577–585.

WILLIAMS TS, CALLEN JP, OWEN LG. Vulvar disorders in the prepubertal female. *Pediatr Ann* 1986;15:588–605.

BUMP RC, SACHS LA, BUESCHING WJ. Sexually transmissible infectious agents in sexually active and virginal asymptomatic adolescent girls. *Pediatrics* 1986;77: 488–494.

HAMMERSCHLAG MR, RETTING PJ, SHIELDS ME. False positive results with the use of chlamydial antigen detection tests in the evaluation of suspected sexual abuse in children. *Pediatr Infect Dis* 1988;7:11–14.

McKay T. *Enterobius vermicularis* infection causing endometritis and persistent vaginal discharge in three siblings. *NZ Med J* 1989;102:56.

Straumanis JP, Bucchini JA Jr. Group A beta-hemolytic streptococcal vulvovaginitis in prepubertal girls: a case report and review of the past twenty years. *Pediatr Infect Dis J* 1990;9:845–848.

64

Chronic pelvic pain

MARK V. SAUER

Chronic pelvic pain is frequently encountered in female patients and represents the chief complaint of approximately one-third of all gynecologic outpatients. A wide variety of illnesses present as pelvic pain, and therefore symptoms alone rarely distinguish one disease state from another. Furthermore, the degree and character of pain are uniquely perceived by each individual, and the response to pain often varies within individuals, depending upon the circumstances surrounding the disorder. Thus, frustration is commonly experienced by both the physician and the patient, since a thorough and complete evaluation requires time, and often ends in negative results. In many instances patients have no organic basis for their complaints and require referral for psychologic consultation. The purpose of this chapter is to outline an approach for investigating pelvic pain patients, and provide guidelines for directing their care.

Pain perception

The perception of pain involves an initial sensation and subsequent reaction. Sensation must first be evoked. Nociceptive stimuli are transmitted by small-diameter nerves, the unmyelinated Aδ and C fibers, originating in the periphery. Through a series of synapses, this information is passed in an ascending fashion to the cortex. The sensation of pain normally elicits an avoidance reaction. Unpleasant stresses may be physical or psychologic.

The understanding of pain perception has changed significantly in recent decades. Several schemas have been proposed to model pain. Early theories, such as the Cartesian theory, are based upon the tenet of a specific stimulus triggering a direct, measured response. In this model peripheral receptors for the sensation of touch, temperature, and pain transmit this information directly to the higher centers to elicit a correct response, usually an avoidance reaction. Although anatomically correct, the simplicity of this theory does little to explain known differences that exist in responses to pain between and within individuals. Furthermore, motivational or affective modification is not accurately portrayed.

The more modern gate theory integrates both peripheral and central nervous system signals, and helps to explain known differences in response to pain by providing a response modulator. In this model, the small nerve fibers which carry pain from the periphery are influenced by other central nervous system activity upon entry into the spinal cord. Bidirectional transmission of information both from the periphery to the brain and from the brain to the spinal cord is thought to occur. Anatomically, this theory is also correct. Rapid-traveling impulses from the periphery to the central nervous system conducted along large myelinated fibers provide a signal to the cortex that precedes the arrival of impulses from smaller unmyelinated tracts carrying the sensation of pain. Individual modulation therefore occurs either consciously or subliminally, with accentuation, dampening, or extinction of evoked stimuli at the level the impulse enters the spinal cord – an opening or closing of the "gate." Modulation is accomplished via descending impulses that control transmission cells within the spinal cord. Among the probable neuromodulators are serotonin and endorphin, both of which are linked to central regulation of mood and pain perception.

Pelvic pain is principally elicited following stimulation of free nerve endings to the reproductive organs and peritoneum. Gynecologic pain is transmitted via one of two routes. In the case of somatic sensory nerves (external genitalia and vagina) perception is rapid and well localized. More commonly, however, pelvic pain is a result of transmission of impulses along the autonomic (visceral) nervous system which innervates the internal reproductive organs. Pain patterns are less well localized. Deep pelvic pain follows the route of the splanchnic nerves throughout the pelvis, synapsing with secondary neurons within the posterior horn of the spinal cord. Referred pain is common since nerves from the pelvis enter into the cord alongside sensory nerves innervating dermatomes of the musculoskeleton. Furthermore, after synapsing within the cord, the message is carried to the higher central nervous system centers along tracts shared with other sensory nerves. Thus, localization of pain complaints along dermatomes may aid in diagnosing pelvic lesions.

Another difficulty in evaluating complaints stems from the shared innervation of other abdominal structures by the same sensory neurons. This explains why pain from the bladder trigone is indistinguishable from the upper vagina, salpingitis mimics appendicitis, and ovarian pain is similar to ureteral complaints. Thus, in general, pelvic pain is poorly localized, usually diffuse, and commonly referred.

Associated conditions

Physicians are trained to regard pain as a symptom of organic disease. In accordance with the specificity theory, pain is felt to be a direct result of sensory fibers being stimulated by damaged tissue in the periphery. Pathologic changes in the internal and external reproductive tract that initiate pain include rupture, ischemia, or destruction of a visceral organ, as well as mechanical, chemical, or microbial inflammation of the pelvic peritoneum. As stated previously, abnormalities that are not associated with the reproductive system are common and must be considered in the differential diagnosis. Table 64.1 lists the most common insults.

Gynecologic pathology tends to present as either episodic or continuous pain, and usually occurs in proximity to an ovulatory or menstrual event. Table 64.2 denotes frequently encountered problems.

Table 64.1 Common causes of pelvic pain not directly associated with the reproductive tract

Appendicitis	Regional enteritis/diverticulitis
Urinary tract infection	Renal and bladder calculi
Mesenteric vascular disease	Rectus hematoma
Aortic aneurysm	Herpes zoster
Porphyria	Sickle cell crisis

Table 64.2 Most common reproductive tract etiologies for pelvic pain

Episodic	
Mittelschmerz	Dysmenorrhea
Endometriosis	Adenomyosis
Salpingitis	Ectopic pregnancy
Adnexal torsion	

Continuous
Adhesions
Pelvic relaxation
Anatomic distortions (e.g., chronic tuboovarian abscess, leiomyomas)

Assessment

A summary assessment should be made as to whether the pain is physiologic or psychologic in origin. Efforts are directed at ruling out all physical reasons for pain before attributing it to a psychologic cause. It is critical to formulate an objective opinion in order to avoid the initiation of empiric therapies.

Evaluation begins with a thorough history and physical examination. The description of pain should include the site, duration, pattern during activity, and association with bodily functions. Common characteristics of chronic pain syndrome include a duration of >6 months, incomplete relief by previous treatments, impaired lifestyle, and depression.

During the physical examination a thorough inspection is essential, with particular attention paid to the presence or absence of vaginismus. Techniques borrowed from relaxation training may aid in the abdominopelvic examination of pain patients. Contraction–relaxation sequences for abdominal and pelvic muscles, combined with deep breathing and a slowly performed, well-explained examination, allow the patient to experience a sense of control while providing the physician with an opportunity to uncover abnormal physical findings in an otherwise uncooperative patient. Palpation of the urethra and bladder base (urethral diverticula; trigonitis), lateral and ventral traction on the cervix (salpingitis; adnexal adhesions), and uterosacral palpation (endometriosis) may aid in localizing subtle pathology.

Laboratory testing should be comprehensive yet specific. Urinalysis, complete blood count, and sedimentation rates are commonly useful. Less frequently considered but equally important is the stool guiaic test which may uncover gastrointestinal disorders such as ulcerative colitis or Crohn's disease. A wet-mount of the cervical mucus will detect *Trichomonas*, which is responsible for many vague abdominopelvic complaints.

Vaginal ultrasonography has proven to be efficient and reliable in screening patients for presumed pelvic pathology. High-frequency probes are often better tolerated and inserted more comfortably than a physician's fingers during bimanual examinations. The enhanced pelvic imaging provided by vaginal ultrasound makes it a useful adjunct in evaluating these patients.

Frequently laparoscopy is required. An outpatient procedure lasting <30 min, laparoscopy represents an invasive but highly effective means to diagnose pathology definitively in these women. Results of diagnostic surgery in patients with pelvic pain are conflicting. In many cases women with chronic complaints have more demonstrable pathology, usually adhesions or endometriosis, than women undergoing laparoscopy for gynecologic reasons not related to pain (e.g., tubal sterilization). However, when compared to pain-free patients known to have a high incidence of pelvic pathology (e.g., infertility patients) undergoing laparoscopy as part of a diagnostic evaluation, no differences between groups have been reported. All studies note that a significant number of women with pelvic pain have no demonstrable pathology (10–50%).

Adolescents with debilitating pelvic pain complaints should be viewed differently than older patients. In this group, the majority of individuals will have visible pathology, usually endometriosis. The frequency of this finding and the importance of early management to avoid the sequelae of infertility and chronic pain make the aggressive investigation of these patients particularly important. Victims of sexual abuse may also present with pelvic pain. This has been noted not only following assaults on the patients themselves, but also subsequent to witnessing abuse of friends, parents, or siblings.

Treatment

Once arriving at a diagnosis, treatment should be specific. Avoidance of empiric therapy prevents the prolongation of the patient's problem while definitively attempting to remedy the malady at hand. Table 64.3 outlines standard treatment plans.

Less conventional approaches to treating pain involve intentionally triggering the release of the brain's β-endorphins to stimulate an endogenous morphine-like response. Such methods have had some success in chronic pain states. Transcutaneous electrical nerve stimulation, injections of dermatomes or anatomic "trigger points" with local anesthetics, and acupuncture all dampen the visceral pain response by increasing levels of β-endorphin centrally, while diminishing peripheral nerve signals at the segmental convergence of visceral and cutaneous nerves.

Table 64.3 Specific course of treatment for discovered pathology

---

Medical therapy
Dysmenorrhea: oral contraceptives, prostaglandin synthetase inhibitors
Endometriosis: gonadotropin-releasing hormone agonist; oral contraceptives, danazol
Salpingitis: antibiotics

Surgical therapy
Adhesiolysis
Organ extirpation
Laparoscopic uterosacral nerve ablation (LUNA)
Presacral neurectomy

Laparoscopically performed ablation of the uterosacral nerves has diminished pain complaints of many women with central pelvic pain. This can be performed during the diagnostic surgery, and gives similar relief to a presacral neurectomy. However, no prospective randomized clinical trials have been completed to assess the clinical efficacy or the placebo effect of this approach.

Psychosomatic pain

In many cases organic pathology is not discovered following the evaluation outlined above. These patients are likely to possess a psychologic reason for their pain complaints. A profile of idiopathic pain patients is listed in Table 64.4. In general, these patients are burdened by a lack of self-esteem and an inability to maintain interpersonal relationships. In many cases a history of prior sexual abuse is elicited. These patients usually have difficulty in externalizing feelings when emotionally stressed. Investigators postulate that the area of psychic conflict and emotional stress may determine the site of pain. Thus, a sexual component to an emotional disturbance is commonly expressed (vaginismus, dyspareunia, anorgasmia).

Treatment should be multidisciplinary to be effective. Initially, the patient is confronted with objective data gained from the evaluation. Emphasis should be placed on the importance of the normal findings to her overall health. Referral to a psychologist or psychiatrist for follow-up care should be offered. Many patients will refuse care and go elsewhere. For those accepting psychologic evaluation, short-term, individualized psychotherapy is initiated. This is usually followed up by long-term group sessions.

Table 64.4 Psychosocial and medical profile of women with idiopathic chronic pelvic pain

Age 25–35 years
Pathology absent
Pain continuous, diffuse, and poorly localized
Positive review of systems (multiple complaints)
History of sexual or physical abuse
Poor self-esteem
Negative attitude toward sex
Poor interpersonal relationships
Previous pelvic surgery
Subjective complaints undocumented by objective testing

Summary

Pelvic pain is a complaint resulting from a multitude of etiologies. The diagnosis and treatment of pain disorders represent a formidable challenge. Pain pathways are shared among many organ systems, making it difficult to differentiate without appropriate adjunctive measures of assessment. Clinical testing should investigate all possibilities for an organic reason to the complaint, understanding the many modulating factors inherently present. Therapy should be directed at specific disease entities, and empiric treatments discouraged. Laparoscopy should be considered in women with long-standing complaints, especially if they are without an obvious source for discomfort. This is particularly true in adolescents, where endometriosis is a common finding. For those without demonstrable disease, integrated physical and psychologic counseling is required.

SUGGESTED READING

CASTELNUOVO-TEDESCO P, KROUT BM. Psychosomatic aspects of chronic pelvic pain. *Psychiatry Med* 1970;1:109–126.

FREDERICK J, PAULSON RJ, SAUER MV. Routine use of vaginal ultrasound in the preoperative evaluation of gynecologic patients. An adjunct to resident education. *J Reprod Med* 1991;36:779–782.

GOLDSTEIN DP, deCHOLNOKY C, EMANS SJ, LEVENTHAL JM. Laparoscopy in the diagnosis and management of pelvic pain in adolescents. *J Reprod Med* 1980;24:251–256.

KRESCH AJ, SEIFER DB, SACHS LB, *et al.* Laparoscopy in 100 women with chronic pelvic pain. *Obstet Gynecol* 1984;64:672–674.

LICHTEN EM, BOMBARD J. Surgical treatment of primary dysmenorrhea with laparoscopic uterine nerve ablation. *J Reprod Med* 1987;32:37–41.

MELZACK R. Neurophysiological foundations of pain. In: STERNBACH RA, ed. *The Psychology of Pain*. 2nd edn. New York: Raven Press, 1986:1–24.

PETERS AAW, VAN DORST E, JELLIS B, VAN ZUUREN E, HERMANS J, TRIMBOS JB. A randomized clinical trial to compare two different approaches in women with chronic pelvic pain. *Obstet Gynecol* 1991;77:740–744.

RAPKIN AJ. Adhesions and pelvic pain: a retrospective study. *Obstet Gynecol* 1986;68:13–15.

TAYLOR PJ, GOMEL V. Pelvic pain. *Curr Probl Obstet Gynecol Fertil* 1987;10:393–437.

WALKER E, KATON W, HARROP-GRIFFITHS J, *et al.* Relationship of chronic pelvic pain to psychiatric diagnoses and childhood sexual abuse. *Am J Psychiatry* 1988;145:75–80.

65

Dysmenorrhea

GAIL MEZROW

Dysmenorrhea is defined as severe pelvic pain occurring before or during menstruation. This pain may be accompanied by headache, nausea, vomiting, diarrhea, lethargy, dizziness, sweating, breast tenderness, tachycardia, and heavy menstrual flow. Dysmenorrhea has been classified as being either primary or secondary. Women with primary dysmenorrhea have no organic cause. In these women painful menstruation usually begins during the teenage years, coinciding with the onset of ovulatory cycles. In all, 75% of women develop primary dysmenorrhea, with 15% having severe symptoms. Some 38% of women with primary dysmenorrhea report the onset of symptoms within 1 year of menarche. Use of oral contraception, smoking, vaginal delivery, and shorter menstrual flow are factors associated with a lower incidence of dysmenorrhea, while women with a positive family history (mother or sister) have a higher frequency. Early pregnancy and menstrual cycle length do not affect the incidence of dysmenorrhea. Secondary dysmenorrhea usually arises later and is a result of pelvic pathology.

Primary dysmenorrhea

Pathophysiology

Patients with primary dysmenorrhea usually have regular menstrual cycles with symptoms beginning just prior to menstruation. Uterine contraction pressure and resting tone are increased in these women. Primary dysmenorrhea occurs only in ovulatory cycles. The pathogenesis is not known; however, the symptoms are all prostaglandin (PG)-induced. The endometrium is the primary site of production of the PGE_2 and $PGF_{2\alpha}$. PGE_2 and $PGF_{2\alpha}$ are produced at higher levels during the luteal phase and are found at increased levels in both the menstrual fluid and plasma of women with dysmenorrhea. Exogenous administration of $PGF_{2\alpha}$ has been shown to cause cramping, nausea, vomiting, diarrhea, headache, uterine contractions with increased amplitude and frequency, and increased resting tone as assessed by intrauterine pressure. The pain is thought to be secondary to ischemia due to reduction in blood flow which accompanies the contractions.

Treatment

PG synthetase inhibitors (PGSIs) alleviate the symptoms of primary dysmenorrhea and decrease the menstrual fluid levels of PG. They reduce uterine contractility, as shown by a reduction in intrauterine pressure. PGSIs block PG formation by inhibiting cyclooxygenase, the enzyme which converts arachidonic acid to endoperoxides. Endoperoxides are then converted to series 2 PG, including PGE_2 and $PGF_{2\alpha}$. PGSIs are classified into two groups: arylcarboxylic acids and arylalkanoic acids. Arylcarboxylic acids include fenamates and acetylsalicyclic acid (aspirin). Arylalkanoic acids (nonsteroidal antiinflammatory drugs; NSAIDs) include the arylpropionic acids: ibuprofen (Motrin), naproxen (Naprosyn), naproxen sodium (Anaprox), and the indoleacetic acids (indomethacin). Ibuprofen is more effective than indomethacin. Recommended dose of ibuprofen is 400–800 mg 4 times a day. There is no difference in effectiveness if treatment is begun before or at the onset of menses. The effective dose for naproxen is 250–500 mg every 6 h. The comparable dose for naproxen sodium is 275–500 mg every 6 h, after an initial dose of 550 mg. Naproxen has a longer duration than the other NSAIDs and naproxen sodium has a more rapid onset of action since it is absorbed quickly due to increased water solubility. Aspirin at normal dosages is no more effective than placebo.

Unlike the other prostaglandin inhibitors, fenamates not only affect prostaglandin synthesis but also block the action of the prostaglandins at the target organ, resulting in more effective pain relief. The effectiveness of treatment is related to the tissue concentration of the drug. Mefenamic acid (Ponstel) is used at a dosage of 250 mg 4 times daily or 500 mg 3 times daily. Meclamen (meclofenamate sodium) is used at a dosage of 100 mg 3 times daily.

Side-effects associated with NSAIDs include autoimmune hemolytic anemia, rash, edema, fluid retention, dizziness, headache, blurred vision, nervousness, and mild elevation of liver enzymes. Indomethacin (Indocid), phenylbutazone (Butazolidin), and oxyphenbutazone (Tandearil) are not approved for the treatment of dysmenorrhea due to serious side-effects. All PGSIs are effective in the relief of primary dysmenorrhea. Unfortunately, few studies have compared the effectiveness of one drug over another. Patients respond differently to different agents, with one PGSI being more effective for one woman and a different one more effective for the next. Therefore if symptoms are not relieved the patient should be switched to a different agent. PGSI use is contraindicated in women with a known hypersensitivity, nasal polyps, angioedema and bronchospasm related to the use of aspirin or NSAIDs, history of chronic ulcer disease, inflammation of the gastrointestinal tract, and chronic renal disease.

Other agents are also effective in the treatment of dysmenorrhea. Oral contraceptives are effective in 90% of women. They inhibit ovulation, suppress PG production, and produce a thinner endometrial lining. Narcotics should only be used in women with severe symptoms who have failed treatment with both PGSIs and oral contraceptives.

Laparoscopic uterosacral nerve ablation has been advocated for women with dysmenorrhea who have failed medical management. This results in transecting afferent pain fibers within the uterosacral ligament. Short-term follow-up has been reported as promising but there are no randomized long-term controlled studies comparing this technique with conventional therapy; therefore, there are inadequate data to justify the routine use of this procedure. Presacral neurectomy is rarely indicated for primary dysmenorrhea. This procedure has been performed laparoscopically but no controlled studies have been performed.

Secondary dysmenorrhea

Pathophysiology

Secondary dysmenorrhea results from pelvic pathology and can occur at any age after menarche and before menopause. A complete history and physical exam will help determine which of the following diagnostic tests may be necessary: laparoscopy, hysteroscopy, ultrasound, and hysterosalpingography.

Cervical stenosis can lead to severe narrowing of the endocervical canal and can result in increased intrauterine pressure. This results in dysmenorrhea and can lead to retrograde menstruation and endometriosis. Cervical stenosis can be a congenital problem, or result from injury (electrocautery, cryotherapy, operative conization, application of caustic substances) or infection. Women with cervical stenosis often have scant menses and suffer pain throughout the menstrual period. The diagnosis is made by either hysterosalpingogram or inability to pass a thin probe through the internal cervical os.

Endometriosis (the presence of ectopic endometrial tissue) is the most common cause of secondary dysmenorrhea. The symptoms are not related to the amount of disease present as women with little disease may have debilitating symptoms and women with severe endometriosis may have minimal or no symptoms. On physical examination nodules may be felt on the uterosacral ligaments; however, the diagnosis can only be made by laparoscopy or biopsy of a cervical or vaginal lesion. Adenomyosis (the presence of endometrium in the myometrial wall) also causes secondary dysmenorrhea. Symptoms occur later in life, the pain is midline, and the uterus is often slightly enlarged and globular.

Pelvic infections due to gonorrhea and *Chlamydia* can lead to inflammation or abscess and result in pelvic adhesions which may cause secondary dysmenorrhea. Endometriosis and previous surgery also can cause adhesions. Whether adhesions are a cause of pelvic pain is still unclear. Some women have severe pain with minimal adhesive disease while others have massive adhesions and relatively little discomfort.

Pelvic congestion syndrome results from engorgement of the pelvic vasculature. On pelvic exam there is vasocongestion and uterine enlargement and tenderness. On laparoscopy there is engorgement of varicosities of the broad ligament and pelvic side wall. This condition is related to tension and stress. There is no evidence that this condition causes pelvic pain.

Intrauterine birth control devices often cause dysmenorrhea. Secondary dysmenorrhea may also be a psychosomatic problem and it is important to consider this in the evaluation of the patient.

Treatment

Cervical stenosis is treated by cervical dilatation. The cervix can be dilated with dilators, laminaria tents, or a stem pessary. This permits more rapid efflux of blood, which causes relief. Unfortunately, cervical stenosis can recur. Cervical obstruction at the internal os can also be caused by endometrial polyps or submucous fibroids which can be removed by operative hysteroscopy.

Dysmenorrhea from endometriosis can be treated with PGSIs. More advanced stages of endometriosis can be treated with surgical resection and/or medically with gonadotropin-releasing hormone agonists or danazol. Presacral neurectomy and amputation of the uterosacral ligaments have been used for dysmenorrhea secondary to endometriosis; however, neither have been proven effective in the long term.

PGSIs should be used as first-line treatment in women suspected of having adenomyosis. If unsuccessful, and after all other possible diagnoses have been excluded, including stress and tension, a hysterectomy should be performed.

If pelvic adhesions are the cause of the dysmenorrhea, treatment consists of lysis of adhesions which usually can be successfully performed through the laparoscope. Pelvic congestion and psychosomatic pain are treated with psychologic counseling and, if necessary, antidepressants and tranquilizers.

Intrauterine device insertion is followed by a rise in PG. PGSIs have been effective in relieving discomfort from insertion as well as dysmenorrhea.

Conclusion

The first line of treatment in primary dysmenorrhea is one of the PGSIs, which are also effective for alleviation of the pain associated with some cases of secondary dysmenorrhea. The last resort in the treatment of dysmenorrhea is hysterectomy. As with any of the surgical treatments, the patient must understand that she may experience postoperative pain. It is important prior to undergoing surgery to exclude gastrointestinal, musculoskeletal, urologic, and psychologic problems which may be causing the dysmenorrhea.

SUGGESTED READING

ANDERSCH B, MILSON I. An epidemiologic study of young women with dysmenorrhea. *Am J Obstet Gynecol* 1982;144:655.

BUDOFF PW. Use of mefenamic acid in the treatment of primary dysmenorrhea. *JAMA* 1979;241:2713.

BUDOFF PW. Mefenamic acid for dysmenorrhea in patients with intrauterine devices. *JAMA* 1979;242:616.

CHAN WY, DAWOOD MY, FUCHS F. Relief of dysmenorrhea with the prostaglandin synthetase inhibitor ibuprofen: effect on prostaglandin levels in the menstrual fluid. *Am J Obstet Gynecol* 1979;135:102.

CUNANAN RG, COUREY NG, LIPPES J. Laparoscopic findings in patients with pelvic pain. *Am J Obstet Gynecol* 1979;135:102.

DINGFELDER R. Primary dysmenorrhea treatment with prostaglandin inhibitors. A review. *Am J Obstet Gynecol* 1981;140:874.

DMOWSKI WP. Visual assessment of peritoneal implants for staging endometriosis. Do number and cumulative size of lesion predict the severity of the systemic disease? *Fertil Steril* 1987;47:382.

HALBERT DR, DEMURS LM. A clinical trial of indomethacin and ibuprofen in dysmenorrhea. *J Reprod Med* 1978;21:219.

HENZL MR, OOTEGA-HERRERA E, RODRIGUEZ C, IZU A. Anaprox in dysmenorrhea: reduction of pain and intrauterine pressure. *Am J Obstet Gynecol* 1979;135:455.

KAUPILLA A, RONNBERG L. Naproxen sodium in dysmenorrhea secondary to endometriosis. *Obstet Gynecol* 1985;65:379.

LICHTEN E, BOMBARD J. Surgical treatment of dysmenorrhea with laparoscopic uterine nerve ablation. *J Reprod Med* 1967;37:18.

LUNDSTROM V, GREEN K. Endogenous levels of prostaglandin $F_{2\alpha}$ and its main metabolites in plasma and endometrium of normal and dysmenorrheic women. *Am J Obstet Gynecol* 1978;130:640.

MILSOM I, ANDERSCH B. Ibuprofen and naproxen-sodium in the treatment of primary dysmenorrhea: a double-blind cross-over study. *Int J Gynaecol Obstet* 1985;23:305.

MUSE KN. Cyclic pelvic pain. *Obstet Gynecol Clin North Am* 1990;17:427.

OWEN PR. Prostaglandin synthetase inhibitors in the treatment of primary dysmenorrhea: outcome trials reviewed. *Am J Obstet Gynecol* 1984;148:96.

PICKLES VR, HALL WJ, BEST FA, *et al.* Prostaglandins in the endometrium and menstrual fluid from normal and dysmenorrheic subjects. *Br J Obstet Gynaecol* 1965;12:185.

ROTH-BRANDEL V, BYGDEMAN M, WIQVIST N. Effect of intravenous administration of prostaglandin E_2 and $F_{2\alpha}$ on the contractility of non-pregnant human uterus *in vivo*. *Acta Obstet Gynecol Scand* (Suppl 5) 1970;49:19.

SMITH RP. The dynamics of nonsteroidal antiinflammatory therapy for primary dysmenorrhea. *Obstet Gynecol* 1987;70:785.

SPEROFF L, RAMWELL P. Prostaglandins in reproductive physiology. *Am J Obstet Gynecol* 1970;107:1111.

TAYLOR HC. Vascular congestion and hyperemia, their effect on the structure and function in the female reproductive system. *Am J Obstet Gynecol* 1949;57:211.

TJADEN B, SCHLAFF, WD KIMBALL A, *et al.* The efficacy of presacral neurectomy for the relief of midline dysmenorrhea. *Obstet Gynecol* 1990;76:89.

VARGYAS JM, CAMPEAU J, MISHELL DRM Jr. Treatment of menorrhagia with sodium meclofenamate. *Am J Obstet Gynecol* 1987;157:944.

VERCELLINI P, FEDELE L, BIANCHI S, CANDIANI GB. Pelvic denervation for chronic pain associated with endometriosis: fact or fancy? *Am J Obstet Gynecol* 1991;165:745.

WILLIAMS EA, COLLINS WP, CLAYTON SG. Studies in the involvement of prostaglandins in uterine symptomatology and pathology. *Br J Obstet Gynaecol* 1976;83:337.

YLIKORKALA O, DAWOOD MY. New concepts in dysmenorrhea. *Am J Obstet Gynecol* 1978;130:833.

66

Premenstrual syndrome: diagnosis and management

DONNA SHOUPE

The clinician is often confronted with female patients complaining of cyclic, unprovoked, and uncontrollable changes in mood and disposition that have adverse effects on family or job. Often these patients are self-diagnosed and are carrying newspaper or magazine articles offering the latest cure-alls for premenstrual syndrome (PMS). Unfortunately, the recent increase in research studies on PMS has not brought a scientific breakthrough on the etiology of PMS and many are either poorly controlled or produce results that are in direct conflict with other studies.

While PMS has gained wide recognition and acceptance, there continues to be controversy regarding the definition, etiology, and treatment. The best approach for the clinician handling PMS problems is simple and nonjudgmental. The treatment plan includes counseling, education, and consideration of one of the methods of ovulation suppression. If these are unsuccessful, medication should be directed at specific symptoms.

Incidence

The incidence of PMS varies depending on the definition used. It is estimated that about 20–30% of women have moderate to severe PMS and around 1–10% have debilitating, severe symptoms. Another 50% of women have what may be considered PMS-like symptoms that do not meet the specific medical diagnosis, but may also respond to treatment.

PMS is most often diagnosed in women in their 30s and 40s, but symptoms usually predate to teenage years. PMS occurs universally with only slight differences between cultural and ethnic groups.

Table 66.1 Symptom groups for premenstrual syndrome

Anxiety	*Water retention*
Nervous tension	Weight gain
Mood swings	Swelling
Irritability	Breast tenderness
Restlessness	Abdominal bloating
Impatience	*Hypoglycemia*
Depression	Headache
Crying	Sweet craving
Confusion	Increased appetite
Social withdrawal	Fatigue
Insomnia	Less coordination
Pain	
Cramps	
Backache	
Breast pain	

Symptoms

There are over 150 symptoms that have been reported in association with PMS. The symptoms can be divided into five major categories: anxiety, water retention, depression, hypoglycemia, and pain (Table 66.1). Most PMS sufferers report symptoms from more than one category.

While difficult to prove scientifically, women self-report increased work absenteeism in the premenstrual phase, an inability to concentrate, lack of interest, decreased coordination, forgetfulness, increased altercations with their spouse, less coital activity, and less patience dealing with children.

Diagnosis

The initial history should include the age of onset of symptomatology, most significant symptoms, number of symptomatic days per cycle, degree and severity of social impact, variations from cycle to cycle, symptoms when using oral contraceptives, psychiatric history, postpartum psychologic changes, and previous treatment for PMS.

A complete physical examination is necessary to rule out any organic causes of secondary dysmenorrhea and chronic pelvic pain. There is no specific physical finding that helps to make the diagnosis of PMS, although breast tenderness may be present in the luteal phase. The differential diagnosis is listed in Table 66.2.

Table 66.2 Differential diagnosis for premenstrual syndrome

Common differential diagnosis
Adjustment disorder with depressed mood
Affective disorders
Anxiety disorder
Substance abuse disorder
Personality disorder
Dysmenorrhea
Postpartum depression

Less common differential diagnosis
Psychosis
Eating disorder
Mastodynia
Manic-depressive disorder

Symptom calendar

In order to clearly establish the diagnosis of PMS, it is necessary to document in a prospective manner for 2 months a relatively asymptomatic follicular phase and an emotional and/or physical laden luteal phase. While most PMS sufferers keep daily diaries, if not available, explanation of a symptom chart is helpful. The patient should list her symptoms on a vertical axis and mark the days of the month on the horizontal. Each day she ranks the severity of each symptom on a 0–5 scale.

If the patient is willing to take a daily basal body temperature, a true follicular phase and luteal phase can be identified. A daily weight record is useful to determine premenstrual weight gain. Days of bleeding, sexual relations, and severity of dysmenorrhea should be recorded.

To firmly establish the diagnosis of PMS, it is necessary prospectively to document a 20–30% increase in luteal score symptoms over 2 months. At least one symptom should negatively impact on lifestyle. It may be helpful to reserve treatment until the diagnosis is firmly established. In some cases, especially milder cases, while addressing other gynecologic needs, such as contraceptive protection or bleeding problems, treatment may be needed immediately. In this case, the relief of bothersome PMS-like symptoms while on treatment can be monitored.

Diagnostic overlap

The rate of psychiatric illness in women with PMS may be as high as 30%. Additionally, the menstrual cycle can intensify other psychiatric disorders such as bulimic episodes, panic attacks, and suicides. Psychiatric admissions during the premenstrual phase are elevated.

Patients with severe depression, drug abuse, suicide threats, violent behavior, severe disruptions of lifestyle, or high follicular-phase scores should be referred to a mental health worker. Treatment with anti-depression drugs may be indicated.

Treatment

With more than 150 symptoms associated with PMS, it is unlikely that there will be a single cure. The clinician must individualize treatment, taking into account other gynecologic problems and needs.

Conservative measures

Initial management of PMS should include emotional support, education, and reassurance. Education about the disorder helps to alleviate stress and increase self-control. Many studies document dietary differences in PMS sufferers and low-salt and refined sugar diets are reported to reduce water retention and hypoglycemia-like symptoms. Limiting alcohol and caffeine intake has been suggested.

Vitamin supplementation has not been shown consistently to reduce PMS symptoms. There are gastrointestinal side-effects associated with vitamin B_6 administration. Calcium supplementation (1000 mg/day) for PMS sufferers has been reported be effective in a few studies.

Medications: ovulation suppression

1 *Oral contraceptives*, especially monophasics, are a first-line treatment. Additional gynecologic benefits include bleeding control, less dys-menorrhea, and contraceptive protection.

2 Inhibition of ovulation can also be achieved with *depo-medroxypro-gesterone acetate* (DMPA) 150 mg im every 3 months. While side-effects include bleeding problems and weight gain, after 1 year 50% of users have amenorrhea. DMPA is now approved by the Food and Drug Administration as a contraceptive agent.

3 *Gonadotropin-releasing hormone (GnRH) agonists* are effective for PMS. Long-term use of GnRH agonist nasal spray (400 µg/day) was effective in 10 of 20 subjects with PMS.

Long-term (1-year) treatment with monthly depo-GnRH and estrogen replacement is effective. Progestin doses may be given every 4 months to minimize side-effects.

Medications: directed at most significant symptoms

1 *Prostaglandin inhibitors* are effective in patients with breast tenderness, low back pain, cramping, headache, or generalized discomfort. Prostaglandin inhibitors may be taken with meals to minimize gastric irritation.

Mefanamic acid (250 mg t.i.d.) for 12 days prior to menses was more effective than a placebo for pain, headache, depression, tension, and irritability (Table 66.3).

2 For symptoms of water retention despite dietary salt restrictions, short-term use of diuretics may be helpful. Spironolactone 25 mg 2 or 3 times daily on symptomatic days may relieve swollen abdomen, generalized bloatedness, migraine and breast discomfort, tension, anxiety, depression, and irritability.

3 *Estradiol* implants 100 mg sc plus 5 mg norethindrone for 7 days each cycle was reported to be successful in over 80% of PMS sufferers. Transdermal estradiol application for 7 days per month is reported to decrease menstrual migraines.

Table 66.3 Symptoms significantly improved by mefanamic acid. (From Mira *et al*. 1986)

	t	P
Physical symptoms		
Fatigue	4.81	<0.001
General aches and pains	3.73	<0.001
Headache	3.63	<0.001
Thirst	2.92	<0.005
Double vision	2.45	<0.05
Mood symptoms		
Tired	5.10	<0.001
Swings in mood	3.15	<0.005
Dissatisfied with everything	2.80	<0.01
Sad	2.74	<0.01
Irritable	2.67	<0.01
Pessimistic	2.65	<0.01
Unattractive	2.65	<0.01
Disinterested in people	2.56	<0.01
Withdrawn	2.54	<0.05
Decreased sexual feeling	2.21	<0.05
Behavior symptoms		
Bad performance	2.58	<0.05
Slow	2.47	>0.05

4 *Bromocriptine* 2.5 mg b.i.d. is useful on days where breast symptomatology predominates. It may be used from the time of ovulation through the onset of menses.

5 For persistent complaints of premenstrual anxiety and irritability, short-acting *antianxiety agents* may be considered. Alprazolam (Xanax) has a rapid onset of action and a short half-life and is ideal for intermittent use. The dose is 0.25 mg 1–3 times daily for only 1–3 days per month.

Other medications

1 *Progesterone* suppositories are no more effective than placebo. There is a great interest in a major ongoing study using oral micronized progesterone.

2 Patients who require *antidepressant medication* should be followed by a psychiatrist. Tricyclic antidepressants are effective in treating PMS exacerbations of depression. Monoamine oxidase inhibitors are used in atypical depression and depression which increases premenstrually. Lithium carbonate is for patients with bipolar components to their depression.

3 The antidepressive *fluoxetine* (Prozac) may have potential for PMS-related depression. There is little information regarding this drug in PMS and the potential for addiction is worrisome.

4 *D-fenfluramine* is an amphetamine-related drug used to treat obesity in Europe. It increases brain levels of serotonin, similar to increases noted after a carbohydrate intake. It is reported to reduce binge eating and emotional symptoms like anxiety, negative mood swings, and depression. Problems with abuse and dependence are of concern. A high-carbohydrate diet may be a substitute, prior to the drug's approval and demonstrated effectiveness in the USA.

5 *Danazol* is associated with a high incidence of side-effects, including weight gain, depression, and androgenic problems. In a recent study, 15 of 21 PMS patients had a "good" response to 6 months of therapy. However, because of the side-effects, danazol is considered only when other drugs have failed. It is most effective in alleviating mastalgia.

6 *RU 486*, a progesterone antagonist, is reported to block ovulation and reduce the symptoms of PMS. It is known widely as the abortion pill and is not yet available in the USA.

Prognosis

There is presently no cure for PMS which, for many patients, means a lifetime of symptoms unless appropriate measures are taken. After a thorough assessment, with careful attention to the differential diagnosis, the appropriate selection of counseling and medication can often be the "right" advice. Suppression of ovulation for PMS sufferers or use of medication directed at specific symptoms can often mean a significant improvement of their symptomatology and quality of life.

SUGGESTED READING

BACKSTROM T, HANSSON-MALMSTROM Y, LINDHE B-A, CAVALLI-BJORKMAN G, NORDENSTROM S. Oral contraceptives in premenstrual syndrome: a randomized comparison of triphasic and monophasic preparations. *Contraception* 1992;46: 253–268.

FREEMAN E. Ineffectiveness of progesterone suppository treatment for premenstrual syndrome. *JAMA* 1990;264:349–353.

HAGAN I, NESHEIM G-I, TUNTLAND T. No effect of vitamin B-6 against premenstrual tension: a controlled clinical study. *Acta Obstet Gynecol Scand* 1985;64: 667–670.

HAMMARBACK S. Induced anovulation as treatment of premenstrual tension syndrome. *Acta Obstet Gynecol Scand* 1988;67:159–166.

HAMMARBACK S, EKHOLM U-B, BACKSTROM T. Spontaneous anovulation causing disappearance of cyclical symptoms in women with the premenstrual syndrome. *Acta Endocrinol (Copenh)* 1991;125:132–137.

HARRISON M. Assessment of premenstrual dysphoria with alprazolam. *Arch Gen Psychiatry* 1990;47:270–275.

MEZROW G, SHOUPE D, SPICER D, LOBO R, LEUNG B, PIKE M. Depot leuprolide acetate with estrogen and progestin addback is effective for long term treatment of premenstrual syndrome. *Fertil Steril* (in review).

MIRA J, McNEIL D, FRASER I, VIZZARD J, ABRAHAM S. Mefanamic acid in the treatment of premenstrual syndrome. *Obstet Gynecol* 1986;68:395.

MORTOLA JF, GIRTON L, FISCHER U. Successful treatment of severe premenstrual syndrome by combined use of gonadotropin-releasing hormone agonist and estrogen/progestin. *J Clin Endocrinol Metab* 1991;71:252A–252F.

O'BRIEN PMS, CRAVEN D, SELBY C, SYMONDS EM. Treatment of premenstrual syndrome by spironolactone. *Br J Obstet Gynaecol* 1979;86:142–147.

STEINBERG S. Minireview: the treatment of late luteal phase dysphoric disorder. *Life Sci* 1991;49:767–802.

THYS-JACOBS S. Calcium supplementation in premenstrual syndrome. *J Gen Intern Med* 1989;4:183–189.

WURTMAN J. Effect of nutrient intake on premenstrual depression. *Am J Obstet Gynecol* 1989;161:1228–1234.

67

Abnormal uterine bleeding: diagnosis

PAUL F. BRENNER

The differential diagnosis of diseases that can cause abnormal uterine bleeding (i.e., excessive or prolonged bleeding or frequent bleeding episodes) covers almost the entire field of gynecology and some diseases that originate outside the reproductive system. When abnormal uterine bleeding is not due to an organic cause, then, by exclusion, the diagnosis of dysfunctional uterine bleeding is assumed.

Excessive uterine bleeding has been defined in quantitative terms, including menses persisting for >7 days, menstrual cycles of <21 days, and total menstrual blood loss >80 ml. Rather than these specific figures, however, abnormal uterine bleeding should be defined in terms of deviation from an individual patient's established menstrual pattern: an increase of two or more sanitary pads per day or menses that last 3 or more days longer than usual. The woman's qualitative description of her blood loss and the number of sanitary pads she uses has a poor correlation with the quantitative measurement of blood loss as determined from photometric quantification of hematin extracted from sanitary pads. Passage of blood clots or bleeding which inconveniences or is socially embarrassing to the woman are better indicators of prolonged or excessive uterine bleeding.

The complaint of abnormal uterine bleeding suggests that the source of the blood is from the pelvic organs. However, blood in the toilet bowl or on a sanitary napkin can originate from the urinary tract or gastrointestinal system. A urinalysis and stool guaiac test should be performed if the anatomic origin of the bleeding is in doubt.

The differential diagnosis of abnormal uterine bleeding includes

Table 67.1 Abnormal uterine bleeding

Organic causes
　　Reproductive tract disease
　　　Complications of pregnancy
　　　Malignancy
　　　Infection
　　　Benign pelvic lesions
　　Systemic disease
　　　Coagulation disorder
　　　Hypothyroidism
　　　Cirrhosis
　　Iatrogenic causes
　　　Steroids
　　　Intrauterine devices
　　　Tranquilizers
Dysfunctional uterine bleeding

---

reproductive tract disease, systemic disease, and iatrogenic causes. The diagnosis of dysfunctional uterine bleeding can be established only by excluding these three categories (Table 67.1).

Reproductive tract disease

This category includes complications of pregnancy, malignancy, infection, and benign pelvic lesions.

Pregnancy complications

Complications of pregnancy are an important cause of abnormal uterine bleeding in women of reproductive age. These complications include threatened, incomplete, or missed abortions, ectopic gestations, trophoblastic disease, placental polyp, and subinvolution of the placental site. Abnormal uterine bleeding in a woman of child-bearing age should be considered the result of a complication of pregnancy until proven otherwise. The history and physical examination must look for symptoms and findings of pregnancy. When appropriate, a pregnancy test is ordered.

When clinical signs and symptoms suggest the possibility of an ectopic pregnancy, a sensitive assay for human chorionic gonadotropin (hCG) and pelvic ultrasonography should be performed. A vaginal transducer is more likely to identify an extrauterine pregnancy than is an abdominal transducer. The absence of an intrauterine gestational sac has been correlated with serum hCG levels as indirect evidence of an extrauterine pregnancy. The level of hCG depends on the type of ultrasound transducer used and the laboratory performing the hCG assay. The presence of an intrauterine gestational sac makes the diagnosis of an ectopic pregnancy unlikely. More reliable in ruling out an ectopic pregnancy is the identification of a fetal pole and/or the presence of fetal cardiac activity within the uterine cavity, as demonstrated by ultrasonography. The very rare possibility of combined intrauterine and extrauterine pregnancies does exist.

Trophoblastic disease must be included in the differential diagnosis for women of reproductive age who have abnormal uterine bleeding, especially in women who have had a recent pregnancy. A sensitive β-hCG assay should be obtained to confirm this diagnosis.

Malignancy

Malignant tumors of the pelvic organs can result in abnormal uterine bleeding. Endometrial cancer, cancer of the cervix, and less frequently vaginal, vulvar, fallopian tube cancers, and estrogen-secreting ovarian tumors can be the source of abnormal genital bleeding.

The incidence of endometrial carcinoma increases with age. All perimenopausal and postmenopausal bleeding should be considered due to malignancy until proven otherwise. Although cancer is not the most common cause of abnormal uterine bleeding in women of this age, it is the most important. Approximately 10% of all abnormal uterine bleeding in perimenopausal women is due to cancer, and about 25% of all women with postmenopausal bleeding will have cancer.

The value of the Papanicolaou test in detecting cervical cancer is well known, but it is considerably less reliable as a diagnostic aid for endometrial cancer. The incidence of endometrial carcinoma in women over the age of 35 years is sufficiently high to recommend that all women in this age group with abnormal uterine bleeding undergo endometrial evacuation with a biopsy or vaginal probe ultrasonography. If examination of an adequate sample of endometrium fails to establish the cause of the bleeding, hysteroscopic directed biopsies or a dilatation and curettage (D&C) should be performed. Women with a long history of oligoovulatory or anovulatory menstrual cycles have a higher incidence of endometrial carcinoma. Eighty percent of women who develop endometrial carcinoma before age 40 have polycystic ovarian disease. When abnormal uterine bleeding occurs in women with a long-standing history or unopposed estrogen, their endometrial histology must be determined if they are 30 years of age or older.

Infection of the upper genital tract

Endometritis with or without salpingitis may cause abnormal uterine bleeding. Uterine and/or adnexal pain on palpation and movement of the pelvic organs, a sensation of increased warmth of the uterus and adnexal structures, and purulent material exuding from the cervical os during bimanual examination should suggest strongly the presence of infection. An elevated temperature, white blood cell count, and erythrocyte sedimentation rate usually indicate infection but do not localize the organs involved in the inflammatory process. Cervical cultures for gonorrhea and *Chlamydia* should be taken. When the possibility of pelvic inflammatory disease is high, a gram stain of the cervical mucus should be prepared to detect gram-negative intracellular diplococci.

Benign pelvic lesions

Benign vaginal disease, including traumatic lesions, severe vaginal infections, and foreign bodies, may cause abnormal uterine bleeding. Benign cervical lesions such as polyps, erosions, and cervicitis may produce genital bleeding. Benign uterine disease involving submucous leiomyoma uteri, adenomyosis, and endometrial polyps may be the source of abnormal uterine bleeding.

Occasionally, a very young patient who has not yet had her desired number of children has recurrent episodes of heavy uterine bleeding at the time of menses. This bleeding can be so copious that the patient's hematocrit falls dramatically. Surgical curettage is necessary to stop the bleeding. This history suggests the presence of a submucous fibroid. If the leiomyoma is not detected during curettage, a hysterosalpingogram or hysteroscopy should be performed several days after the bleeding has ceased.

Systemic disease

This category includes coagulation disorders, hypothyroidism, and cirrhosis.

Coagulation disorders

Disorders associated with platelet deficiency (leukemia, severe sepsis, idiopathic thrombocytopenic purpura, hypersplenism), disorders of defective platelet activity (von Willebrand's disease), and prothrombin deficiency are blood dyscrasias that rarely first present clinically as abnormal uterine bleeding. Women with a blood dyscrasia usually can be identified by a history of easy bleeding or bruising, a family history of a bleeding disorder, bleeding from other orifices, and excessive bleeding associated with minor trauma, minor surgery, or dental surgery. In addition, they may have ecchymoses or petechiae. Teenage patients with abnormal uterine bleeding that produces a significant reduction in hemoglobin (below 10 g/100 ml) and that requires hospitalization or starts at menarche and is repetitive should be investigated for a blood dyscrasia. A blood dyscrasia was found in approximately 20% of adolescent females who were hospitalized for excessive uterine bleeding. A platelet count, examination of the stained blood smear, bleeding time, and partial thromboplastin time are ordered when the history indicates a blood dyscrasia is likely or when therapy for dysfunctional uterine bleeding fails.

Cirrhosis

Estrogens are metabolized in the liver. Advanced hepatic disease may cause a reduction in the liver's ability to conjugate estrogen, leading to increased estrogen in the circulation, which results in abnormal uterine bleeding. A history of liver disease or excessive alcohol ingestion and the physical findings of jaundice, hepatomegaly, spider hemangiomas, palmar erythema, and ascites indicate the need to order liver function tests.

Hypothyroidism

Women with myxedema usually have amenorrhea, but women with lesser degrees of thyroid hypofunction have a disruption of their menstrual cycles expressed as abnormal uterine bleeding. Weight gain, marked fatigue, cold hands and feet, and failure to perspire in warm weather are symptoms and signs of hypothyroidism. Some women who have abnormal pelvic bleeding and were clinically euthyroid were found to have hypothyroidism when baseline thyroid-stimulating hormone (TSH) levels were measured and thyrotropin-releasing hormone (TRH) stimulation tests were performed. When the baseline TSH levels were normalized in these women with thyroid replacement therapy, the bleeding irregularities were corrected. A TSH assay or a TRH stimulation test should be performed when therapy for dysfunctional uterine bleeding fails.

Iatrogenic causes

Iatrogenic causes of abnormal uterine bleeding include steroids, intrauterine devices, digitalis, anticoagulants, and hypothalamic depressants. Steroids which may lead to genital bleeding include oral contraceptives, estrogen replacement therapy, androgens, anabolic agents, and corticosteroids. There is no specific laboratory test that can determine an iatrogenic cause of abnormal uterine bleeding. A careful history is required to make the correct diagnosis.

Evaluation

It is important in every patient with abnormal uterine bleeding to consider the entire differential diagnosis. Failure to make the correct diagnosis usually is the result of a hasty evaluation that did not include all of the diagnostic possibilities. All women of child-bearing age with abnormal uterine bleeding should have a careful history and physical examination, Papanicolaou smear (if not done in the previous 12 months), complete blood count, and an assay for hCG. A single-passage endometrial biopsy from a site at the top of the fundus or a vaginal probe ultrasound study should be obtained from adult women but is not required in the teenager with menstrual irregularities. Thyroid function tests, liver function tests, studies of the clotting mechanism, gram stain of the cervical mucus, pelvic ultrasonography, and hysteroscopic-directed biopsies or a D&C are performed only when indicated by the history and physical examination. Hysteroscopy provides the opportunity for direct visualization of the endometrial cavity and therefore is a more reliable diagnostic procedure for identifying endometrial lesions than a D&C. A D&C will miss 10–25% of the endometrial lesions found with hysteroscopy.

Menorrhagia is excessive and/or prolonged uterine bleeding that occurs at regular intervals. Metrorrhagia is uterine bleeding that occurs at irregular but frequent intervals. Heavy cyclic menstruation, referred to as menorrhagia, is more likely to be indicative of organic gynecologic disease than the irregular bleeding episodes described as metrorrhagia.

If a diagnosis of dysfunctional uterine bleeding is considered, the presence or absence of ovulation should be documented by use of a basal body temperature record, serum progesterone concentration, or endometrial biopsy. A biphasic basal body temperature curve, a serum progesterone level >3 ng/ml, or a biopsy interpreted as secretory endometrium indicates that the patient is ovulatory, that the cause of bleeding is probably organic, and that the endometrial cavity must be investigated by hysteroscopy. Besides evidence of ovulation, anemia and long-standing complaints of abnormal bleeding are indications for a study of the endometrial cavity. Submucous leiomyomas and endometrial polyps may be the cause of the bleeding in as many as half of these patients. If the patient is anovulatory, or if she is ovulatory and the endometrial cavity is found to be normal, dysfunctional uterine bleeding may be diagnosed.

SUGGESTED READING

ANDERSON MM, IRWIN CE Jr, SNYDER DL. Abnormal vaginal bleeding in adolescents. *Pediatr Ann* 1986;15:697–707.

CLAESSENS EA, COWELL CA. Acute adolescent menorrhagia. *Am J Obstet Gynecol* 1981;139:277–280.

COUPEY SM, AHLSTROM P. Common menstrual disorders. *Pediatr Clin North Am* 1989;36:551–571.

GIMPELSON RJ, RAPPOLD HO. A comparative study between panoramic hysteroscopy with directed biopsies and dilatation and curettage. *Am J Obstet Gynecol* 1988;158:489–492.

KIVIKOSKI AI, MARTIN CM, SMELTZER JS. Transabdominal and transvaginal ultrasonography in the diagnosis of ectopic pregnancy: a comparative study. *Am J Obstet Gynecol* 1990;163:123–128.

LOFFER FD. Hysteroscopy with selective endometrial sampling compared with D&C for abnormal uterine bleeding: the value of a negative hysteroscopic view. *Obstet Gynecol* 1989;73:16–20.

MENCAGLIA L, PERINO A, HAMOU J. Hysteroscopy in perimenopausal and postmenopausal women with abnormal uterine bleeding. *J Reprod Med* 1987;32:577–582.

VAN EIJKEREN MA, CHRISTIAENS GCML, SIXMA JJ, HASPELS AA. Menorrhagia: a review. *Obstet Gynecol Surv* 1989;44:421–429.

WILANSKY DL, GREISMAN B. Early hypothyroidism in patients with menorrhagia. *Am J Obstet Gynecol* 1989;160:673–677.

68

Treatment of dysfunctional uterine bleeding

GAIL MEZROW

Dysfunctional uterine bleeding (DUB) is defined as abnormal bleeding that has no organic cause.

Pathophysiology

The vast majority of women with DUB are anovulatory, which results in prolonged estrogen stimulation to the endometrium without the influence of progesterone. This results in a thickened proliferative endometrium without structural support. The endometrium outgrows its blood supply. There is release of prostaglandin, resulting in vasospasm of spiral arterioles and ischemia, and increased development of Golgi–lysosomal complexes with elevated levels of hydrolytic enzymes. These events result in superficial breaks in the fragile endometrium with random portions bleeding at various times.

Anovulation with DUB is seen most frequently in perimenopausal women (50% of cases) and postmenarchal adolescent girls (20% of cases). The adolescent fails to ovulate since there has not been full maturation of the hypothalamic–pituitary–ovarian axis, while in the perimenopausal woman the ovary is less responsive to gonadotropin stimulation, resulting in decreased estrogen and elevated follicle-stimulating hormone levels. Women with polycystic ovarian disease and obesity also are frequently anovulatory and at high risk for DUB. These women have high levels of unopposed estrogen due to increased conversion of androstenedione to estrogen.

A few women with ovulatory menstrual cycles develop DUB. Most have an abnormality of the corpus luteum, including persistence of the corpus luteum (Halban's syndrome), premature senescence of the corpus luteum, or insufficient progesterone production (luteal-phase deficiency). Other causes of ovulatory DUB include an overactive fibrinolytic system and an abnormality or deficiency of estrogen or progesterone receptors in the endometrium.

Treatment

If the first episode of DUB is not excessive and the hemoglobin is within the normal range the patient may be observed; otherwise, hormonal therapy is indicated. Acute bleeding must be treated with a regimen that includes estrogen or, if the patient is unstable, dilatation and curettage (D&C). Estrogen must be used if there is minimal tissue obtained by an endometrial biopsy or if the patient is using a progestin. Estrogen causes endometrial growth and stabilizes lysosomal membranes but has no effect on hemostasis. Intravenous, intramuscular, and oral estrogen administration are equally effective. Conjugated estrogens, 2.5 mg, can be given orally 4 times a day for 21 days. If the bleeding persists after 3 days of therapy the estrogen dose should be increased to 5 mg. If the bleeding continues, a hysteroscopy and D&C should be performed. Medroxyprogesterone acetate, 10 mg, is given daily for the last 5 days of estrogen therapy. The progestin has an antiestrogenic, antimitotic, and antigrowth effect on the endometrium. It stops endometrial growth and stabilizes the endometrium. The withdrawal of hormones allows for an organized slough.

An alternative regimen is to use oral contraceptives (OCs), one tablet, 4 times a day. This regimen will stop acute bleeding but there is a higher rate of recurrent bleeding when therapy is discontinued. The first regimen mimics the normal cycle and may induce a more complete sloughing on the endometrium than OCs.

Androgens are as effective as estrogen in stopping uterine bleeding but have no advantage over estrogen. Their use is associated with androgenic side-effects. Danazol has been shown to be effective in dosages of 200–400 mg daily and is most effective in women with ovulatory DUB.

Long-term therapy for DUB is based on age and the need for contraception or desire for pregnancy. If the patient is not sexually active and anovulatory, she may be treated with medroxyprogesterone acetate for the first 10 days of each month or cyclic OCs. Progestin therapy is only used for long-term therapy as it does not stop acute bleeding. Side-effects of progestin-only therapy include premenstrual-type symptoms, fatigue, moodiness, and weight gain. Chronic use may be detrimental to the lipid profile. Local progesterone treatment can decrease bleeding without side-effects or changes in the lipid profile. The progesterone-releasing intrauterine device has been shown to be effective in women with ovulatory DUB.

The women who need contraception should receive OCs. Birth-control pills decrease menstrual flow by 60% in normal women. If a patient is having bleeding and anovulatory cycles a prolactin level should be obtained prior to treatment and yearly thereafter, since the pill will mask signs of hyperprolactinemia, namely amenorrhea and galactorrhea. If the patient is anovulatory and pregnancy is desired, then treatment with clomiphene citrate is indicated. The perimenopausal woman may be treated with either OCs, if she is a nonsmoker with no vascular disease, or started on a cyclic hormonal replacement regimen similar to that used in the treatment of menopause (conjugated equine estrogen or estradiol and medroxyprogesterone acetate).

Nonsteroidal antiinflammatory drugs (NSAIDs) have been shown to be effective in reducing menstrual blood loss. They inhibit platelet aggregation and block prostaglandin production, both thromboxane and prostacyclin, by blocking the enzyme fatty acid cyclooxygenase. Prostacyclin relaxes vessel walls and reverses the platelet aggregation stimulated by thromboxane. There are no NSAIDs that selectively block prostacyclin production. NSAIDs have been shown to decrease menstrual blood loss by 30–50% in women with ovulatory menorrhagia. Some of these women have been found to have increased levels of prostacyclin. A greater reduction in blood loss is seen when NSAIDs are used in conjunction with either OCs or a progestin. NSAIDs are not very successful in treating anovulatory DUB. They are reported to be successful, however, in controlling abnormal bleeding secondary to endometritis and the intrauterine device.

Antifibrinolytic agents block fibrinolysis and have been shown to be effective in women who ovulate with DUB. Their use has been limited due to side-effects. Similar to NSAIDs, they work best in combination with OCs or a progestin.

Ergot derivatives are not effective in the treatment of DUB. Furthermore, they are associated with a high incidence of side-effects.

Women with DUB secondary to hypothyroidism should be treated with L-thyroxine. Women without documented hypothyroidism should not be treated with thyroid hormone.

Gonadotropin-releasing hormone (GnRH) agonists produce a medical menopause and therefore can be used to treat severe cases of DUB refractory to medical therapy. These agents are very expensive, produce menopausal side-effects, and can cause bone loss. Addback therapy with estrogen and progestin will prevent side-effects and may help to prevent bone loss.

D&C will stop acute bleeding but bleeding recurs in 60% of women. This procedure is indicated if the patient is medically unstable, has failed medical management, is older with risk factors for endometrial carcinoma, or the endometrial biopsy is abnormal or inadequate. The D&C can be done under hysteroscopic guidance to insure that pathology is not missed. Blind D&C has been shown to miss pathology in 10–25% of cases. This treatment is not successful in women with ovulatory DUB.

Hysterectomy used to be the last resort for women with DUB. Now there is an alternative procedure, endometrial ablation. The endometrial lining is destroyed with this procedure using the operating hysteroscope with either electrocautery or laser photovaporization with the neodymium-YAG laser. Long-term follow-up is not known. These women still need progestin if estrogen replacement therapy is instituted at the time of menopause.

Conclusion

Treatment for DUB must be individualized based on age, desire for contraception or pregnancy, and ovulatory status. A combination of more than one agent may be necessary to control bleeding adequately.

SUGGESTED READING

BERGQVIST A, RYBO G. Treatment of menorrhagia with intrauterine release of progesterone. *Br J Obstet Gynaecol* 1983;90:255.

DECHERNEY AH, DIAMOND MP, LAVY G, POLAN ML. Endometrial ablation for intractable uterine bleeding: hysteroscopic resection. *Am J Obstet Gynecol* 1986; 155:574.

DEVORE GR, OWENS O, KASE N. Use of intravenous premarin in the treatment of dysfunctional uterine bleeding: a double-blind randomized control study. *Obstet Gynecol* 1982;59:265.

DOCKERAY CJ, SHEPPARD BL, BONNARD J. Comparison between mefenamic acid and danazol in the treatment of established menorrhagia. *Br J Obstet Gynaecol* 1989;96:840.

FRASER IS. Treatment of ovulatory and anovulatory dysfunctional uterine bleeding with oral progestogens. *Aust NZ J Obstet Gynecol* 1990;30:353.

FRASER IS, MCCARRON G, MARKHAM R, *et al*. Long-term treatment of menorrhagia with mefenamic acid. *Obstet Gynecol* 1983;61:109.

GARRY R, ERIAN J, GROCHMAL SA. A multi-centre collaborative study into the treatment of menorrhagia by Nd-YAG laser ablation of the endometrium. *Br J Obstet Gynaecol* 1991;98:357.

GIMPELSON RJ, RAPPOLD HO. A comparative study between panoramic hysteroscopy with directed biopsies and dilation and curettage. *Am J Obstet Gynecol* 1988;158:489.

GOLDRATH MH, FULLER TA, SEGAL S. Laser photovaporization of endometrium for the treatment of menorrhagia. *Am J Obstet Gynecol* 1981;140:14.

HALL P, MACLACHLAN N, THORN N, *et al*. Control of menorrhagia by the cyclo-oxygenase inhibitors naproxen sodium and mefanamic acid. *Br J Obstet Gynaecol* 1987;94:554.

HALLBERG L, HOGDAHL AM, NILSSON L, RYBO G. Menstrual blood loss—a population study: *Acta Obstet Gynecol Scand* 1966;45:320.

HAMMOND RH, OPPENHEIMER LW, SAUNDERS PG. Diagnostic role of dilation and curettage in the management of abnormal premenopausal bleeding. *Br J Obstet Gynaecol* 1989;96:496.

LOFFER FD. Hysteroscopy with selective endometrial sampling compared with D&C for abnormal uterine bleeding: the value of a negative hysteroscopic view. *Obstet Gynecol* 1989;73:16.

MAGOS AL, BAUMANN R, TURNBULL AC. Transcervical resection of endometrium in women with menorrhagia. *Br Med J* 1989;298:1209.

MAKARAINEN L, YLIKORKALA O. Ibuprofen prevents IUD-induced increases in menstrual blood loss. *Br J Obstet Gynaecol* 1986;93:285.

MARCH CM. The endometrium in the menstrual cycle. In: Mishell DR Jr, Davajan V, eds. *Infertility, Contraception, and Reproductive Endocrinology*. 3rd edn. Oradell, NJ: Medical Economics Books, 1991.

MENCAGLIA L, PERINO A, HAMOU J. Hysteroscopy in perimenopausal and post-menopausal women with abnormal uterine bleeding. *J Reprod Med* 1987;32:577.

NILSSON L, RYBO G. Treatment of menorrhagia. *Am J Obstet Gynecol* 1971;110:713.

PARMER J. Long-term suppression of hypermenorrhea by progesterone intra-uterine contraceptive devices. *Am J Obstet Gynecol* 1984;149:578.

PETRUCCO OM, FRASER IS. The potential for the use of GnRH agonists for treatment of dysfunctional uterine bleeding. *Br J Obstet Gynaecol* 1992;99:34.

SHAW RW, FRASER HM. Use of a superactive luteinizing hormone releasing hormone (LHRH) agonist in the treatment of menorrhagia. *Br J Obstet Gynaecol* 1984;9:913.

THOMAS EJ, OKUDA KJ, THOMAS NM. The combination of a depot gonadotrophin releasing hormone agonist and cyclic hormone replacement therapy for dysfunctional uterine bleeding. *Br J Obstet Gynaecol* 1991;98:1155.

TOWNSEND DE, RICART RM, PASKOWITZ RA, WOOLFORD RE. Rollerball coagulation of the endometrium. *Obstet Gynecol* 1990;76:310.

VAN EIJKEREN MA, CHRISTIANS GC, SIXMA JJ, HASPELS AA. Menorrhagia: a review. *Obstet Gynecol Surv* 1989;44:421.

VARGYAS JM, CAMPEAU JD, MICHELL DA. Treatment of menorrhagia with meclofenamate sodium. *Am J Obstet Gynecol* 1987;157:944.

WILANSKY DL, GREISMAN B. Early hypothyroidism in patients with menorrhagia. *Am J Obstet Gynecol* 1989;160:673.

69

Evaluation and management of asymptomatic adnexal masses

JOHN B. SCHLAERTH

Examination and evaluation

Proper preparation of the patient is necessary for a pelvic examination to exclude a mass lesion. A full urinary bladder and a rectum that contains stool can limit the quality of the examination and also masquerade as pathologic masses themselves. There are other impediments to an adequate examination that are not so easily corrected, e.g., pain, tenderness, psychologic unpreparedness, and obesity. Pelvic ultrasound, computed tomography (CT), magnetic resonance imaging, or pelvic examination under anesthesia are the usual alternatives in these situations.

The technique of the examination is also important. An adnexal mass usually is situated in the posterior pelvis behind the uterus. Bimanual abdominal–vaginal examination will detect only those masses large enough to fill the posterior pelvis and extend out of the cul-de-sac. The only proper means of clinically evaluating the adnexa for mass lesions is the bimanual abdominal–rectovaginal examination.

The diagnostic work-up and therapy for adnexal masses depend on the stage of reproductive life in which they occur: the premenarchal, reproductive, or postmenopausal years.

Premenarchal years

Because pelvic examinations are not routine in this age group, small adnexal masses rarely are detected in premenarchal girls. Most commonly, it is a pelvic–abdominal mass that gives rise to symptoms (abdominal enlargement, pain, and perception of a mass). Physiologic causes of ovarian enlargement are rare prior to menarche. Consequently, all pelvic abdominal masses must be presumed to be neoplastic and require a laparotomy without delay.

About 60% of ovarian neoplasms in this age group are malignant germ cell tumors (dysgerminoma, endodermal sinus tumor, embryonal carcinoma, immature teratoma, choriocarcinoma, or mixed types). The benign germ cell tumor (the dermoid cyst) and the gonadal stromal tumors (thecoma, granulosa cell tumor, arrhenoblastoma) are next most common and occur with roughly equal frequency (approximately 20% each).

The preoperative evaluation should address the possible origin of the mass in the adrenal glands or kidney (adrenoblastoma, Wilms tumor). Similarly, preoperative determination of the status of retroperitoneal lymph nodes and for hepatic or lung metastasis is strongly advised. CT of the chest, abdomen, and pelvis is probably the best way to obtain this information.

As germ cell malignancies are so common in this age group and often arise in dysgenetic gonads, preoperative karyotyping to determine the presence of a Y chromosome may be worthwhile. If Y chromosome is present, it is advisable to remove all gonadal tissue. This is important because a germ cell tumor can develop in remaining dysgenetic gonadal tissue later. Furthermore, dysgenetic gonads, which contain no oocytes, render a patient infertile.

Malignant germ cell tumors can secrete glycoproteins, which can serve as tumor markers and may exert hormonal effects. Classically, human chorionic gonadotropin (hCG) is elaborated by choriocarcinoma or embryonal carcinoma elements. Cases of precocious puberty have been associated with increased serum levels of hCG produced by these neoplasms. α-Fetoprotein is secreted by endodermal sinus and embryonal carcinoma elements. Dysgerminomas can produce elevated levels of lactic dehydrogenase (LDH). The gonadal stromal tumors can also, at times, secrete hormonal substances. These are usually sex steroids and, in particular, estrogens. The presence of estrogens or androgens should be clinically obvious in this age group and easily confirmed by serum estradiol or testosterone determinations.

Reproductive years

It is of the utmost importance that physiologic causes be considered in the fertile woman with an adnexal mass. It has long been known that an early intrauterine pregnancy can enlarge the uterine fundus and soften the lower uterine segment so as to create the impression of a mass distinct from the cervix/uterus (Hegar's sign).

Physiologic cystic enlargement of the ovaries is common in women who ovulate. These are either follicle or corpus luteum cysts that can become as large as 10 cm and are invariably unilateral. At times, they cause pain secondary to rupture, hemorrhage, or torsion. Because these physiologic cysts are self-limiting and more common than pathologic cysts, a conservative course is advisable. Thus, a unilateral cystic adnexal mass <10 cm in an ovulating woman should be followed for 4–8 weeks to determine if regression occurs.

Some suggest that pituitary gonadotropins be inhibited with oral contraceptives during this observation period, although a recent randomized study of young women with small (mean 3.0 cm) cysts suggests this is of no benefit. If the mass has not disappeared at the end of this observation period, it can no longer be considered physiologic, and laparotomy should be performed. If a woman develops a unilateral, cystic adnexal mass while taking oral contraceptives, the mass is assumed to be neoplastic, and an observation period is unlikely to lead to disappearance of the cyst. A solid ovarian tumor, bilateral cystic ovarian tumors, and adnexal cysts >10 cm all are presumed to be pelvic neoplasms, and surgical removal is advised.

Another "physiologic" event, although clearly a pathologic entity, can present as an adnexal mass: ectopic (tubal) pregnancy. Ectopic pregnancy is a most important entity which can present as a pelvic mass, as it is imminently life-threatening. The presence of an adnexal mass in a young woman should automatically arouse this suspicion, and at least a quantitative serum hCG level should be determined. Both patient and physician should remain alerted until this diagnosis has been excluded.

Two anatomic variants have been noted in the literature on pelvic masses with some frequency: the ectopic (pelvic) kidney and sacral meningocele. An intravenous pyelogram would disclose the kidney and reveal a defect in the sacrum as well.

The common clinical pathologic entities presenting as pelvic masses in adult women are listed in Table 69.1. Of importance to premenopausal women are the ovarian tumors. Most commonly, the neoplasms are benign; dermoid cysts and serous and mucinous cystadenomas are the most common types. Malignant germ cell neoplasms peak in incidence in the teenage years and are a distinct rarity after age 30. Ovarian adenocarcinoma accounts for most of the ovarian malignancies in this age group (30 years and older), with a frequency that increases as menopause approaches. Gonadal stromal neoplasms are uncommon throughout the reproductive years.

Table 69.1 Adnexal mass: differential diagnosis

Nonpathologic
Full bladder
Stool in rectosigmoid colon
Pelvic kidney
Intrauterine pregnancy
Functional ovarian cyst

Pathologic

Nongenerative organs
   Diverticulosis/diverticulitis
   Appendiceal abscess
   Colon carcinoma

Generative organs
   Salpingo-oophoritis, inflammatory lesions
   Endometriosis
   Leiomyoma uteri
   Ectopic pregnancy
   Ovarian neoplasms
   Tumor-like conditions of the ovary
      Polycystic ovaries
      Pregnancy luteoma
      Hyperplasia of ovarian stroma and hyperthecosis
      Massive edema
      Multiple luteinized follicle cysts
      Surface epithelial inclusion cysts
      Simple cysts
      Paraovarian cysts

Postmenopausal years

With cessation of ovarian function, the ovaries gradually grow smaller over a period of several months. Because physiologic cysts cannot develop in these atrophic ovaries, an adnexal mass in postmenopausal women is presumed to be neoplastic. Furthermore, as women in this age range have the highest incidence of ovarian carcinoma, prompt evaluation and surgical treatment are indicated.

The concept of a postmenopausal palpable ovary (PMPO) has become popular. The basis for this concept is that ovaries involute over several months to a few years after the menopause. Therefore, small masses, including those consistent in size with a premenopausal ovary, must be viewed with suspicion. Although there are few data on operative findings in women in this category, the advanced stage and high mortality of most cases of ovarian cancer at the time of diagnosis emphasize the need for early diagnosis. We therefore prefer to perform a laparoscopy or laparotomy when a PMPO is found, as it could represent an early, curable ovarian carcinoma. How to proceed becomes more difficult when a small mass appears in a woman of advanced age who has other medical problems that make anesthesia a significant risk, e.g., heart, lung, or kidney disease or diabetes. In this setting culdocentesis or paracentesis, with peritoneal lavage to obtain samples for cytology, determination of serum CA-125 level, and/or serial pelvic and ultrasound examinations to detect enlargement of the mass may be more appropriate.

Preoperative work-up

If a patient has an adnexal mass that requires surgery, a number of diagnostic tests bear mention. A chest X-ray and EKG are routine pre-anesthetic tests. The chest X-ray may reveal a hydrothorax, which may accompany a benign or malignant ovarian neoplasm.

It is essential that the presence or absence of a pregnancy be determined prior to surgery for a pelvic mass. Timing of surgery, choice of anesthesia, and supportive measures for the pregnancy are important decisions to be made.

Intravenous pyelogram generally is indicated preoperatively. Possible exceptions are smaller, mobile, unilateral cystic masses where compromise of the urinary tract by the mass is unlikely.

Determination of the presence of occult blood in the stool and barium enema/sigmoidoscopy generally is recommended to exclude colonic causes for a pelvic mass in women over 35 years of age.

An upper gastrointestinal series is recommended if upper abdominal signs and symptoms warrant or if there is clinical suspicion that the mass is malignant, i.e., bilateral masses, solid masses, ascites, palpable intra-abdominal metastases.

CA-125

CA-125 is a glycoprotein found in elevated levels in the serum of 80% of women with ovarian epithelial carcinomas. Elevated serum levels can also be seen in some other cancers (gastrointestinal, breast), benign ovarian neoplasms, benign gynecologic conditions (endometriosis, adenomyosis), and, rarely, with a variety of other medical conditions. To date its most important use has been to monitor the response of ovarian carcinoma to treatment. Efforts to apply it as a screening test have been plagued by high rates of false positivity. There may be some value, however, in using serum CA-125 levels as a diagnostic aid for pelvic masses. The sensitivity and specificity of serum CA-125 alone as a diagnostic test are not high enough for routine use in this regard. However, there may be benefit when used together with other diagnostic aids such as ultrasound.

Ultrasound

Preoperative ultrasound examination of pelvic masses has become a common practice, although the results seldom substantially influence management. Ultrasound examination certainly benefits the physician–patient relationship as there is commonly an aura of disbelief on the part of the patient and an immediate desire to know more details when the discovery of cystic pelvic mass is made in an asymptomatic woman. The sensitivity and specificity of ultrasound in distinguishing nonovarian from ovarian masses and physiologic versus benign versus malignant ovarian cysts are unacceptably low to be used alone as a diagnostic tool. Ultrasound is, however, an important tool when the pelvic examination is of suboptimal quality. It also can detect occult bilateralism of ovarian masses, fluid in the cul-de-sac, and internal characteristics of the cysts that may help to make clinical decisions. Ultrasound also can detect the presence of masses/cysts whose size is below the sensitivity of clinical examination (2–5 cm). Transvaginal ultrasound offers a better detailed examination of the internal pelvic genitalia than transabdominal ultrasound. Using the color-flow Doppler technique, changes in blood flow to the adnexa can be detected and may provide evidence of malignancy or benignity.

Laparoscopy

Laparoscopy for diagnosis can prevent an unnecessary laparotomy for pelvic masses which do not require removal. Instances where, in retrospect, laparotomy for a pelvic mass might have been avoided include asymptomatic hydrosalpinx, endometriosis, postoperative adhesions, and small serosal uterine fibroids. The clinical history should be very helpful in suggesting these entities, except perhaps with the fibroid tumors.

Occasionally laparoscopy will reveal an incidental cystic enlargement of the ovary. There is a school of thought advising puncture of these cysts, with cytologic analysis of the cystic contents. Experience with laparoscopic aspiration of follicles with *in vitro* fertilization suggests this can be done safely. There are questions that arise, however. Considering the possible causes (physiologic, congenital, inflammatory, endometriotic, neoplastic) it can be expected that these cysts either will disappear on their own or reform. Therefore, no treatment at all or surgical removal is indicated. Aspiration of sebaceous material or old blood may allow for removal of a dermoid cyst or endometrioma during the same anesthetic but otherwise puncture via laparoscope is superfluous. There are other concerns that may outweigh this occasional advantage. Cytologic analysis of cystic contents has proved difficult at times, particularly between physiologic, benign epithelial cysts and malignant cysts, and undercalls and overcalls have been made. Torsion or rupture could be avoided by aspiration, but these risks are very unlikely in small cysts and of short-term duration. Possible harm from laparoscopic aspiration includes the possibility of delay in diagnosing a neoplasm, the risk of contaminating the peritoneal cavity with malignant cells, and bleeding. As a general rule, puncturing cysts without biopsy or removal at laparoscopy is not recommended.

There is continuing debate whether spilling intracystic contents of an ovarian cancer harms the patient. There is no definitive evidence that it is either innocuous or harmful. The issue becomes most important when a cystic ovarian cancer is spilled and there are no risk factors, except for the iatrogenic spill, that would necessitate postoperative therapy. Then if postoperative treatment is decided upon, the risks, complications, and costs are all a direct result of the spill.

In premenopausal women laparoscopic removal of persistent adnexal cystic masses which have no suspicion for malignancy is a rapidly expanding area of surgery. Preoperatively, transvaginal ultrasonography with color-flow Doppler assistance and serum CA-125 determinations can reinforce the impression on benignity to the mass. Small (<5 cm) sonolucent cysts with normal color-flow Doppler examinations in women with normal serum CA-125 levels are invariably benign. It is unclear at the present time to what degree the risk for malignancy or the capabilities of laparoscopy will change as cyst size, ultrasound complexity, and serum CA-125 levels also increase.

In postmenopausal women who are found to have incidental sub-clinical persistent sonolucent masses 2–5 cm in size, laparoscopy offers a simpler approach than laparotomy. Adnexectomy or bilateral adnexectomy via laparoscopy seems to be a convenient solution to this problem. A nonsurgical alternative which has received some support is to follow such women with transvaginal ultrasound examinations and serum CA-125 levels indefinitely.

SUGGESTED READING

BARBER HRK, GRABER GA. The PMPO syndrome (postmenopausal palpable ovary syndrome). *Obstet Gynecol* 1971;38:921–923.

FINKLER NJ, BENACERRAF B, LAVIN PT, WOJCIECHOWSKI C, KNAPP RC. Comparison of serum CA 125, clinical impression, and ultrasound in the preoperative evaluation of ovarian masses. *Obstet Gynecol* 1988;72:659–664.

GOLDSTEIN S, SUBRAMANYAM B, SUYDER JR, BELLER U, RAGHAVENDRA N, BECKMAN EM. The postmenopausal cystic adnexal mass: the potential role of ultrasound in conservative management. *Obstet Gynecol* 1989;73:8–10.

JACOBS I, BAST RC Jr. The CA 125 tumour-associated antigen: a review of literature. *Hum Reprod* 1989;4:1–12.

MAIMAN M, SELTZER V, BOYCE J. Laparoscopic excision of ovarian neoplasms subsequently found to be malignant. *Obstet Gynecol* 1991;77:563–565.

PARKER WH, BEREK JS. Management of selected cystic adnexal masses in postmenopausal women by operative laparoscopy: a pilot study. *Am J Obstet Gynecol* 1990;153:1574–1577.

SCHWARTZ LB, SEIFER DB. Diagnostic imaging of adnexal masses. *J Reprod Med* 1992;37:63–71.

SPANOS WJ. Preoperative hormonal therapy of cystic adnexal masses. *Am J Obstet Gynecol* 1973;116:551.

STEINKAMPF MP, HAMMOND KR, BLACKWELL RE. Hormonal treatment of functional ovarian cysts: a randomized, prospective study. *Fertil Steril* 1990;54:755.

70

Ectopic pregnancy: diagnosis

MARK V. SAUER

Ectopic pregnancy occurs when a zygote implants and grows outside the uterine cavity. Although rarely observed in mammals, extrauterine gestations are relatively common in humans. The number of ectopic pregnancies in the USA continues to increase annually. Suggested reasons for the increase in cases include the higher prevalence of risk factors in the general population, improvements in diagnostic methods used in evaluating suspected patients, and the postponement of child-bearing until later reproductive life, at which time ectopic pregnancy rates are considered highest.

Despite the increased incidence, mortality rates remain low. The case-fatality rate is approximately 4.9 deaths per 10 000 cases of ectopic pregnancy, a decline of 86% from the 35.5 deaths per 10 000 cases reported to the Centers for Disease Control in Atlanta, Georgia in 1970. This improvement is largely attributable to the advances in the diagnostic methods employed in managing patients at risk for ectopic gestations. When deaths have occurred, they are usually secondary to exsanguination following the rupture of the fallopian tube of a misdiagnosed ectopic pregnancy. A diagnostic delay of 7–10 days was common in fatal cases.

This chapter reviews current modalities used in the investigation of patients suspected of having an ectopic pregnancy. Recognizing the patient at risk and obtaining timely serologic and ultrasonographic tests for evaluating the status of the early pregnancy expedite the delivery of life-saving care. Integrating hormone measurements with ultrasound imaging provides an algorithmic framework from which the clinician can manage most cases.

Risk determinants

Risk factors for ectopic gestations should be elicited during the initial interview. Known associations include a history of salpingitis, low socio-economic status, previous tubal surgery, minority race, *in utero* exposure to diethylstilbestrol, advanced maternal age, progestin-only contraceptives, postcoital estrogen contraceptives, progesterone-containing intra-uterine devices, ovarian hyperstimulation, and prior *in vitro* fertilization and embryo transfer. Patients who have previously experienced an ectopic pregnancy are at increased risk of a recurrent event in approximately 12–15% of subsequent pregnancies.

The presentation of ectopic pregnancy is heterogeneous. Patients may appear acutely ill with severe abdominal pain or may have minimal signs and symptoms. The triad of lower abdominal pain, amenorrhea, and vaginal bleeding has been reported in 80–100% of patients. However, as diagnostic testing has improved, increasing numbers of ectopics are discovered prior to the onset of clinical illness.

Laboratory testing

The history and physical examination still constitute the basis upon which most ectopic pregnancies are diagnosed. However, if relying on these methods alone, a correct impression is at best established in 50% of cases. Laboratory and ultrasonographic testing has become integral in evaluating early pregnancy. Established algorithms utilizing serologic measurements of human chorionic gonadotropin (hCG) and other hormones provide defined parameters that aid in identifying and tracking normal and abnormal gestations.

Human chorionic gonadotropin

The measurement of β-hCG is essential for fully evaluating women of reproductive age for pregnancy. Qualitative enzyme immunoassays (EIAs) measure β-hCG levels in the urine as low as 50 mIU/ml (Inter-National Reference Preparation, IRP), EIAs are easy to perform, and do not require expensive equipment. Results are colorimetric, and obtained within minutes of performing the test. Pregnancy may be diagnosed prior to the missed menstrual period.

Unfortunately, the EIA has limited clinical utility. It only diagnoses pregnancy and does not define the normalcy of the gestation under study. The assay is qualitative, and monitoring the progress of the pregnancy requires serial quantitative measures. However, the likelihood of an ectopic pregnancy in any woman testing negative on a urine EIA is exceedingly small, and essentially rules out the diagnosis in such cases. Thus, the value of universal pregnancy screening lies in the detection of positive results. In women testing positive, intensified surveillance for ectopic pregnancy is warranted.

Traditionally serum β-hCG has been used to track the course of early pregnancy states. Levels of serum β-hCG are known to rise exponentially in early gestation. Evaluation using serial estimations has been based on the linear regression of log-transformed values. However, changes in β-hCG levels occur in a curvilinear manner and a simple linear model is only applicable during the first 6 weeks of gestation. Serial serum β-hCG measurements have been shown to be of diagnostic value when the serum β-hCG is approximately <6500 mIU/ml (IRP). During this time period β-hCG values normally increase by at least 66% every 2 days and more than double every 3 days. Pregnancies that demonstrate variation to this pattern are typically abnormal. Beyond 6 weeks of pregnancy the normal rate of increase for levels of β-hCG is slower, and may take more than a week to double. However, ectopic pregnancies generally demonstrate a slower rise in levels of β-hCG than is seen in normal pregnancies.

Serial β-hCG measurements can only be used in clinically stable patients. The use of a single-value discriminatory zone for diagnosing ectopic pregnancy requires ultrasound visualization of normal landmarks for early pregnancy. Single critical values of β-hCG reported for a number of ultrasound growth parameters in fact represent but an estimate of the upper value of the discriminatory zone. If therefore remains imperative to ascertain the approximate gestational age when solely relying upon β-hCG measurement. Since one-third to one-half of all women presenting with ectopic gestations are uncertain of their last menstrual period, the clinical utility of a single value for β-hCG is limited.

Progesterone

Studies suggest that the measurement of serum progesterone using a rapid, direct radioimmunoassay (RIA) or its urinary metabolite pregnanediol 3-α-glucuronide (PDG) by EIA provides an alternative method for evaluating early pregnancies. Difficulties exist using this approach since normal intrauterine gestations have been detected with levels as low as 6 ng/ml. Furthermore, reassurance cannot be gained with elevated levels of progesterone since 33–50% of patients presenting with ectopic pregnancies demonstrate levels >10 ng/ml.

PDG measurements are commonly depressed in women with abnormal gestations. However, dilute specimens provided by women with normal intrauterine pregnancy lessen the specificity of the assay, thus limiting its clinical usefulness.

The role of serum progesterone and urinary PDG in the evaluation of ectopic pregnancy remains undefined. Based upon the current published studies it appears these tests offer little advantage in diagnosing ectopic pregnancy over that of serial hCG determinations. However, in cases where values of progesterone are depressed, measurements may complement other studies such as hCG and ultrasound in establishing a diagnosis.

Other biochemical tests

A variety of other serum proteins and hormones have been investigated for adjunctive tests for ectopic pregnancy. These include Schwangerschafts protein 1 (SP1), pregnancy-associated plasma protein A (PAPP-A), human placental lactogen (hPL), prolactin, α-fetoprotein (AFP), CA-125, α-amylase, active renin, and estradiol. None of these assays to date has demonstrated superiority over serial measurements of hCG in accurately identifying ectopic pregnancy.

Ultrasound

Ultrasound imaging has been used in conjunction with serum measurements of hCG to track the course of the developing pregnancy. Using a standard 5-mHz vaginal probe, visualization of the gestational sac becomes possible at the time of the missed menstrual period (2-mm sac size). The diameter of the sac normally continues to increase daily and by 40 days from the last menstrual period approximates 10 mm. More importantly, a yolk sac normally becomes visible at 5 weeks of pregnancy within the developing gestational sac, confirming the presence of embryonic tissue within the uterine cavity. Thus, even prior to the appearance of an embryonic heartbeat, the intrauterine location of the pregnancy can be discerned.

Typically, pathologic pregnancies deviate from this pattern of development. Other important signs include a complex cystic mass in the adnexa or cul-de-sac, free fluid in the peritoneal cavity, or the lack of a gestational sac in the uterus normally visualized using transvaginal ultrasound when serum levels of β-hCG are >1500 m IU/ml (IRP).

Culdocentesis

Culdocentesis has traditionally been considered an important test in the evaluation of ectopic pregnancy. The diagnosis of hemoperitoneum in a pregnant patient as ascertained by culdocentesis is highly predictive of an ectopic gestation. However, a negative or nondiagnostic tap does not exclude a tubal pregnancy, and can also occur in the presence of a ruptured ectopic gestation. Furthermore, a positive tap does not correlate with tubal rupture, and may be present in 1–2% of women evaluated with intrauterine pregnancies. The combination of data obtained from vaginal ultrasound and serum pregnancy tests is generally more helpful, and much less invasive, in establishing the diagnosis. Thus, culdocentesis should probably only be performed when ultrasound is unavailable or in cases of emergency in order best to triage care.

Uterine curettage

Uterine curettage is often performed following the documentation of an abnormal pregnancy state. When villi are recovered, the risk of ectopic pregnancy is virtually eliminated, since the likelihood of a concomitant ectopic and intrauterine pregnancy is quite remote. Therapeutically, the curettage also removes degenerating trophoblast within the intrauterine cavity, resulting in a fall in hCG titers and a completed abortion.

Although endometrial sampling aids in distinguishing intrauterine from extrauterine pregnancies, the histologic appearance of the endometrium is of little value unless chorionic villi are present in the specimen. Decidualized and nondecidualized endometria may be encountered. Proliferative endometrium may also be obtained in up to 25% of tubal gestations.

Laparoscopy

Laparoscopy has the highest positive predictive value for diagnosing ectopic pregnancy as a single test, and provides a correct diagnosis in >90% of cases. Aggressive use of the laparoscopy has resulted in a decrease in the proportion of tubal pregnancies in which the diagnosis is delayed or in which tubal rupture has occurred. Increasingly, the diagnostic laparoscope is used therapeutically, with operative intervention performed immediately following visualization of the tubal pregnancy.

Clinical assessment

Hormonal measurements, ultrasound imaging, and uterine curettage may be integrated into a diagnostic algorithm to diagnose ectopic pregnancy (Fig. 70.1). Improved detection expedites the delivery of care and allows for a greater degree of treatment options, ranging from the traditional surgical approach to the more recent nonsurgical remedies. For symptomatic patients in need of acute care, serial examinations may not be

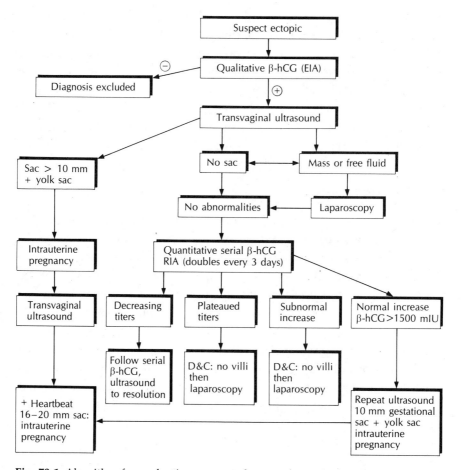

Fig. 70.1 Algorithm for evaluating suspected cases of ectopic pregnancy. β-hCG, β-Human chorionic gonadotropin; EIA, enzyme immunoassay; RIA, radioimmunoassay; D&C, dilatation and curettage.

possible. In such emergencies a rapid urine pregnancy test followed by transvaginal ultrasound or culdocentesis frequently establishes the diagnosis. Laparoscopy is definitive and, although invasive, should be used liberally.

SUGGESTED READING

DAYA S. Human chorionic gonadotropin increase in normal early pregnancy. *Am J Obstet Gynecol* 1987;156:286–290.

DORFMAN SF, GRIMES DA, CATES W, BINKIN NJ, KAFRISSEN ME, O'REILLY KR. Ectopic pregnancy mortality, United States, 1979 to 1980: clinical aspects. *Obstet Gynecol* 1984;64:386–390.

FOSSUM GT, DAVAJAN V, KLETZKY OA. Early detection of pregnancy with transvaginal ultrasound. *Fertil Steril* 1988;49:788–791.

LAWSON HW, ATRASH HK, SAFTLAS AF, FINCH EL. Ectopic pregnancy in the United States, 1970–1986. *MMWR* 1990;38:1–10.

SAUER MV, RODI IA. Utility of an algorithm to diagnose ectopic pregnancy. *Int J Gynecol Obstet* 1990;31:29–34.

SAUER MV, GORRILL MJ, RODI IA, *et al.* Nonsurgical management of unruptured ectopic pregnancy: an extended clinical trial. *Fertil Steril* 1987;48:752–755.

SAUER MV, VERMESH M, ANDERSON RE, VIJOD AG, STANCZYK FZ, LOBO RA. Rapid measurement of urinary pregnanediol glucuronide to diagnose ectopic pregnancy. *Am J Obstet Gynecol* 1988;159:1531–1535.

SAUER MV, SINOSICH MJ, YEKO TR, VERMESH M, BUSTER JE, SIMON JA. Predictive value of a single serum pregnancy associated plasma protein A or progesterone in the diagnosis of abnormal pregnancy. *Hum Reprod* 1989;3:331–334.

VERMESH M, GRACZYKOWSKI JW, SAUER MV. Reevaluation of the role of culdocentesis in the management of ectopic pregnancy. *Am J Obstet Gynecol* 1990;162:411–413.

YEKO TR, GORRILL MJ, HUGHES LH, RODI IA, BUSTER JE, SAUER MV. Timely diagnosis of early ectopic pregnancy using a single blood progesterone measurement. *Fertil Steril* 1987;48:1048–1050.

71

Ectopic pregnancy: treatment

MICHAEL VERMESH

The traditional catastrophic presentation of a ruptured ectopic gestation and hemoperitoneum no longer is common. Today this condition is typically diagnosed before a rupture occurs, while the patient is hemodynamically stable. Accordingly, treatment has shifted from an immediate life-saving intervention to conservative methods of management, directed at preserving fertility and reducing morbidity. While the repeat ectopic rates after radical and conservative management are similar, the intrauterine pregnancy rate seems to be higher after conservative tubal surgery. Thus, the patient's desire for future fertility should play a major role in management design. For women not desiring future fertility, a salpingectomy is performed, whereas the objective of conservative treatment of ectopic pregnancy is removal of the products of conception while inflicting as little damage to the involved tube as possible. This can be attempted either surgically or nonsurgically.

Surgical treatments

Diagnostic laparoscopy should always be considered when the diagnosis of ectopic gestation is contemplated, except when the patient is hemodynamically unstable. At the time of laparoscopy, a definitive diagnosis of tubal gestation is usually possible. In a patient who desires future fertility, the most conservative procedure should be attempted whenever possible. The choice of surgical technique will be determined by various considerations: (1) condition of the tube (ruptured, unruptured); (2) location of the gestation within the tube (interstitium, isthmus, ampulla); (3) size of the gestation; (4) accessibility (presence of adhesions); and (5) complications (uncontrollable bleeding).

Based on these considerations the surgeon can choose to perform one of the following procedures by laparoscopy or laparotomy: linear salpingostomy, segmental resection, or salpingectomy. Linear salpingostomy is the procedure of choice for treatment of unruptured isthmic or ampullary gestation in patients who desire future fertility. Subsequent conception rate is about 60% (versus 40% after salpingectomy) and recurrent ectopic rate is about 13%, not significantly different from the rate following salpingectomy. The procedure can be performed through the laparoscope with viable pregnancy rates and recurrent ectopic pregnancy rates similar to those obtained when laparotomy is performed. However, laparoscopy is more economic and requires a shorter recovery period. Another conservative surgical method, termed fimbrial expression or milking, consists of evacuation of a distal ampullary or fimbrial gestation by either digital expression or suction through the infundibular end of the tube. Unfortunately, this technique has been associated with continued bleeding from the implantation site, unacceptably high rates of recurrent ectopic gestation, and persistence of trophoblastic tissue. Whenever a patient with an ectopic pregnancy is treated with conservative surgery via laparoscopy or laparotomy she should be monitored postoperatively with serial β-human chorionic gonadotropin (β-hCG) titers every 3 days until the levels are below the sensitivity of the assay. An increase in serum β-hCG after an initial decline is highly suggestive of persistent ectopic pregnancy, i.e., the continued proliferation of the trophoblast after the conservative treatment. The choice of management of persistent ectopic pregnancy should be based on serum β-hCG levels, patient's symptoms, and surgeon's experience. Management options include observation, surgical approach, and methotrexate therapy (see the section on non-surgical treatment, below).

Segmental resection is recommended for treatment of ruptured isthmic or ampullary gestation, especially when the contralateral tube is irreversibly damaged or absent. Reanastomosis of the proximal and distal segments can be performed after a period of time, when tissues are less edematous. Salpingectomy should only be performed if future fertility is not desired or the tube cannot be salvaged. Elective ipsilateral oophorectomy is not advocated. If the remaining ovary following ipsilateral oophorectomy requires extirpation at a later date, the patient will be left without any functional ovarian tissue. At the present time there is no evidence that fertility is improved or the incidence of ectopic pregnancy is reduced by performing an ipsilateral oophorectomy in the treatment of ectopic pregnancy. Hysterectomy should not be performed, except for some cases of ruptured cornual pregnancy, or cervical pregnancy, even if both tubes have been removed. Contrary to previous recommendations, corrective surgery on the contralateral tube may include lysis of adhesions, fimbrioplasty, and salpingoneostomy for hydrosalpinx and may be performed at the time of the ectopic pregnancy surgery. However, microsurgical reanastomosis should be deferred, and performed under optimal conditions.

Nonsurgical treatment

Despite the recent improvement in pregnancy rates, and a decrease in morbidity after conservative surgery for ectopic pregnancy, the outcome is still far from ideal. Recently, several nonsurgical methods have been employed, with varying degrees of success, in the treatment of a small unruptured tubal gestation. The emergence of these methods has been boosted by the development of sensitive and rapid assays for hCG, and improved ultrasound technology, that facilitate early diagnosis and accurate monitoring of ectopic gestation. These modalities include: (1) expectant management; (2) methotrexate; (3) antiprogesterone drugs; and (4) prostaglandins. Expectant management is based on the observation that in many patients with tubal pregnancies and declining hCG levels, resorption or spontaneous abortion of the ectopic pregnancy occurs. Expectant management or nonintervention may be considered when hCG titers are falling, there is no active bleeding, no evidence of rupture observed by transvaginal scanning, and the greatest diameter of the ectopic pregnancy and surrounding mass is not >3 cm. About 67% of small ectopic pregnancies undergo spontaneous resolution, tubal patency is maintained in 85%, and the subsequent pregnancy rate is 52%. These results are similar to those obtained with other conservative surgical and nonsurgical methods. The potential advantages of expectant therapy include the avoidance of surgery, lower cost, and improved fertility potential. However, nonintervention requires very close vigilance and the risk of rupture and bleeding is an impediment.

Methotrexate has been known for years to be effective in the treatment of trophoblastic disease. A considerable experience with the use of this folinic acid antagonist in the treatment of tubal gestation now exists and its value in the treatment of early and persistent ectopic pregnancy is being realized. Methotrexate may be given systemically or locally. Systemic treatment consists of intramuscular or intravenous administration of multidose or single-dose methotrexate. When using the multidose protocol, citrovorum factor should be given on the day after the methotrexate dose. Patients are instructed to refrain from sexual intercourse until complete resolution of the ectopic pregnancy (hCG < 15 m IU/ml), to avoid vitamins containing folic acid, and to abstain from alcohol while receiving methotrexate. Absolute contraindications include active liver or renal disease and tubal rupture. The single-dose protocol consists of intramuscular methotrexate ($50\,mg/m^2$) without citrovorum factor rescue. The reported side-effects from systemic methotrexate therapy include dermatitis, stomatitis, gastritis, liver enzyme elevations, bone marrow suppression, and pleuritis. Local injection of methotrexate (salpingocentesis) appears to have the advantage of minimizing side-effects associated with the parenteral protocols while maximizing the cytotoxic effect of the drug on the trophoblast because of high local tissue concentrations. While reports of local injection via laparoscopy appear to be promising, the reports on transvaginal treatment using ultrasound guidance have mixed results. Methotrexate is also useful for the treatment of persistent ectopic pregnancy. It seems that oral methotrexate ($0.4\,mg/$ kg body weight per day $\times$ 5 days) or a single dose of intramuscular methotrexate administration ($50\,mg/m^2$) is the practical way to treat persistent ectopic pregnancy.

RU-486, a progesterone receptor blocker, has been demonstrated effective in terminating intrauterine pregnancy in the first trimester. Attempts to interrupt tubal pregnancies with this drug were not promising. The drug also failed when it was used to treat a patient with persistent ectopic pregnancy.

Prostaglandins (PGE_2 or $PGF_{2\alpha}$) or hyperosmolar glucose may be injected into the amniotic sac at laparoscopy. Side-effects of the laparoscopic injection of prostaglandins have included cardiac arrhythmia and transitory hypertension, with pulmonary edema and atrioventricular block. These may be related to intravasation of $PGF_{2\alpha}$ into surrounding blood vessels. Transvaginal injection of prostaglandins and of KCl have also been described.

In conclusion, surgical treatment of ectopic pregnancy remains the method of choice and can be safely done by laparoscopy. Methotrexate administration is a promising treatment modality in patients with early or persistent ectopic pregnancy. Alternate treatments should be further evaluated.

SUGGESTED READING

DeCherney AH, Boyers SP. Isthmic ectopic pregnancy: segmental resection as the treatment of choice. *Fertil Steril* 1985;44:307.

Feichtinger W, Kemeter P. Conservative treatment of ectopic pregnancy by transvaginal aspiration under sonographic control and methotrexate injection. *Lancet* 1987;1:381.

Fernandez H, Rainhorn JD, Papiernik E, Bellet D, Frydman R. Spontaneous resolution of ectopic pregnancy. *Obstet Gynecol* 1988;71:171.

GARCIA AJ, AUBERT JM, SAMA J, JOSIMOVICH JB. Expectant management of presumed ectopic pregnancies. *Fertil Steril* 1987;48:395.

KOVACS L, SAS M, RESCH BA, *et al.* Termination of very early pregnancy by RU 486-antiprogestational compound. *Contraception* 1984;29:399.

LANG P, WEISS PAM, MAYER HO. Local application of hyperosmolar glucose solution in tubal pregnancy. *Lancet* 1989;2:922.

LEVIN JH, D'ABLAING III G, LACARRA M, GRIMES DA, VERMESH M. Mifepristone (RU 486) failure in an ovarian heterotopic pregnancy. *Am J Obstet Gynecol* 1990; 163:543.

LINDBLOM B, KALKFELT B, HAHLIN M, *et al.* Local prostaglandin F_2 injection for termination of ectopic pregnancy. *Lancet* 1987;1:776.

POULY JL, MAHNES H, MAGE G, CANIS M, BRUHAT MA. Conservative laparoscopic treatment of 321 ectopic pregnancies. *Fertil Steril* 1986;46:1093.

SHERMAN D, LANGER R, HERMAN A, BUKOVSKY I, CASPI E. Reproductive outcome after fimbrial evacuation of tubal pregnancy. *Fertil Steril* 1987;47:420.

STOVALL TG, LING FW, GRAY LA. Methotrexate treatment of unruptured ectopic pregnancy: a report of 100 cases. *Obstet Gynecol* 1991;77:749.

TIMOR-TRISCH I, BAXIS L, PEISNER DB. Transvaginal salpingocentesis: a new technique for treating ectopic pregnancy. *Am J Obstet Gynecol* 1989;160:459.

VERMESH M. Conservative management of ectopic gestation. *Fertil Steril* 1989;51: 559–567.

VERMESH M, PRESSER SC. Reproductive outcome after linear salpingostomy for ectopic gestation: a prospective three year follow-up. *Fertil Steril* 1992;57:682.

VERMESH M, SILVA PD, SAUER MV, VARGYAS JM, LOBO RA. Persistent tubal ectopic gestation: patterns of circulating human chorionic gonadotropin and progesterone, and management options. *Fertil Steril* 1988;50:584.

VERMESH M, SILVA PD, ROSEN GF, STEIN AL, FOSSUM GT, SAUER MV. Management of unruptured ectopic gestation by linear salpingostomy: a prospective, randomized clinical trial of laparoscopy versus laparotomy. *Obstet Gynecol* 1989; 73:400–404.

72

Uterine leiomyomas

CHARLES M. MARCH

Leiomyomas of the uterus are a familiar problem to gynecologists because they are the most common uterine tumor and occur in 25% of women past the age of 35. The majority of patients with myomas are asymptomatic and have multiple firm-tumors of varying size that are easily palpated by bimanual pelvic examination. Although there is no good explanation for their frequency, estrogen is an important growth factor. Leiomyomas are of clinical importance only during the reproductive years and tend to enlarge during pregnancy and shrink after menopause. This estrogen dependency has formed the basis of newer treatment strategies.

Myomas range in size from microscopic lesions to huge tumor masses filling the entire abdomen. They are classified according to location as submucous, intramural, or subserous and can be found extending between the leaves of the broad ligament or in the cervix and round ligaments. They are surrounded by a pseudocapsule of areolar tissue from which they derive their blood supply. Usually one can identify a primary blood supply consisting of one or two major vessels and multiple small arteries arranged in random fashion. The tumors themselves consist of tightly compacted muscle and fibrous tissue arranged in a whorled pattern and are relatively avascular.

Diagnosis

Pelvic pressure and heaviness, urinary frequency, hypermenorrhea, dysmenorrhea, pelvic pain, abdominal enlargement, premature labor, first-

and second-trimester abortion, and even infertility may all be complaints of the patient with one or more leiomyomas.

The diagnosis of myomas can usually be made by a pelvic examination, but other causes of uterine enlargement and asymmetry, such as pregnancy, adenomyosis, and congenital anomalies, must be considered. In addition, other kinds of pelvic masses, including ovarian cysts, hydrosalpinges and endometriosis, can be confused with myomas. Calcified myomas can be diagnosed by X-ray, and submucous tumors can be detected by hysteroscopy or suspected by hysterography or curettage. In puzzling cases, ultrasonography and pelvic pneumogynegraphy have been helpful.

The presence of smooth, circular or crescent-shaped defects which persist after the entire uterine cavity has been filled with contrast media, suggests the presence of a submucosal myoma. Occasionally, however, the radiographic defect noted by hysterography cannot permit the gynecologist to differentiate a submucosal myoma from a polyp or a gestational sac. Another value of the hysterosalpingogram is that it provides information about the fallopian tubes. This is extremely important if the patient wishes to preserve her child-bearing capacity. The definitive diagnosis of a submucosal myoma can be made by hysteroscopy. Direct inspection of the lesion permits the surgeon to know the diagnosis with certainty. In addition, the size, location, and relation to the tubal ostia and internal os can be determined.

Treatment

Conservative management

The majority of women with myomas require no treatment and can be observed by means of periodic pelvic examinations every 6 or 12 months to detect evidence of tumor growth. Ultrasonography may be used to monitor tumor growth more precisely than by pelvic examination. The need for intervention is dictated by symptoms and the patient's age and desire for pregnancy as well as the size, location, and growth pattern of the tumor(s).

Myomectomy

The effect of myomas upon reproduction is not certain. Infertility, first- or second-trimester abortion, premature labor, and abnormal presentations have all been associated with submucosal myomas. Rarely a submucosal myoma may markedly distort the external cervical os, thereby excluding it from the seminal pool. Thus, sperm transport would be hindered. A myoma near the cervix could obstruct labor.

Infertility is an occasional indication for myomectomy if no other cause for infertility can be demonstrated and if one or more myomas appear to be in a location that might interfere with nidation. Although some recent reports have suggested that myomectomy for even relatively small intramural myomas may result in conceptions, these are not controlled studies and therefore are difficult to interpret.

On the other hand, the role of the submucosal myoma is easier to understand because the endometrium immediately adjacent to the myoma does not undergo the normal cyclic changes as does the endometrium which is in contact with normal myometrium. Patients who have symptomatic myomas and wish to retain their child-bearing capacity should undergo myomectomy. In addition, those asymptomatic women who have uterine enlargement of 12 weeks' gestational size or greater and wish further fertility should have a myomectomy because of the greater chance of uterine conservation when the uterine enlargement is only moderate.

Estrogen deprivation has been utilized as primary therapy for myomas as well as short-term (2–3 months) preoperative therapy to facilitate the surgical procedure by producing tumor shrinkage and reducing uterine blood flow. If the patient is anemic, the amenorrhea induced by the drug will allow iron stores to be replenished. Gonadotropin-releasing hormone agonists can induce a 25–50% reduction in the size of the myomas. Maximum shrinkage occurs within 3 months of therapy. As the sole modality of treatment, these agents are of limited value because within 6 months of discontinuing the medication, the myomas will return to their original size. Treatment with an agonist for longer than 6–9 months is not warranted because the profound estrogen deficiency can lead to osteoporosis.

Small submucous myomas (<5–6 cm) may be resected at the time of hysteroscopy using a scissor, a resectoscope, or a laser under direct vision. Those which are pedunculated may be excised completely. For myomas which have a significant intramural component, the line of resection stops at a point even with the normal adjacent endometrium. Often the remaining intramural component of the myoma is expelled during the first 2 postoperative months. Long-term results of hysteroscopic myomectomy are excellent.

Myomectomy performed at the time of laparotomy for the treatment of infertility, or as an alternative to hysterectomy, is a relatively simple procedure that gives good results if a few precautions are followed. First, it is important to minimize blood loss by local injection of a solution containing 20 U vasopressin (Pitressin) in 20–40 ml of saline. Vasopressin is more effective than a clamp or tourniquet but has the theoretic disadvantage of masking inadequate hemostasis. Second, whenever possible, the uterine incisions should be made on the anterior uterine surface to minimize the development of postoperative adhesions involving the adnexa. Third, an attempt should be made to remove multiple myomas through one incision. Pregnancy may be attempted in 3 or more months following the operation.

Following myomectomy, about 40% of patients with prior reproductive problems will achieve a successful pregnancy and 20% will have a recurrence of myomas necessitating subsequent hysterectomy.

Some submucous myomas become pedunculated and extend through the cervical canal. If the pedicle is elongated, as is usually the case, the myoma can be removed per vaginam by means of a snare or by twisting until the pedicle breaks. The risk of hemorrhage from the base is small, and additional surgery, such as hysterectomy, should be deferred for 6–8 weeks to minimize the risk of operative infection. Often the myomectomy is curative.

Myomas in pregnancy

A pregnant patient with myomas has a risk of hemorrhage and infarction. If the tumor is submucous or intramural, the patient should be treated with analgesics with reasonable expectation that the process will subside without having produced premature labor. Only pedunculated subserous myomas that have become infarcted should be surgically removed from a pregnant uterus. But if myomectomy becomes necessary at the time of an abdominal delivery, hemostasis is usually better than anticipated because of myometrial contraction.

Hysterectomy

Submucous myomas frequently necessitate hysterectomy because of associated hypermenorrhea, which is probably due to a combination of increased endometrial surface, interference with uterine contractility, increased venular ectasia, and incomplete regeneration of the endometrium. In planning therapy it should be kept in mind that the bleeding of a myomatous uterus can also be due to other organic causes, such as endometrial polyps, an undetected cancer, or pregnancy, as well as hormonal dysfunction, and these possibilities should first be ruled out by appropriate diagnostic procedures. The medical management of bleeding associated with submucous myomas is unrewarding. Hormonal therapy is unsatisfactory, and irradiation produces menopausal symptoms and causes an increase in the risk of subsequent uterine cancer in these patients.

A second indication for hysterectomy is pain produced by infarction, torsion, infection, or impaction of the myomas within the bony pelvis.

A third indication is obstruction producing urinary retention, ureteral dilatation, or excessive constipation.

Size of itself is an important consideration for hysterectomy because an enlarged uterus can mask the diagnosis of coexisting pelvic disease, such as ovarian neoplasms, particularly if the uterus is larger than the size of a 12–14-week pregnancy. In a patient with a uterus of that size which is otherwise asymptomatic, assessment of ovarian size by annual or semiannual ultrasound study may obviate that concern.

Rapid growth is another indication for hysterectomy both because additional delay increases the likelihood of operative complications and because of the possibility of uterine sarcoma. The risk of sarcoma associated with myomas is quite small, probably a fraction of 1%, and there is no conclusive evidence that sarcomatous degeneration of preexisting myomas occurs.

In preparing the patient for surgery, the need for special diagnostic procedures, such as an intravenous pyelogram or barium enema, must be considered, particularly if the diagnosis is uncertain. Intravenous pyelography (including a lateral view) is of particular value in demonstrating ureteral displacement by an intraligamentous myoma or even a rare pelvic kidney. But the surgeon must remember that most ureteral injuries are due to failure to expose and identify the ureter in complicated cases rather than failure to order an intravenous pyelogram.

When surgical exposure is adequate, there are few operative complications. On occasion it is useful to gain better exposure by enucleating one or more large myomas prior to hysterectomy, or to perform a subtotal hysterectomy before removing the cervical stump. Because many patients having a hysterectomy for any reason will be in their 40s, a decision regarding ovarian preservation will be necessary. The appropriate age for prophylactic oophorectomy is still a matter of opinion, although age 45 seems to be the national consensus. The risk of dying from ovarian cancer must be balanced against the risk of dying from a complication of estrogen deprivation, such as myocardial infarction or a fractured hip secondary to osteoporosis. If the decision is to preserve the ovaries, the uterine cavity should be inspected before the abdomen is closed to rule out an undetected malignancy.

SUGGESTED READING

BABAKNIA A, ROCK JA, JONES HW. Pregnancy success following myomectomy for infertility. *Fertil Steril* 1978;30:644.

BROOKS GG, STAGE HM. The surgical management of prolapsed pedunculated submucous leiomyomas. *Surg Gynecol Obstet* 1975;141:397.

BURTON CA, GRIMES DA, MARCH CM. Surgical management of leiomyomata during pregnancy. *Obstet Gynecol* 1989;74:707.

BUTTRAM VC, REITER RC. Uterine leiomyomata: etiology, symptomatology and management. *Fertil Steril* 1981;36:433.

DERMAN SG, REHNSTROM J, NEUWIRTH RS. The long-term effectiveness of hysteroscopic treatment of menorrhagia and leiomyomas. *Obstet Gynecol* 1991; 77:591.

FRIEDMAN AJ, HARRISON-ATLAS D, BARBIERI RL, *et al.* A randomized, placebo-controlled, double-blind study evaluating the efficacy of leuprolide acetate depot in the treatment of uterine leiomyomata. *Fertil Steril* 1989;51:251.

MALONE MJ, INGERSOL FM. Myomectomy in infertility. In: Behrman SJ, Kistner RW, eds. *Progress in Infertility*. 2nd edn. Boston, Little, Brown, 1975.

NEUWIRTH RS. A new technique for an additional experience with hysteroscopic resection of submucous fibroids. *Am J Obstet Gynecol* 1978;131:91.

RAMSEY B, FREDERICK I. The occasional need for myomectomy. *Obstet Gynecol* 1979;53:437.

ROSENFELD DL. Abdominal myomectomy for otherwise unexplained infertility. *Fertil Steril* 1986;48:328.

73

Breast disease

WILLIAM H. HINDLE

Introduction

The major breast problem in obstetrics and gynecology is the evaluation of a dominant breast mass. Women, fearful of dying of breast cancer, anxiously present in the office with a perceived breast mass or symptoms they believe may represent an underlying breast cancer. These patients deserve an empathetic hearing, careful examination, and expedient diagnosis. The diagnostic triad of clinical breast examination, fine-needle aspiration, and mammography will usually yield a specific diagnosis which can expedite prompt treatment or, if no significant abnormality is found, thoughtful reassurance can be given to the patient. Continuing follow-up is important.

Symptoms

The common breast symptoms are: (1) a perceived mass; (2) pain; (3) nipple discharge; and (4) evidence of infection (erythema, fever, and tenderness).

Mass

A persistent dominant palpable breast mass must be diagnosed. After complete bilateral breast examination and diagnostic mammography, fine-needle aspiration with an adequate cell sample will usually give a specific definitive cytologic diagnosis of any of the benign or malignant breast neoplasms. When there is congruence of these three diagnostic techniques, the accuracy of the specific diagnosis approaches certainty. When there is doubt, an open surgical biopsy should be done for definitive histologic diagnosis.

Cysts are immediately identified by fine-needle aspiration. Grossly bloody fluid should be sent for cytology but nonbloody fluid may be discarded. All the fluid in the cyst should be removed by aspiration and then the area examined for any residual mass or lesion that may have been concealed by the cyst. Follow-up breast examinations in 1 month and then 2 months later will insure that the cyst has not reformed and that no residual mass is present. Then, the patient returns to routine annual follow-up. If a cyst reforms, it should be reaspirated. However, if it reforms again, cystography or a biopsy should be performed to rule out an intracystic cancer, which is reported to occur in about 1:1000 cyst aspirations.

Fine-needle aspiration

The technique of fine-needle aspiration of a solid palpable breast mass is illustrated in Figure 73.1. Utilizing a 22-gauge $1\frac{1}{2}$-in (4-cm) needle with a transparent hub, attached to a 10-ml syringe, the aspirator applies negative pressure only while the needle tip is in the mass. Otherwise, the

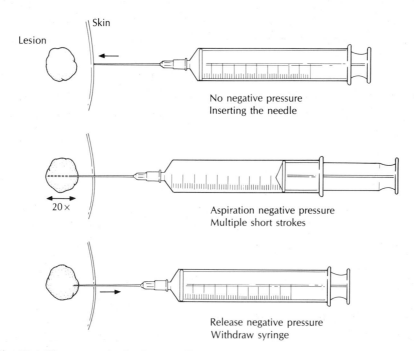

Fig. 73.1 Three steps in the fine-needle aspiration of a solid palpable breast mass for cytology.

Table 73.1 American College of Obstetricians and Gynecologists breast examination guidelines

---

Breast self-examination
    Monthly beginning at age 18
Clinical breast examination
    Annually beginning at age 18

Table 73.2 American College of Obstetricians and Gynecologists screening mammography guidelines

---

Baseline (initial) mammogram
    Between the ages of 35 and 40
Mammogram every 1–2 years
    Between the ages of 40 and 50
Annual mammogram
    Age 50 and every year thereafter

---

small amount of tissue juice within the bore of the needle is sucked up into the syringe and cannot be recovered for cytologic evaluation. Immediately after the aspiration, the needle is detached and about 10 ml of air drawn up in the syringe; the needle is reattached; and the air is ejected forcefully down the needle, producing a drop of tissue juice on the slide. The drop is then smeared like a hematology smear and rapidly fixed (like a Pap smear). Then the slide can be stained and read at leisure.

Many aspirators prefer to use one of the commercially available pistol-type syringe holders or a three-finger control syringe to assist in maintaining the negative pressure during the aspiration.

After definitive cytologic diagnosis, benign lesions such as fibroadenomas can be followed or excised at the patient's request. Unless the patient perceives a distinct change in the character or size of the lesion being followed (such as hardness or sudden growth) by her breast self-examinations, she can be followed, as should all women over 40, with annual clinical breast examinations and mammography (Tables 73.1 and 73.2).

Mastalgia

Because of the morbid fear of breast cancer, any pain in the anterior chest wall area may be thought of as an ominous breast symptom by the patient. Cervical radiculitis, costochondritis, myalgia, neuritis, and referred shoulder pain can be perceived as "in the breast." More than 40% of menstruating women have cyclic mastalgia. Women presenting with breast pain require understanding and complete breast evaluation and then firm reassurance if no pathologic entity is found. Breast clinics in England have found that 75% of women presenting with mastalgia, after complete evaluation, require no other treatment than reassurance. A well-fitted supportive bra, premenstrual salt restriction, nonsteroidal analgesics, and suppression of ovulation should be sequentially tried, and coupled with supportive care, counseling, and reassurance. Danazol is the only Food and Drug Administration-approved medication for the pharmacologic treatment of mastalgia but bothersome masculinizing side-effects make the treatment unacceptable to most women. Low-dose birth-control pills are effective for controlling breast pain in about 80% of women with cyclic mastalgia. Noncyclic mastalgia does not respond as well to any of the treatment regimens. Restriction of methylxanthines has no more effect than placebos when tested in double-blind crossover studies. Similarly, thyroid, vitamin A, vitamin B_1, vitamin B_6, and vitamin E have no documented pharmacologic effectiveness in the treatment of mastalgia.

Nipple discharge

Nipple discharge is pathologic if it is spontaneous, unilateral, and from a single duct opening on the nipple. Most women can elicit some nipple discharge by repeatedly squeezing the nipples. Physiologic nipple discharge (and galactorrhea) comes from multiple duct openings on the nipple and is often bilateral. Intraductal papillomas are the etiology of most watery, serous, or bloody spontaneous single-duct nipple discharge. Galactography (ductography) can usually outline the intraductal lesions and the extent of the duct involvement, allowing precise surgical excision of the portion of the duct involved. Single intraductal papillomas tend to be subareolar and are almost always benign. Usually they are nonpalpable. Multiple peripheral intraductal lesions may represent papillary carcinoma. All intraductal papillary lesions should be excised and a definitive histologic diagnosis confirmed. Nipple discharge was found to be due to underlying carcinoma in 6% of serous single duct discharge and 13% of grossly bloody nipple discharge (nonpregnant) in a large Swedish study.

Mastitis

Mastitis should be treated urgently and empirically, and then followed every 3 days until completely resolved. Mastitis is most common during pregnancy or lactation and is usually caused by *Staphylococcus aureus* or occasionally *Peptostreptococcus magnus*. Dicloxacillin 500 mg orally every 6 h for 7 days is usually effective. If there is localized flocculation suggesting early abscess formation, it should be drained by 18-gauge needle aspiration under local anesthesia. Repeated aspirations may be necessary. A large abscess should be opened and completely drained; this usually requires general anesthesia to be certain all the loculi have been broken. Dependent Penrose-type drains should be placed to facilitate complete drainage of the abscess cavity.

If a breast infection is not responding, cultures for bacterial identification and antibiotic sensitivity studies should be taken and biopsy considered in order to rule out inflammatory carcinoma, a clinical manifestation of ductal carcinoma invading the dermal lymphatics.

Lactating women should continue nursing their infants during treatment for mastitis. If an abscess forms, the affected breast should be pumped.

Nonpuerperal mastitis may be caused by *Staph. aureus*, *P. magnus* or *Bacteroides fragilis* and should be empirically treated with amoxycillin/clavulanate 400 mg orally every 8 h for 7 days. Chronic mastitis is usually due to mixed aerobes and anaerobes with *Staphylococcus* coagulase-negative and *P. proprioni* being the most common organisms. The treatment is dicloxacillin 500 mg orally every 6 h and metronidazole 500 mg orally every 8 h for 10 days. Recurrent subareolar abscesses and fistulas require surgical excision.

Mammography

Only screening mammography reliably detects suspicious nonpalpable breast lesions. The clinically significant mammographic findings are: (1) a spiculated stellate mass; (2) a circumscribed mass; (3) clustered irregular microcalcifications; (4) asymmetric density; and (5) skin thickening and/or retraction. The mammogram should be reported as showing no abnormality, or a specific lesion that is mammographically benign, indeterminate, suspicious, or malignant. Usually additional views, e.g., cone compression or magnification, are necessary to complete the mammographic evaluation. Even when reported as negative, a mammogram does not rule out cancer. With current methods of treatment, mammographically detected nonpalpable breast cancers have an overall 90% 10-year disease-free survival compared to an overall 50% 10-year disease-free survival for palpable breast cancers.

Cancer treatment

When cancer is diagnosed, the patient and family should be counseled and promptly referred to a comprehensive multidisciplinary treatment planning conference (center). Cancer patients are keenly appreciative of continuing follow-up by their obstetrician–gynecologist. Throughout their treatment, they will have legitimate medical questions and seek authoritative reassurance.

For stage I and II breast cancer, equivalent results as measured by disease-free survival, overall survival, local and regional recurrences, distant metastasis, contralateral breast cancer, and second nonbreast cancer are obtained by breast-conserving surgery (lumpectomy, axillary lymph node dissection, and radiation therapy) or modified radical mastectomy. In 1990, the National Institutes of Health Consensus Development Conference on Early-Stage Breast Cancer recommended breast conservation treatment as the preferred method of primary therapy for women with stage I and II breast cancer.

In spite of all the improvements in therapy, only screening mammography, with its ability to detect small nonpalpable lesions, has been proven to decrease the overall mortality from breast cancer. Breast cancers are not "cured" by extended or radical surgery, axillary lymph node dissection, radiation therapy, chemotherapy, or hormonal manipulation.

Oral contraceptives

Numerous published studies and multivariant analyses have not shown any consistent or significant influence of oral contraceptive therapy upon the risk of breast cancer. Benign breast conditions are often suppressed by oral contraceptive therapy.

Estrogen replacement therapy

Reviews of the effect of estrogen replacement therapy (ERT) on the relative risk of breast cancer reveal an increased epidemiologic "weak association" (relative risk 1.2). There is no documented proof that ERT causes breast cancer. Though it is possible that an estrogen-sensitive residual nidus of breast cancer could be stimulated by ERT in a patient who is estrogen-deficient and has been treated for breast cancer, the documented benefits of ERT upon the risk of osteoporosis and coronary artery disease are impressive. However, if ERT is offered to such a patient, the potential risks and benefits should be objectively outlined, her quality of life decisions evaluated, and her detailed informed consent clearly documented and signed by the patient in her medical record.

SUGGESTED READING

AMERICAN COLLEGE OF OBSTETRICIANS AND GYNECOLOGISTS. *Standards for Obstetric-Gynecologic Services*. 7th edn. Washington DC: American College of Obstetricians and Gynecologists, 1989.

AMERICAN COLLEGE OF OBSTETRICIANS AND GYNECOLOGISTS. *Carcinoma of the Breast*. Technical bulletin 158. Washington DC: American College of Obstetricians and Gynecologists, 1991.

HARRIS JR, HELLMAN S, HENDERSON IC, *et al*. *Breast Diseases*. 2nd edn. Philadelphia: Lippincott, 1991.

HINDLE WH. *Breast Disease for Gynecologists*. Norwalk, CT: Appleton & Lange, 1990.

LOVE SM, LINDSEY K. *Dr Susan Love's Breast Book*. New York: Addison-Wesley, 1990. [Available in paperback for patients.]

PAGE DL, ANDERSON TJ. *Diagnostic Histopathology of the Breast*. New York: Churchill Livingstone, 1987.

TABAR L, DEAN PB. *Teaching Atlas of Mammography*. New York: Georg Thieme Verlag, 1985.

74

Rectovaginal injuries

SUBIR ROY

The great majority of rectal injuries encountered in gynecologic practice are due to previous obstetric trauma and consist of either complete perineal tears extending into the rectal wall or rectovaginal fistulas. The successful surgical correction of rectovaginal injuries depends on healthy tissues at the site of injury and good surgical technique, as well as the avoidance of postoperative infection. Under adverse circumstances, even the simplest of operative repairs can fail.

If the fistula or tear is the result of recent trauma or the breakdown of a surgical repair, the operation must be delayed until the injured tissues are free of edema and induration or other evidence of residual infection. This process takes at least 8 weeks and often longer. On the average, the appropriate waiting period appears to be 12 weeks. Steroids to hasten the disappearance of the inflammatory reaction are not recommended because they interfere with wound healing.

Preoperative preparation

Preoperative preparation of patients with either perineal tears or rectovaginal fistulas is an important part of the total management of these injuries. Preoperative preparation includes evacuation of the bowel by instituting a variety of measures, beginning with a clear liquid diet 3 days prior to surgery. On the day before surgery she should ingest 4 l of Golytely (each liter containing 105 g of polyethylene glycol + electrolytes) over 4 h and one 10 oz bottle of magnesium citrate (at a concentration of 1.745 g/oz) at 23:00 h. In addition, the patient should receive an antibiotic bowel preparation and a regimen of antibiotic prophylaxis. One antibiotic bowel preparation consists of Flagyl 1 g with neomycin 1 g taken orally at 11:00, 20:00, and 23:00 h the day prior to surgery. Tap-water enemas should be administered until clear at bedtime.

In most situations antibiotic prophylaxis is preferable not only because it is simpler and requires less preoperative hospitalization, but also because the perfect method of antibiotic bowel preparation has yet to be devised. Effective antibiotic prophylaxis should provide broad aerobic and anaerobic coverage such as is provided by cefoxitin (Mefoxin) 2 g iv on call to surgery and then 2 g iv every 6 h twice, then 1 g every 6 h for 3–5 days. Other antibiotic regimens give similar results. The use of antibiotics is extremely important because of the considerable risk of postoperative infection, leading to operative failure.

At examination under anesthesia, a rectal examination should be performed. If any stool or fecal liquids are encountered, they should be removed and the patient should be treated with povoiodine enemas until clear before beginning the repair procedure.

Complete perineal tear

A complete perineal tear can be effectively repaired by a layer closure or the Warren flap procedure. Nonabsorbable sutures should be avoided because they can form a nidus of infection and secondary fistula formation. Either chromic catgut or polyglycolic sutures are satisfactory. It does not matter whether a submucosal or through-and-through stitch is used to close the rectal mucosa. What is important is that the muscular coat of the rectum and its fascia be reapproximated with a second layer of sutures. Repair of the rectal sphincter usually requires that some time be devoted to recovering the well-retracted torn ends. The use of a paradoxical incision, partial or complete, in the reapproximated sphincter is occasionally necessary so that the repaired sphincter admits a single digit tightly. The pubococcygeal muscles should be reapproximated because they contribute to fecal continence. In addition, the perineal body and vaginal sphincter should be repaired to restore normal vaginal function.

Rectovaginal fistula

A rectovaginal fistula can be repaired either by excision with a three-layer closure of vagina, rectal muscular coat, and rectal mucosa or by laying open the fistulous tract by means of an episioproctotomy, followed by excision of the tract and a three-layer closure. The latter technique is usually to be preferred whenever the fistula involves the perineal body or multiple fistulous tracts are suspected. But with either procedure, as with the repair of a complete perineal tear, careful approximation of the muscular coat of the rectum is the single most important step. Irrespective of the location of the rectovaginal fistula, the use of a diverting colostomy is not indicated as a primary procedure.

Reoperation

When the first operation for correction of a rectovaginal injury has failed, the success of a second or third operation can be greatly enhanced by the use of a Martius graft to reinforce the area of closure. A Martius graft consists of a flap of bulbocavernous muscle and its surrounding fat that has been isolated through a longitudinal incision in the labia majora, detached at its anterior pole, brought through a tunnel under the lateral vaginal wall, and fixed in place between the rectum and posterior vagina. The Martius graft should always be used whenever healing is uncertain because of previous scarring or multiple operative failures. The use of a diverting colostomy is never indicated as a primary procedure and is rarely needed following operative failures. Before resorting to colostomy, a repair incorporating a Martius graft should first be tried.

Postoperative care

The postoperative care of these patients requires some special measures in order to minimize the likelihood of operative site infection with subsequent failure of the surgery. Generally speaking, particulate matter in the surgical field is undesirable because of the relatively poor blood supply in this region. Therefore, a variety of strategies can be adopted in an attempt to keep the bowel empty until the operative tissues have a chance to heal: clear liquids with Vivonex for up to several weeks or peripheral intravenous administration of total parenteral nutrition for 5–7 days. Should any loose stools occur during the first few days, Lomotil can be used. Alternatively, simply prescribing stool softeners until normal bowel function has been restored has also been recommended.

SUGGESTED READING

HIBBARD LT. Surgical management of rectovaginal fistulas and complete perineal tears. *Am J Obstet Gynecol* 1978;130:139.

MARTIUS M. *Martius' Gynecologic Operations.* Boston: Little Brown, 1956:328.

MILLER NF, BROWN W. The surgical treatment of complete perineal tears in the female. *Am J Obstet Gynecol* 1937;34:196.

RUSSELL TY, GALLAGHER DM. Low rectovaginal fistulas. *Am J Surg* 1977;134:13.

75

Prepubertal vulvar lacerations and hematomas, labial adhesions, and prolapse of the urethra

PAUL F. BRENNER

Vulvar lacerations

Vulvar lacerations occur when a child falls on a pointed object or is injured with a foreign body. Frequently, when a physician attends a young child who has recently sustained a vulvar laceration, a single vessel is identified as the source of the bleeding. It is very tempting to secure hemostasis and repair the child's vulvar laceration using local anesthesia. However, repair can seldom be accomplished under these conditions. Most children do not remain sufficiently immobile for the sutures to be properly placed and the operative field kept sterile. Instead of achieving hemostasis, attempts to repair vulvar lacerations in children under local anesthesia may create increased bleeding. The best advice is to repair all vulvar lacerations in prepubertal children under general anesthesia, even when the laceration is small and a single pumping vessel is identified as the source of the bleeding. The laceration should be irrigated, all bleeding vessels identified and ligated, and the edges of the wound closed. If the location of the laceration suggests that the vagina, urethra, bladder, or rectum might be involved in the injury, these structures are examined while the patient is anesthetized. A vulvar abrasion may be the source of bleeding which can be controlled with the application of Gelfoam or Surgigel, avoiding the placement of sutures.

Vulvar hematomas

The most common cause of vulvar hematomas in children is "straddle" injuries. While riding a bicycle or climbing on a jungle-gym or falling from or on to furniture the child sustains blunt trauma to the vulva. A prepubertal child with a vulvar hematoma presents with a swollen, ecchymotic, tender labial lesion. Vulvar hematomas are usually small in size, well-localized, and do not present a life-threatening event. The single most important feature in the management of a child with a vulvar hematoma is to identify the lesion's full extent. Inspection and palpation of the vulva and perineum are not sufficient to define the borders of the collection of blood. A rectal examination must be performed, as there is a large space along the lateral walls of the vagina for the collection of concealed blood, which might be incorrectly interpreted as a small hematoma if only the perineum is examined. Very rarely, the amount of bleeding is so great that the child goes into shock.

If the hematoma has not expanded after a minimum of 4 h of observation, the patient has spontaneously voided clear urine, and the hematoma is not large enough to cause her undue distress, a nonsurgical approach may be used. Application of ice packs to the hematoma for an interval of 8–12 h from the time of the trauma is all the treatment necessary.

A hematoma that enlarges, causes considerable pain, and/or obstructs the urethra must be treated surgically. The hematoma should be incised, the blood clots evacuated and actively bleeding vessels identified and ligated. When complete hemostasis is secured the use of a drain is not necessary. The cavity is then closed in layers. If the bed of the hematoma continues to ooze then the use of a pack and drain for 24 h may be considered.

Labial adhesions

In young girls at any age prior to puberty, the labia can become fused as the result of adhesions. This is also called labial fusion or labial agglutination. Fusion may be partial or it may completely occlude the vaginal orifice. Fusion usually starts at the posterior fourchette and progresses toward the clitoris. The adhesions may be so extensive that only a minute aperture remains for the passage of urine. It may be very difficult to identify this small opening upon initial inspection of the perineum. Usually a pale, translucent vertical raphe is present in the midline, demarcating the site of fusion. Labial adhesions are usually the result of local inflammation and chronic irritation to hypoestrogenized vulvar tissue. Most commonly children with fused labia are asymptomatic. Infrequently the child may report difficulty voiding.

The need for treatment is based on the patient's ability to void spontaneously. As long as the child can urinate without discomfort, and is free of urinary tract symptoms, there is no need to initiate therapy. The patient and parents should be counseled that in most cases the labia separate spontaneously in early puberty as the concentration of endogenous estrogen in the peripheral circulation increases. Attempts to separate the labia manually are rarely indicated as these manipulations are guaranteed to cause both physical and emotional trauma. Almost always these attempts fail and even more scarring occurs as the labia fuse once again. Occasionally, when the line of fusion is very thin, the adhesions may be separated by use of a blunt probe following the administration of a local anesthetic ointment. These attempts should be terminated immediately if they cause the child any discomfort.

If labial adhesions cause problems in voiding or recurrent urinary tract infections, active treatment must be started. Improved perineal hygiene and the topical application of estrogen cream to the labia once or twice a day for 10–14 days is almost always successful in bringing about separation of the labia. Once the labia separate, the estrogen cream is continued for another 7 consecutive days so that the new edges of the labia have a chance to reepithelialize. This reduces the chance that the labia will fuse again when the estrogen cream has been discontinued.

Labial adhesions may be confused with vaginal agenesis. When the vagina is congenitally absent the vulva appears normal except for the absence of an opening into the vagina. The urethra has a normal anatomic location and appearance and the urethral meatus is easily identifiable. With vaginal agenesis the opening to the vagina is replaced by vulvar tissue which has some minor folds.

Prolapse of the urethra

Prolapse of the urethra results in the urethral mucosa protruding through the external urethral orifice as an annular mass reddish or reddish-blue in color. The tissue may be friable or even necrotic in nature. Urethral prolapse is usually first noted after a sudden increase in intraabdominal pressure from crying, coughing, or straining, although rarely it can occur spontaneously. Injury is almost never a significant etiologic factor. Support of the distal urethra is in part estrogen-dependent and prolapse of the urethra may be related to hypoestrogenism. This disorder most commonly occurs in childhood with a peak incidence observed between the ages of 5 and 9 years. For unknown reasons it is observed more frequently in black girls. Children with prolapse of the urethra may complain of vulvar pain, bleeding, or dysuria. Diagnosis is usually made by recognizing the urethral orifice in the center of the mass, which to some degree may be friable. Passage of a catheter into the urinary bladder will confirm the diagnosis. At times the diagnosis may be more difficult, especially when the mass of prolapsed tissue is quite large and edematous. Examination under anesthesia, vaginoscopy, and even biopsy may rarely be necessary to distinguish a prolapse of the urethra from a mesodermal mixed tumor, condylomata, papilloma, periurethral cyst, and periurethral abscess.

Prolapse of the urethra usually responds to nonsurgical treatment. Sitz baths, topical application of estrogen, antibiotics, and saline compresses have all been successfully used to reduce the edema and return the prolapsed tissue to its normal anatomic location. There is some disagreement whether a catheter should be left in the bladder for several days to reduce the possibility of recurrence and it is not used in our medical center. Indications for surgical intervention would include the presence of necrotic prolapsed tissue, failure of nonsurgical methods to achieve return of the prolapsed tissue to its normal site, and frequent recurrence. Surgery involves excising the redundant prolapsed mucosa, and suturing the mucosal edge to the skin using fine sutures. Cauterization is not recommended as a treatment modality for prolapse of the urethra.

SUGGESTED READING

ADDUCCI JE, FISCHBACH AL, ADDUCCI CJ. Microsurgical repair of pediatric vulvar trauma. *J Reprod Med* 1985;30:792–794.

BERKOWITZ CD, ELVIK SL, LOGAN MK. Labial fusion in prepubescent girls: a marker for sexual abuse? *Am J Obstet Gynecol* 1987;156:16–20.

JENKINSON SD, MACKINNON AE. Spontaneous separation of fused labia minora in prepubertal girls. *Br J Med* 1984;289:160–161.

KHANAM W, CHOGTU L, MIR Z, SHAWL F. Adhesion of the labia minora – a study of 75 cases. *Obstet Gynecol Surv* 1978;33:364–365.

MCCANN J, VORIS J, SIMON M. Labial adhesions and posterior fourchette injuries in childhood sexual abuse. *Am J Dis Child* 1988;142:659–663.

MURAM D. Genital tract injuries in the prepubertal child. *Pediatr Ann* 1986;15: 616–620.

RIMSZA ME. Gonorrheal vulvovaginitis, labial fusion; imperforate hymen. *Am J Dis Child* 1989;143:381–382.

WHEELER RA, BURGE DM. Urinary obstruction due to labial fusion. *Br J Urol* 1991;67:102.

WILLIAMS TS, CALLEN JP, OWEN LG. Vulvar disorders in the prepubertal female. *Pediatr Ann* 1986;15:588–605.

Gynecologic Urology

76

Diagnosis and treatment of urinary incontinence

ARIEH BERGMAN & CHARLES A. BALLARD

Urinary incontinence in the female is very common and not necessarily pathologic. Questionnaires given to a large number of young, nulliparous women reveal that half have experienced incontinence at one time or another and 16% suffer from this problem daily. Parous women in their 30s or 40s give positive replies even more frequently. Only when the incontinence has progressed to the point where it is socially embarrassing should it be considered pathologic.

Urinary incontinence is caused by lowered urethral resistance (stress incontinence), inappropriate elevation of bladder pressure (detrusor instability), or when anatomically urethral resistance is bypassed (fistula, diverticula, or ectopic ureter). Accurate diagnosis of each of these conditions is crucial, since treatment of each of them is completely different.

Stress urinary incontinence

Definition

Stress urinary incontinence (SUI) is the involuntary loss of urine from the urethra at the time of stress in the absence of bladder contraction.

Diagnosis

The diagnosis is established in three phases. The first two phases can be done as office diagnostic procedures and should provide enough information to establish the diagnosis in 80–85% of patients. Phase III is the sophisticated urodynamic testing and is required for only 15% of patients (previous surgical failures, combined SUI and unstable bladder, following radical surgery, or negative preoperative (Q-tip) test).

Phase I

1 Urine culture and sensitivity: a midstream urine culture should be taken at the time of evaluation. Incontinence evaluation should be looked at as inaccurate, if it is performed at the time of an unsuspected urinary tract infection. Urinary infection can simulate any lower urinary tract pathology, either detrusor instability or SUI. Diagnosis of incontinence established at the time of unsuspected urinary tract infection is inaccurate in 50% of patients.

2 History and physical examination: a detailed questionnaire completed by the patient, followed by history taking, can guide the physician, but one should never rely totally on the history, which may be misleading. In various studies it has been shown that the history of "pure" SUI was confirmed in 70–75% of cases, while the history of "pure" bladder instability was urodynamically confirmed in only 50% of cases. The physical examination should include the neurologic evaluation of the S2–S4 lower micturition center, since urinary incontinence may be secondary to central nervous system lesions. This evaluation includes testing the sensation in the inner thighs, perirectal, and vulvar areas (sensory dermatomes representing S2–S4) and bulbocavernous reflex (when a gentle squeeze to the clitoris should result in reflectory contraction of the perirectal muscle) which represents the motor component of S2–S4, where the lower micturition center is located.

Phase II: simple office diagnostic procedures

1 Cystourethroscopy: cystourethroscopy is performed without topical anesthesia, using either carbon dioxide or a water medium. The urethroscope is introduced into the urethra, and the mucosa examined. The bladder and trigone are examined for gross pathology. The urethrovesical junction (UVJ) is dynamically examined, as per the response to "hold urine" (when UVJ is expected to close, in the absence of peripheral neuropathy) and the response to cough and the Valsalva maneuver (where the UVJ should close, as opposed to SUI and weak urethral sphincter where UVJ funnels and opens). The urethroscope is slowly withdrawn along the urethra (which is distended with gas or water), allowing a thorough examination for diverticula (since urethral diverticula can simulate SUI) or exudate (since urethritis may simulate detrusor instability).

2 Q-Tip test: a sterile Q-tip, lubricated with Xylocaine jelly, is introduced into the urethra and advanced to the UVJ. Using the orthopedic goniometer, the resting and straining angles of the Q-tip to the horizontal are measured. A change of greater than 35% is indicative of a poor support of the UVJ. A negative Q-tip test should raise doubt on the diagnosis on SUI and the more sophisticated urodynamic tests should then be ordered.

3 Simplified cystometry: cystometry is performed in the standing position with periodic cough provocations. The bladder is filled with water or gas and detrusor pressures are measured during the procedure. Bladder contractions of >15 cmH$_2$O are indicative of an unstable bladder. Detrusor instability should always be ruled out before the diagnosis of SUI is established since bladder contractions induced by cough (detrusor instability) can result in symptoms and clinical findings of stress urinary incontinence.

In cases of pure SUI where urethrocystoscopy demonstrates a weak sphincter and no other pathology, Q-tip test (>35°) demonstrates poor support to the UVJ, and cystometry demonstrates a stable bladder, the diagnosis of SUI can be established with certainty, and the phase III evaluation is not required. If any of these tests is inconsistent with SUI, phase III urodynamic evaluation is necessary.

Phase III

1 Sophisticated urodynamics evaluation: urethrocystometry is used to record concomitant pressures in the bladder, urethra, and abdomen (estimated by vaginal recording) while filling the bladder. This test will detect minor degrees of bladder instability as well as urethral instability.

2 Urethral pressure profiles: profiles are performed along the urethra, while bladder and abdominal pressures are concomitantly recorded. This test is performed at rest (rest profile) and repeated while the patient coughs continuously (cough profile). The test measures urethral pressures at stress, abdominal pressure transmission to the urethra, and distinguishes between the component of bladder instability and a weak sphincter as contributors to urinary incontinence, in cases of mixed pathology. A diagnosis of SUI and low urethral pressure (rest profile of ≤20 cmH$_2$O) requires an obstructive surgical procedure (sling) rather than a "physiologic" (Burch, Marshall–Marchetti–Krantz (MMK), Pereyra) one.

Bladder instability

Definition

Bladder instability is the appearance of uninhibited detrusor contraction of ≥15 cmH$_2$O during bladder filling or detrusor pressure increase of ≥15 cmH$_2$O during cystometry.

Diagnosis

Cystometry is performed using either water or gas. The test performed in the supine position will diagnose 85% of patients with bladder instability. The test performed in the standing position with cough provocation will diagnose 98% of patients with bladder instability.

Pathophysiology

Bladder instability can be secondary to a central nervous system lesion. If a primary central nervous system lesion is identified, the bladder condition is defined as detrusor dyssynergia. It accounts for 10% of cases. If no neurologic abnormality can be identified, the condition is defined as idiopathic bladder instability. It accounts for 90% of cases. Neurologic screening test of S2–S4 lower micturition center (sensory dermatomes of lower extremities and the bulbocavernous reflex, described earlier) are essential to rule out central neuropathy that may result in bladder instability.

Bypass urinary incontinence

A fistula or ectopic ureter is easily identified by observing the loss of urine through the vagina. In case of any doubt, the vagina is packed with pads and bladder filled with methylene blue. Once the diagnosis is established, the treatment is surgical closure of the fistula (details in Chapter 74). Urethral diverticula are diagnosed by urethroscopy and confirmed by urethrography (using a Tratner catheter). A surgical correction is needed only if the diverticula are symptomatic.

Treatment of urinary incontinence

Stress urinary incontinence

The primary treatment of SUI should be surgical, either abdominally or vaginally, to correct the anatomic defect. The aims of surgery are: (1) relocate the proximal urethra in the intraabdominal pressure sphere; (2) support the bladder base, so it does not descend at the time of coughing; and (3) increase the tension of the periurethral striated muscle. The cure rate following primary surgery is usually >85%. The various procedures available for stress incontinence include the MMK, Burch, and Pereyra operations and a fascial sling. If a vaginal approach is necessary for uterine descensus plus a cystocele and a rectocele, one may do a Pereyra procedure. The endopelvic fascia is detached from the pubic rami bilaterally. A helical suture is placed through this fascia, incorporating the pubourethral ligament, and then tied over the rectus fascia.

If there is no need for a vaginal repair or if a primary abdominal hysterectomy is to be performed, an MMK or Burch procedure is carried out. The MMK is a vesicourethral suspension. The space of Retzius is entered, with sutures placed in the periurethral tissue and the posterior periosteum of the pubis. This procedure has had widespread use with a high success rate. It has been especially useful as a secondary procedure in patients who have failed a prior operation for stress incontinence.

We believe that the Burch procedure offers some technical advantages over the original MMK procedure. Cooper's ligament is a more reliable tissue than the periosteum, and the vagina allows a more sturdy purchase than the periurethral tissue. After the space of Retzius has been entered using a nonabsorbable suture, the vagina lateral to the bladder neck is transfixed to the iliopectineal ligament. This effectively creates a sling out of the patient's anterior vagina and leaves the bladder neck and urethra alone so that excessive scarring will not interfere with the delicate mechanism of voiding and continence. The bladder neck is identified with a large transurethral Foley catheter and, if there is any doubt as to the placement of the sutures in relationship to the bladder, the bladder is opened. We have achieved the highest success rate using the Burch procedure as the primary approach in women with incontinence.

The fascial sling operation has been performed as the ultimate effort where other procedures have failed. Numerous modifications in materials and the placement of the support sling have been made. The most successful versions are those using homologous tissues such as the anterior abdominal fascia or fascia lata.

The nonsurgical treatment for SUI should be offered to patients who are poor surgical candidates or who do not desire surgery.

Estrogen treatment

Estrogen treatment affects the urethral mucosa factor, thickening of the urethral mucosa and engorgement of blood vessels beneath. This treatment results in an increase of urethral pressure and improvement or cure of SUI in 60% of postmenopausal patients. Estrogen can be administered as a vaginal cream (Premarin vaginal cream, 2 g every other day) or orally (0.625 mg daily of Premarin or the equivalent) for an indefinite period of time.

α-Sympathomimetics

α-Sympathomimetics increase the tone of the smooth periurethral muscle. α-Adrenergic receptors are located in the urethra and trigone affecting urethral tone, by causing contraction of the smooth periurethral muscles. Sudafed 60 mg t.i.d. and imipramine 50 mg t.i.d. for 3 months give good results in 50% of patients.

Kegel exercises

Kegel exercises promote hypertrophy and thickening of the striated periurethral muscle. This passive exercise is performed many times a day and should be continued for a few months. The patient tightens her pubococcygeal muscle (which she learns to identify by starting and stopping her urine stream without moving her legs) 20–30 times a day, continued for a period of 3–4 months. A significant improvement or cure is reported in >50% of patients.

Electrical stimulation

Electrical stimulation of the pudendal nerve through the vagina or rectum causes reflectory contraction of the striated periurethral muscle. The mechanism of action and treatment duration are similar to Kegel exercises.

Vaginal pessary

A vaginal pessary mechanically supports the bladder base and restores the urethra to an intraabdominal position. Since the mechanism of the pessary is similar to that of surgery, it was recently suggested as a preoperative test.

Bladder instability

The treatment of idiopathic bladder instability is primarily medical.
1 Anticholinergic drugs: Pro-Banthine (15 mg t.i.d.) for 6 months; Ditropan (5 mg t.i.d.) for 6 months; imipramine (50 mg t.i.d.) for 6 months.
2 Muscle relaxant (local): Cistospas (0.15 mg b.i.d.).
3 Prostaglandin inhibitors: Naprosyn 250 mg t.i.d. for 6 months.
   The overall success rate of these medical treatment modalities is about 60%, and medications should be continued for at least 6 months.
4 Behavioral modification (bladder drills), biofeedback, and hypnotherapy. The aim of this treatment is to regain cortical inhibitory control over the bladder. These treatments are effective in >70% of patients, but require prolonged treatment and dedicated personnel.

5 Bladder overdistention: this treatment is designed to break the "cell-to-cell junctions" causing relative bladder hypotonicity. Distention is done under anesthesia, filling the bladder to 600–800 ml.

6 Electrical stimulation of the pudendal nerve through the vagina or rectum causes reflectory inhibition of the pelvic nerve (which innovates the detrusor muscle) through inhibition of the lower micturition center.

7 Interruption of innovation, by peripheral denervation through the vagina (Hodgkinson technique), through the abdomen, or by sacral rhizotomy. A major disadvantage of this technique is the possibility of bladder hypotonicity requiring permanent intermittent self-catheterization.

Bypass urinary incontinence

Fistula

Urethrovaginal or vesicovaginal fistulas, which are not secondary to irradiation or tumor, can be corrected vaginally or abdominally. The technique is described in Chapter 74.

Ectopic ureter

The collecting system can be connected end-to-side to the other ureter. An intravenous pyelogram is required prior to such a procedure.

Diverticula

Diverticula are treated only if they are symptomatic. If the diverticulum is distal to the area of maximal urethral pressure, a simple Spence procedure (marsupialization) is adequate. If a diverticulum is proximal to the area of maximal urethral pressure, a diverticulectomy is indicated, to prevent secondary stress incontinence.

SUGGESTED READING

BATTCOCK TM, CASTLEDEN CM. Pharmacological treatment of urinary incontinence. *Br Med Bull* 1990;46:147.

BERGMAN A. Office work-up of lower urinary tract dysfunctions and indications for referral for urodynamic testing. *Obstet Gynecol Clin North Am* 1989;16:787.

BERGMAN A, BHATIA NN. Effect of urinary tract infection upon urethral and bladder function. *Obstet Gynecol* 1985;66:366.

BERGMAN A, MATTHEWS L, BALLARD CA, ROY S. Suprapubic vs. transurethral bladder drainage after surgery for stress urinary incontinence. *Obstet Gynecol* 1987;69:546.

BERGMAN A, BALLARD CA, KOONINGS PP. Comparison of three different surgical procedures for genuine stress incontinence: prospective randomized study. *Am J Obstet Gynecol* 1989;160:1102.

BHATIA NN, BERGMAN A, KARRAM M. Effect of estrogen on urethral functions in women with urinary incontinence. *Am J Obstet Gynecol* 1989;160:176.

KARRAM MM, BHAITA NN. The Q-tip test: standardization of the technique and interpretation in women with urinary incontinence. *Obstet Gynecol* 1988;71:807.

77

Bladder injuries and vesicovaginal fistulas

ARIEH BERGMAN & CHARLES A. BALLARD

Bladder injuries

Bladder injuries are common complications of pelvic surgery despite the best of operative techniques. Fortunately, such injuries heal rapidly and securely if promptly recognized and appropriately repaired.

Injuries to the bladder dome

The dome of the bladder can be either lacerated or deliberately opened during the course of an abdominal operation. Accidental lacerations are commonly associated either with an anatomic distortion as a result of previous operations or tumors, or with adhesions as a result of surgery, infection, or endometriosis. Elective cystotomy is usually performed to assist in dissecting the bladder free of dense adhesions, or as an aid in evaluating suspected ureteral injury. Cystotomy can also be utilized in techniques to correct urinary stress incontinence. While accidental bladder injury can be minimized by good technique, including intrafascial rather than extrafascial hysterectomy and sharp rather than blunt dissection, it is equally important to disprove a suspected injury by filling the bladder with dye or even opening the dome of the bladder to inspect its mucosal surface.

Closure of accidental or intentional cystotomy is best accomplished utilizing 2-0 chromic suture, which holds its tensile strength better than polyglycolic or polyglactin suture, particularly in the presence of infected urine. While several closure techniques are satisfactory, animal experimentation has demonstrated that continuous unlocking sutures produce a better closure. Paradoxically, continuous locking sutures result in excessive leakage and should be avoided. If a two-layer closure is employed, the first layer should include both the mucosa and muscularis. There is no advantage in attempting to avoid the mucosa because chromic sutures that penetrate this layer will be covered by epithelium in 3 days. In addition, closure of the mucosa eliminates the possibility of subsequent bleeding from its free edge as a result of the lytic action of urine. A second layer of continuous inverting suture provides reinforcement.

Testing a two-layer continuous closure by distending the bladder with 500 ml of fluid is reassuring, but probably not necessary because such a repair is invariably watertight. Prolonged postoperative decompression of the bladder by catheter drainage is also unnecessary: we find 5 days of catheter drainage more than adequate. Drainage of the space of Retzius is not required.

Injuries to the bladder base

Accidental injuries to the bladder base are more complicated, for several reasons. First, they are apt to be unrecognized. Second, healing may be impeded because the immediate operative field is infected. Third, one or both ureters may be involved by either the injury or the repair. The most common cause of injury to the bladder base is a laceration occurring during vaginal entry of the anterior cul-de-sac. Such a misadventure is likely to be due to forceful blunt dissection by jabbing with a gauze-wrapped finger. The site of injury is usually in the midline, permitting repair without encroaching on the ureters. A two-layer repair, as described above, should be utilized. The second layer of suture may be interrupted rather than continuous. If there is any question of ureteral involvement, cystoscopy should be performed following closure and the ureteral orifices observed for the prompt bilateral appearance of indigo carmine dye after intravenous administration.

If the insult to the bladder occurs during anterior colporrhaphy then ureteral involvement is very likely since the ureteral orifice is at the level of the mid vaginal anterior wall. In these cases the surgeon should always determine that there is ureteral patency by cystoscopy and visualizing indigo carmine (given intravenously) or by passing ureteral stents through the cystoscope.

Because of the uncertainty of healing, postoperative urethral or suprapubic catheter drainage should be continued for at least 10 days. In addition, transvaginal drainage of the proximal area of the repair can be considered. If the closure is less than satisfactory, the area of repair shold be reinforced with a bulbocavernous fat pad (Martius) graft. Injury to the bladder base during the course of an abdominal procedure, if recognized, should be managed in a similar fashion.

Vesicovaginal fistulas

Vesicovaginal fistulas can be categorized as being due to surgery, radiation, obstetric trauma, or a miscellany of rare causes such as tuberculosis, syphilis, trauma, electrocautery, malignancy, or bladder neck resection. Obstetric trauma is no longer a significant factor in developed countries, and the incidence of radiation fistulas has been greatly reduced with the advent of more sophisticated techniques. At the M.D. Anderson Hospital, the incidence of vesicovaginal fistulas resulting from radiation therapy for cervical carcinoma is only 1.2%. The great majority of vesicovaginal fistulas currently encountered are the result of pelvic surgery for benign disease.

Three-quarters of vesicovaginal fistulas follow an abdominal operation, and the vast majority of these are the result of unrecognized trauma at the time of the operation. The most common error is misplacement of a suture through the bladder wall at the time of closure of the vaginal cuff. The resulting focal devascularization supplemented by an inflammatory response results in a small vesicovaginal fistula just anterior to the line of vault closure. Vesicocervical or vesicouterine fistulas can occur if these structures have not been removed.

Fistulas can also result from the presence of a foreign body draining an open vaginal cuff or from an infected vault hematoma.

The diagnosis of a postoperative vesicovaginal fistula can be suspected by unexplained fever, persistent bloody urine, or heavy vaginal discharge. If the diagnosis is suspected, cystoscopy can be considered, although the additional trauma of the procedure may make matters worse. Constant or intermittent leakage of urine is usually observed on the fifth postoperative day, or later, depending on the size and length of the fistula tract.

Once the fistula has developed the diagnosis may be obvious, depending on its size and location. Even so, excretory urography is mandatory to rule out coincidental involvement of the upper urinary tract. If the opening is small or the tract is long or tortuous, cystoscopy and the instillation of methylene blue dye into the bladder may not be adequate to confirm the diagnosis, particularly in the presence of mucosal edema. In this event, the triple-swab test of Moir is helpful. Following dye instillation into the bladder, three dry cotton swabs are inserted deep into the vagina, and the patient is instructed to ambulate for 20–30 min. If, at the end of this period, only the innermost swab is wet but not blue, the diagnosis is urethrovaginal fistula. If only the outermost swab is wet (and blue), the diagnosis is urinary incontinence. If the upper swabs are both wet and blue, the diagnosis is a vesicovaginal or high urethrovaginal fistula. Occasionally, ingenious methods must be employed to locate an elusive fistula. As recommended by Robertson, the "flat tire test" consists of placing the patient in the knee–chest position, filling the vaginal vault with water, insufflating the bladder with carbon dioxide, and observing the water for the appearance of bubbles.

Whenever a diagnosis of vesicovaginal fistula is strongly suspected or established, prolonged bladder drainage is indicated, in the hope of spontaneous closure. Suprapubic drainage may be more convenient, particularly if the patient is sent home. In addition, the urine is acidified by means of ascorbic acid 500 mg twice daily, and sterilized utilizing an appropriate antibiotic. Once it is apparent that the tract is epithelialized, the possibility of spontaneous closure no longer exists.

While cauterization of a small, persistent fistulous tract is occasionally successful, the majority will require a surgical repair. Immediate combined transabdominal–transvesical repair has its advocates, but there is the risk of failure with a resulting larger defect and a more difficult secondary repair. Early closure following a 10-day course of glucocorticoids has been recommended by Collins and Raz, mainly when the injury site in the bladder appears to be not inflamed and well healed, but the majority opinion is that it is better to wait at least 3–6 months to allow all inflammatory changes to subside before attempting a repair. Experience proves that delayed closure has the greatest chance of success.

When the optimal time for surgical repair is reached, preoperative preparation should include acidification and sterilization of the urine, local estrogens when indicated, and correction of any coexisting vaginal infection. A regimen of prophylactic antibiotics such as cefoxitin (Mefoxin) 2 g on call to surgery and 6 and 12 h later may enhance the chances of successful closure.

Indications for use of the abdominal approach are: (1) fistulas with a diameter >2 cm; (2) fistulas affecting the ureteric orifices; (3) multiple fistulas; (4) vesicocervical fistulas; (5) recurrence of a fistula; and (6) poor quality of local tissues (for example, following irradiation, chronic infection, or in diabetes mellitus).

In 95% of cases or better, vaginal repair of a fistula is preferable. Indwelling ureteral catheters should be placed prior to surgery if the fistula is in close proximity to a ureter. As an aid to palpation, the wire stents should then be replaced in the catheters. Principles of repair include adequate mobilization, tension-free sutures at the fistula edges, and a three-layer closure using delayed absorbable sutures. Excision of the fistula's tract is not always necessary and the tract can be left intact. In these cases the sutures of the first layer may include the tract and partial thickness of the vaginal wall. Insertion of a small Foley catheter through the fistula to the bladder and pulling of the catheter ease intraoperative identification of the fistula's opening.

For fistulas at the apex of the vaginal vault, Latzko's technique, including a partial colpocleisis, is particularly effective. Regardless of the approach, most repairs of vesicovaginal fistulas should be successful if the surgeon is able to obtain a tension-free closure of viable tissue, avoid overlapping suture lines, and insure good uninterrupted postoperative catheter drainage.

When poor healing is a possibility, the area of repair should be reinforced with a Martius graft. In cases of large radiation fistulas, even better reinforcement is provided by a myocutaneous graft utilizing the gracilis muscle. A Martius graft is a simple procedure and it should be in the repertoire of every pelvic surgeon. A gracilis muscle graft is a relatively formidable undertaking.

SUGGESTED READING

ELKINS TE, DELANCY JOL, McGUIRE EJ. The use of the modified Martius graft as an adjunctive technique in vesicovaginal fistula. *Obstet Gynecol* 1990;75:727.

GANNON MJ. The three swab test using knots for urovaginal fistula. *Surg Gynecol Obstet* 1990;170:171.

LATZKO W. Postoperative vesicovaginal fistulas. *Am J Surg* 1942;58:211.

MANDAL AK, SHARMA SK, VAIDYANATHAN S, GOSWAMI AK. Urethrovaginal fistula: summary of 18 years experience. *Br J Urol* 1990;65:453.

WANG Y, HADLEY HR. Nondelayed transvaginal repair of high lying vesicovaginal fistula. *J Urol* 1990;144:34.

78

Surgical injury to the ureter

CHARLES A. BALLARD & ARIEH BERGMAN

Introduction

Although surgical injury to the ureter is uncommon, its potential medical and legal complications are most serious. The injury occurs most often during an abdominal hysterectomy. Surgical injury to the ureter is six times more frequent during an abdominal than a vaginal hysterectomy. Ureteral injury occurs more commonly when other pelvic disease, such as tuboovarian abscess, ovarian neoplasm, endometriosis, or a broad-ligament leiomyoma are present. The highest incidence of damage to the ureter occurs with a radical hysterectomy, but this operation usually is performed by gynecologic oncologists. The incidence of ureteral injuries associated with major gynecologic surgical procedures is 0.5–2.0%. One-half to three-quarters of all iatrogenic ureteral injuries occur during gynecologic operations. Because most injuries are asymptomatic, the actual incidence of injury may even be higher.

The most frequent site of injury is in the region of the uterine vessels. Other common sites of ureteral injury are at the level of the pelvic brim and at the ureterovesical junction. With the increased use of the laparoscope ureteral injuries have occurred during laparoscopic surgical procedures. Iatrogenic ureteral injuries have been reported during laparoscopy-assisted vaginal hysterectomy, operative laparoscopy for the treatment of pelvic endometriosis, laparoscopic lysis of adhesions, laparoscopic coagulation of the uterosacral ligaments, and laparoscopic tubal sterilization. The types of injuries to the ureters during surgery include ligation, transection, laceration, devascularization, excision of a portion of the ureter, and crush injuries.

Prevention

As a preventive measure, a preoperative intravenous pyelogram (IVP) has been recommended, but its value in preventing injury is questionable, except with a ureter displaced anteriorly by a retroperitoneal mass. To detect this malposition, a lateral film is necessary, which may be helpful also in diagnosing anomalies such as double ureter or absent kidney. Preoperative placement of a ureteral catheter also has been recommended for difficult cases, the only problems being: (1) that this may lead to a false sense of security; and (2) the catheter is not always palpable throughout the entire course of the ureter. For a difficult dissection, the bladder may be opened at the dome, and either a ureter catheter is inserted or the patient may be given intravenous indigo carmine.

The primary procedures in preventing ureter damage are precise knowledge of the pelvic anatomy and specifically the course of the ureter, adequate surgical exposure during the operation and identification of the ureter, even if this means opening the broad ligament and following the course of the ureter. Also, careful dissection of adherent masses and removal of broad ligament leiomyomas before hysterectomy will reduce the incidence of ureter damage.

Diagnosis

Approximately one-third of ureter injuries are recognized intraoperatively. If an injury is suspected at the time of surgery, the ureter is identified and followed to the site of potential damage. Patency is demonstrated with the intravenous administration of indigo carmine, performing a cystotomy in the dome of the bladder, and observing for active spurting of urine and dye bilaterally from ureteral orifices. If urine or dye appear to be impaired, a number 4 or 5 ureteral catheter can be passed in a retrograde fashion to rule out an obstruction.

Frequently, the discovery of iatrogenic ureteral injury occurs later. Ureteral injuries may be present in patients who also have a vesicovaginal fistula. Bilateral ureteral injuries may be present when initial studies suggest injury to only one ureter. Other conditions, such as hematuria, flank pain, abdominal discomfort, ileus, anuria, or urinary tract infection should suggest a possible ureter injury. An IVP or dye excretory cystoscopy using intravenous indigo carmine is helpful in making the diagnosis. Ultrasonography also has been used to demonstrate hydronephrosis.

Treatment: ureteral injuries recognized intraoperatively

Prompt intraoperative recognition of ureteral injuries and the immediate surgical repair result in an increased incidence of good renal function, reduced ureteral complications, and reduced morbidity.

The ureter can be clamped, crushed, ligated, lacerated, transected, or denuded of its sheath. The management of these injuries depends principally upon their extent and location. When a clamp or suture is discovered on a ureter during the course of an operation, it should be removed immediately and the ureter inspected carefully. If ureteral peristalsis is present, no further care may be necessary. Some suggest placement of a retroperitoneal Penrose drain or ureteral catheter for possible urinary extravasation around the site of injury. Tears in the ureteral sheath can be repaired with 5-0 chromic suture. If the ureter is transected, the mobility of the ureter and bladder and the location of the injury dictate the type of repair.

The laparoscopic repair of a ureter injured during operative laparoscopy has been reported. During laparoscopic surgery to treat extensive endometriosis located on the pelvic side wall, a 1.5 cm portion of ureter was resected. Laparoscopic anastomosis of the ureter was successfully accomplished. In a second case a transverse laceration of the ureter was sutured through the laparoscope.

The ideal repair should preserve normal kidney function and restore function of the ureter. The ureter can be repaired by an end-to-end anastomosis or implanted in the bladder dome. The implantation is probably the better operation. Unfortunately, this can be performed only when the injury to the ureter is low. If the injury occurs in the upper or mid-portion of the ureter, a ureteroureteral anastomosis is performed. The cut ends of the ureter are spatulated and reapproximated over a ureteral catheter by five or six loose sutures of 5-0 catgut, and the area is drained by a retroperitoneal flank drain. The ureteral catheter is left *in situ* for 10–12 days. A flank drain is left in place until all drainage stops.

When bladder implantation is selected, the distal ureteral stump is ligated with nonabsorbable suture, and the proximal ureter is brought through a stab wound in the bladder, its spatulated ends fixed to the bladder wall with 5-0 catgut suture. A reinforcing outer layer of suture unites the adventitia of the ureter to the bladder surface. Whenever possible, tension on the line of anastomosis can be reduced by hitching the bladder to the psoas muscle. A retroperitoneal flank drain also should be inserted.

Treatment: ureteral injuries recognized postoperatively

Unfortunately, most ureteral injuries are not recognized at the time of surgery. Bilateral ligation becomes apparent by the appearance of anuria. Ureteral catheters are placed to demonstrate an obstruction but rarely overcome an obstruction. Bilateral nephrostomy or deligation may be performed. If a nephrostomy is performed, a laparotomy may be undertaken 4–6 weeks later, at which time ureteral plastic work may be completed.

Unilateral ureteral injury may become apparent following a hysterectomy when the patient develops pyelitis, fever, flank pain, ileus, peritonitis, distention, or urinary leakage from the vaginal vault, or by a ureterovesicovaginal fistula. Ureteral catheterization is performed. Usually it is impossible to pass the catheter past the fistula; however, if it is done and the catheter can pass the site of obstruction, it is left in for several days.

Commonly, the surgical repair of ureteral injuries sustained during gynecologic procedures which are not recognized until the postoperative period is delayed for an interval up to 3 months. Ureteral injuries sustained during a clean operation and recognized in the early postoperative period can be repaired as soon as the diagnosis is made with results equal to those of a delayed repair. Immediate reconstruction of the ureter would not be attempted in patients who are septic or are considered a poor surgical candidate. In addition the successful passage of a ureteral catheter or stent eliminates the need for immediate surgery. Unfortunately, with most iatrogenic ureteral injuries stent placement is not feasible, with the possible exception of ureterovaginal fistulas.

It is always necessary to differentiate between a vesicovaginal and ureterovaginal fistula. Cotton balls are placed in the vagina, and a weak solution of methylene blue is placed in the bladder. If the cotton balls remain free of dye, a ureterovaginal fistula is present. If a complete obstruction is present, a nephrostomy may be performed, and 4–6 weeks later a reparative procedure is undertaken. Not infrequently, occlusion of one ureter is asymptomatic, leading to renal atrophy. If a hydronephrosis kidney mass is found several months after surgery, a nephrostomy may be necessary.

SUGGESTED READING

BLANDY JP, BADENOCH DF, FOWLER CG, JENKINS BJ, THOMAS NWM. Early repair of iatrogenic injury to the ureter or bladder after gynecological surgery. *J Urol* 1991;146:761–765.

GOMEL V, JAMES C. Intraoperative management of ureteral injury during operative laparoscopy. *Fertil Steril* 1991;55:416–419.

GRAINGER DA, SODERSTROM RM, SCHIFF SF, GLICKMAN MG, DeCHERNEY AH, DIAMOND MP. Ureteral injuries at laparoscopy: insights into diagnosis, management and prevention. *Obstet Gynecol* 1990;75:839–843.

LEE RA. Vesicovaginal and ureterovaginal fistulae. In: Ostergard DR, Bent AE, eds. *Urogynecology and Urodynamics*. 3rd edn. Baltimore, MD: Williams & Wilkins, 1991:296–305.

NEUMAN M, EIDELMAN A, LANGER R, GOLAN A, BUKOVSKY I, CASPI E. Iatrogenic injuries to the ureter during gynecologic and obstetric operations. *Surg Gynecol Obstet* 1991;173:268–272.

NEWTON M. Intraoperative complications. In: Newton M, Newton ER, eds. *Complications of Gynecologic and Obstetric Management*. Philadelphia, PA: WB Saunders, 1988:36–57.

NEZHAT C, NEZHAT F. Laparoscopic repair of ureter resected during operative laparoscopy. *Obstet Gynecol* 1992;80:543–544.

ST LEZIN MA, STOLLER ML. Surgical ureteral injuries. *Urology* 1991;38:497–506.

TARKINGTON MA, DEJTER SW Jr, BRESETTE JF. Early surgical management of extensive gynecologic ureteral injuries. *Surg Gynecol Obstet* 1991;173:17–21.

THOMPSON JD. Operative injuries to the urinary tract. In: Nichols DH, ed. *Reoperative Gynecologic Surgery*. St Louis, MO: Mosby Year Book, 1991:163–210.

WOODLAND MB. Ureter injury during laparoscopy-assisted vaginal hysterectomy with the endoscopic linear stapler. *Am J Obstet Gynecol* 1992;167:756–757.

79

Urinary tract infection

ARIEH BERGMAN & CHARLES A. BALLARD

Urinary tract infection is a very common problem among women. For the obstetrician–gynecologist, infections of the urinary tract are among the most common seen in both office and hospital practice. The prevalence increases with age from 1% in young schoolgirls, to 4% in young women, 5–7% in pregnant women, and 8–10% in postmenopausal women. In pregnancy, bacteriuria is as common as among nonpregnant women, but it seldom remits spontaneously, whereas in nonpregnant women spontaneous remission is very common.

The assessment and management of culture-documented urinary tract infection should be based on three infection patterns: first infection (symptomatic), recurrent infection, and persistent urinary tract infection.

Acute cystitis

Acute (symptomatic) cystitis is a very common problem. First infections are generally caused by common gram-negative organisms (*Eschericha coli* in approximately 85% of cases), although gram-positive staphylococci and streptococci are not uncommon. The source of the pathogen is usually the patient's bowel flora. The microscopic examination of urinary sediment avoids the 24–48-h delay of the culture results, but there are a few problems with this method. The presence of pyuria (10 leukocytes per high power field) is not a reliable sign of infection. These white cells may be present in women with urethritis and urethral syndrome, and they can be a normal finding in postpartum patients. Furthermore, pyuria is absent in 50% of patients with significant bacteriuria. There is a much better correlation between the presence of bacteria in the microscopic examination of the uncentrifuged urine and positive bacterial cultures. All of these microscopic evaluations should be confirmed by results of a urine culture. Significant bacteriuria has traditionally been based on quantitative urine cultures demonstrating 100 000 or more CFU/ml. It is now clear that <100 000 bacteria per ml can be associated with significant urinary tract infection. In most cases a count of 10 000 CFU/ml of voided or catheterized urine specimen should be indicative of urinary tract infection. Urine collection by transurethral catheterization avoids surface contamination, but does carry with it a 1–2% chance of resulting bacteriuria in a patient previously free of infection.

A clean voided urine sample with poor cleansing of the introitus before voiding or a poor collection technique will increase the contamination of the urine specimen by lower genital tract bacteria. One clean voided specimen of urine with a colony count of 100 000 or higher has an 80% chance of accuracy. Two consecutive clean voided specimens with recovery of the same organism have a 91% chance of indicating urinary tract infection. In cases where a urine culture is unavailable, the use of dip slides or similar devices provides accurate quantitative urine culture at a relatively low cost. Another low-cost office test is the Greiss test that measures the reduction of nitrate to nitrite in the urine, which is caused by the presence of a significant number of enterobacteria. The two major short-comings of the test are that it may not yield positive results in some women with significant bacteriuria, particularly when gram-positive aerobes are involved, and some incubation in the bladder is needed for the nitrate reduction.

Although single-dose therapy appears to be effective, many patients continue to have symptoms for several days after initiating therapy and 7–10 days of treatment is preferred. The following drugs are recommended for a first uncomplicated urinary tract infection.

1 Nitrofurantoin 100 mg orally 4 times a day. Nitrofurantoin is usually active against *E. coli*, *Streptococcus faecalis*, and *Staphylococcus aureus*. It is active against most strains of *Proteus*. The nitrofurantoins sufficiently concentrate in the urine to be effective, yet they do not mask signs and symptoms outside the urinary tract since they do not penetrate soft tissue sites in a high enough concentration to be effective.

2 Penicillin G, 250 mg (400 000 U) orally 4 times daily. Ampicillin 250 mg orally 4 times daily is as effective as penicillin, but more costly. These regimens are effective against most strains of *E. coli*, *Proteus mirabilis*, *Strep. faecalis*, and 25% of *Klebsiella*.

3 Sulfonamides: trimethoprim 80 mg and sulfamethoxazole 400 mg (Bactrim) orally twice daily for 7 days; sulfisoxazole (Gantrisin) 500 mg 4 times daily for 1 week orally. *E. coli* is the most susceptible species, followed by *Klebsiella* species, *P. mirabilis*, *Pseudomonas*, and *Staph. aureus*.

4 Trimethoprim-sulfamethoxazole (Bactrim or Septra) two tablets regular strength or one tablet double-strength orally twice daily for 1 week. Almost half of the women with the complaints of urgency, frequency, dysuria, and nocturia do not have a culture-proven bacterial cystitis. These women may have urethritis or urethral syndrome. They should be evaluated urethroscopically to have the diagnosis confirmed and treated with tetracycline 2 g daily for 10 days or urethral dilatation (three dilatations on a weekly basis). Other possible etiologies for these complaints are atopy that resolves after desensitization, atrophic urethritis that responds to estrogen therapy (Premarin vaginal cream, 1 g daily for 6 weeks), vulvovaginitis, or cervicitis.

Recurrent urinary tract infections

Recurrences at long intervals (usually longer than 2 weeks) and with different bacterial strains are characteristic of reinfection. In the presence of upper urinary tract infection, hemorrhagic cystitis or renal calculus, a thorough urologic evaluation is warranted. In the absence of these risk factors, intravenous pyelography may be deferred.

The etiology of recurrent urinary tract infection is unknown in most cases. Stamey and colleagues have reported that the female vaginal vestibule is the primary reservoir for recurrent infections. These women have a significantly greater degree of colonization of the vestibule with Enterobacteriaceae compared to the control group. In the same study, Stamey and colleagues demonstrated that bacterial adherence to the vaginal mucosa was significantly greater in women with a history of recurrent urinary tract infection than in normal controls. The authors concluded that biologic suceptibility to recurrent urinary tract infection is related to a defect at the cellular level that favors bacterial adherence.

Over 95% of all recurrent infections in women are caused by reinfection due to the spread of bacteria from the rectum to the vaginal vestibule and then to the urethra and bladder, often with coitus as a participating episode. Looking into the toilet habits of these women it was found that in many of them, wiping the rectum after a bowel movement was performed from the anus forward to the introitus. In addition to the trauma and milking action induced by coitus, improper hygiene may play a significant role in the process of recurrent infection.

If the patient's history suggests that reinfections are preceded by intercourse, it is suggested that the patient takes a single antimicrobial tablet of Macrodantin 50 mg routinely before or after intercourse. Many patients will have a minimal number of reinfections using this form of preventive therapy.

The most effective form of therapy is continuous low-dose prophylaxis. The ideal agents for chronic urinary prophylaxis should have three characteristics. First, they should be drugs to which the common infecting organisms (i.e., Enterobacteriaceae) are sensitive; second, they should cause minimal change in the sensitivity pattern of the fecal flora; and third, they should be well tolerated by the patient. Once a urine culture shows no bacterial growth, a nightly therapy of either 50 mg nitrofurantoin or half a tablet of regular-strength trimethoprim-sulfamethoxazole is recommended. Because most urinary infections are caused by bacteria from the fecal reservoir, it is important to minimize the impact of antimicrobial therapy on the bowel flora and prevent development of transferable drug resistance. Nitrofurantoin does not produce fecal resistance because of its complete absorption in the upper intestinal tract and its excretion in high concentration in the urine. Likewise, trimethoprim-sulfamethoxazole rarely causes development of resistant strains. This low-dosage prophylactic treatment should be discontinued after 6 months and the patient should then simply be followed with frequent cultures. At least 30% of women will have spontaneous remission for at least 6 months after such a treatment regimen. Unfortunately, a remission is not a cure. Long infection-free intervals are often followed by reinfections, and intermittent or continuous therapy must be reinstituted.

Persistent infection

In some patients, infections tend to recur rapidly and are caused by the same species. It is important to establish whether the first infection was actually eradicated by antimicrobial therapy. Even if infection was adequately treated and the interval between infections is more than a few days but the infective organism is the same in all infective episodes, the urinary infection should be considered and evaluated as persistent urinary infection. The most common cause for infection are stones, resulting from urea-splitting organisms, such as *P. mirabilis*. A congenital or acquired anomaly such as caliceal diverticulum or stones can become a nidus for infection, showering repeatedly the same organism. Evaluation of persistent urinary infection should include a thorough urologic work-up, including cystoscopy and intravenous pyelography.

Surgical therapy plays a pivotal role in management of women with recurrent urinary tract infections. When the focus of bacterial persistence has been localized it should be removed or the responsible defect corrected. If surgical removal of the focus is not possible, or no focus of infection is found, long-term suppressive antimicrobial therapy is required and is similar to that recommended for recurrent urinary tract infections.

SUGGESTED READING

BERGMAN A. Urinary tract infections in women. *Curr Opin Obstet Gynecol* 1991; 3:541.

BUMP RC. Urinary tract infection in women: current role of single dose therapy. *J Reprod Med* 1990;35:785.

KINGDOM JCP, KITCHENER MC, MACLEAN AB. Prospective urinary tract infection in gynecology: implications for antibiotic prophylaxis policy. *Obstet Gynecol* 1990;76:636.

KRIEGER JN. Urinary tract infections in women: causes, classification, and differential diagnosis. *Urology* 1990;35:4.

LEIBOVIC L, WYSENBEEK AJ. Single-dose antibiotic treatment for symptomatic urinary tract infections in women: a meta analysis of randomized trials. *Q J Med* 1991;78:43.

SANT GR, WAINSTEIN M. Therapy of urinary tract infections in the elderly. *Urology* 1990;35:19.

PART 5

Gynecologic Oncology

80

Preinvasive disease of the lower genital tract

LYNDA D. ROMAN

Vulvar intraepithelial neoplasia

Etiology

Vulvar intraepithelial neoplasia (VIN) unassociated with vulvar dystrophy is generally severe enough to be classified as VIN III or carcinoma-*in-situ*. Approximately one-half of the patients present with pruritus; the remaining cases are usually found incidentally at the time of routine gynecologic examination.

VIN may be unifocal or multifocal in distribution. Color ranges from white through gray, red, and brown, depending on the degree of keratinization, the patient's race or complexion, and the type of lesion. VIN usually is sharply demarcated and slightly elevated. The surface may be shiny, smooth, granular, rough, or keratinized. Multifocal extensive lesions of bowenoid papulosis are found in a younger age group and more often are associated with, and sometimes confused with, condylomata acuminata. The multifocal lesions appear to have a smaller chance of progressing to invasive carcinoma.

Evaluation

Evaluation consists of careful inspection of the entire perineum. VIN is often inapparent to the casual observer or may be disarmingly insignificant in appearance. The most common locations are the labia minora and the introitus between 3 and 9 o'clock. Bowenoid papulosis is often confluent, involving predominantly the glabrous (nonhairy) mucosa. Disease involving the anal canal and intergluteal cleft, which occurs in up to 30% of cases, frequently is overlooked. VIN of the glans clitoris is uncommon and urethral involvement is rare.

Whereas colposcopic examination can aid in defining the extent of VIN, the first requirement is an awareness of the disease combined with a familiarity with its visual characteristics. Acetic acid and toluidine blue staining are useful adjuncts. Lugol's solution applied to the well-estrogenized posterior fourchette and adjacent mucosa will fail to stain areas of squamous neoplasia. Multiple biopsies may be required to define the extent of the disease and to exclude invasion. Squamous dysplasia and carcinoma tend to involve all organs of the lower genital tract sequentially or simultaneously. Consequently, the cervix and vagina must also be evaluated for squamous neoplasia whenever the vulva is involved.

Treatment

The treatment of significant VIN has undergone major changes in the past decade. The most important difference is the general recognition that total or even simple vulvectomy is seldom warranted and usually is contraindicated. In addition, the documentation that spontaneous regression can occur requires recognition of this behavior in the treatment plan. Thus, the premenopausal woman who has newly diagnosed non-keratinized, multifocal, or extensive VIN should be observed for at least 6 months after the most recent pregnancy for evidence of regression unless biopsy indicates that the lesion is aneuploid by the presence of abnormal mitosis. The older the patient and the more severe the dysplasia, however, the greater is the risk of cancer being already present or developing subsequently. For these patients, prolonged observation is proportionately less acceptable.

The two options for treatment of VIN are laser ablation and wide local excision. The former is generally the preferred method of treatment as it gives excellent cosmetic results in an area where preservation of appearance is clearly important. It is essential to rule out invasive disease before laser ablation is performed. As invasive disease in association with VIN is more likely to occur in a postmenopausal patient as compared to a younger woman, the preferred treatment method has been excision for the older woman and laser ablation for the younger woman. However, there is room for individualization. Though rare, invasive cancer of the vulva has been reported even in very young women (<25 years old), where it has frequently been misdiagnosed as condyloma. It is essential to biopsy thoroughly, if not excise, suspicious (markedly papillary, ulcerated, or indurated) vulvar lesions in young women prior to laser ablation. In postmenopausal women, laser ablation may be used in conjunction with excision so as to allow primary closure and to avoid excision at problematic sites such as the urethral or clitoral areas. It should also be kept in mind that the sites most likely to harbor invasive disease are the posterior perineal and perianal areas; both should be thoroughly examined prior to laser treatment. The failure rate of both excision and laser treatment in VIN ranges from 15% up to 40%.

Vaginal intraepithelial neoplasia (VAIN)

Etiology

Preinvasive lesions of the vaginal squamous epithelium occur in only 1–3% of the patients with cervical neoplasia. The majority of women with this lesion, however, have had cervical intraepithelial neoplasia (CIN). In a series of over 50 cases of VAIN reviewed at the Los Angeles County–University of Southern California Medical Center, 40% had prior and 15% coexisting cervical or vulvar neoplasia. Human papillomavirus is thought to be a major etiologic factor in VAIN, as well as in CIN and VIN. Other predisposing causes of VAIN are radiation and immunosuppressive therapy. It has been suggested that postmenopausal atrophy of the vagina is also conducive to the development of VAIN; however, it is more likely that exfoliated cells from the atrophic vaginal epithelium often are interpreted incorrectly as intraepithelial neoplasia, exaggerating the true association of these factors.

Detection and evaluation

The Papanicolaou (Pap) smear is the single most important means of bringing the preinvasive vaginal lesion to the attention of the physician. A saline-moistened, cotton-tipped applicator or a moistened wooden spatula is used for cytologic sampling of the vaginal mucosa as the speculum is withdrawn and rotated. Vaginal cytology is suggested yearly for patients who have had a hysterectomy for preinvasive cervical disease and every 3–5 years if the hysterectomy was done for a benign condition in patients not epidemiologically at high risk for VAIN.

Colposcopy is helpful in evaluating the patient with VAIN. Before performing colposcopy, a Pap smear is obtained and the vaginal tube is then moistened thoroughly with vinegar. To provide an end-on view of the tissues, the speculum is withdrawn and rotated, causing the vaginal muscosa to fold over the end of the speculum blades. Biopsy specimens of lesions that appear to be invasive (raised, ulcerated) are taken immediately. Intraepithelial lesions are generally white, sharply bordered, and finely granular, often with areas of punctation. Mosaic structure rarely is seen.

If invasive disease is not suggested, half-strength aqueous Lugol's solution is applied to the vaginal mucosa. Excess iodine is removed to prevent burning. Lugol's iodine dehydrates the epithelium, so it may be necessary to add a thin film of lubricating jelly to reinsert the speculum. Again, the speculum is withdrawn and rotated. The most significant lesions usually stain a light yellow and have sharp borders, in contrast to the mahogany color of the normal mucosa. Less significant lesions have a variegated iodine uptake with indistinct borders.

After the number and distributions of the lesions are determined, biopsies are taken of representative areas. This is seldom painful; but if pain is a problem, a vaginal tampon soaked in a topical anesthetic is placed in the vagina for 3–5 min before proceeding. The patient with postmenopausal or postradiation atrophy of vaginal mucosa should use intravaginal estrogen cream daily for 2 weeks before colposcopy, as the atrophic epithelium is often difficult to interpret colposcopically and does not stain well with Lugol's solution. Moreover, if the abnormal cytology is due to atrophic cells, topical estrogen cream will convert the cytology to normal.

The most common location of VAIN is the upper third of the vagina; the middle and lower thirds are involved <10% of the time. The lesions are often multifocal and may be found within the vaginal folds. The post-hysterectomy recesses at the 3 and 9 o'clock "corners" are especially common sites for VAIN. In this situation, the fold can be everted with an iris hook or exposed with an endocervical speculum to obtain a satisfactory view.

Treatment

For limited focal VAIN, surgical excision is an effective means of treatment. Shortening of the vagina can result, however, if the excision is very large and the defect is closed. An excisional biopsy is recommended for those patients with only one or two small lesions or in whom invasion is suspected. For many cases of vaginal dysplasia, however, the carbon dioxide laser provides a simple and effective means of treatment.

The posthysterectomy patient may present a difficult management problem if the VAIN lesions involve the corners of the vaginal cuff. When this situation exists, surgical excision is the treatment of choice, although the laser can be used successfully in favorable situations. Excision of lesions in this location must take into account the close proximity of the ureter. In the postmenopausal patient, intravaginal estrogen for 3–4 weeks can reverse early euploid VAIN lesions in about 50% of cases. As a consequence, a trial of intravaginal estrogen cream is warranted in postmenopausal women after invasive cancer has been ruled out.

Perhaps the most challenging clinical problem among women with VAIN is multifocal disease that involves many levels of the vagina. Total vaginectomy and skin grafting have been used with success, as has radiation therapy. Laser ablation is difficult to use in this situation as it is extremely hard to encompass the entire vagina. Also, diffuse lasering of the vagina may lead to adherence of the vaginal walls during healing, resulting in a shortened vagina. Topical 5% 5-fluorouracil (Efudix) has gained popularity for use in cases of diffuse VAIN because it offers a relatively simple and effective method of eradicating the dysplastic lesions on an outpatient basis without compromise of vaginal function. Approximately 80% can expect to have all clinical and cytologic evidence of vaginal dysplasia remit after one or two courses of local therapy. Several regimens have been tried ranging, from half an applicator nightly for 7 days to half an applicator nightly once a week for 10 weeks. While both regimens appear to be equally effective, the latter may cause less vulvitis. The perineum is protected by applying a coat of zinc oxide paste before each treatment and every morning. Because of its simplicity, we recommend topical 5-fluorouracil as the treatment of choice for this group of patients. Laser therapy may be tried when the 5-fluorouracil treatment is unsuccessful.

CIN

Etiology

In the 1970s, the prime suspect for the genesis of CIN and invasive cervical cancer was herpes simplex virus type 2 (HSV-2). More recent studies have stripped HSV-2 of its status as the premier etiologic suspect. It has been replaced by various serotypes of the human papillomavirus (HPV), particularly 16 and 18. Herpes may be a cocarcinogen. Other suspected cocarcinogens include smegma, repeated infections, smoking, and certain chemicals.

Detection

The best detection technique for CIN is cytology, but there are numerous sources of error. The generally accepted false-negative rate for the Pap smear is 10–20%. Sampling error accounts for the greatest number of misses. The most effective method of cervical sampling is sampling of the canal with a cytobrush coupled with an ectocervical scape.

Another source of error in cervical cytology is the failure to fix the slide properly. Once the cervical mucus and free-floating cells have been placed on to the glass slide, this material should be cytofixed within a few seconds. Air drying can lead to misinterpretation of subtle details, unless the laboratory requests air-dried smears. Laboratory error accounts for a very small number of cytology misses. Consequently, correct Pap smear procedure and rapid fixation are critical steps in insuring optimal results. A last source of error is the performance of a Pap smear too soon after a previous Pap smear. It takes approximately 3–4 months after a Pap smear for enough cellular exfoliation to occur to produce an adequate sample.

The class II or atypical Pap smear

Although the presence of inflammatory cells is the most frequent reason for the class II designation, squamous and glandular atypia also are included in this Pap smear category. Several investigations have documented that in 20% of patients with a class II Pap smear, the cause is squamous dysplasia and, on rare occasions, invasive carcinoma. Patients with inflammatory atypia should be evaluated and treated for specific causes of vaginitis (*Gardnerella, Monilia, Trichomonas, Chlamydia*, atrophic) prior to colposcopy assessment and biopsy. Patients in all other categories should undergo colposcopy immediately, as up to 50% will have dysplasia.

Evaluation

Colposcopy is an important technique in office evaluation of women with an abnormal Pap smear, an abnormal-looking cervix, and any abnormalities of the vulva, vagina, or anus. It permits the physician to determine easily the precise nature of most squamous lesions of the lower genital tract, and up to 95% of the time it will eliminate the need for diagnostic conization of the cervix. The colposcopic examination employs 10–20× magnification combined with a green filter and vinegar (acetic acid) to accentuate the colposcopic findings. The standard examination consists of the following:
1 gross examinations of the vulva, vagina, and cervix;
2 repeat cytology if there is no access to the preceding abnormal Pap smear;
3 cleaning the cervix with vinegar (3–5% acetic acid);
4 colposcopic examination;
5 endocervical curettage (ECC; not performed in pregnant patients);
6 colposcopically directed punch biopsies of the most suspicious lesions.

Colposcopy is considered to be satisfactory in patients in whom the entire limits of the dysplastic lesion and the squamocolumnar junction are visible. In patients with an adequate colposcopic exam, an ECC should be performed routinely, as assessment errors have been documented repeatedly. As a consequence, failure to perform the ECC has led to a missed diagnosis of invasive cancer. In addition, early asymptomatic and cytologically negative adenocarcinoma has been detected by routine ECC.

Management (Table 80.1)

Colposcopy satisfactory, negative endocervical curettage

A negative ECC means that there is no evidence in the ECC specimen of squamous dysplasia, atypical glandular cells, or malignancy. When colposcopic examination is satisfactory, the ECC is negative, and there is no evidence on colposcopic-directed biopsy or the Pap smear of invasive carcinoma or glandular atypia, the patient is eligible for outpatient or office therapy by cryosurgery or laser vaporization (Table 80.1) as the presence of invasive cancer should have been ruled out.

Table 80.1 Outline for management of cervical dysplasia

Cone biopsy (knife or laser)
Cervical punch biopsy diagnosis of dysplasia with colposcopically unevaluable canal disease
Cervical punch biopsy diagnosis of microinvasion or colposcopic suspicion of invasion
Dysplasia on ECC
Atypical glandular epithelium on biopsy or ECC
Negative evaluation with persistent Pap smears indicative of dysplasia or carcinoma

Destructive therapy (cryotherapy, laser, cautery)
Exclusion of invasion is an absolute prerequisite
Colposcopic evaluation, biopsies, ECC, Pap smears, and gross appearance of cervix concordant
Squamocolumnar junction entirely visualized and ECC negative
Cryotherapy most effective for small CIN I and II lesions with gland duct or canal involvement
Laser therapy is preferred for large lesions, and lesions extending into the canal but colposcopically evaluable. Laser also is recommended for cryotherapy failures

Hysterectomy (vaginal or abdominal)
Dysplasia at cone tip
Past reproductive age with other indications for hysterectomy (fibroids, prolapse, carcinoma-*in-situ*, etc.)
Other preinvasive disease of the lower genital tract

ECC, Endocervical curettage; CIN, cervical intraepithelial neoplasia.

Colposcopy satisfactory, positive endocervical curettage

The ECC is positive up to 15% of the time even when the colposcopist finds that the entire limits of the lesion are easily visible. A careful review of these curettings often will reveal a single fragment of neoplastic epithelium, which is usually a contaminant inadvertently dislodged from the visible component of the dysplasia. If the ECC is done before the directed biopsies, the false-positive rate may be reduced. A repeat ECC in 3–4 weeks (to permit healing) should be negative. If the repeat ECC is positive, however, cone biopsy is indicated. If review of the initial ECC specimen reveals many fragments of dysplasia or if glandular atypia or any areas suspicious for invasive cancer are present then conization must be performed to exclude the possibility of significant disease in the endocervix.

Colposcopy unsatisfactory

If the dysplastic lesion extends into the endocervical canal so that it cannot be fully evaluated by colposcopy and invasion cannot be ruled out, a conization should be performed. Therefore, local destructive therapy is contraindicated. Unless there is clinical suggestion of frankly invasive endocervical carcinoma (bleeding, enlarged, nodular, or hard cervix), it is preferable not to do an ECC before cone biopsy because invasion in this circumstance is diagnosed only occasionally. On the other hand, the ECC disrupts the very epithelium to be removed by cone biopsy for microscopy, potentially complicating the diagnosis of microinvasion and preventing an accurate assessment of the cone-tip margin. When there is no ectocervical lesion, ECC is always necessary.

In patients undergoing a conization biopsy, further management depends on the pathologic findings in the conization specimen. If only dysplasia is present and the conization biopsy has cleared the lesion (surgical margins negative), treatment is complete. If the cone biopsy has not cleared the lesion, repeat conization, simple vaginal hysterectomy, or abdominal hysterectomy is recommended, depending on the patient's reproductive status, when there is evidence on the follow-up examination that CIN is still present. This decision is based upon a repeat ECC and cytology 12 weeks after the cone biopsy. In most cases, there is no residual dysplasia, and observation is the treatment of choice during the reproductive years. If invasive cancer is discovered in the conization specimen the patient is generally treated with hysterectomy, the extent of which depends on the amount of invasion present.

Recently, the loop electrosurgical excision procedure (Leep) has been introduced in the USA as an alternative to cryotherapy and laser ablation.

Using an electrodiathermy current passed through a thin wire electrode the transformation zone and any abnormal lesions are excised. The usual size of the electrode varies from 1×1 to 2×0.8 cm. Reported success rates after short-term follow-up have been 90–94% and the rate of post-procedure bleeding has been 2–9%. The advantages of Leep are that it is easy to perform, it can be done in a single outpatient setting, and it results in a specimen. Thus invasive cancers may be discovered that would otherwise have been missed had ablative therapy been performed. Possible disadvantages are that, as compared to ablative procedures, more tissue may be removed and the rate of postprocedure bleeding may be higher.

Future studies will hopefully provide information on the long-term success and complication rates of Leep. Other unanswered questions are: how often do specimens removed by Leep have margins positive for dysplasia and what is the risk of persistent disease in such cases? Lastly, though Leep is being tried in some centers as an alternative to conization biopsy, the exact role of Leep in such a setting is as yet unclear.

SUGGESTED READING

ANDERSON MC. Treatment of cervical intraepithelial neoplasia with the carbon dioxide laser: report of 543 patients. *Obstet Gynecol* 1982;59:720.

BAGGISH MS. Improved laser techniques for the elimination of genital and extra-genital warts. *Am J Obstet Gynecol* 1985;153:545.

BERNSTEIN SG, KOVACS BR, TOWNSEND DE, et al. Vulvar carcinoma-*in-situ*. *Obstet Gynecol* 1983; 61:304.

CAPEN CV, MASTERSON BJ, MAGRINA JF, et al. Laser therapy of vaginal intra-epithelial neoplasia. *Am J Obstet Gynecol* 1982;142:973.

COPPLESON M, PIXLEY E, REID B. *Colposcopy*. 2nd edn. Springfield, IL: Charles C Thomas, 1978.

CRUM CP, LEVINE RU. Human papillomavirus infection and cervical neoplasia: new perspectives. *Int J Gynecol Pathol* 1984;3:376.

FERENCZY A, MITAO M, NAGAI N, et al. Latent papillomavirus and recurring genital warts. *N Engl J Med* 1985;313:784.

HATCH KD, SINGLETON HM, ORR JW Jr, et al. Role of endocervical curettage in colposcopy. *Obstet Gynecol* 1985;65:403.

KIRWAN PH, SMITH IR, NAFTALIN NJ. A study of cryosurgery and the CO_2 laser in treatment of carcinoma *in situ* (CIN III) of the uterine cervix. *Gynecol Oncol* 1985;22:195.

KOHAN S, NOUMOFF J, BECKMAN EM, et al. Colposcopic screening of women with atypical Papanicolaou smears. *J Reprod Med* 1985;30:383.

LARSSON G, GULLBERG B, GRUNDSELL H. A comparison of laser and cold knife conization. *Obstet Gynecol* 1983;62:213.

LENEHAN PM, MEFFE F, LICKRISH GM. Vaginal intraepithelial neoplasia: biologic aspects and management. *Obstet Gynecol* 1986:68–333.

LEUCHTER RS, TOWNSEND DE, HACKER NG, et al. Treatment of vulvar carcinoma *in situ* with the CO_2 laser. *Gynecol Oncol* 1984;19:314.

MORROW CP. Advances in the treatment of preinvasive and invasive carcinoma of the vulva. In: Bonnar J, ed. *Recent Advances in Obstetrics and Gynecology,* vol 15. London: Churchill Livingstone, 1987:215–235.

REID R, SCALZI P. Genital warts and cervical cancer. VII. An improved colposcopic index for differentiating benign papillomavirus infection from high-grade cervical intraepithelial neoplasia. *Am J Obstet Gynecol* 1985;153:611.

SCHLAERTH JB, MORROW CP, NAICK RH, *et al.* Anal involvement by carcinoma *in situ* of the perineum in women. *Obstet Gynecol* 1984;64:406.

TOWNSEND DE, LEVINE RU, CRUM CP, *et al.* Treatment of vaginal carcinoma *in situ* with the carbon dioxide laser. *Am J Obstet Gynecol* 1982;143:565.

TOWNSEND DE, RICHART RM. Cryotherapy and carbon dioxide laser management of cervical intraepithelial neoplasia: a controlled comparison. *Obstet Gynecol* 1983;61:75.

TOWNSEND DE, LEVINE RU, RICHART RM, *et al.* Management of vulvar intraepithelial neoplasia by carbon dioxide laser. *Obstet Gynecol* 1984;60:406.

WEBB MJ. Invasive cancer following conservative therapy for previous cervical intraepithelial neoplasia. *Colposc Gynecol Laser Surg* 1985;1:245.

WRIGHT TC, GAGNON S, RICHART RM, FERENCZY A. Treatment of cervical intraepithelial neoplasia using the loop electrosurgical excision procedure. *Obstet Gynecol* 1992;79:113.

81

Evaluation and management of the patient with vulvar carcinoma

C. PAUL MORROW

Vulvar carcinoma is predominantly a disease of postmenopausal women; the average age at diagnosis is 68 years. Although the etiology is unknown, vulvar cancer tends to occur in women with a history of chronic vulvar disease, including lymphogranuloma venereum, lichen sclerosus, and condyloma acuminatum. There also appears to be an increased frequency of this malignancy among women who are obese. The most common symptoms are vulvar pruritus, pain, and a lump or mass. Occasionally the patient with vulvar malignancy presents with bleeding or spotting, burning with urination, or vaginal discharge.

Pathophysiology

Approximately 90% of all carcinomas of the vulva are squamous. They usually arise from the clitoral prepuce, the labia minora, the interlabial sulcus, the Bartholin's gland area, or the posterior fourchette. The growth pattern of vulvar squamous carcinoma may be endophytic and ulcerative, or exophytic and polypoid. As the tumor enlarges, it extends to the adjacent vagina, urethra, anus, rectum, levators, or pubic ramus. There may be a concurrent invasive carcinoma or carcinoma-*in-situ* of the cervix or vagina. The lymphatics of the vulva, from the perineal body to the clitoral prepuce, drain in an orderly fashion anteriorly to the mons pubis and then laterally to the inguinal and femoral lymphatics. Under normal circumstances the vulvar lymphatics do not cross the labial–crural fold on to the medial thigh. From the inguinal nodes, the lymphatics drain to the pelvic wall nodes and then to more distant sites. The orderly lymphatic spread of squamous vulvar carcinoma is one of its most characteristic features.

Diagnosis

The diagnosis of vulvar carcinoma depends on patient cooperation and physician alertness. Management of this disease still suffers from patients' reluctance to seek medical attention and from physicians' reluctance to examine or biopsy the vulva. When a mass is present, directed biopsy is indicated immediately. Patients with a diffuse lesion of the vulva may require multiple biopsies. If a mass is small (≤ 1 cm), excisional rather than incisional biopsy is done.

The work-up begins with a careful physical examination. Since many of these patients are elderly, medical problems are common and may require attention before definitive treatment for the malignancy is carried out. In addition to a detailed evaluation of the primary lesion and the peripheral lymph nodes, colposcopic and cytologic study of the cervix and vagina are recommended.

Treatment

Broadly speaking, the treatment of choice for invasive squamous carcinoma of the vulva is radical excision and groin lymphadenectomy, bilateral unless the lesion is well lateralized and not >2 cm. If the groin nodes are positive, pelvic lymphadenectomy should be carried out on the side of the involved groin nodes. If more than one or two groin nodes are involved, radiation therapy is given postoperatively. The so-called superficial groin dissection is ineffective, as is radiation only to the groin nodes. If the disease is locally advanced with involvement of the vagina, urethra, anus, levators, or pubic ramus, more extensive surgery is necessary. Preoperative radiation therapy with or without chemotherapy often provides satisfactory control of the disease and may avoid ultraradical surgery. In the elderly or debilitated patient, wide resection alone may be warranted. Malignant melanoma is treated the same as squamous carcinoma if the thickness of the lesion is >0.75 mm. Certain sarcomas and basal cell carcinoma of the vulva can be managed by wide local excision.

Microinvasive

The recent literature has several reports on the prognosis and treatment of microinvasive carcinoma of the vulva. By definition this is an invasive lesion so early that it is adequately treated by partial vulvectomy (wide excision) without lymph node dissection. This treatment is applicable to stage I (≤2 cm) lesions with ≤1 mm of invasion and no vascular space involvement.

Prognosis

As with other malignancies, the prognosis for squamous carcinoma of the vulva is related to the extent of disease at the time of diagnosis. Lesions >3 cm in size, particularly if they extend to the urethra, vagina, or anus, are associated with a significant risk of local recurrence, and clitoral lesions have a high risk of nodal metastases. Patients with inguinal and/or pelvic node involvement are likely to have both local recurrence and distant metastases. Most recurrences are identified within 2 years of treatment. The corrected 5-year survival rate for patients with squamous carcinoma of the vulva and negative groin nodes is approximately 90%. Patients with positive groin nodes have a 5-year cure rate of about 40%, while pelvic node metastases reduce the probability of surviving 5 years to 20%.

Complications

Although radical operation and bilateral groin dissection are relatively extensive and disfiguring, they are surprisingly well tolerated by even elderly patients. Operative mortality has been <5% and usually results from pulmonary thromboembolism, stroke, or myocardial infarction. Pulmonary embolism can be minimized by the prophylactic use of low-dose heparin or pneumatic calf compression. Other postoperative complications include infection and necrosis of the groin skin flaps, and lymphocysts. Long-term postoperative problems include chronic lymphedema, genital prolapse, and urinary incontinence. Chronic lymphedema may be complicated by intermittent bouts of streptococcal cellulitis if long-term antibiotic prophylaxis is not utilized. Less radical surgery, which has become the standard of practice in recent years for lesions ≤2 cm, results in proportionately less morbidity and less disfigurement.

SUGGESTED READING

Barnes AE, Crissman JD, Schellhas HF, Azoury RS. Microinvasive carcinoma of the vulva: a clinicopathologic evaluation. *Obstet Gynecol* 1980;56:234.

Boronow RC. Combined therapy as an alternative to exenteration for locally advanced vulvovaginal cancer: rationale and results. *Cancer* 1982;49:1085.

Boyce, J, Fruchter RG, Kasambilides E, Nicastri AD, Sedlis A, Remy JC. Prognostic factors in carcinoma of the vulva. *Gynecol Oncol* 1985;20:364.

CHU J, TAMIMI HK, EK M, FIGGE DC. Stage I vulvar cancer: criteria for micro-invasion. *Obstet Gynecol* 1982;59:716.

HACKER NF, BEREK JS, LAGASSE LD, NIEBERG RK, LEUCHTER RS. Individualization of treatment for stage I squamous cell vulvar carcinoma. *Obstet Gynecol* 1984;63:155.

HOMESLEY HD, BUNDY B, SEDLIS A. Randomized study of radiation therapy (regimen I = reg. I) versus pelvic node resection (regimen II = reg. II) for patients with invasive squamous cell carcinoma of the vulva having positive groin nodes. Presented at the 16th Annual Meeting of the Society of Gynecologic Oncologists, Miami, Florida, February 3–6, 1985.

MAGRINA JF, WEBB MJ, GAFFEY TA, SYMMONDS RE. Stage I squamous cell cancer of the vulva. *Am J Obstet Gynecol* 1979;134:432.

MORLEY GW. Infiltrative carcinoma of the vulva: results of surgical treatment. *Am J Obstet Gynecol* 1976;124:874–888.

MORROW CP, RUTLEDGE FN. Melanoma of the vulva. *Obstet Gynecol* 1972;39:745.

NORI D, CAIN JM, HILARIS BS, JONES WB, LEWIS JL. Metronidazole as a radio-sensitizer and high-dose radiation in advanced vulvovaginal malignancies, a pilot study. *Gynecol Oncol* 1983;16:117.

82

Carcinoma of the vagina

LAILA I. MUDERSPACH

A primary vaginal malignancy is one arising *de novo* in the vagina without evidence of lesion continuity with the vulva distally or with the cervix proximally. Before a vaginal lesion can be considered a primary malignancy, metastases from the cervix, endometrium, ovary, gastrointestinal tract, and urinary tract must be excluded. This exclusion is very important, as metastases to the vagina are much more common than primary vaginal carcinoma. The vagina ranks fifth among primary genital organ cancer sites behind uterine, cervical, ovarian, and vulvar carcinomas. Primary carcinoma of the vagina accounts for 1–2% of all gynecologic malignancies.

Incidence

Approximately 90% of vaginal tumors have squamous cell histology. Adenocarcinoma, sarcoma, melanoma, and other rare tumors make up the remaining 8–10%. There appears to be a predominant histologic cell type for a given age level. Squamous-cell carcinoma and melanoma frequent the postmenopausal group, whereas sarcoma botryoides and a rare endodermal sinus tumor occur in infancy. The diethylstilbestrol (DES)-related clear-cell adenocarcinoma is found in the teenage years, with a peak age of 19. Leiomyosarcoma occurs in the 30–50-age group.

Etiology

Most epidemiologic studies of vaginal cancer have sought to outline the etiology of squamous-cell carcinoma, as it is the most common cell type. Although many predisposing factors have been suggested and numerous etiologic agents incriminated, no cause–effect documentation is known to date. However, the growing association between certain human papillomavirus subtypes and squamous-cell neoplasia of the cervix and vulva may become applicable to the vagina as well. There is, however, a strong association between maternal DES ingestion and clear-cell adenocarcinoma in the vagina in young women.

Diagnosis

The diagnosis of vaginal carcinoma usually is entertained because of abnormal cytology or patient symptomatology. Abnormal vaginal cytology is investigated in the same manner as abnormal cervical cytology. Vaginal bleeding and discharge of various quantities and characteristics are the most common symptoms. Less frequent symptoms include dyspareunia, urinary frequency, pelvic pain, and postcoital spotting. Few patients are asymptomatic at the time of diagnosis. Usually, the more severe the symptoms, the higher the stage and extent of tumor spread.

Actual diagnosis is made by vaginal inspection, palpation, and direct biopsy of any gross lesion. The most common tumor location is the upper posterior vagina. The lesions are usually exophytic, papillary, spongy, and friable. In the absence of gross lesions, areas of abnormality by colposcopy or nonstaining after application of Lugol's iodine solution should be biopsied.

Staging

When malignancy is confirmed, the disease should be staged (Table 82.1). Minimum investigation should include a detailed pelvic exam, cystoscopy, proctoscopy, sigmoidoscopy, intravenous pyelography, and chest X-ray. The pelvic examination should include meticulous inspection and palpation of the vulva, perineal area, vagina, and cervix. In addition to outlining uterine and ovarian pathology, the bimanual examination should detail any tumor infiltration of the paravaginal and parametrial tissues. The lymph nodes in both inguinal areas should be palpated.

Computed tomography (CT) scans of the chest, abdomen, and pelvis are indicated when the lesion is sarcomatous or locally advanced. Biopsy of palpable inguinal lymph nodes should be performed. Percutaneous fine-needle aspiration or lymph node biopsy at laparotomy may be indicated for suspicious lymph nodes seen on CT scan to determine the correct treatment choice.

Table 82.1 International Federation of Gynecology and Obstetrics (FIGO) staging for vaginal carcinoma

Stage I	The carcinoma is limited to the vaginal wall
Stage II	The carcinoma has involved the subvaginal tissue but has not extended to the pelvic wall
Stage III	The carcinoma has extended to the pelvic wall
Stage IV	The carcinoma has extended beyond the true pelvis or has involved the mucosa of the bladder or rectum. A bullous edema, as such, does not permit a case to be allotted to stage IV
Stage IVa	Spread of the carcinoma to adjacent organs
Stage IVb	Spread of the carcinoma to distant organs

Treatment

The treatment modality depends on histologic cell type, tumor location and volume, potential for spread, age of the patient, desire to retain sexual function, and proximity of the tumor to the bladder and rectum. Surgery is the treatment of choice for melanoma, sarcoma, and adenocarcinoma (including the DES-related clear-cell variety), and early stage squamous-cell lesions. Surgical procedures range from partial vaginectomy to total pelvic exenteration, depending on size, location, stage, and prognosis. Radiation therapy is the treatment of choice for large or advanced squamous-cell tumors. Irradiation treatment usually entails 4000–5000 cGy of whole-pelvis radiation therapy and two intravaginal applications. The intravaginal applications consist of placing radioactive sources in the vagina (tandem and ovoids), placing radioactive sources in the paravaginal tissues (interstitial needle implants), or a combination of both. When necessary, a radiation boost dose via a smaller treatment field can be given to the involved area.

Prognosis

Prognostic data indicate an approximate overall 5-year survival rate of 5% for melanoma, 35% for sarcoma, 60% for clear-cell adenocarcinoma, and 35–45% for squamous-cell carcinoma. The 5-year survival rates for early-stage, clear-cell adenocarcinoma and squamous-cell carcinoma are significantly higher than the collective survival rate.

SUGGESTED READING

CHU AM, BEECHINOR R. Survival and recurrence patterns in radiation treatment of carcinoma of the vagina. *Gynecol Oncol* 1984;19:298.

KUCERA H, LANCER M, SMEKA LG, *et al*. Radiotherapy of primary carcinoma of the vagina: management and results of different therapy schemes. *Gynecol Oncol* 1985;21:87.

MORROW CP, CURTIN JP, TOWNSEND DE (eds). *Tumors of the Vagina in Synopsis of Gynecologic Oncology*. 4th edn. New York: Churchill Livingstone 1993.

PEREZ CA, CAMEL HM. Long term follow up in radiation therapy of carcinoma of the vagina. *Cancer* 1982;49:1308.

83

Cancer of the cervix uteri

JOHN B. SCHLAERTH

Epidemiology

Multiple sexual partners and beginning sexual intercourse at an early age are generally accepted as high-risk criteria for cervical cancer. Recently, evidence that certain subtypes of the human papillomavirus may be causally related to cervical cancer has been accumulating. This finding, if true, would confirm the long-held suspicion that cervical cancer is a sexually transmitted disease. Cigarette smoking is also identified as increasing the risk for cervical carcinoma.

Clinical features

Age

Cervical cancer is rare before age 20. Recent data suggest that the mean age is decreasing – from the mid 50s a few decades ago to the 40s now. In fact, in a National Cancer Institute study, it was the most common invasive cancer in women aged 25–29 and second most common among those aged 30–34. There is a suggestion that the younger the patient, the more virulent the cancer.

Symptoms

Abnormal vaginal bleeding, especially contact (postcoital) bleeding, and vaginal discharge are the usual presenting symptoms. Pain usually denotes advanced, neglected cases. Some cases are asymptomatic and these are usually detected by Pap smear screening.

Signs

Unfortunately, the combination of the sequelae of childbirth, the contrasting squamous and mucinous epithelia on the portio of the cervix, and varying degrees of cervicitis can impart a gross appearance to an otherwise normal cervix that is highly suggestive of cancer. Because this appearance is so commonly encountered, missing or misinterpreting early cancers as normal is a scenario that is repeated too often. Ulcerative, granular, friable, exophytic, and necrotic are the terms most often used to describe the typical visual appearance of cancer of the cervix.

As a cancer grows, a mass involving both the cervix and vagina and then the paravaginal, parametrial, vesicovaginal, or rectovaginal tissues becomes apparent on inspection and palpation.

Diagnosis

Pap smears can detect clinically occult cervical cancers and their precursors. Unfortunately, they are accompanied by a false-negative rate as high as 20%. This false negativity is especially true for cancerous as compared with precancerous changes. Unawareness of this false negativity may account for misunderstanding the place of the Pap smear in clinical medicine. The Pap smear is a screening test for cervical cancer and its precursors for asymptomatic women who have no signs compatible with cervical neoplasia. Abnormal vaginal bleeding, persistent or nonspecific vaginal discharge, and an abnormal-appearing cervix are all indications for colposcopy and biopsy, not a Pap smear by itself.

Pathology

Of cervical cancers, 90% are of the squamous-cell variety. The squamous-cell subtypes are the keratinizing large cell, nonkeratinizing large cell, small cell, mucoepidermoid, and verrucous, with the majority belonging to two large-cell varieties. Adenocarcinomas comprise 5–10% of cervical cancers and include mucinous (most common), endometrioid, clear-cell, adenoid cystic, and glassy cell types. Adenocarcinomas seem to have a poorer prognosis than squamous cell cancer.

Adenosquamous, a mixed variety, is well known. Probably depending on their own interests and thoroughness, different authors have reported that this variety accounts for 5–30% of all cervical cancer. Melanomas, carcinoids, sarcomas, and lymphomas are rare histologic types.

Degree of differentiation and involvement of lymphatic spaces are also features that may be present in biopsy material and that confer a poorer prognosis.

Natural history

Typically, cervical cancer arises from the squamocolumnar junction at or near the portio of the cervix. It can arise from a focus of dysplastic epithelium which has preexisted for months or years at this site or can arise *de novo*. The diagnosis of cancer depends on the neoplasm penetrating the basement membrane and invading the underlying stroma or vasculature. Two growth phenomena are then possible, separately or together.

First, expansive geographic spread is possible in all directions. Besides expanding the cervix, the cancer can spread to and down the vagina. It can spread laterally to the paracervical, parametrial, and paravaginal tissues and then to the pelvic walls. It can spread anteriorly to the bladder and posteriorly to the rectum. Finally, it can penetrate the posterior cervix or uterine fundus and then disseminate intraperitoneally.

Second, access to lymphatic spaces can be gained in the cervical stroma. Metastasis to lymph nodes then can take place. Lymph node involvement tends to be sequential, beginning with the groups closest to the cancer. Lymph node groups in this sequence are the parametrial, the obturator, the hypogastric and external iliac, the common iliac and presacral, and the paraaortic lymph nodes. Lymphatic drainage then passes to the thoracic duct and from there to the scalene lymph nodes. Thereafter, venous access is attained, and widespread visceral metastasis is possible.

The typical advanced case exhibits lymphedema of the legs from lymphatic obstruction, leg pain from sciatic nerve involvement, and uremia from ureteral obstruction. The uncontrolled tumor mass produces a disagreeable odor and bloody discharge. Vesicovaginal or rectovaginal fistulas may be present, which add to the pain and odor. Cachexia and fever are evident, and death classically comes from uremia.

Staging

The staging system for cervical cancer was revised in 1985 and is given in Table 83.1. This is a clinical staging system, and the only information allowed for determining stage is from history and physical examination, biopsy, chest X-ray, intravenous urography, barium enema, cystoscopy, and sigmoidoscopy. Information from computed tomography scans or other imaging techniques or laparotomy may be useful for directing

Table 83.1 Stages of carcinoma of the cervix – FIGO

Stage	Definition
Stage 0	Carcinoma-*in-situ*, intraepithelial carcinoma. Cases of stage 0 should not be included in any therapeutic statistics for invasive carcinoma
Stage I	The cervical carcinoma is confined strictly to the cervix (extension to the corpus should be disregarded)
Ia	The carcinoma is confined strictly to the cervix (extension to the corpus should be disregarded)
Ia1	Minimal microscopically evident stromal invasion
Ia2	Lesions detected microscopically that can be measured. The upper limit of the measurements should not show a depth of invasion of >5 mm taken from the base of the epithelium, either surface or glandular, from which it orginates, and a second dimension, the horizonatal spread, must not exceed 7 mm. Larger lesions should be staged as Ib
Ib	Lesions of greater dimensions than stage Ia2, whether seen clinically or not. Preformed space involvement should not alter the staging but should be specifically recorded so as to determine whether it should affect treatment decisions in the future.
Stage II	The carcinoma extends beyond the cervix, but it has not extended on to the pelvic wall. The carcinoma involves the vagina, but not as far as the lower third
IIa	No obvious parametrial involvement
IIb	Obvious parametrial involvement
Stage III	The carcinoma has extended to the pelvic wall. On rectal examination, there is no cancer-free space between the tumor and the pelvic wall. The tumor involves the lower third of the vagina. All cases with a hydronephrosis or nonfunctioning kidney should be included, unless they are known to be due to other causes
IIIa	No extension on the pelvic wall, but involvement of the lower third of the vagina
IIIb	Extension on the pelvic wall or hydronephrosis or nonfunctioning kidney
Stage IV	The carcinoma has extended beyond the true pelvis or has clinically involved the mucosa of the bladder or rectum
IVa	Spread of the growth to adjacent organs
IVb	Spread to distant organs

Table 83.2 Diagnostic tests in cervical cancer

Routine
History + physical examinations
Biopsy
Chest X-ray
Intravenous pyelogram

To clarify questions raised by routine tests
Cystoscopy, urinary cytology
Sigmoidoscopy, barium enema, stool for occult blood
Bone scan

Potentially useful
Computed tomography scan, pelvis and abdomen
Laparotomy for staging
Serum tumor markers CEA, SCCA

CEA, Carcino embryonic antigen; SCCA, squamous-cell carcinoma antigen.

therapy but is not admissible for staging. The diagnostic work-up is listed in Table 83.2.

Treatment

Radiation therapy

Radiation therapy is potentially curative, has general applicability to all stages of cervical cancer, and is generally without severe side-effects.

Radiation therapy is directed not only at the visible cancer, but also to the entire pelvis, as this is the location of the tissues at risk for the earliest metastases. Usually there are two parts to this therapy. First, external beam pelvic radiation therapy is administered as an outpatient procedure daily on weekdays for 4–6 weeks (approximately 4000–5000 rad or cGy). About 2 weeks thereafter, the first of two intracavitary treatments is given. Under general anesthesia, a tandem and ovoids are packed in place in the uterus and vagina. Following this, X-rays are taken to insure correct positioning relative to the tumor, bladder, rectum, and bony pelvis. Radioactive cesium (^{137}Cs) or radium (^{224}Ra) then is loaded into the tandem and ovoids. The radioactive sources remain in place with the patient at bedrest for 2–3 days. A second intracavitary application is repeated about 2 weeks later. Diarrhea, fatigue, and urinary urgency accompany radiation therapy.

About 60% of all patients with cervical cancer will be cured by radiation therapy, and approximately 5% will experience severe morbidity, i.e., vesicovaginal or rectovaginal fistula, small bowel obstruction, or necrosis. Later, symptoms of proctosigmoiditis, hemorrhagic cystitis, and vaginal necrosis also can occur. Death from therapy or from complications of therapy can occur.

Surgery

It is only in the earliest stages of cervical cancer (stage Ia1, Ia2, Ib, and some stage IIa) that surgical removal of affected and at-risk tissues can be accomplished with cure rates equal to radiation therapy and with acceptable morbidity and disability. The standard operation for early-stage cancers is the radical abdominal hysterectomy and bilateral pelvic lymphadenectomy. An exception to this is considered later in the section on microinvasion. The benefits of surgical therapy are most apparent in, but by no means confined to, the young. The ovaries can be retained, and vaginal shortening is usually minimal, whereas radiation therapy destroys ovarian function and has a somewhat unpredictable tendency to shorten and narrow the vagina. Perhaps the greatest feature of the surgery is the detailed examination of the resected tissues it allows. Death from pulmonary embolus, infection, or hemorrhage, however, can occur. Urinary tract fistula and lymphocyst formation may lead to further surgery. Most women experience temporary dysfunction of the urinary bladder.

Combined therapy

There has been recent interest in the possible improvement in survival of patients with large (>6 cm) bulky cervical cancers confined to the cervix or with minimal vaginal or parametrial extension. It is suggested that pelvic external beam radiation and one intracavitary application followed by hysterectomy not only decrease the incidence of local recurrences in the pelvis, compared with radiation therapy or surgery as sole treatment modalities, but also improve overall survival rates from the disease. There is also great interest in improving cure rates for cervical cancer treated by radiation therapy without increasing toxicity. There are indications that combining radiation therapy with drugs such as hydroxyurea and perhaps 5-fluorouracil or cisplatin will improve cure rates. There are suggestions that adding hyperthermia to radiation therapy also may be beneficial.

Posttreatment surveillance

Most recurrences appear within 2 years of treatment. Essentially all, with few exceptions, appear within 5 years of treatment. Follow-up examinations every 2 or 3 months during the first 2 years and every 4–6 months during the following 3 years are recommended. Inspection of the vagina and cervix, bimanual rectovaginal/abdominal examination, palpation of inguinal and cervical lymph nodes, and examination of the abdomen and legs are particularly important. A Pap smear should be done. Yearly chest X-rays and intravenous pyelograms every 6 months for 2 years are recommended. There is growing evidence that elevations of the serum tumor markers, CEA and SCCA, can be the first hint that the cancer is recurring. Conversely, normal levels may support the opinion that all is well. At this time, it seems reasonable to include these markers in the plan of post-treatment surveillance.

Recurrence

In most patients whose disease recurs after therapy, the problems mentioned under the section on natural history will develop. There are, however, clinical situations in which a cure is possible after recurrence.

A recurrence confined to the central pelvis following radical hysterectomy and bilateral pelvic lymphadenectomy can be treated with external pelvic radiation followed by vaginal intracavitary radiation therapy. Late-appearing (>2 years) lung metastasis as the sole site of recurrence can be treated by wedge resection/lobectomy with some hope of cure. Most patients with recurrence are incurable and palliative measures, i.e., systemic chemotherapy or focal radiation therapy, may be indicated.

Some patients with pelvic recurrence after radiation therapy can be cured by pelvic exenteration. This most radical pelvic surgery has seen numerous changes and improvements in recent years. The development of continent urinary diversions, neovaginal constructions with the use of grafts, low rectal anastomoses via stapling devices, and reconstruction of the pelvic floor have markedly improved morbidity and disability from this operation and provided the only chance for cure for these women.

Special situations

Microinvasion

Microinvasion is the concept of a cancer so small and/or early in its development that simple excision of the organ of origin is the standard curative therapy. Criteria for the diagnosis of microinvasion are that the cancer penetrates <3 mm beneath the basement membrane of origin, there is no lymph/vascular space involvement, and there are no confluent, interanastomosing cords of neoplasm. Equally important is that the diagnosis be made on a cone biopsy or hysterectomy specimen with clear margins. Sectioning and step sectioning, beyond the standard amount, should be done to rule out the presence of a more advanced lesion. Standard therapy for microinvasion is a simple hysterectomy.

Unfortunately, the diagnostic standards that have evolved for the concept of microinvasion are not reflected in the current International Federation of Gynecology and Obstetrics (FIGO) staging system. This double standard leads to understandable confusion. Most but not all cases of stage Ia1 and some cases of Ia2 cervical cancers will qualify as microinvasion. This is so because vascular space involvement is not included in the staging but is important in the concept of microinvasion and because the invasive depth criteria differ.

Occasionally, a patient is interested in preserving fertility. In this case, review of all pathologic material with a consultant who is familiar with microinvasive lesions may result in a decision that no further treatment is required after the conization. Some time – 4–6 months – should pass after the cone biopsy to reveal that there is no persistent neoplasia before pregnancy is attempted.

Pregnancy

In the first half of pregnancy, cervical cancer management is the same as in the nonpregnant state. If radiation therapy is used, it may be necessary to remove the nonviable products of conception before intracavitary therapy is performed, either by curettage or hysterotomy. In the later part of pregnancy, cesarean section is advised when fetal maturity is assured. At the time of cesarean section, radical hysterectomy and bilateral pelvic lymphadenectomy can be performed for treatment of early cancers. For advanced cancers, radiation therapy begins shortly after cesarean section has been performed. Delivery through a cancerous cervix should be avoided because the potential for lacerations and hemorrhage exists. There is also a possibility that dissemination of the cancer can occur through vaginal delivery.

Pregnancies with cervical cancer diagnosed from the mid second trimester on are difficult management problems. Commonly, a judgment is required whether or not to await fetal maturity. A wait of 8 weeks traditionally has been the maximum delay permitted to allow for fetal maturity. With advances in neonatal nurseries, the rate of fetal survival once expected for a 36-week gestation now applies to earlier gestations. Granting this, cervical cancer now diagnosed earlier in pregnancy may be managed expectantly. It is reasonable to assume that this trend in expectant management of cervical cancer in the second trimester will continue as advances in neonatal medicine continue.

The extent of the tumor also may play a role in decision-making. A cone biopsy with clear margins showing early stromal invasion in the first trimester can allow further treatment to be deferred until postpartum.

Paraaortic lymph node metastasis

It appears that some patients with cervical cancer whose only extrapelvic site of metastasis is the paraaortic lymph nodes can be cured. Patients most likely to have paraaortic lymph node metastases are those with large (>6 cm) stage I lesions and stage II, III, and IV cancers.

Computed tomography scans as diagnostic tools have limitations in this setting. At the extremes, they diagnose very well large metastatic nodes that cannot be treated for cure, and they miss small metastatic nodes that can be treated for cure. Lymph node biopsy via laparotomy is the best diagnostic technique, but it is expensive and risky. The patients most likely to benefit from an aggressive diagnostic and therapeutic approach are those with small aortic lymph node metastases, with no tumor in the scalene lymph nodes or other sites of metastasis, and with a potentially curable cancer in the pelvis.

SUGGESTED READING

HOLLOWAY RW, TO A, MORADI M, BOOTS L, WATSON N, SHINGLETOM NY. Monitoring the course of cervical carcinoma with the squamous cell carcinoma serum radioimmunoassay. *Obstet Gynecol* 1989;74:944–949.

SIMON NL, CORE H, SLINGLETON HM, SOONG SJ, ORR JW, HATCH KD. Study of superficially invasive carcinoma of the cervix. *Obstet Gynecol* 1986;68:19–24.

STEHMAN FB, BUNDY BN, KEYS H, CURRIE JL, MORTEL R, CREASMAN WT. Randomized trial of hydroxyurea versus misonidazole adjunct to radiation therapy in carcinoma of the cervix. *Am J Obstet Gynecol* 1988;159:87–94.

WALKER J, BLOSS JD, LIAO SY, BERMAN M, BERGEN S, WILCZYNSKI SP. Human papillomavirus genotype as a prognostic indication in carcinoma of the uterine cervix. *Obstet Gynecol* 1989;74:781–785.

84

Endometrial hyperplasia

JOHN B. SCHLAERTH

Endometrial hyperplasia is a spectrum of alterations of the endometrial glands and stroma, ranging from physiologically normal endometrium to endometrial carcinoma. Until recently the terminology for these disorders had not been standardized. In 1985 Kurman *et al.* proposed a classification system based on histologic architecture and cellular atypism. In a relatively short period of time this system has gained acceptance. There are three subdivisions in this classification: simple, complex, and atypical. In *simple hyperplasia* there is a benign proliferation in the number of endometrial glands. *Complex hyperplasia* is characterized by glands with irregular outlines that demonstrate marked structural complexity and back-to-back crowding. *Atypical hyperplasia* designates a proliferation of glands exhibiting cytologic atypia in which varying degrees of nuclear atypia and loss of polarity are present.

This system reflects the progression that hyperplasias are capable of and each type represents a state of disease with an increased likelihood of resultant cancer if therapy is not undertaken.

Endometrial hyperplasia is clinically important because not only can it develop into endometrial cancer, but also it can result in heavy bleeding, can occur with and complicate infertility, and it can be secondary to estrogen-producing diseases of the ovaries. The management of endometrial hyperplasia depends on the woman's age relative to her reproductive life, the histologic severity of the endometrial lesion, and her future reproductive expectations.

Postpubescent women

Endometrial hyperplasia usually presents as a menstrual cycle irregularity and may culminate in heavy vaginal bleeding. The diagnosis then becomes apparent when a endometrial biopsy or cervical dilatation and curettage (D&C) is performed. If an endometrial biopsy reveals any degree of hyperplasia, a diagnostic D&C should be done to evaluate completely the hyperplasia and exclude carcinoma. A serum estradiol also should be obtained to exclude an autonomous subclinical source for estrogen.

Following the D&C, simple and complex hyperplasias can be treated with monthly cyclic progestins, such as medroxyprogesterone acetate 10 mg for 10 days. This will prevent further episodes of heavy bleeding and insure regular withdrawal bleeding.

For the patient in this group who has atypical hyperplasia, the therapy is more involved. Long-term progestin therapy is given to reverse the hyperplasia. Many regimens have been used with some success. Our preference is to use megestrol acetate 20 mg/day. We obtain a follow-up endometrial biopsy after 3 months of progestin therapy to confirm regression of the hyperplastic lesion. Treatment is then discontinued if responsiveness to progestins is documented. At that time these women should continue to receive monthly cyclic progestin therapy, using medroxyprogesterone acetate 10 mg daily for 10 days to insure regular shedding of the endometrium. The usual stimulus for the hyperplasia in these patients is unopposed estrogen from anovulation.

These women should not be presumed to be infertile, as ovulation may resume spontaneously. Once the endometrial hyperplasia has regressed, it presents no contraindication to the use of oral contraceptives as an alternative to monthly cyclic progestin therapy.

Infertile women

Another group presenting with endometrial hyperplasia are infertile women of reproductive age. The association of infertility, anovulation, and endometrial hyperplasia makes an endometrial biopsy an important step in evaluating these patients. Endometrial hyperplasia is usually secondary to unopposed estrogen from disordered ovulation. Nevertheless, before embarking on a costly and involved infertility work-up, exclusion of an autonomous estrogen source by serum estradiol determination is wise. For patients with simple or complex hyperplasia, the routine therapy is to induce ovulation after a D&C is done to exclude carcinoma. For patients with atypical hyperplasia diagnosed by biopsy and D&C, it is important to document histologically that regression has occurred before attempting to induce ovulation. Ovulation may not occur for several months, and during this time the endometrium would continue to be stimulated by endogenous estrogens. Also, pregnancy can occur even if the premalignant lesion does not revert to a normal pattern. Regression almost always can be accomplished with megestrol 20 mg daily for 3 months. The endometrium then is biopsied to confirm regression.

Perimenopausal women

As a woman ends her reproductive years and ovulation tends to become less regular, endometrial hyperplasia may occur due to the presence of unopposed estrogen. Any abnormal bleeding in perimenopausal women should be evaluated to rule out the presence of endometrial or endocervical carcinoma.

With a fractional D&C diagnosis of simple or complex hyperplasia, the patient can be maintained on monthly progestins such as medroxyprogesterone acetate 10 mg for 10 days a month to insure regular withdrawal bleeding. However, at times, perimenopausal patients with simple or complex hyperplasia have difficulties complying with progestin therapy, which they may have to continue for several years. In addition, these patients continue to be at increased risk for developing endometrial cancer after the menopause. Therefore hysterectomy may be a suitable alternative for these patients.

If atypical hyperplasia is present, hysterectomy is indicated in the medically suitable patient. These women appear to be at higher risk for eventually developing endometrial carcinoma after cessation of menses. Also the sensitivity of the hyperplasia to progestins declines with age.

If a woman cannot be treated surgically, megestrol acetate 20 mg daily is indicated. Histologic regression should be documented 3 months later, and therapy should continue until the menopause. Again, excluding autonomous subclinical sources of estrogen by serum estradiol determination is worthwhile.

Postmenopausal women

Postmenopausal patients not on estrogen therapy who present with vaginal bleeding should have a fractional D&C to rule out endometrial and endocervical carcinoma. If simple hyperplasia is found in women who are <5 years postmenopausal, an endometrial biopsy should be performed 3 months after the D&C to confirm regression.

The presence of hyperplasia in a woman more than 5 years after menopause or who has persistence of these lesions after D&C should not be followed expectantly. An endogenous estrogen source (granulosa–theca-cell tumors, ovarian cortical stromal thecosis, other gonadal stromal or metastatic neoplasms to the ovary) should be considered by serum estradiol measurements. Although there is some evidence that further observation or progestin therapy may suffice for these women, we have preferred hysterectomy and bilateral salpingo-oophorectomy.

The presence of complex hyperplasia in this age group is a significant problem. Occasionally, surgery is contraindicated in such patients. Daily megestrol acetate 20 mg indefinitely is a reasonable treatment in such patients, and a follow-up biopsy is indicated after 3 months of treatment. Interestingly, only a minority of patients exhibit regression of the hyperplasia. Most show that the hyperplasia is still present but under the retarding effects of the progestin. In these cases especially, therapy should continue indefinitely with serial biopsies to insure that hormonal control is not lost. Lastly, the hyperplasia in some patients will be resistant to progestins and will cause reconsideration of not operating or the use of intrauterine radiation therapy.

The postmenopausal patient on estrogen replacement therapy who has endometrial hyperplasia also should have a fractional D&C to rule out endometrial carcinoma. In the absence of atypical hyperplasia, estrogen replacement therapy can be resumed with the addition of progestins, i.e., medroxyprogesterone acetate 10 mg/day for the last 10 days of each month's estrogen treatment. Withdrawal bleeding will then follow. Other acceptable alternatives include estrogen and progestin (medroxyprogesterone acetate 5 mg) every day or Mondays through Fridays. If progestins were already being utilized with the estrogens, consideration should be given to increasing the progestin dose, increasing the duration of progestin use each month, or both. Atypical hyperplasia occurring during postmenopausal estrogen replacement therapy is treated best by hysterectomy and bilateral salpingo-oophorectomy.

Basic principles

The management of all patients presenting with endometrial hyperplasia is facilitated by keeping in mind a few principles. The cause of endometrial hyperplasia is unopposed estrogen. A firm understanding of the source of and indications for estrogen is a prerequisite to definitive therapy. Patients with endometrial hyperplasia may be harboring an endometrial carcinoma, and until the endometrial cavity is thoroughly evaluated by D&C, one cannot disregard this possibility. Finally, the synthetic oral progestins have a major role in the management of these patients and, especially in young women, the progestins can eliminate most endometrial hyperplasias.

New possibilities

Diagnosis

Transvaginal ultrasound examinations have proven very useful in evaluating the adnexa and the uterus. There is much interest in screening women for endometrial cancer and in evaluating women for abnormal uterine bleeding with this techinique. The thickness of the endometrium can be measured and it may be that significant endometrial pathology can be ruled out by this test. Hysteroscopic examination at the time of elective D&C is becoming popular. The hysteroscope adds precision to the sampling and can insure that all endometrial pathology present has been sampled. Some have suggested that hysteroscopy should be an integral part of every elective D&C.

Therapy

Uncommonly, a woman will be seen with hyperplasia resistant to standard progestin therapy who wishes to retain her fertility. Higher doses of progestins (megestrol acetate 20–320 mg/day), antiestrogen therapy (tamoxifen 10–20 mg b.i.d.), and gonadotropin-releasing hormone agonist therapy seem to be forms of treatment with the possibility of benefit for these women.

SUGGESTED READING

FERENCZY A, GELFAND M. The biologic significance of cytologic atypia in progestogen treated endometrial. *Am J Obstet Gynecol* 1989;160:126–131.

GAL D. Hormonal therapy for lesions of the endometrium. *Semin Oncol* (Suppl 4) 1986;13:33–36.

GAL D, EDMAN CD, VELLIOS F, *et al*. Long term effect of megesterol acetate in the treatment of endometrial hyperplasia. *Am J Obstet Gynecol* 1983;146:316.

GAMBRELL RD. The prevention of endometrial cancer in postmenopausal women with progestins. *Maturitas* 1978;1:107.

KURMAN RJ, KAMINSKI PF, NORRIS HJ. The behavior of endometrial hyperplasia. A long term study of "untreated" hyperplasia in 170 patients. *Cancer* 1985;56: 403–412.

VARNER RE, SPARKS JM, CAMERON CD, ROBERTS LL, SOONG SJ. Transvaginal sonography of the endometrium in postmenopausal women. *Obstet Gynecol* 1991;782:195–199.

85

Evaluation and management of endometrial carcinoma

C. PAUL MORROW

Incidence

Endometrial carcinoma is the most common malignancy of the female genital tract in the USA. Among all malignancies in women, it is exceeded in frequency only by breast and colorectal cancer. According to American Cancer Society projections, 33 000 new cases of endometrial carcinoma are expected annually, and each year 5500 women will die from it. The average age at the time of diagnosis is 58 years. The incidence at age 40 is <10 cases per 100 000 women per year. The incidence rises to 60:100 000 at age 50 and reaches a peak of 125:100 000 at age 70.

Risk factors

Constitutional factors associated with an approximately twofold increase in the risk of developing endometrial cancer are obesity, infertility, late menopause, and diabetes mellitus. Several studies have shown an association between the use of postmenopausal estrogens and a two- to sixfold increased risk for developing endometrial cancer. Although over 90% of cases occur in postmenopausal women, the obese, infertile, pre-menopausal woman characterized by the polycystic ovary syndrome is also at relatively high risk.

Endometrial carcinoma is predominantly a disease of middle- and upper-class women, and studies have suggested an associated risk with breast, ovarian, and colon carcinoma. There have been a few reported instances of the familial occurrence of endometrial cancer.

Symptoms

The first sign of endometrial carcinoma is usually abnormal vaginal bleeding after or around the time of the menopause. Methods of evaluation are discussed in detail in Chapter 67. Any woman with abnormal and perimenopausal or postmenopausal bleeding requires a careful evaluation for genital tract cancer.

Common presumptions regarding postmenopausal bleeding that can lead to a delay in diagnosis are: (1) that the bleeding is due to supplemental estrogens in women receiving such therapy; (2) that the bleeding is of vaginal origin in women with atrophic vaginitis; (3) that the bleeding is from the endometrium, when it may be arising from cervical, vaginal, or ovarian carcinoma; and (4) that the bleeding is not sufficient to require evaluation. Less commonly, the patient with endometrial carcinoma may present with enlargement of the uterus without bleeding, or with chronic vaginal discharge (pyometra).

Prognostic factors and spread pattern

Prognosis and, therefore, survival are related to the histologic degree of differentiation, the extent of disease at the time of diagnosis, the quality of the therapy, and the patient's medical status. Pretreatment evaluation is directed toward the definition of these factors.

The histology of endometrial carcinoma is often not straightforward. Distinguishing between severe atypical hyperplasia and very well-differentiated adenocarcinoma is a frequent problem. At the other end of the spectrum it can be difficult to distinguish between poorly differentiated endometrial carcinoma and endometrial sarcoma. As with many cancers, the degree of histologic differentiation may vary from one area of tumor to another. If the tumor is not adequately sampled, an error in assessing the histologic grade may occur. In addition to the poorly differentiated lesions, papillary serous and clear-cell carcinomas have a poorer than average prognosis.

Endometrial carcinoma usually arises in the fundus and tends to remain localized. Initially it spreads by extension within the endometrium and then invades the myometrium, advancing toward the isthmus and cervix. It can invade the full thickness of the uterine musculature and disseminate within the peritoneal cavity. Occasionally, it presents with parametrial invasion or metastases to the vagina, particularly the suburethral area.

Less well appreciated is the proclivity of this disease to spread via the lymphatics. Approximately 10% of patients with clinical stage I endometrial carcinoma have pelvic lymph node metastasis. The probability of pelvic node involvement increases as the tumor becomes less differentiated, and also increases as the tumor invades the myometrium more deeply. Other common, clinically occult sites of spread are the adnexa, cervix, paraaortic nodes, and peritoneal cavity.

Work-up and diagnosis

Based on this preceding information, the preoperative evaluation should include the following: a general physical examination with special attention to the supraclavicular and inguinal lymph nodes, and abdominal masses. After inspection and palpation of the introitus, the suburethral area, the vaginal walls, and the cervix, a Papanicolaou smear is taken. On bimanual rectovaginal examination, the uterus, adnexa, and parametria are evaluated. The uterine cavity is sounded. A fractional curettage is performed, submitting the endocervical and endometrial specimens separately. (This can usually be done in the office.)

In terms of a metastatic survey, only a chest X-ray is needed unless the patient has a poorly differentiated cancer or evidence of extrauterine spread. In these cases computed tomogram scan or magnetic resonance imaging of the abdomen and pelvis is recommended. Many of these patients have medical problems related to age and obesity; evaluation for diabetes, hypertension, and renal disease is required.

Management of clinically localized cases

The cornerstone in the management of endometrial carcinoma apparently confined to the uterine corpus is total hysterectomy, including removal of the tubes and ovaries. In most instances, an abdominal procedure should be done through a vertical incision in order further to evaluate the extent of disease. The aortic and pelvic areas are palpated for evidence of retroperitoneal node metastases. Enlarged or suspicious nodes should be removed or biopsied. Cytologic washings are taken from the pelvis, and the abdomen is carefully explored.

Removal of the adnexa is part of the therapy, as they may be sites of occult metastases. In addition, the ovaries may contain an occult ovarian tumor or produce estrogen that might stimulate residual, occult disease. It is not necessary to remove a margin of vaginal cuff, nor does there appear to be any benefit to freeing up the ureters and taking extraparametrial tissue. The entire cervix, however, should be excised with the uterus.

The pathologist's evaluation of the specimen is very important. The least differentiated area of the tumor, the greatest depth of myometrial invasion, vascular space invasion, and the proximity of the tumor to the isthmus or cervix must be identified. Each of these factors has prognostic as well as therapeutic implications. In addition, accurate study of the peritoneal cytology, lymph nodes, and adnexa is crucial.

If the lesion is grade 2 or 3 and there is deep (>50%) myometrial invasion or extension to the isthmus on frozen section, selective pelvic and paraaortic lymph node dissections are performed. The dissections are not meant to be therapeutic but are rather a selected sampling of the nodes.

Postoperatively, all patients with deep (>33%) myometrial invasion or a poorly differentiated cancer should have pelvic radiation, 4000–5000 rad. Documented aortic node or pelvic node metastasis is an indication for extended field radiation. Should more extensive disease be encountered, adjunctive hormonal therapy (e.g., Megace 320 mg/day orally) is indicated for patients with measurable levels of progesterone receptor, while chemotherapy is recommended for patients with negative receptors.

Preoperative radiation

Contraindications

Those who employ preoperative radiation should be familiar with the contraindications to its use, i.e., the indications for surgery first. The most common is the presence of a stage I, grade 1 lesion, which seldom requires adjuvant therapy. Other contraindications are the presence of an adnexal mass, a history of or concurrent pelvic abscess (tuboovarian, appendiceal, diverticular), the presence of pyometra, numerous prior abdominal surgical procedures, previous abdominal–perineal resection, and pelvic kidney. The patient who fears radiation, who is unable to cooperate during a prolonged treatment course, or who has had prior radiation (cervical cancer) is also not a candidate for radiation therapy. Preoperative intracavitary radiation (single implant) is a reasonable way of managing patients with a grade 2 or 3 lesion, but there is no established indication for preoperative whole-pelvis radiation.

Radiation–hysterectomy interval

If a course of preoperative radiation is undertaken, it is common practice to wait several weeks before hysterectomy is carried out. The reasons for waiting are generally as follows: (1) resolution of radiation reaction; (2) regression of a large, carcinomatous mass lesion; and (3) eradication of the uterine cancer ("sterilization" of the uterus). The first two are presumed to facilitate the surgical procedure, while the last is thought to provide maximum if not absolute protection against intraoperative tumor spread. None of these reasons has any compelling data to support it. What seems to be of greater relevance is that delay may be deleterious, since it provides additional time for any residual viable uterine tumor (present in 25–50% of cases) to involve extrauterine sites. Since there is no way to identify preoperatively those cases that have total eradication of the uterine tumor, individualization of the radiation–hysterectomy time interval would not be reliable. The waiting policy is probably most unsuited to high-grade cancers, considering they are the most rapidly growing and most aggressive. The poorly differentiated tumors are also the most difficult to destroy by preoperative radiation. To avoid the problem of delay and to utilize the surgical staging data, only preoperative intracavitary therapy should be employed. This can be followed by hysterectomy within a week.

Special management problems

Postoperative diagnosis of endometrial cancer

Occasionally endometrial cancer is an unexpected finding in the hysterectomy specimen. This situation usually arises after a vaginal hysterectomy. If the uterus is routinely opened in the operating suite, most such problems can be avoided. Our recommendation is to reoperate to remove the adnexa and surgically stage the patient when the lesion is deeply invasive or is poorly differentiated.

Medically inoperable patient

Severe cardiopulmonary disease is the primary reason why a patient with endometrial carcinoma is deemed medically inoperable. Obviously, clinical judgment will vary a great deal in these cases. Nevertheless, in everyone's experience there will be patients for whom the risk of anesthesia and surgery exceeds the likely benefits of hysterectomy. For the patient with a grade 1 lesion and a temporary contraindication to general anesthesia or who is altogether unsuited to radiation therapy or surgery, high-dose progestin is the treatment of choice. All other cases are given radiation therapy. If the uterus is small, tandem, and ovoid, intracavitary therapy alone is used. The patient with a large uterus probably stands a better chance of cure by the Heyman packing technique. Whether radiation or hormonal therapy is administered, endometrial biopsy or curettage should be performed after 3 months. If the cancer is still present, the contraindications to surgery must be reassessed.

The young woman

The diagnosis of endometrial carcinoma during the reproductive years should always be viewed with skepticism since the malignancy is uncommon and confusion with hyperplasia is frequent. The histologic distinction between atypical hyperplasia, which can be treated hormonally, and well-differentiated carcinoma, which should be treated surgically, is to some extent subjective. When preservation of fertility is a significant clinical factor, the diagnosis of well-differentiated carcinoma should be based on endometrial curettings, and consultation with a recognized authority in the field of endometrial pathology is recommended. Equivocal lesions should be managed in the same manner as atypical hyperplasia, i.e., continuous high-dose progestin (medroxyprogesterone acetate 20–40 mg by mouth daily) should be administered for 3 months. Endometrial biopsy is done at that time to demonstrate that the lesion is responding. If the lesion has been reversed within 6 months (based upon dilatation and curettage), ovulation induction can proceed. After the woman has completed her child-bearing, hysterectomy should be performed.

Vaginal hysterectomy

The vaginal approach to hysterectomy for endometrial carcinoma is seldom used today because it compromises surgical staging and often surgical treatment as well. Removal of the adnexa is more difficult through the vagina; exploration of the pelvis and abdomen cannot be done; the validity of transvaginal peritoneal cytology would be questionable; and node sampling cannot be carried out. Nevertheless, there are instances in which vaginal hysterectomy may be preferable to the abdominal approach: (1) in the obese, parous woman with a well-differentiated carcinoma; (2) in the young woman with significant pelvic relaxation and grade 1 endometrial carcinoma; and (3) in the case of the patient who for medical reasons may tolerate vaginal hysterectomy but not abdominal hysterectomy. In some centers staging can be completed laparoscopically.

Estrogen replacement

Many women after treatment for endometrial cancer will suffer the effects of estrogen insufficiency, i.e., hot flushes, the dyspareunia of vaginal dryness, and rapid loss of calcium from bone. Such women also are concerned about recurrent cancer and reasonably exhibit fear with respect to taking estrogens. Most will experience symptomatic improvement by taking medroxyprogesterone acetate 20–30 mg daily by mouth or 150 mg intramuscularly every 3 months. Should this prove ineffective, a low dose of conjugated estrogens, e.g., 0.3 or 0.625 mg dialy, can be given in addition to the progestin. The progestin will prevent or minimize the possibility of a growth-enhancing estrogenic effect should there be any residual carcinoma. If the estrogen is not administered for 2–3 years after treatment, the risk of residual disease is very small. The risks and benefits should be discussed with each patient and management individualized.

SUGGESTED READING

AALDERS JG, ABELER V, KOLSTAD P, ONSRUD M. Postoperative external irradiation and prognostic parameters in stage I endometrial carcinoma. *Obstet Gynecol* 1980;56:419.

BORONOW RC, MORROW CP, CREASMAN WT, *et al.* Surgical staging in endometrial cancer: clinicopathologic findings of a prospective study. *Obstet Gynecol* 1984;63:825.

CHRISTOPHERSON WM, ALBERHASKY RC, CONNELLY PJ. Carcinoma of the endometrium. I. A clinicopathologic study of clear-cell carcinoma and secretory carcinoma. *Cancer* 1982;49:1511.

CHRISTOPHERSON WM, ALBERHASKY RC, CONNELLY PJ. Carcinoma of the endometrium. II. Papillary adenocarcinoma: a clinical pathological study of 46 cases. *Am J Clin Pathol* 1982;77:534.

EHRLICH CE, YOUNG PCM, CLEARY RE. Cytoplasmic progesterone and estradiol receptors in normal, hyperplastic, and carcinomatous endometria: therapeutic implications. *Am J Obstet Gynecol* 1981;141:539.

MALKASIAN GD Jr. Carcinoma of the endometrium: effect of stage and grade on survival. *Cancer* 1978;41:996.

MORROW CP. Specific management problems in endometrial carcinoma. In: Morrow CP, Bonnar J, O'Brien TJ, Gibbons WE, eds. *Recent Clinical Developments in Gynecologic Oncology.* New York: Raven Press, 1983:83.

MORROW CP, SCHLAERTH JB. Surgical management of endometrial carcinoma. *Clin Obstet Gynecol* 1982;25:82–92.

PODRATZ KC, O'BRIEN PC, MALKASIAN GD Jr, DECKER DG, JEFFRIES JA, EDMONSON JH. Effects of progestational agents in treatment of endometrial carcinoma. *Obstet Gynecol* 1985;66:106.

POTISH RA, TWIGGS LB, ADCOCK LL, SAVAGE JE, LEVITT SH, PREM KA. Para-aortic lymph node radiotherapy in cancer of the uterine corpus. *Obstet Gynecol* 1985;65:251.

86

Management of ovarian carcinoma

LYNDA D. ROMAN

Ovarian carcinoma ranks fourth among all cancers as a cause of death in women and is responsible for more deaths than any other gynecologic cancer. The risk at birth of eventually developing ovarian cancer is 1.5% among white women in the USA and 1.0% for nonwhite women. On an annual basis, there are approximately 20 700 new cases of ovarian carcinoma diagnosed and 12 000 deaths due to this disease. Epidemiologically, ovarian carcinoma is predominantly a malignancy of industrialized countries. Women at greatest risk are those of low parity and high social status. A few instances of familial occurrence have been documented. No means of early detection have been discovered; consequently, more than two-thirds of the malignancies are unresectable when first diagnosed. The overall 5-year survival rate is 35%, but this rate ranges from <5% to >90%, depending on the stage, histology, and treatment.

Operative treatment

Surgery is the most important phase of treatment for all types of ovarian cancer and should be undertaken as soon as the diagnostic survey has been completed. A low transverse incision is inappropriate with a presumptive diagnosis of ovarian carcinoma. The surgeon selecting this incision should forewarn the patient that an upper abdominal incision may be required if carcinoma is found. Upon entering the abdomen, the surgeon performs a thorough exploration to evaluate the disease extent. Ovarian carcinoma spreads predominantly by intraperitoneal implantation and retroperitoneal lymphatic metastasis. The undersurface of the diaphragm, surface of the liver, omentum, retroperitoneal nodes, paracolic gutters, parietes, pelvic peritoneum, pelvic cul-de-sacs, and small and large bowel surfaces are inspected and palpated for signs of spread. Findings suggestive of malignancy include: bilateral ovarian tumors, ascites (especially bloody ascites), surface papillations, and a multicystic or solid tumor. None of these is, however, diagnostic of malignancy.

After exploration of the abdomen and in the absence of ascites or obvious extraovarian spread, cytologic specimens should be obtained from over the liver, the posterior *cul-de-sac*, and both paracolic gutters. They may be submitted as a single specimen. The surgeon must guard against rupturing a malignant cyst if intraperitoneal spread is not already apparent.

The surgical procedure most appropriate for epithelial ovarian carcinoma depends largely on the patient's age and the extent of disease. In a young woman desirous of fertility with an ovarian carcinoma apparently limited to one ovary, unilateral salpingo-oophorectomy is appropriate. In all other cases total abdominal hysterectomy and bilateral salpingo-oophorectomy should be performed. If there is no evidence of extrapelvic disease, multiple peritoneal biopsies (including pelvic, right and left paracolic gutters, and right diaphragmatic), greater omentectomy, and pelvic and aortic nodal sampling should be performed. If the disease is widespread, the goal is to remove as much of the tumor as possible. Ideally, the patient should be left with no residual disease. If this is not possible, leaving <2 cm of tumor seems to result in an improved disease-free survival.

At times, the malignancy is too extensive to permit more than exploration of the abdomen and biopsy of the cancer. Resection of bowel is generally not advisable unless 90% or more of the tumor burden can be removed. It is recommended that the abdominal incision be closed with a monofilament, nonabsorbable suture employing the Smead–Jones internal retention stitch. This is particularly important in individuals with incompletely resected cancer.

Pathological study of the surgical specimen(s) is a very important phase in the evaluation of ovarian neoplasms. Epithelial malignancies and germ cell tumors both are notorious for the histologic variability within a single tumor. Without adequate sampling, the most malignant portion of the tumor may remain undiagnosed, which may lead to undertreatment. Consultation with a pathologist who is knowledgeable in this area is recommended whenever there is a diagnosis of a benign solid teratoma, a germ cell tumor in a woman over age 30, a poorly differentiated carcinoma in a woman under age 30, or a granulosa cell tumor. The 1985 International Federation of Gynecology and obstetrics (FIGO) staging scheme for ovarian cancer is given in Table 86.1.

Table 86.1 Stages for primary carcinoma of the ovary FIGO, 1985*

Stage I	Growth limited to the ovaries
Ia	Growth limited to one ovary; no ascites. No tumor on the external surface; capsule intact
Ib	Growth limited to both ovaries; no ascites. No tumor on the external surface; capsules intact
Ic†	Tumor either stage Ia or Ib but with tumor on surface of one or both ovaries; or with capsule ruptured; or with ascites present containing malignant cells or with positive peritoneal washings
Stage II	Growth involving one or both ovaries with pelvic extension
IIa	Extension and/or metastases to the uterus and/or tubes
IIb	Extension to other pelvic tissues
IIc†	Tumor either stage IIa or IIb, but with tumor on surface of one or both ovaries; or with capsule(s) ruptured; or with ascites present containing malignant cells or with positive peritoneal washings
Stage III	Tumor involving one or both ovaries with peritoneal implants outside the pelvis and/or positive retroperitoneal or inguinal nodes. Superficial liver metastasis equals stage III. Tumor is limited to the true pelvis but with histologically proven malignant extension to small bowel or omentum
IIIa	Tumor grossly limited to the true pelvis with negative nodes but with histologically confirmed microscopic seeding of abdominal peritoneal surfaces
IIIb	Tumor of one or both ovaries with histologically confirmed implants of abdominal peritoneal surfaces not exceeding 2 cm in diameter. Nodes are negative
IIIc	Abdominal implants >2 cm in diameter and/or positive retroperitoneal or inguinal nodes
Stage IV	Growth involving one or both ovaries with distant metastases. If pleural effusion is present, there must be positive cytology to allot a case to stage IV. Parenchymal liver metastasis equals stage IV

*Stages are based on findings at clinical examination and/or surgical exploration. The histology is to be considered in the staging, as is cytology concerning effusions. It is desirable that a biopsy be taken from suspicious areas outside of the pelvis.

†To evaluate the impact on prognosis of the different criteria for allotting cases to stage Ic or IIc, it would be valuable to know: (1) if rupture of the capsule was (a) spontaneous or (b) caused by the surgeon; or (2) if the source of malignant cell detected was (a) peritoneal washings or (b) ascites.

Table 86.2 Ovarian carcinoma chemotherapy regimens

Drug	Dosage	Frequency
Cytoxan	$750 \, mg/m^2$ ⎫	Intravenously every 3 weeks
Cisplatin	$75 \, mg/m^2$ ⎭	
Cytoxan	$500 \, mg/m^2$ ⎫	
Adriamycin	$50 \, mg/m^2$ ⎬	Intravenously every 3 weeks
Cisplatin	$50 \, mg/m^2$ ⎭	
Melphalan	$7 \, mg/m^2$ per day	Orally for 5 days every 4 weeks

Postoperative management

Borderline ovarian carcinoma is managed surgically because neither chemotherapy nor radiation therapy has proved to be of therapeutic value. Thus, surgery is the primary therapy and the preferred treatment for recurrence. In the face of unresectable, progressive disease, chemotherapy with cytoxan and cisplatinum (CP) with or without Adriamycin is recommended (Table 86.2).

For a patient with a true carcinoma (serous, mucinous, endometrioid), no postoperative therapy is required if the patient has a stage Ia grade 1 lesion. For all other stage I and II cases, six cycles of chemotherapy with cytoxan and CP is recommended, although intraperitoneal ^{32}P or whole-abdomen radiation appears to be similarly effective. For all other cases, a total of 6–12 cycles of platinum-based multiagent chemotherapy is recommended. The most commonly used regimens are CP or cytoxan, Adriamycin and CP (PAC). A restaging laparotomy is performed after six cycles to assess the response. If multiagent chemotherapy is contraindicated or the patient is unwilling to accept such rigorous therapy, treatment with melphalan is appropriate.

Second-look surgery

The second-look operation has received much attention in the management of ovarian carcinoma. It is generally agreed that certain patients may benefit from a second laparotomy at the completion of 6–12 months of chemotherapy. The primary objective is to document as accurately as possible, prior to discontinuing chemotherapy, that no carcinoma remains or to remove resectable residual carcinoma. The knowledge gained from second-look surgery can be used to aid in a decision regarding the need for and the nature of further therapy.

Only patients with residual disease following initial surgery or those with a relatively high risk of early recurrence are candidates for second-look surgery. Patients treated with whole-abdomen radiotherapy or intra-peritoneal nuclides are at greater risk for bowel complications. Patients with stage I–II ovarian tumors of low malignant potential or grade 1 differentiation are likely not benefited by a second-look operation. Second-look surgery involves numerous biopsies of the peritoneal surfaces and retroperitoneal nodes, resection of the residual omentum, and multiple cytologic specimens.

Conservative management in ovarian cancer

Surgical therapy consisting of a unilateral salpingo-oophorectomy without adjuvant chemotherapy often can be adequate treatment for early ovarian cancer in the young woman who wishes to retain her reproductive potential. The requirements for such conservative management include a unilateral, encapsulated grade 1 or borderline epithelial carcinoma with negative peritoneal cytology (stage Ia). The contralateral ovary either must be known to be normal, or it must be biopsied to confirm normality. After the patient's reproductive years have been completed, the residual ovary can be removed as an elective procedure. If the epithelial ovarian cancer is grade 2 or 3, adherent, ruptured, or metastatic, but the contralateral ovary and uterus are normal, conservative surgery may still be feasible, but 6 months of postoperative chemotherapy is recommended.

Similarly, conservative treatment may be undertaken if the unilateral ovarian tumor is a Sertoli–Leydig cell tumor, granulosa cell tumor, or germ cell tumor.

Serous effusion

Ascites and plural effusion commonly are associated with ovarian carcinoma. Preoperative removal of these fluids is not recommended unless the patient is experiencing respiratory embarrassment or pain. This policy minimizes the likelihood of rupturing a large, malignant ovarian cyst. Often ascites formation is a problem in the immediate postoperative period. In this circumstance, intravenous chemotherapy is initiated promptly to stop the loss of fluid and protein into the abdominal cavity. This also helps to avert the complications related to abdominal distention and oliguria. When serous effusions are refractory to systemic chemotherapy, instillation of colloidal chromium phosphate or tetracycline may be therapeutic.

Follow-up

Follow-up evaluation for ovarian carcinoma should be frequent (every 2–3 months) during the first 2 years; the majority of recurrences will appear during this time. Long-term follow-up is also recommended, as this malignancy may recur 5 or more years posttreatment.

History and physical examination are of primary importance in follow-up evaluation, as few laboratory tests or X-rays are useful. Serial serum CA-125 measurements can be helpful, as a rising titer is almost universally associated with recurrence. Recurrences often are heralded by partial large- or small-bowel obstruction, indigestion, a palpable pelvic mass, an enlarged peripheral lymph node, evidence of ascites, or increase in CA-125 level. It should be remembered that these women are epidemiologically similar to women at high risk for breast cancer. Regular breast examination and mammography should be part and parcel of follow-up care.

SUGGESTED READING

COLGAN TJ, NORRIS HJ. Ovarian epithelial tumors of low malignant potential: a review. *Int J Gynecol Pathol* 1983;1:367.

COPELAND LJ, GERSHENSON DM, WHARTON JT, *et al*. Microscopic disease at second-look laparotomy in advanced ovarian cancer. *Cancer* 1985;55:472.

DEMBO AJ. Abdominopelvic radiotherapy in ovarian cancer. *Cancer* 1985;55:2285.

GERSHENSON DM, COPELAND LJ, WHARTON JT, *et al*. Prognosis of surgically determined complete responders in advanced ovarian cancer. *Cancer* 1985; 55:1129.

GRIFFITHS CT, PARKER LM, FULLER AF Jr. Role of cytoreductive surgical treatment in the management of advanced ovarian cancer. *Cancer Treat Rep* 1979;63: 235.

HRESHCHYSHYN MW, PARK RC, BLESSING JA, *et al*. The role of adjuvant therapy in stage I ovarian cancer. *Am J Obstet Gynecol* 1980;138:139.

LAVIN PT, KNAPP RC, MALKASIAN G, WHITNEY CW, BEREK JS, BAST RC Jr. CA-125 for the monitoring of ovarian cancer during primary therapy. *Obstet Gynecol* 1987;69:223.

MORROW CP, TOWNSEND DE. *Synopsis of Gynecologic Oncology*. 3rd edn. New York: Wiley, 1987:231–303.

OMURA GA, MORROW CP, BLESSING JA, *et al*. A randomized comparison of melphalan versus melphalan plus hexamethylmelamine versus adriamycin plus cyclophosphamide in ovarian carcinoma. *Cancer* 1983;51:783.

OMURA GA, BLESSING JA, EHRLICH CE, *et al*. A randomized trial of cyclophosphamide and adriamycin with or without cisplatin in advanced ovarian carcinoma: a gynecologic oncology group study. *Cancer* 1986;57:1725.

OMURA GA, BUYSE M, MARSONI S, *et al*. Cyclophosphamide plus cisplatin versus cyclophosphamide, doxorubicin, and cisplatin chemotherapy of ovarian carcinoma: a meta-analysis. *J Clin Oncol* 1991;9:1668–1674.

THIGPEN JT. Principles of chemotherapy. In: Morrow CP, Townsend DE, eds. *Synopsis of Gynecologic Oncology*, 3rd edn. New York: Wiley, 1987:409–458.

YOUNG RC, WALTON LA, ELLENBERG SS, *et al*. Adjuvant therapy in stage I and stage II epithelial ovarian cancer. *N Engl J Med* 1990;322:1021.

87

Special tumors of the ovary

LAILA I. MUDERSPACH

Germ cell tumors

Proper management of germ cell tumors of the ovary is important because many are malignant and occur in young women. It is possible in many cases to treat these tumors without loss of fertility. The benign dermoid cyst may be the most common ovarian neoplasm while the malignant germ cell tumors are distinctly uncommon: immature teratoma, dysgerminoma, endodermal sinus tumor, embryonal carcinoma, and choriocarcinoma.

Teratomas

Dermoid cyst

More than 95% of teratomas are mature cystic teratomas, commonly referred to as dermoid cysts. These tumors can occur throughout a woman's reproductive life and frequently give rise to symptoms of an acute abdomen secondary to either torsion or rupture. Most commonly, dermoid cysts are detected on routine pelvic examination or during the investigation of minor complaints. More than half can be diagnosed by ultrasonography or X-ray through the identification of calcifications, tooth formation, a specific fat-halo sign on X-ray, or the characteristic density appearance on ultrasound.

In a young woman, the surgical procedure of choice for a dermoid cyst is enucleation with preservation of as much ovarian tissue as possible. The opposite ovary should also be evaluated by inspection and palpation for the presence of a dermoid tumor. Dermoid cysts have an overt bilateralism rate approaching 15%. However, bilateralism is not always expressed at the time of surgery and may not be detected until months or years later. Consideration has been given to bivalving the opposite, normal-appearing ovary, and removing a wedge for biopsy; but if the contralateral ovary is normal to inspection and palpation, we do not recommend this procedure. The risk of infertility from bivalving the ovary probably outweighs any potential benefit.

Approximately 1% of dermoid cysts will contain a malignancy. Usually these malignancies occur in postmenopausal women and are squamous cell carcinomas. However, a variety of other malignancies also may occur. These tumors usually are found in the solid papilla on the inside of the cyst, the so-called Rokitansky protuberance.

Immature teratoma

Malignant ovarian teratomas are called immature teratomas because their malignant behavior is exhibited by tissues that are embryonic or fetal in appearance. The more immature the tissue, the more malignant is its behavior.

A microscopic grading system for immature teratomas has been proposed by Norris and Benson and seems to correlate well with prognosis. In the past, confusion has arisen from use of the terms solid or cystic to describe teratomas because these terms are purely descriptive. Whether a tumor is solid, cystic, or both has no bearing on its degree of malignancy.

Most immature teratomas occur in adolescent girls and involve only one ovary. In these patients, the operative treatment consists of unilateral salpingo-oophorectomy. Bilateral extension requires bilateral salpingo-oophorectomy and metastasis requires removal of as much tumor as possible.

A patient with higher-grade or metastatic immature teratoma needs additional treatment after surgery with chemotherapy. Radiotherapy has not been proved beneficial. Impressive results (cures) have been obtained with combination chemotherapy using vincristine, dactinomycin, and cyclophosphamide (VAC). Equally good, possibly superior, results have occurred with vinblastin, bleomycin, and cisplatin (VBP), or bleomycin, etoposide, and cisplatin (BEP).

Dysgerminoma

The dysgerminoma is the most common malignant germ cell tumor of the ovary. It usually occurs before age 30, often in females with dysgenetic gonads. Most often, it is confined to one ovary at the time of diagnosis. In 15% of cases, the dysgerminoma is not a pure tumor. Therefore, it is important that dysgerminomas be sampled extensively for microscopic study, particularly in areas of hemorrhage or necrosis, to rule out the presence of a more malignant element.

A suggested treatment plan for dysgerminoma is as follows: if a patient is young and desirous of future child-bearing, the dysgerminoma involves only one ovary, is <10 cm in diameter, unruptured, and without malignant ascites or positive peritoneal cystology, a unilateral salpingo-oophorectomy should be performed. A wedge biopsy of the opposite, normal-appearing ovary should be performed, as the opposite ovary may contain a subclinical focus of tumor. If tumor is present in both ovaries then a bilateral oophorectomy is indicated. At laparotomy, particular attention should be paid to pelvic and paraaortic lymph nodes, as this is the primary route of metastasis. Ipsilateral pelvic and aortic lymph nodes should be sampled. Peritoneal washings and omental biopsy should also be performed. Routine postoperative radiation is unnecessary. A karyotype should be obtained to rule out the presence of a Y chromosome. The presence of a uterus and a nonstreak gonad does not necessarily rule out the presence of a Y chromosome and dysgenetic gonads. If a Y chromosome is found, bilateral gonadectomy is indicated because prospects for fertility are nil, and malignant risk is present in both gonads.

If the tumor is >10 cm, or accompanied by rupture or malignant ascites, the likelihood of metastasis mandates performance of pelvic and aortic lymph node biopsies, omental biopsy, peritoneal washings, and target biopsies. Surgery should be followed by chemotherapy or radiation therapy to the abdomen with a boost to the pelvis. The radiation dosage considered curative in this disease is within the range that is tolerable for the abdomen and pelvis. If metastases are found in the aortic nodes, radiation therapy should be extended to include the mediastinum and supraclavicular areas. Postoperative lymphangiography or computed tomography (CT) should be done to monitor for retroperitoneal lymph node metastases or recurrence. There is some recent evidence suggesting that chemotherapy (VAC or VBP) can replace radiation therapy, especially in patients with remaining functional ovarian tissue and a uterus whose dysgerminoma was confined to the ovary but accompanied by high-risk features (large size, ruptured, ascites). A great benefit to this approach is the maintenance of fertility. If chemotherapy were to fail, radiation therapy is an option for treatment.

Follow-up of patients with ovarian dysgerminoma should include a chest X-ray every 3 months and consideration of a repeat CT of the chest, abdomen, and pelvis at 1 year. Serum lactate dehydrogenase (LDH) may be elevated with dysgerminomas and can subsequently be followed as a tumor marker. Serum studies of α-fetoprotein (AFP) and human chorionic gonadotropin (hCG) should be performed every 3 months to monitor patients for the appearance of another type of metastatic germ cell tumor that may have been missed at the time of the initial examination of the tumor. Its presence would be an indication for chemotherapy. Essentially, all recurrences become manifest within 5 years.

Endodermal sinus tumor

The endodermal sinus tumor (or yolk-sac carcinoma) is perhaps the most malignant ovarian neoplasm. It is rare, occurring usually in female children or young adults (age 10–30), and is characterized by rapid growth. AFP is secreted by most, if not all, endodermal sinus tumors.

When only one ovary is involved, a unilateral salpingo-oophorectomy is appropriate. When intraabdominal metastases are encountered, it seems most reasonable to remove as much tumor as possible without risking delayed postoperative recovery. The ultimate fate of these patients, whether the tumor seems confined to one ovary or not, rests on the success of chemotherapy, which should be initiated as quickly as possible postoperatively. Intensive combination chemotherapy with bleomycin, etoposide, and cisplatin (BEP) is indicated. Serial assays for hCG and AFP should be included in the management of patients to confirm tumor progression or regression.

Embryonal carcinoma

This neoplasm only recently has been recognized as a distinct entity in women. It shares many features with endodermal sinus tumors, with which it undoubtedly had been grouped in the past; but it differs most significantly from endodermal sinus tumors in that it usually produces both hCG and AFP. Aggressive behavior is the rule for this neoplasm. The same treatment guidelines apply for this tumor as for endodermal sinus tumors.

Choriocarcinoma

Pure choriocarcinoma arising in the ovary is indeed a rare tumor. It is virulent and is reported to have a high death rate. Because of this, most patients have been treated postoperatively with chemotherapy regimens similar to those used for gestational choriocarcinoma, i.e., MAC, a combination of methotrexate, dactinomycin, and an alkylating agent, cyclophosphamide or chlorambucil. The EMA/CO regimen — etoposide, methotrexate, dactinomycin, cyclophosphamide, and vincristine — may prove to be as effective. These tumors secrete hCG, which should be used as a tumor marker.

Gonadoblastoma

The gonadoblastoma occurs almost exclusively in dysgenetic gonads. The affected females usually have a Y chromosome. The gonadoblastoma is included here because nearly 30% are associated with the development of malignant germ cell tumors. The gonadoblastoma is a benign tumor composed of two cell types: primitive germ cells and a sex-cord stromal element. There also may be cells resembling luteinized theca cells or Leydig cells. Because of the high risk for development of dysgerminomas, endodermal sinus tumors, etc., in gonadoblastomas, the appropriate therapy is bilateral gonadectomy.

Mixed germ cell tumors

Not uncommonly, malignant germ cell tumors contain more than one histologic type. Usually, routine examinations of the primary tumor and sampling of metastases, if present, will make the mixture apparent. However, the detection of elements may be difficult due to the presence of only small foci in a large tumor mass. Therefore, it is recommended that thorough and painstaking microscopic investigation be carried out for all germ cell malignancies.

The detection of a mixed germ cell tumor also may be indirect. The presence of elevated hCG or AFP levels in the serum of a patient presumed to have an immature teratoma or a dysgerminoma is evidence for the presence of choriocarcinoma or embryonal or endodermal sinus tumor elements as well.

One example of a situation in which precise diagnosis may be critical is the patient with an apparently pure dysgerminoma. Postsurgical management for pure dysgerminoma consists of adjuvant chemo- or radiation therapy or no further treatment. But, if the tumor is actually a mixture of dysgerminoma and one or more other germ cell elements, these therapy choices could prove to be fatal errors. In this setting, chemotherapy (BEP), not radiation or observation, should be considered.

Gonadal stromal neoplasms

Roughly 5% of ovarian neoplasms is derived from the ovarian stroma. Neoplasms of the stroma unique to the ovary are called specialized gonadal stromal tumors and are known clinically as granulosa cell, theca cell tumors (alone or in combination), and Sertoli–Leydig tumors (arrhenoblastomas). The only common neoplasm of the nonspecialized ovarian stroma is the fibroma.

Granulosa–theca tumors

Granulosa and theca cell tumors as pure cell types occur in equal numbers. It is more common, however, to find them combined in a neoplasm. Neoplastic granulosa cells are malignant, whereas the theca cell tumor component is invariably benign. Both granulosa and theca cells are capable of autonomous production of sex steroids, usually estrogens but occasionally androgens. Therefore, at times, these neoplasms can present with symptoms of precocious puberty, menorrhagia, amenorrhea, postmenopausal vaginal bleeding, or virilization. Because of this estrogen production, 5–15% of granulosa–theca tumors have been associated with endometrial adenocarcinoma.

Granulosa cell tumors usually are confined to one ovary and represent a low-grade malignant risk. Of the cases that recur, a significant percentage relapse 10 or even 20 years after surgical removal. When confined to one ovary in a young woman, removal of the ovary is sufficient; however in a woman near menopause or older, removal of both ovaries and the uterus is recommended. If conservative surgery is performed, the uterus should be sampled to rule out endometrial pathology. If the tumor has spread beyond one ovary, removal of both ovaries and the uterus, together with postoperative therapy – usually pelvic and abdominal radiation therapy – is indicated.

In the past few years, some success with combination chemotherapy has been achieved in advanced cases. Both the VAC regimen and VBP have been shown to be effective.

There has been a suggestion that a group of granulosa cell tumors clinically confined to one ovary with a high risk of recurrence can be identified by certain factors, such as number of mitoses, degree of atypia, size, spontaneous rupture, and/or ascites. Patients who have tumors with these risk factors deserve intensive follow-up and, as more information becomes available, may be candidates for postoperative therapy as well.

Theca cell tumors are unilateral and benign. Treatment is surgical – usually unilateral oophorectomy in the young woman; hysterectomy and bilateral oophorectomy in women at or near menopause.

Sertoli–Leydig cell tumor (arrhenoblastoma)

The term arrhenoblastoma is being replaced in the medical literature by the more informative designation of Sertoli–Leydig cell tumor. Classically the Sertoli–Leydig cell tumor produces testosterone, which in turn produces defeminization then virilization. Rarely, these neoplasms produce estrogen instead. These neoplasms have a low-grade malignant potential. In young women with the neoplasm confined to one ovary, unilateral salpingo-oophorectomy is sufficient treatment. In women at or near menopause, hysterectomy and bilateral salpingo-oophorectomy are indicated. If metastasis or recurrence occurs, there is some evidence that chemotherapy with VAC or BEP is effective. There is recent evidence that the malignant behavior of Sertoli–Leydig cell tumors can be predicted from the degree of cellular dedifferentiation or by the presence of heterologous elements. This information may allow for selection of some women with Sertoli–Leydig cell tumors clinically confined to one ovary to receive postoperative therapy such as BEP or VAC.

Fibroma

The fibroma is the most common neoplasm of the nonspecific mesenchyme of the ovary. Not uncommonly it is found incidentally in ovaries removed for other reasons. Occasionally, these tumors are bilateral. Fibromas frequently cannot be distinguished easily from theca cell tumors and vice versa. The fibroma of the ovary is well known as the prime causative factor for Meigs syndrome: benign ovarian tumor, ascites, and hydrothorax. These findings usually indicate advanced metastatic ovarian cancer, which in the past was regarded as hopeless. The existence of Meigs syndrome meant that all such patients had to be evaluated carefully, as simple removal of the fibroma is curative. Due to advances in preoperative, intraoperative, and postoperative techniques and treatment, all such patients now stand to benefit from a surgical approach and the original clinical significance of the syndrome is diminished somewhat.

Most fibromas do not produce effusions, however, and are treated by unilateral oophorectomy in the young woman and bilateral oophorectomy and hysterectomy in the woman at or near menopause.

SUGGESTED READING

BJORKHOLME E, SILFERSWARD C. Prognostic factors in granulosa cell tumors. *Gynecol Oncol* 1981;11:261.

COLOMBO N, SESSA C, LANDONI F, *et al.* Cisplatin, vinblastine and bleomycin combination chemotherapy in metastatic granulosa cell tumor of the ovary. *Obstet Gynecol* 1986;67:265.

EVANS AT, GAFFEY TA, MALKASIAN GD, *et al.* Clinicopathologic review of 118 granulosa and 82 theca cell tumors. *Obstet Gynecol* 1980;155:231.

GERSHENSEN DM, MORRIS M, CANGIR A, *et al.* Treatment of malignant germ cell tumors of the ovary with bleomycin, etoposide and cisplatin. *J Clin Oncol* 1990; 8:715.

KREPART G, SMITH JP, RUTLEDGE F, *et al.* The treatment for dysgerminoma of the ovary. *Cancer* 1978;41:986.

NORRIS HJ, BENSON WL. Immature (malignant) teratoma of the ovary. *Cancer* 1976;37:2359.

SCHWARTZ PLG. Combination chemotherapy in the management of ovarian germ cell malignancies. *Obstet Gynecol* 1984;64:654.

SLAYTON RE. Management of germ cell and stromal cell tumors of the ovary. *Semin Oncol* 1984;11:299.

STENWIG JT, HAZEKAMP JT, BEECHAM JB. Granulosa cell tumors of the ovary: a clinicopathological study of 118 cases with long term follow-up. *Gynecol Oncol* 1979;7:136.

TAYLOR MH, DEPETRILLO AD, TURNER AR. Vinblastin, bleomycin and cisplatin in malignant germ cell tumor of the ovary. *Cancer* 1985;56:1341.

88

Diagnosis and management of trophoblastic neoplasia

LAILA I. MUDERSPACH

Hydatidiform or hydatid mole is an abnormal pregnancy characterized by gross vesicular swelling of the placental villi and the absence of a fetus or embryo. In the USA, its prevalence is approximately 1:1500 live births. Historically, the patient presents with a clinical picture of threatened abortion with a uterus larger than 12 weeks' gestational size. In addition to the absence of fetal heart tones, other evidence supporting the diagnosis of hydatid mole includes hyperemesis gravidarum, a uterus large for gestational age, and toxemia.

Because molar pregnancy is uncommon, in the past the diagnosis was often overlooked until the patient aborted the pathognomonic vesicles. Due to the advances and common use of ultrasonography, molar pregnancies are now being diagnosed earlier. The patient with a molar pregnancy is at high risk for serious complications that tend to worsen with time, making an early diagnosis desirable. Chronic and acute blood loss, hypervolemia, toxemia, and thyrotoxicosis are some of the likely complications of molar pregnancy. High-output heart failure accompanied by acute pulmonary edema may result. Another serious potential complication is infection of the uterine contents accompanied by sepsis, which occurs in approximately 10% of cases.

When a molar pregnancy is suggested, an ultrasound examination usually will confirm or rule out the diagnosis. In the past when ultrasound was unavailable or equivocal, a transabdominal amniocentesis with amniography was employed to confirm the diagnosis. Ultrasound examination is also useful in the unusual case in which a fetus coexists with a molar pregnancy, called a partial molar gestation. This serious condition of partial mole may be characterized by toxemia and a large uterus.

In the past, measurement of urinary human chorionic gonadotropin (hCG) often was used to help identify patients with molar pregnancies. Although a urinary concentration exceeding 500 000 IU/l is highly suggestive of the presence of hydatid mole, it is not diagnostic. A multifetal gestation also may be associated with unusually high levels of urinary hCG. The easy access to serum hCG levels now makes urinary measurement less useful.

The differential diagnosis of hydatid mole includes multifetal gestation, polyhydramnios, uterine fibroids (which may enlarge rapidly in early pregnancy), and ovarian tumor during early pregnancy.

Management

Termination of molar pregnancy

As soon as the diagnosis of hydatid mole is confirmed, the pregnancy should be terminated by vacuum curettage. Conventional sharp curettage is adequate in patients who have spontaneously evacuated part of the mole so that the uterus is less than 12 weeks' gestational size. Suction curettage is carried out under general anesthesia in the operating room. If the patient is bleeding heavily on admission, an oxytocin infusion is started at the time; otherwise, none is given until the curettage is under way or completed. Oxytocin or prostaglandin induction is indicated only in the patient with a coexistent fetus. A better option would be hysterotomy and the evacuation of the coexistent fetus and mole.

Complications

During the immediate postoperative period, the most common and important complications are sepsis and acute pulmonary crisis. The latter is due to trophoblastic embolization or fluid overload with heart failure. This syndrome appears within a few hours of evacuation and is characterized by dyspnea, tachycardia, and hypotension. Rarely, heart failure appears prior to evacuation. This complication may be life-threatening.

Unilateral or bilateral enlargement of the ovaries due to multiple theca lutein cysts is clinically detectable in approximately 30% of patients with hydatid moles. In some cases, they are not noted until the first or second week after evacuation. These cysts apparently result from the high levels of hCG. They regress slowly as the hCG titer diminishes postevacuation. The presence of these cysts should not lead to surgical intervention or the mistaken belief that they represent an ovarian neoplasm. It is recommended that RhoGAM be given to Rh⁻ mothers, although hydatid mole has not been documented as a cause of Rh-sensitization.

Surveillance

Approximately 15% of patients with molar pregnancies will have either invasive mole or choriocarcinoma. Invasive mole is histologically similar to noninvasive mole, but is distinguished by its ability to invade the uterine muscle and metastasize, usually to the lungs or lower genital tract. Uterine perforation and hemorrhage may occur with invasive mole or choriocarcinoma.

Evaluation for neoplastic complications begins during the initial hospitalization when a chest X-ray and gynecologic examination are performed. Mole patients with a uterus large for dates or clinically detectable theca/lutein cysts are more likely to have invasive mole or choriocarcinoma than other mole patients.

The high incidence of postmolar trophoblastic disease and its potentially serious sequelae requires follow-up surveillance for every patient. Weekly measurements of serum hCG for the β subunit should begin 1 week after the mole is delivered and continue until the titer becomes normal (<5 mIU/ml). A normal value should occur within 15 weeks of evacuation. Titers then are repeated monthly for a year. If no rise occurs, no further follow-up is necessary. Pregnancy should be prevented with oral contraceptives during follow-up to avoid difficulties in interpreting a rise in hCG titer.

Treatment

There are three indications for treatment after molar pregnancy: (1) the presence of metastases; (2) a titer rising or unchanged over a 3-week period; and (3) a rise in titer after titer remission. It is not necessary to have a tissue diagnosis prior to initiating treatment. A diagnosis of trophoblastic neoplasia is based on the clinical history and hCG titer. Early detection based on postevacuation serial hCG titers insures a virtually 100% cure rate of these potentially lethal growths.

During the period of surveillance with serial hCG titers, no other test or examinations need to be carried out unless the patient develops symptoms or the hCG titer fails to fall. The most common associated problem is vaginal bleeding which may require curettage. In the absence of vaginal bleeding or an enlarging uterus, uterine curettage is not indicated and is of neither diagnostic nor therapeutic value.

The patient who develops stable or rising hCG titers should be evaluated for evidence of metastasis by physical examination and chest X-ray.

Table 88.1 Staging for gestational trophoblastic tumors (GTT). (From FIGO)

Stage	Definition
Stage I	Disease confined to the uterus
IA	Disease confined to the uterus with no risk factors
IB	Disease confined to the uterus with one risk factor
IC	Disease confined to the uterus with two risk factors
Stage II	GTT extends outside the uterus but is limited to the genital structures (adnexa, vagina, broad ligament)
IIA	GTT involves genital structures without risk factors
IIB	GTT extends outside the uterus but limited to genital structures with one risk factor
IIC	GTT extends outside the uterus but limited to genital structures with two risk factors
Stage III	GTT extends to the lungs with or without known genital tract involvement
IIIA	GTT extends to the lungs with or without genital tract involvement and with no risk factors
IIIB	GTT extends to the lungs with or without genital tract involvement and with one risk factor
IIIC	GTT extends to the lungs with or without genital tract involvement and has two risk factors
Stage IV	All other metastatic sites
IVA	All other metastatic sites without risk factors
IVB	All other metastatic sites with one risk factor
IVC	All other metastatic sites with two risk factors

The following factors should be considered and noted in reporting.
1 Prior chemotherapy.
2 Placental site tumors should be reported separately.
3 Histologic verification of disease is not required.
   Risk factors affecting staging include the following:
1 Human chorionic gonadotropin 100 000 m IU/ml.
2 Duration of disease >6 months from termination of the antecedent pregnancy.

In the case of rising hCG titers, an intrauterine pregnancy should be excluded by ultrasonography. The most common sites of metastases are the lungs and lower genital tract. If metastases are noted on these studies, additional work-up is necessary. The work-up and the management of metastatic disease are discussed later in this chapter. Included in Table 88.1 is the 1991 International Federation of Gynecologists and Obstetricians (FIGO) staging of gestational trophoblastic tumors.

Nonmetastatic trophoblastic neoplasia

The treatment of choice for postmolar nonmetastatic disease is simple hysterectomy for those women who wish to be sterilized. The ovaries need not be removed. Patients treated by hysterectomy still must be monitored postoperatively by monthly hCG titers until the titers have been normal for 12 months. Titer remission, as this is called, must be confirmed by β-hCG serum measurement, which has a sensitivity of at least 5 mIU/ml.

Most women with a molar pregnancy wish to retain their child-bearing capacity, and the treatment of choice is systemic chemotherapy. Chemotherapy should be carried out only by an experienced physician who is also knowledgeable in the treatment of trophoblastic disease. Single-agent therapy, using weekly methotrexate, intravenously or in-tramuscularly or biweekly actinomycin D, is the treatment of choice.

Chemotherapy is continued to one course past the first normal hCG titer. The average number of treatments required to induce titer remission is four. Patients must use effective means of contraception during treat-ment to avoid the confusion of a rising hCG titer due to an intercurrent pregnancy. Following titer remission, patients are monitored by monthly hCG assays until a minimum of 1 year of remission has been observed.

Chemotherapy has not been associated with a detectable increase in congenital anomalies in subsequent pregnancies, but these women may have a higher probability of spontaneous abortion. However, patients with a history of molar gestation have a greater frequency of infertility and spontaneous abortions than women without such a history. Any woman who has had one molar pregnancy has an approximately 2% risk of having another molar pregnancy during her reproductive life.

Metastatic trophoblastic neoplasia

In contrast to trophoblastic neoplasia confined to the uterus, metastatic trophoblastic disease is, in the great majority of cases, choriocarcinoma rather than invasive mole. Because of the important differences in prog-nosis and management, these two clinical situations are presented separa-tely. Metastatic trophoblastic neoplasia usually has a latency period of several months following the culpable pregnancy. During this time, the patient invariably has low but detectable levels of hCG, which neither cause symptoms nor interfere with normal, cyclic menstruation. She may, in fact, ovulate and conceive during this latency period. Occasionally, metastases from choriocarcinoma appear during a molar or nonmolar gestation, particularly a normal intrauterine pregnancy.

Metastatic choriocarcinoma is a great mimic, often presenting with symptoms entirely unrelated to the genital tract. It must be considered in women of reproductive age who have any of the following presumptive diagnoses: stroke, intracerebral hemorrhage, brain or spinal cord tumor, hepatitis, gastrointestinal bleeding, hematuria, nodular or diffuse pulmonary disease, and any malignancy of uncertain histology and origin. It is good policy to screen all women admitted with these diagnoses using a sensitive pregnancy test.

The patient with choriocarcinoma also may have signs and symptoms of eclampsia, hemoperitoneum, threatened or missed abortion, ectopic pregnancy, or delayed postpartum hemorrhage. The patient with intrauterine choriocarcinoma presenting with the symptoms of threatened or missed abortion has a typical history of amenorrhea followed by uterine enlargement, vaginal spotting, and a positive pregnancy test. A high suspicion should be aroused if there is a history of molar pregnancy. The diagnosis is made when the uterus fails to enlarge further; curettage is performed, and trophoblast without fetal or placental tissue is obtained.

Hemoperitoneum may be secondary to a ruptured liver, bleeding ovarian metastases, ruptured theca–lutein cysts, or perforation of the uterus by tumor. Understandably, these patients often undergo laparotomy, with a presumptive diagnosis of ruptured ectopic pregnancy. Every patient with delayed postpartum bleeding should be screened for choriocarcinoma by pregnancy testing, even though the yield will be small.

The importance of the hCG titer in the diagnosis of choriocarcinoma cannot be overemphasized. This test and the medical history are sufficient to make the diagnosis in virtually every case. Tissue diagnosis is almost always unnecessary, sometimes dangerous, and often misleading.

On physical examination, special attention is given to the genital tract, as choriocarcinoma often metastasizes to the cervix, vagina, urethra, and vulva. There may be parametrial extension and ovarian metastases. In addition to a chest X-ray, computed tomography (CT) scan of the brain and abdomen should be performed as a part of the work-up. If the chest X-ray is negative, a CT scan of the thorax is warranted in the presence of a high hCG titer or other metastases.

Management

The management of metastatic choriocarcinoma will depend to some extent upon the site of the metastases. Patients with metastases only in the lung have the most favorable prognosis; those with metastases in the liver are the most difficult to cure.

All cases with metastases should have combination chemotherapy, usually with dactinomycin, methotrexate, and chlorambucil for 5 days each treatment cycle. Intravenous cyclophosphamide may be substituted for chlorambucil if nausea and vomiting make oral therapy difficult. The 5-day course is repeated approximately every other week. Another option is the EMA/CO regimen (etoposide, methotrexate, actinomycin D, cyclophosphamide, and vincristine) which reportedly has fewer side-effects.

When the patient with metastatic choriocarcinoma presents in poor condition, combination drug therapy may not be feasible. In this situation, it has been our practice to initiate treatment with actinomycin D alone.

The most common reason for treatment failure is bone marrow and gastrointestinal toxicity, rather than drug resistance. Toxicity can result in a prolonged interval between treatment courses, during which the tumor recovers along with the normal tissues. If the 5-day regimen cannot be given more frequently than every 3 weeks, cure is unlikely.

To monitor tumor response, hCG titers are obtained weekly. The drugs are continued on an every-other-week schedule until three consecutive weekly β-hCG serum values of less than 1 mIU/ml are reported. Because of an approximately 10% relapse rate after titer remission, continuing treatment is recommended for a minimum of three courses after the first normal titer.

The presence of central nervous system metastases requires special management because of the threat of intracranial hemorrhage. The brain is also thought to be a sanctuary for cancer, because the blood–brain barrier protects it from cytotoxic agents. Although choriocarcinoma is sometimes initially diagnosed at craniotomy, surgery usually can be avoided if the diagnosis is made earlier. Nevertheless, decompression craniotomy may be a necessity.

As soon as the presence of brain metastases has been demonstrated by clinical symptoms, physical examination, or CT scan, whole-brain irradiation should be initiated. A total dose of 2000–3000 cGy is given over 2 weeks. This has the immediate effect of preventing hemorrhage, and it is therapeutic as well.

Liver metastases are a most difficult problem. To prevent hemorrhage and eradicate tumor, some authorities have recommended whole-liver irradiation to approximately 2000 cGy. However, this has not been proven effective. We reserve it for cases with extensive or subcapsular metastases. We recommend chemotherapy alone for all other cases with liver involvement.

The prognosis is excellent for patients with lung metastases only. Approximately 90% can be expected to have a sustained remission. For those with central nervous system metastases, a 50% cure rate can be anticipated. Those with liver metastases have a significantly poorer prognosis – perhaps 25% of them survive.

The curability of metastatic choriocarcinoma is to a great extent dependent on the therapist's understanding of this cancer, the role of surgery, radiation, and chemotherapy in its management, and the nuances of hCG testing. Consequently, referral to a treatment center is advisable. Metastatic trophoblastic disease is so extraordinarily uncommon that few physicians, even specialists, have the experience required to manage this malignancy optimally.

SUGGESTED READING

BAGSHAWE KD, BAGENT RHJ. Trophoblastic tumors: clinical features and management. In: Coppleson M, ed. *Gynaecologicial Oncology*. London: Churchill Livingstone, 1981:757–772.

BREWER JI, HALPERN B, TOROK EE. Gestational trophoblastic disease: selected clinical aspects and chorionic gonadotropin test methods. In: Hickey RC, Clark RL, Benfield JR, eds. *Current Problems in Cancer*, vol 3. Chicago: Yearbook Medical Publishers, 1979:2.

BUCKLEY JD. The epidemiology of molar pregnancy and choriocarcinoma, *Clin Obstet Gynecol* 1984;27:153.

DUBUC-LISSOIR J, ZWEIZIG S, SCHLAERTH JB, MORROW CP. Metastatic gestational trophoblastic disease: a comparison of prognostic classification systems. *Gynecol Oncol* 1992;45:40.

GOLDSTEIN DP, BERKOWITZ RS (eds). Gestational trophoblastic neoplasms: clinical principles of diagnosis and management. In: *Major Problems in Obstetrics and Gynecology*, vol 14. Philadelphia: WB Saunders, 1982.

GOLDSTEIN DP, BERKOWITZ RS, COHEN SM. The current management of molar pregnancy. *Curr Probl Obstet Gynecol* 1979;2:1.

GOLDSTEIN DP, BERKOWITZ RS, BERNSTEIN MR. Reproductive performance after molar pregnancy and gestational trophoblastic tumors. *Clin Obstet Gynecol* 1984; 27:221.

HAMMOND CB, SOPER JT. Poor-prognosis metastatic gestational trophoblastic neoplasia. *Clin Obstet Gynecol* 1984;27:228.

HAMMOND CB, WEED JC Jr, CURRIE JL. The role of operation in the current therapy of gestational trophoblastic disease. *Am J Obstet Gynecol* 1980;136:844.

KOVACS BW, SHAHBAHRAMI B, TAST DE, CURTIN JP. Molecular genetic analysis of complete hydatidform moles. *Cancer Genet Cytogenet* 1991;54:143.

LURAIN JR, BREWER JI. Treatment of high-risk gestational trophoblastic disease with methotrexate, actinomycin D, and cyclophosphamide chemotherapy. *Obstet Gynecol* 1985;65:830.

LURAIN JR, BREWER JI, TOROK EE, et al. Gestational trophoblastic disease: treatment results at the Brewer Trophoblastic Disease Center. *Obstet Gynecol* 1982; 60:354.

LURAIN JR, BREWER JI, TOROK EE, et al. Natural history of hydatidiform mole after primary evacuation. *Am J Obstet Gynecol* 1983;145:591.

MORROW CP. Postosmolar trophoblastic disease: diagnosis, management and prognosis. *Clin Obstet Gynecol* 1984;27:211.

MORROW CP, SCHLAERTH JB. Recent advances in trophoblastic disease. In: Morrow CP, Bonnar J, O'Brien TJ, et al., eds. *Recent Clinical Developments in Gynecologic Oncology*. New York: Raven Press, 1983:532–567.

NEWLAND ES, BAGSHAWE KD, BEGENT RHJ, *et al.* Developments in chemotherapy for medium- and high-risk patients with gestational trophoblastic tumours (1979–1984). *Br J Obstet Gynaecol* 1986;93:63.

PETTERSSON F. Staging rules for gestational trophoblastic tumors and fallopian tube cancer. *Acta Obstet Gynecol Scand* 1992;71:224.

SCHLAERTH JB. Methodology of molar pregnancy termination. *Clin Obstet Gynecol* 1984;27:192.

SCHLAERTH JB, MORROW CP, KETZKY OA. Prognostic characteristics of serum human chorionic gonadotropin titer regression following molar pregnancy. *Obstet Gynecol* 1981;58:478.

SZULMAN AE, SURTI V. The syndromes of partial and complete molar gestation. *Clin Obstet Gynecol* 1984;27:199.

WEED JC Jr, HAMMOND CB. Cerebral metastatic choriocarcinoma: intensive therapy and prognosis. *Obstet Gynecol* 1980;55:89.

YORDAN EL, SCHLAERTH JB, GADDIS O, *et al.* Radiation in the management of gestational choriocarcinoma metastatic to the central nervous system. *Obstet Gynecol* 1987;69:627.

PART 6

Reproductive Endocrinology and Infertility

89

Diagnosis and management of sexual ambiguity in the newborn

DANIEL R. MISHELL, JR

The sex of an individual can be identified by four anatomic characteristics: (1) sex chromosomes; (2) gonadal histology; (3) morphology of the external genitalia; and (4) morphology of the internal genitalia. When all these characteristics are not consistently male or female, the condition of hermaphroditism, or intersexuality, exists. The psychologic characteristics of sex, which include sex of rearing, are usually related to the morphology of the external genitalia. When intersexuality exists in a newborn, it is very important to determine and designate the individual's future sex soon after birth to avoid a change in gender role later in life, with its accompanying psychologic trauma.

When intersexuality exists, the Krebs classification is used to provide definitions. When there is inconsistency among the four anatomic characteristics just described and the gonads are masculine, the individual is designated as a male pseudohermaphrodite. Likewise, when the histology of the gonads is feminine, the individual is designated as a female pseudohermaphrodite. If both male and female elements are present in one or both gonads, the individual is classified as a true hermaphrodite.

Disorders of sexual ambiguity can be further divided into two major categories on the basis of their etiology: (1) disorders of gonadal development, in which the basic defect is usually a major chromosomal lesion that occurs by chance and is not hereditary; and (2) disorders of fetal endocrinology, in which the individual has normal chromosomes corresponding to his or her gonadal sex but usually has a genetic (and often hereditary) defect.

Disorders of gonadal development

When a disorder of gonadal development occurs, the major chromosomal lesion can be due to an error in either meiosis or mitosis. Since these lesions occur by chance, they are neither hereditary nor more likely to occur in siblings. Errors in meiotic division can cause aneuploidy, which produces an incorrect number of sex chromosomes or structural abnormalities in sex chromosomes. Abnormalities in mitotic division can also occur. In this instance, both divided cells remain in the organism and mosaicism results. Mosaicism is a condition in which the individual has cells of different karyotypes but of one genetic origin.

The most common disorders of gonadal development, Klinefelter's syndrome and gonadal dysgenesis, do not cause problems of sexual differentiation in the newborn. Klinefelter's syndrome with a 47,XXY karyotype produces aspermia, and infertility is the most common presenting complaint.

Gonadal dysgenesis is associated with involution of the germ cells soon after they migrate into the undifferentiated gonad during early embryonic life. Thus, the gonads fail to develop and persist only as bilateral streaks of fibrous tissue that do not produce hormones. This syndrome is associated with normal female genitalia at birth and a wide range of karyotypes. It has been estimated that about half of the individuals with gonadal dysgenesis have a total absence of an X chromosome, while mosaicism is present in one-third. The gonads fail to develop and persist only as bilateral streaks. Phenotypically, individuals with gonadal dysgenesis appear as females with normal external and internal genitalia. With the lack of estrogen production, they fail to develop secondary sex characteristics usually and present with the complaint of primary amenorrhea and/or lack of any breast development.

The other disorders of gonadal development include true hermaphroditism and male pseudohermaphroditism. The disorders will cause problems in identifying the sex of the newborn. In true hermaphroditism, there are both male and female elements in the gonads. A uterus is nearly always present, and the differentiation of the internal genitalia corresponds closely to the histology of the adjacent gonad. Cryptorchidism is frequently present, together with some deficiency in labioscrotal fusion. The external genitalia are generally more male than female, but at puberty about three-fourths of true hermaphrodites develop gynecomastia and more than half menstruate. Therefore, it is important to make the diagnosis at birth so that these individuals are not raised as males.

There are two types of male pseudohermaphrodites with problems of gonadal development. The first has a primary gonadal defect with no gonads present and a normal 46,XY karyotype. The external genitalia are ambiguous, a vagina is present, and there is no evidence of female internal genitalia. The other is a Y chromosomal defect, which causes the syndrome of asymmetric gonadal differentiation, mixed gonadal dysgenesis. These patients have a testis on one side and a streak on the other. The external genitalia are most often ambiguous at birth, ranging from a normal male type with hypospadias to a normal female type with clitoromegaly. The internal genitalia usually are normal female. Cytogenetically, X chromosomal mosaicism is almost always involved, and the most frequent sex chromosome combination is X/XY.

Disorders of fetal endocrinology

Female pseudohermaphroditism with partial virilization

The second major category, disorders of fetal endocrinology, can be subdivided into female pseudohermaphroditism with partial virilization and male pseudohermaphroditism with partial failure of virilization. Female pseudohermaphroditism is usually due to congenital adrenal hyperplasia (CAH), although some forms have a nonadrenal etiology. CAH is the most frequent cause of ambiguous genitalia in the newborn. This is the only type of intersexuality with the possibility of entirely normal sexual function, including the capability of conception, as the virilization involves only the external genitalia. The gonads and internal genitalia are completely normal female, and the external genitalia can be surgically reconstructed to those of a normal female. This is the only intersex disorder than can jeopardize survival, and it is imperative to make the diagnosis at birth.

CAH is a recessive disorder that produces one of three enzyme deficiencies, which in turn cause lack of cortisol synthesis with a resultant increase in adrenocorticotropic hormone (ACTH) production. The increased ACTH causes increased production of adrenal androgens, which masculinize the external genitalia. Because the androgen production can vary according to the enzymatic defect, the virilization seen in these patients is variable in degree and can range from clitoromegaly with minimal labial fusion to complete scrotal fusion with the urethra opening at the tip of the phallus. In the latter case, the infant may resemble a completely normal male with cryptorchidism. It is therefore very important for the obstetrician to examine every male newborn and palpate the scrotum. If no testes are palpable, CAH should be suspected and appropriate diagnostic tests should be performed as soon as possible.

11β-Hydroxylase deficiency is the form of CAH least dangerous to the patient's life but is associated with hypertension. 21-Hydroxylase deficiency with salt-wasting and 3β-ol dehydrogenase deficiency may cause death. Once the diagnosis of CAH is suspected, it can be confirmed by measuring the levels of 17-hydroxyprogesterone in the serum. This steroid is elevated in all forms of CAH. The nonadrenal type of female pseudohermaphroditism is caused by excess exogenous or endogenous androgen stimulation of the fetus during pregnancy. Exogenous androgen can come from maternal ingestion of androgenic drugs. Endogenous androgen can be produced by a virilizing maternal ovarian tumor such as a luteoma.

Male pseudohermaphroditism with partial failure of virilization

There are three categories of male pseudohermaphroditism with partial failure of virilization. The most common is due to a defect in testosterone action. This is most frequently caused by a complete or partial defect of the androgen cellular receptor in the target organs. The terms androgen insensitivity syndrome and testicular feminization syndrome have been applied to this disorder. These individuals are genetically gonadal males with completely normal external female appearance and normal growth and development, including breast development. They usually present to the clinician after puberty with primary amenorrhea, scanty or absent pubic and axillary hair, absent internal genitalia, and female external genitalia with a short or absent vagina. These individuals have to be differentiated from females with normal ovaries and congenital absence of the uterus. The latter have normal pubic and axillary hair. If there is only a partial defect in the receptor protein, there may be varying degrees of ambiguity in the external genitalia, ranging from females with partial labioscrotal fusion through males with only minimal hypospadias. All of these individuals develop breasts at puberty, and varying degrees of development of the male internal genitalia are also seen.

Another type of defect of testosterone action is a deficiency of the 5α-reductase enzyme. This defect is an autosomal recessive disorder found in certain families. Males with this disorder are born with ambiguity of the external genitalia with bilateral undescended testes and lack of a phallus. Puberty brings marked virilization, phallic growth, and descent of the testes into the scrotum. Gynecomastia does not occur. In certain instances, individuals with this disorder can be raised as males, as they can ultimately have adequate male sexual function.

The second category of male pseudohermaphroditism is abnormality of Müllerian inhibitory factor synthesis, which leads to males with bilateral testes and normal male internal and external genitalia; however, they also have a uterus and oviducts. The latter are frequently present in inguinal hernia.

The third category includes those rare patients with various defects of biosynthesis of testosterone due to an autosomal recessive deficiency of certain enzymes. They have male gonads, ambiguous external genitalia, and no female internal genitalia, and may develop breasts at puberty. They constitute the nonvirilizing form of the adrenogenital syndrome.

Diagnosis and management

The newborn infant with ambiguous genitalia represents a medical emergency. Regardless of the complexity of the anomaly, appropriate and rapid gender assignment at the time of delivery, or soon thereafter at referral hospitalization, will often determine the success of the final outcome for the child and the family. Gender assignment is based on the existing anatomy and a full understanding of the pathologic and endocrine reasons for the sexual ambiguity. It should be stressed that the objective is to assign a gender concordant with the child's best future anatomic and sexual functioning. The sex chromosome pattern and gonadal histology are entirely immaterial with regard to gender assignment.

It is imperative that the parents be informed immediately in a non-traumatic manner. They should be told that the baby's sex organs are incompletely developed and that this birth defect precludes immediate gender assignment. However, diagnostic studies will commence at once to determine the gender of the baby. Until then, the sex of the child should not be announced and a birth certificate cannot be completed. Giving the baby a name that would suit a girl as well as a boy can only reinforce the idea of sexual ambiguity, which should be avoided under all circumstances. The parents should be allowed to examine the baby and its genitalia with the physician. It is important not to convey to the parents the idea of sexual ambiguity. The physician assigns the gender based on the following considerations and presents the assigned gender as the *de facto* diagnosis.

The diagnostic work-up should begin immediately. If inspection of the external genitalia reveals a transposition of the phallus and scrotum (i.e., if the phallus originates posterior to the scrotum), the physician should at once search for additional malformations that may be life-threatening, such as tracheoesophageal fistula, imperforate anus, or cardiac anomalies. In such instances, the extragenital malformations may be much more serious than the abnormal sexual development, or even incompatible with life.

In the absence of genital transposition, the physician should direct attention to the size of the phallus, the position of the urethral orifice, the degree of hypospadias if present, and the extent of labioscrotal fusion. Following inspection, the most important part of the physical examination is the palpation for gonads. Gonads palpable in the inguinal canal, in the labioinguinal area, or the labioscrotal folds are virtually always testes. Thus, the presence of one or two palpable gonads rules out virilization of an otherwise normal female, the most common form of ambiguous genitalia. Conversely, the infant born with ambiguous genitalia without palpable gonads most often represents virilization of a genetic female, usually as the result of CAH. Thus, determining the presence or absence of palpable gonads is the key in the initial evaluation.

The initial anatomic evaluation of the infant without palpable gonads is designed to establish whether a cervix and uterus are present. This can be accomplished by ultrasonography and/or genitography. It should be noted that ultrasonography is best performed within 24–48 h of delivery, because the estrogens of pregnancy that stimulate endometrial growth disappear rapidly in the neonatal period. Infants with a cervix and uterus should almost always be assigned the female gender irrespective of phallus size, because they are virilized genetic females with full reproductive potential (CAH, exogenous androgens, maternal virilizing disorders), individuals with mixed (asymmetric) gonadal dysgenesis, or true hermaphrodites.

Infants without a cervix and uterus (consistent with the presence of mullerian inhibiting substance of testicular origin) present a problem. Their gender assignment will often depend on the adequacy of the phallic structure. The infant with cryptorchidism or anorchia usually has an adequate phallus and should be assigned the male gender. Hormonal studies and surgical exploration can be performed later; exogenous testosterone therapy at the time of puberty will assist appropriate development and function as a male. Infants with an inadequate phallus and/or severe hypospadias are best assigned the female gender unless there is good potential for phallic reconstruction, as determined by a competent urologic surgeon. Errors in testosterone action tend to preclude adequate virilization, and infants born with these disorders usually should be assigned the female gender. The same holds true for most infants with 5α-reductase deficiency.

When an infant with ambiguous genitalia does have palpable gonads, the assessment should be as follows. First, one should distinguish between infants with unilaterally and those with bilaterally palpable gonads. A unilaterally palpable gonad may indicate asymmetric development of the internal genitalia and be consistent with either mixed gonadal dysgenesis or true hermaphroditism. A genitourogram may show unilateral or complete Müllerian duct development. Such infants are best assigned the female gender. But infants with ambiguous genitalia and symmetric labioscrotal or inguinal gonads usually represent cases of incomplete androgen insensitivity of type I or II or defects in testosterone biosynthesis. It is imperative to rule out deficiency of 3β-hydroxysteroid dehydrogenase, because this disorder could result in early salt loss, dehydration, and death. No infant with bilateral palpable gonads will have a cervix or uterus. Usually, infants with ambiguous genitalia resulting from type I or II incomplete androgen insensitivity or defects in testosterone biosynthesis should be assigned the female gender.

It is unnecessary to obtain a karyotype before gender can be assigned. The karyotype is helpful only when it confirms the clinical and anatomic findings.

All intraabdominal gonads or gonadal streaks in patients with intersex disorders and a Y chromosome have a relatively high potential for becoming malignant. The two most common tumors are dysgerminoma and gonadoblastoma. Tumor incidence markedly increases about the time of puberty in all intersex disorders with a Y chromosome other than androgen insensitivity disorders. These include gonadal dysgenesis, asymmetric gonadal differentiation (mixed gonadal dysgenesis), and other types of male pseudohermaphroditism. Therefore, the gonads should be removed before puberty from individuals with these disorders and a Y chromosome. Tumors are uncommon before the age of 20 in individuals with testicular feminization. Since the gonadal secretion of these individuals induces normal pubertal feminization, including breast development, removal of their gonads may be delayed until about age 18 with relative safety. Intersex patients without a Y chromosome rarely develop gonadal tumors, so their gonads or streaks should not be removed.

Disorders such as pure gonadal dysgenesis and androgen insensitivity usually do not become manifest until after the time of puberty, when affected individuals present with primary amenorrhea.

SUGGESTED READING

DONAHOE PK, HENDRAN WM. Evaluation of the newborn with ambiguous genitalia. *Pediatr Clin North Am* 1976;23:361.

IMPERATO-MCGINLEY J, PETERSON RE. Male pseudohermaphroditism. The complexities of male phenotypic development. *Am J Med* 1976;61:251.

MANUEL M, KATAYAMA KP, JONES HW. The age of occurrence of gonadal tumors in intersex patients with a Y chromosome. *Am J Obstet Gynecol* 1976;124:293.

PARK IJ, AIMAKHU VE, JONES HW. An etiologic and pathogenic classification of male hermaphroditism. *Am J Obstet Gynecol* 1975;123:505.

REINDOLLAR RH, LEWIS JB, WHJITE PC, et al. Prenatal diagnosis of 21-hydroxylase deficiency by the complementary deoxyribonucleic acid probe for cytochrome P-450^{C-210H}. *Am J Obstet Gynecol* 1988;158:545.

ROSEN GF, KAPLAN B, LOBO RA. Menstrual function and hirsutism in patients with gonadal dysgenesis. *Obstet Gynecol* 1988;71:677.

SIMPSOM JL. Genetics of sex determination. In: Iizuka R, Semm K, eds. *Human Reproduction: Current Status/Future Prospect.* New York: Elsevier, 1988:19.

WALSH PC, MADDEN JD, HARROD MJ, *et al.* Pseudohermaphroditism type II. *N Engl J Med* 1974;291:944.

WILSON JD, HARROD MJ, GOLDSTEIN JL, *et al.* Familial incomplete male pseudo-hermaphroditism, type I. Evidence of androgen resistance and variable clinical manifestations in a family with Reifenstein syndrome. *N Engl J Med* 1974;290: 1097.

90

Precocious puberty

PAUL F. BRENNER

Precocious puberty in the genetic, gonadal, and phenotypic female is defined as the presence of breast development prior to the age of 8 years or menarche prior to the age of 9 years.

A girl who feminizes early is defined as having isosexual precocious puberty; her secondary sex characteristics are in agreement with her genetic and phenotypic sex. A girl who virilizes early is defined as having heterosexual or contrasexual precocious puberty; her secondary sex characteristics are in disagreement with her genetic and phenotypic sex. The classification of the etiology of precocious puberty is listed in Table 90.1.

Incomplete precocious puberty

Isosexual precocious puberty is incomplete if only one pubertal change is clinically apparent without any evidence of a systemic estrogen effect. Absence of superficial cells desquamated from the vaginal mucosa or failure of the roentgenologic bone age to exceed the chronologic age is evidence for the absence of a systemic estrogen effect. The remaining pubertal events occur at a normal age. Incomplete forms of precocious puberty include premature thelarche, premature adrenarche, and premature pubarche.

Premature thelarche

Premature thelarche is the appearance of breast development prior to the age of 8 years without the presence of any other pubertal change or

Table 90.1 Classification of female precocious puberty

Isosexual precocious puberty
Incomplete precocious puberty
    Premature thelarche
    Premature adrenarche
    Premature pubarche

Complete precocious puberty
    Central (gonadotropin-dependent) precocious puberty
      Idiopathic
      Organic brain disease
    Peripheral (gonadotropin-independent) precocious puberty
      Ovarian
      Adrenal
      Iatrogenic
      Hypothyroidism
      McCune–Albright syndrome
      Hemihypertrophy syndrome
    Combined precocious puberty

Heterosexual (contrasexual) precocious puberty

evidence of systemic estrogen. This condition is benign and therapy is not required. Premature thelarche occurs most commonly between 1 and 4 years of age. A long-term follow-up of young girls with premature thelarche reveals that most have no progression of their breast development, one-third have regression of their breast changes, and one-tenth have progressive breast enlargement. Young girls with premature thelarche have low prepubertal (<20 pg/ml) estradiol levels, low levels of luteinizing hormone (LH) measured by bioassay (rat interstitial cell), and an increase in serum follicle-stimulating hormone (FSH) but not LH following gonadotroropin-releasing hormone (GnRH) stimulation.

Premature adrenarche

Premature adrenarche is the appearance of axillary hair prior to the age of 8 years without the presence of any other pubertal change or evidence of systemic estrogen. Premature adrenarche is also a benign condition and therapy is not required.

Premature pubarche

Premature pubarche is the appearance of pubic hair prior to the age of 8 years without the presence of any other pubertal change or evidence of systemic estrogen. Premature pubarche is the result of a functional increase in the production of adrenal androgens. Some children with premature pubarche have an exaggerated response of 17-OH-progesterone following adrenocorticotropic hormone (ACTH) stimulation, suggesting that heterozygosity for 21-hydroxylase deficiency may explain the clinical presentation of premature pubarche. Some series report that approximately one-half of all children with premature pubarche have organic brain disease. The reason for this association is unknown.

Complete isosexual precocious puberty

Complete isosexual precocious puberty is classified into three groups: central, peripheral, and combined. In all groups there is an increase in circulating estrogen levels which leads to the appearance of secondary sex characteristics, pubertal changes which may progress to menarche, rapid acceleration of linear growth, and premature closure of the distal epiphyses. Thus children who may be taller than their peers when the precocious development is first apparent will ultimately be of short stature if they are not treated.

Central isosexual precocious puberty

Central isosexual precocious puberty has also been referred to as true isosexual precocious puberty, cerebral isosexual precocious puberty, and gonadotropin-dependent precocious puberty. Ninety percent of all children with complete isosexual precocious puberty will have the central form. In the central form there is a cyclic release of gonadotropins and fertility is possible. The etiology of this form of isosexual precocious puberty always involves the central nervous system. Central isosexual precocious puberty is divided into two diagnostic subgroups: (1) idiopathic; and (2) organic brain disease.

Idiopathic disease is the most common etiology for female central precocious puberty, accounting for 70% of the children with this problem. The underlying etiology for the premature activation of the reproductive axis is unknown. In idiopathic precocious puberty the progression of endocrine events of normal puberty occurs at an early age. These endocrine events are appropriate for the child's pubertal stage of development and are advanced with respect to the child's chronologic age. Children with idiopathic precocious puberty have a growth spurt which is rapid but of short duration. At first, they are much taller than their peers but ultimately they will be very short in stature. The earlier the disease begins, the shorter will be the child's final height. About one-third of these children have alterations in EEG patterns consistent with epilepsy.

The onset of symptoms may occur at any age prior to 8 years but is quite uncommon in the first year of life. The rate of progression and the sequence of symptoms can vary greatly. Spontaneous remissions are extremely rare.

The general health of children with idiopathic precocious puberty is not impaired but the pubertal changes may create emotional conflicts for both the child and her family. These children may have an increase in minor psychopathologic symptoms but do not manifest an increase in severe psychiatric disorders. Children with idiopathic precocious puberty may have functional follicular ovarian cysts identified by a pelvic ultrasonographic exam. Problems of infertility and premature ovarian failure are not increased in children with idiopathic precocious puberty. The diagnosis of idiopathic precocious puberty is made by excluding all other causes of precocious puberty.

The development of imaging modalities of high resolution has resulted in an increase in the identification of organic brain disease as a cause of central isosexual precocious puberty. Approximately 30% of children with central precocious puberty have organic brain disease which includes tumors, obstructive disease, congenital defects, neurofibromatosis, cranial irradiation, postinfective lesions, and posttraumatic brain injury. All children with central precocious puberty must have a thorough evaluation, including a complete neurologic examination and computed tomography (CT) scan or magnetic resonance imaging (MRI) before central nervous system disease can be excluded.

Peripheral isosexual precocious puberty

Peripheral isosexual precocious puberty has also been referred to as pseudoisosexual precocious puberty, and gonadotronpin-independent precocious puberty. Children with peripheral precocious puberty do not attain cyclic function of the reproductive axis, follicular maturation and ovulation do not occur, and they are not fertile. Peripheral isosexual precocious puberty is divided into six diagnostic subgroups: (1) ovarian; (2) adrenal; (3) iatrogenic; (4) hypothyroidism; (5) McCune–Albright syndrome; and (6) hemihypertrophy syndrome.

The most common cause of peripheral isosexual precocious puberty is an *ovarian tumor* that produces estrogen (granulosa–theca cell tumors). These tumors are almost always palpable on rectoabdominal examination and can be identified by ultrasonography. Most granulosa–theca cell tumors are benign and are confined to one ovary. The usual treatment is unilateral salpingo-oophorectomy. Choriocarcinoma, of ovarian or extragonadal origin, secretes human chorionic gonadotropin (hCG) which may stimulate ovarian estrogen secretion and cause precocious puberty.

An estrogen-secreting *adrenal tumor* is a very rare cause of isosexual precocious puberty. Clinically virilizing symptoms and signs have preceded the clinical manifestations of excess estrogen.

Oral or topical administration of estrogens (cosmetics, powders, creams, medications) may cause peripheral precocious puberty. A complete history and careful review of all possible *iatrogenic sources* of estrogen in the home is the only means of identifying iatrogenic sources of estrogen.

Children who are markedly hypothyroid lose the negative feedback of thyroxin on the hypothalamus and pituitary. As thyroid-stimulating hormone secretion is increased by the pituitary there is a concomitant indiscriminate increase in gonadotropins. The rise in gonadotropins produces clinical signs of precocious puberty and may stimulate the growth of ovarian cysts. With thyroid replacement therapy the children will become euthyroid and the ovarian cysts will regress. Children with *hypothyroidism* are short in stature and their bone age is retarded. Hypothyroidism as a cause of precocious puberty is limited almost entirely to girls.

McCune–Albright syndrome is composed of the triad of precocious puberty, multiple areas of fibrous dysplasia of bone, and *café-au-lait* spots on the skin. Facial asymmetry and/or skeletal deformities are pathognomonic of polyostotic fibrous dysplasia. The diagnosis can be derived from the identification of dysplastic lesions of bone seen on X-ray. This rare disease is found more frequently in girls. Most commonly, children with McCune–Albright syndrome have widely fluctuating estrogen levels and low gonadotropin concentrations which are independent of GnRH stimulation.

The *hemihypertrophy syndrome* of Wilkins is the appearance of both unilateral sexaual precocity and vascular anomalies in the same child. The diagnosis of this very rare condition is made by physical examination.

Combined peripheral and central precocious puberty

Children with combined isosexual precocious puberty initially present with peripheral precocious puberty. As the disease progresses the reproductive hormonal axis is activated and central gonadotropin-dependent precocious puberty is present. Congenital adrenal hyperplasia is the most common cause of combined precocious puberty. Other causes include McCune–Albright syndrome and a virilizing adrenal tumor.

Diagnosis

Heterosexual precocious puberty can be distinguished from isosexual precocious puberty by a history and physical examination that identify male secondary sex characteristics in a genetic, gonadal, and phenotypic female. These children with symptoms and signs of virilization are evaluated in a manner identical to all female patients who present with androgen excess, as described in Chapter 95.

All children with isosexual precocious puberty should have their stage of pubertal development determined by the method of Tanner based on the stage of breast development and the stage of pubic hair growth. The child's height should be determined accurately using a stadiometer at each visit. The child's growth chart should be reviewed to determine the age of onset of increase in rapid growth velocity. The incomplete forms of precocious puberty (premature thelarche, premature adrenarche, premature pubarche) are diagnosed when serial observations at least 6 months apart reveal that only one pubertal change has occurred, and that the bone age corresponds with the chronologic age. Other diagnostic tests to distinguish premature thelarche from central idiopathic precocious puberty include serum estradiol and prolactin, bioassay of LH, and a GnRH stimulation test. Children with premature thelarche have prepubertal levels of serum estradiol and prolactin, low quantities of bioassayable LH, and an increase of FSH but not LH 30–60 min following the intravenous bolus injection of 50–100 μg of GnRH. Children with idiopathic precocious puberty have increased concentrations of estradiol and prolactin above the prepubertal range in their peripheral circulation, elevated quantities of LH determined by bioassay, and an increase in FSH and LH in response to GnRH stimulation. An increase in FSH and LH to GnRH excludes the diagnosis of premature thelarche. An increase in FSH only to GnRH administration may occur in premature thelarche and the very early manifestations of idiopathic precocious puberty. Children with premature pubarche should be further evaluated with a cranial CT scan and the determination of 17α-hydroxyprogesterone levels at baseline and following intravenous ACTH stimulation.

Children who are hypothyroid and present with precocious puberty have a retarded bone age compared to their chronologic age. Thyroid function tests will confirm the diagnosis and serve as a baseline from which the effects of therapy can be judged. Hypothyroidism is the only etiology of precocious puberty for which the bone age is significantly less than the chronologic age of the child.

The advancement of bone age above the 95th percentile for the chronologic age indicates a peripheral estrogen effect. A GnRH stimulation test differentiates central precocious puberty from peripheral precocious puberty. Children with peripheral precocious puberty have an advanced bone age and fail to manifest a change in gonadotropins following GnRH stimulation. A rectoabdominal examination and pelvic ultrasonography will identify granulosa–theca cell tumors. Serum hCG concentrations are elevated in the presence of trophoblastic disease. Adrenal tumors are diagnosed with the use of adrenal sonograms. Iatrogenic sources of estrogen can only be detected by a thorough medical history and a careful search of the child's environment. McCune–Albright syndrome is diagnosed by physical examination denoting facial asymmetry, skeletal deformities and *café-au-lait* spots. A radiographic skeletal survey or technetium bone scan will confirm the presence of dysplastic bone lesions. The diagnosis of hemihypertrophy syndrome is established by physical examination.

Children with central precocious puberty have an advanced bone age and demonstrate an increase in gonadotropin levels in response to GnRH. Central nervous system disease is confirmed with the use of neurologic and ophthalmologic examinations, skull X-ray, EEG, and CT cranial scan or MRI study of the brain. The diagnosis of idiopathic precocious puberty is made by the exclusion of all other causes of precocious puberty.

Treatment

The treatment of precocious puberty depends upon the specific etiology. Incomplete forms of isosexual precocious puberty are usually self-limited and do not require treatment. The hypothyroid child is managed with thyroid replacement therapy. Once iatrogenic sources of estrogen are identified they should be eliminated from the child's environment. Ovarian and adrenal tumors causing precocious puberty should be removed surgically. Testolatone, an aromatase inhibitor, has been successfully used in the treatment of children with McCune–Albright syndrome. Testolactone is started with a total daily oral dose of 20 mg/kg body weight in four divided doses. Over a 3-week interval the total daily dose is increased to 40 mg/kg body weight. Estrogen concentrations in the peripheral circulation are reduced, ovarian volume measured by ultrasound is reduced, and the frequency of menses diminished with testolactone therapy. There is little effect of testolactone on the regression of breast development or pubic hair growth. The effect of this therapy on skeletal growth has been difficult to assess. Diarrhea and abdominal cramping are side-effects attributed to testolactone. There is no treatment for hemihypertrophy syndrome.

Medroxyprogesterone acetate, danazol, and cyproterone acetate have been used to treat idiopathic precocious puberty. All three treatment modalities inhibit gonadotropin secretion and uniformly suppress ovulation. The suppression of menstruation and the regression of secondary sex characteristics are less consistent with any of these therapies. The accelerated rates of linear growth and premature epiphyseal closure fail to respond to any of these agents. None of these agents has been able to improve the potential for linear growth in these patients.

Long-acting GnRH agonists have become the treatment of choice for idiopathic precocious puberty. After an initial rise, pituitary secretion of gonadotropins decreases, estrogen levels decline to the prepubertal range, ovarian volume and uterine size as determined by ultrasound regress, breast development is halted or regresses, menstruation ceases, and the rates of linear growth and skeletal maturation decrease. Children with idiopathic precocious puberty treated with GnRH agonists will achieve a greater height as the result of their therapy. Recovery of the reproductive axis is prompt when the GnRH agonists are discontinued.

Several long-acting GnRH analogs are available for the treatment of idiopathic precocious puberty. Deslorelin 4–8 µg/kg, leuprolide acetate 20–60 µg/kg, and buserelin 20–30 µg/kg are administered once daily as a subcutaneous injection. Buserelin 1200–1800 µg/day and nafarelin 800–1200 µg/day have been administered intranasally. Leuprolide contained in microcapsules is administered as a 60 µg/kg intramuscular injection every 4 weeks. GnRH analogs are reported as being successful in the treatment of idiopathic precocious puberty and in the treatment of central nervous system disease resulting in gonadotropin-dependent precocious puberty. GnRH agonists have not been proven efficacious for peripheral, gonadotropin-independent precocious puberty. Side-effects observed with the use of GnRH agonists to treat precocious puberty include allergic reactions at the injection site, allergy symptoms of the lungs with intranasal administration, and vasomotor symptoms. Therapy should be started as early in the clinical presentation of the endocrinopathy as possible, in order or maximize the opportunity of the child to achieve her full height potential. GnRH agonist therapy should be continued until children with central precocious puberty reach at least the mean age for pubertal development.

SUGGESTED READING

FEUILLAN PP, FOSTER CM, PESCOVITZ OH, *et al.* Treatment of precocious puberty in the McCune–Albright syndrome with the aromatase inhibitor testolactone. *N Engl J Med* 1986;315:1115–1119.

KOEHLER B, KOEHLER M, OSUCH-JACZEWSKA R. Intranasal LH-RH analogue treatment of precocious puberty. *Exp Clin Endocrinol* 1988;92:252–256.

LEIPER AD, STANHOPE R, KITCHING P, CHESSELLS JM. Precocious and premature puberty associated with treatment of acute lymphoblastic leukaemia. *Arch Dis Child* 1987;62:1107–1112.

OERTER KE, MANASCO P, BARNES KM, JONES J, HILL S, CUTLER GB Jr. Adult height in precocious puberty after long-term treatment with Deslorelin. *J Clin Endocrinol Metab* 1991;73:1235–1240.

PESCOVITZ OH, HENCH KD, BARNES KM, LORIAUX DL, CUTLER GB Jr. Premature thelarche and central precocious puberty: the relationship between clinical presentation and the gonadotropin response to luteinizing hormone-releasing hormone. *J Clin Endocrinol Metab* 1988;67:474–479.

RIDDLESBERGER MM Jr, KUHN JP, MUNSCHAUER RW. The association of juvenile hypothyroidism and cystic ovaries. *Radiology* 1981;139:77–80.

ROGER M, CHAUSSAIN J-L, BERLIER P, *et al.* Long-term treatment of male and female precocious puberty by periodic administration of a long-acting preparation of D-Trp^6-luteinizing hormone-releasing hormone microcapsules. *J Clin Endocrinol Metab* 1986;62:670–677.

SIEGEL SF, FINEGOLD ND, URBAN MD, McVIE R, LEE PA. Premature pubarche: etiological heterogeneity. *J Clin Endocrinol Metab* 1992;74:239–247.

SOCKALOSKY JJ, KRIEL RL, KRACH LE, SHEEHAN M. Precocious puberty after traumatic brain injury. *J Pediatr* 1987;110:373–377.

STARCESKI P-J, LEE PA, ALBRIGHT AL, MIGEON CJ. Hypothalamic hamartomas and sexual precocity. *Am J Dis Child* 1990;144:225–228.

91

Differential diagnosis of primary amenorrhea

DANIEL R. MISHELL, JR & VAL DAVAJAN

The diagnosis of primary amenorrhea is made when a patient has had no spontaneous uterine bleeding by the age of 17. However, a diagnostic work-up should be initiated at age 15 if the patient develops no secondary sex characteristics or if 2 years or more have elapsed following the onset of secondary sex development but this is not followed by menarche.

Individuals with primary amenorrhea can be classified into four groups based on the presence or absence of breast development and uterus: group 1, those without breast development and with a palpable uterus; group 2, those with breast development and no uterus; group 3, those with neither breast development nor a uterus; group 4, those with breast development and palpable uterus (Table 91.1).

Group 1

Individuals without breast development and with a palpable uterus may have either hypogonadotropic hypogonadism or gonadal dysgenesis. The correct differential diagnosis can be made easily by measuring serum follicle-stimulating hormone (FSH), which is elevated consistently in patients with gonadal dysgenesis. Although serum luteinizing hormone (LH) usually is elevated, it can on occasion be within the normal range.

Individuals with hypogonadotropic hypogonadism have either low or normal serum values of both LH and FSH. Some of these also may present with anosmia (Kallmann syndrome). Therefore, all women in this group (without elevated FSH) should have at least a qualitative test for olfaction with coffee, tobacco, orange, and cocoa. If one wishes to

Table 91.1 Classification of disorders in primary amenorrhea with normal external genitalia

Group	Definition
Group 1	Primary amenorrhea without breast development; uterus present
(a)	Hypothalamic failure secondary to inadequate GnRH release
(b)	Pituitary gonadotropin insufficiency
(c)	Gonadal failure
(i)	45,X (Turner syndrome)
(ii)	46,X, abnormal X (e.g., short or long arm deletion)
(iii)	Mosaicism (e.g., X/XX, X/XX/XXX)
(iv)	46,XX or 46,XY pure gonadal dysgenesis
(v)	17α-hydroxylase deficiency with 46,XX karyotype
(d)	Central nervous system lesions
Group 2	Primary amenorrhea with breast development; uterus absent
(a)	Androgen insensitivity (testicular feminization)
(b)	Congenital absence of uterus
Group 3	Primary amenorrhea without breast development; uterus absent
(a)	17,20-desmolase deficiency
(b)	Agonadism
(c)	17α-hydroxylase deficiency with 46,XY karyotype
Group 4	Primary amenorrhea with breast development; uterus present
(a)	Hypothalamic causes
(b)	Pituitary causes
(c)	Ovarian causes
(d)	Uterine causes

identify further the etiology of the hypogonadotropic hypogonadism, patients may be tested with gonadotropin-releasing hormone (GnRH). Hypothalamic or higher central nervous system disorders are the most common cause of hypogonadotropic primary amenorrhea. Additional causes can be craniopharyngioma, tuberculous granuloma, sequelae of menigoencephalitis, thalassemia major, retinitis pigmentosa, or non-secreting pituitary adenoma. Therefore, a computed tomography or magnetic resonance imaging of the sella turcica should be obtained. A karyotype is not necessary, as all these patients have 46,XX. Women with hypogonadotropic hypogonadism have good potential for successful reproduction with the administration of exogenous gonadotropins or GnRH administered with a pulsatile pump. If pregnancy is not desired, 0.625 mg of conjugated estrogen should be given daily to induce breast development. During the first 12 days of each month a progestin should be added to prevent endometrial hyperplasia or adenocarcinoma.

Individuals with gonadal dysgenesis have elevated gonadotropins and need chromosome analysis. Karyotype is important because the presence of a Y chromosome is an indication to remove the gonads. It has been estimated that the risk of developing a gonadal tumor with a Y chromosome present is over 25% by age 30. However, if the karyotype does not contain a Y chromosome, the gonads need not be removed unless there is clinical evidence of androgen production. Women with gonadal dysgenesis need estrogen replacement to induce breast development and to prevent osteoporosis. In short patients, the conjugated estrogen at first dose should not be more than 0.3 mg/day in order to avoid premature closure of the epiphyses. Patients of normal height should be given 0.625 or 1.25 mg/day of conjugated estrogen to induce menses. A daily dosage of 0.625 mg of conjugated estrogen is sufficient to produce adequate breast development. Higher doses of estrogen do not enhance breast development. During the first 12 days of each month 5 mg of oral medroxyprogesterone acetate is added in order to differentiate and cause cyclic sloughing of the endometrium. These women cannot conceive, but they can receive an ovum from a donor, which is fertilized *in vitro* with the patient's husband's sperm and then transferred to her uterus, which has been appropriately stimulated with steroids.

Individuals with hypogonadotropic hypogonadism or gonadal dysgenesis should be differentiated from those with 17α-hydroxylase deficiency which have a similar phenotype. They have the same clinical features as individuals with a 46,XX karyotype and a low-serum FSH, but they have hypertension and hypokalemia. Thus, individuals with primary amenorrhea, no breast development, and a palpable uterus must have their blood pressure measured and, if elevated, serum electrolytes should be ordered and, if abnormal, 17α-hydroxylase deficiency must be ruled out. In addition to estrogen/progestagen, these patients should be treated with an adequate replacement dose of corticosteroids.

Group 2

Individuals with primary amenorrhea with normal breast development but no uterus have either congenital absence of the uterus or androgen insensitivity syndrome (testicular feminization). Women with absence of the uterus usually ovulate and have normal pubic hair. Individuals with androgen insensitivity syndrome do not ovulate and have no or minimal pubic hair. The presence of ovulation can be determined by taking the basal body temperature or weekly measurements of serum progesterone. If ovulation is documented, no further diagnostic testing is necessary because the woman obviously does not have androgen insensitivity.

Because women with congenital absence of the uterus have normal ovarian function, no hormonal replacement is necessary.

Another approach to differentiate these two types of individuals is to measure serum testosterone. With congenital absence of the uterus, serum testosterone levels are within the normal female range. Individuals with androgen insensitivity have serum testosterone levels within the normal male range. With an elevated testosterone level a karyotype examination should be performed. An individual with this syndrome has 46,XX chromosomes, testes, and female phenotype. Abnormal clinical features in these patients include the lack of axillary and pubic hair with normal breast development and a blind vaginal pouch (absence of the uterus).

All patients with androgen insensitivity should have the gonads surgically removed after puberty because of the high incidence of malignancy. The incidence of gonadal tumors in patients over 30 years of age with this syndrome is approximately 25%. It is usually recommended that the testes not be removed until the patient has undergone full sexual development with her own endogenous testicular steroids since most tumors have been reported to develop after the patient is older than 20. Following gonadectomy, the patient should be placed on 0.625 mg of conjugated estrogen replacement daily to prevent osteoporosis. Progestins should not be administered to these patients as they have no uterus. It is our recommendation to tell patients with this syndrome that there is an abnormal sex chromosome and not specifically refer to the abnormality as a Y chromosome, as most of the patients know that an XY karyotype is indicative of being a male. The term gonad should be used instead of testis when referring to the gonadal abnormality. The patient also should be told that she cannot become pregnant and that she may require vaginoplasty in order to have normal sexual function. Patients with congenital absence of the uterus also may need a vaginoplasty as some may have a short or absent vagina.

Group 3

Patients with primary amenorrhea who have neither breast nor uterus development are very rare, and the differential diagnosis is difficult to make. These individuals all have a male karyotype, elevated gonadotropin levels, and testosterone values in the normal female range. They differ from patients with gonadal dysgenesis because they do not have a uterus and from patients with androgen insensitivity because they do not have breast development and their serum testosterone levels are in the normal female range. The etiology for the abnormality can be a 17,20-desmolase deficiency, testicular regression, or 17α-hydroxylase deficiency.

If the patient has gonads, they should be removed; if no gonads are present or after the gonads are removed, estrogen should be replaced in order to induce breast development in doses and forms previously recommended.

Patients with the 17α-hydroxylase deficiency have a 46,XY karyotype, no secondary sex characteristics, no uterus, and hypertension. Management is similar to those patients with the same enzymatic defect but with a uterus and a 46,XX karyotype.

Group 4

The presence of primary amenorrhea in women with spontaneous breast development and a normal uterus indicates that a disturbance of the hypothalamic–pituitary–ovarian axis occurs after the initiation but before the completion of puberty. Women with primary amenorrhea with breast development and an intact uterus should have a careful breast examination to detect the presence of galactorrhea and a serum prolactin determination to rule out a prolactin-secreting pituitary adenoma. Patients with normal serum prolactin levels have the same features as the patients with secondary amenorrhea. Their work-up is discussed in detail in Chapter 92.

SUGGESTED READING

ABAD L, PARRILLA JJ, MARCOS J, et al. Male pseudohermaphroditism with 17 alpha-hydroxylase deficiency: a case report. *Br J Obstet Gynecol* 1980;87:1162.

CHANG RJ, DAVIDSON BJ, CARLSON HE, et al. Hypogonadotropic hypogonadism associated with retinitis pigmentosa in a female sibling: evidence of gonadotropin deficiency. *J Clin Endocrinol Metab* 1981;53:1179.

FRISCH RE, REVEL RR. Height and weight at menarche and a hypothesis of menarche. *Arch Dis Child* 1971;46:695.

KLETZKY OA, NICOLOFF JT, DAVAJAN V, et al. Idiopathic hypogonadotrophic primary amenorrhea. *J Clin Endocrinol Metab* 1978;46:808.

KLETZKY OA, MARRS RP, COSTIN G, et al. Gonadotropin insufficiency in patients with thalassemia major. *J Clin Endocrinol Metab* 1979;48:901.

MANUEL M, KATAYAMA KP, JONES HW Jr. The age of occurrence of gonadal tumors in intersex patients with a Y chromosome. *Am J Obstet Gynecol* 1976;124:293.

MASHCHAK CA, KLETZKY OA, DAVAJAN V, et al. Clinical and laboratory evaluation of patients with primary amenorrhea. *Obstet Gynecol* 1981;57:715.

REINDOLLAR RH, BYRD JR, MCDONOUGH PG. Delayed sexual development: a study of 252 patients. *Am J Obstet Gynecol* 1981;140:a371.

ROSEN GR, KAPLAN B, LOBO RA. Menstrual function and hirsutism in patients with gonadal dysgenesis. *Obstet Gynecol* 1988;17:677.

ROSEN GF, VERMESH M, D'ABLAING G, WACHTEL S, LOBO RA. The endocrinologic evaluation of a 45,X true hermaphodite. *Am J Obstet Gynecol* 1987;157:1272.

TURNER HH. A syndrome of infantilism, congenital webbed neck and cubitus-valgus. *Endocrinology* 1938;23:566.

WENTZ AC, JONES GS. Prognosis in primary amenorrhea. *Fertil Steril* 1978;29:614.

92

Differential diagnosis of secondary amenorrhea

DANIEL R. MISHELL, JR & VAL DAVAJAN

Secondary amenorrhea is usually defined as a 6-month interval without menses in a nonpregnant woman of reproductive age. Amenorrhea is a symptom of various disorders. To establish the diagnosis, it is appropriate to divide the patients with these symptoms into various groups. Patients with amenorrhea and no clinical evidence of excess cortisol (Cushing syndrome), androgen production, or hyperprolactinemia can be divided into two groups based on whether or not they have uterine bleeding following intramuscular injection of 100 or 200 mg of progesterone in oil or a serum estradiol level above or below 40 pg/ml.

The positive or negative response of the endometrium to progesterone correlates well with the levels of serum estradiol. No uterine bleeding will usually occur if the level of estradiol is below 40 pg/ml. Any amount of uterine bleeding is considered a positive test (from minimal dark-brown staining to a normal menstrual flow). When uterine bleeding does occur, it usually occurs 2–14 days after the progesterone injection. The etiology of amenorrhea in individuals with normal breast development and an intact uterus without evidence of androgen or cortisol excess or galactorrhea can be due to a hypothalamic, pituitary, ovarian, or uterine factor (Table 92.1).

Uterine causes

The integrity of the endometrium always should be considered first before initiating the endocrine evaluation. To determine whether intrauterine synechiae (Asherman syndrome) are present any patient with amenorrhea who has had a prior curettage, especially in pregnancy, should have the uterus sounded or, even better, a hysterosalpingogram and/or hysteroscopy. If synechiae are found, appropriate therapy should be performed as discussed in Chapter 106.

Hypothalamic causes

Hypothalamic dysfunction without exercise, stress, weight loss, or medication

One of the most common causes of amenorrhea is anovulation secondary to hypothalamic dysfunction (euestrogenic amenorrhea) without any

Table 92.1 Responses to progesterone

Step 1

Progesterone in oil (100 mg im) (or oral medroxyprogesterone 30 mg/day × 3)

Uterine bleeding (positive response)	Allow 2–14 days	No uterine bleeding Return for progesterone 200 mg im
		No uterine bleeding (negative response)

Step 2

Progesterone in oil
|
Positive uterine bleeding
|
LH

High (>25 mIU/ml)	Normal
Polycystic ovary disease, hyperandrogenic chronic anovulation	Hypothalamic dysfunction (drug-related) (stress-related) (exercise-related)
Testosterone DHEA-S	PRL

		Normal	High

Induce bleeding every 2 months or use OC, dexamethasone. or spironolactone if androgens are elevated	Induce uterine bleeding every 2 months with progestins (medroxyprogesterone 5 mg/day × 12 days)	Workup

Continued on p. 606.

Table 92.1 *Continued*

Step 3

Intramuscular progesterone
|
Negative response
|
FSH

Normal or low*	Elevated
Hypothalamic–	Ovarian failure
pituitary failure*	If <25 years, karyotype
	If <35 years, thyroid antibodies,
1 CT scan or MRI	24-h urine free cortisol
2 PRL (if elevated workup)	Serum calcium/phosphorus
3 T3, T4, free thyroxine index	ANA/rheumatoid factors.
4 ACTH reserve test†	

* Patients with simple weight loss, history of drug intake, stress or exercise, who do not have hyperprolactinemia do not need CT or MRI scan.
† Only in patients with history of postpartum hemorrhage or abnormal MRI or CT scan.
OC, Oral contraceptive.

history of stress or drug intake. These individuals have disorders of frequency of the normal pulsatile release of GnRH.

Hypothalamic dysfunction due to drugs or stress

Drugs most commonly associated with amenorrhea are the phenothiazide derivatives and some hypertensive agents. Some patients will develop amenorrhea when a stress situation is encountered (e.g., going away to school, divorce in the family, etc.). These patients have levels of estradiol of at least 40 pg/ml and therefore have uterine bleeding following progesterone administration. Random sampling of follicle-stimulating hormone (FSH) and luteinizing hormone (LH) levels is in the normal range.

Hypothalamic dysfunction (euestrogenic) or failure (hypoestrogenic) resulting from exercise

The incidence of amenorrhea among women engaged in running exercise increases as weekly training mileage increases. This increase in incidence is not always related to weight loss but cannot be separated from stress as the major contributing factor. The pathophysiology of exercise-induced amenorrhea may be mediated via the increase in the levels of catechol estrogens which in turn reduces the rate of catecholamine degradation.

This results in increased levels of dopamine which can suppress the release of gonadotropin-releasing hormone (GnRH) and thus the gonado-tropins. Another possible explanation of this syndrome may be via the increase in levels of natural opiates (endorphins) during exercise which in turn have a direct negative effect on GnRH secretion and in addition a positive effect on dopamine secretion.

Hypothalamic dysfunction or failure due to weight loss

This includes simple weight loss and anorexia nervosa. Patients with simple weight loss are those individuals who become amenorrheic after losing 15–20% of ideal body weight (usually referred to as being under-weight) or those with >25% weight loss who are labeled severely under-weight. These individuals may have normal or low gonadotropins and normal or low estrogen, depending upon the degree of weight loss. Patients with anorexia nervosa, in addition to having severe weight loss (>25% of ideal body weight), have the added complaints of constipation, hypotension, bradycardia, and hypothermia. They invariably have an abnormal ideation concerning their body image and an aversion to food intake. They have low serum gonadotropin and low estrogen levels. In addition, most patients with anorexia nervosa, in contrast to those with simple weight loss, have a low serum triiodothyronine level (T3) by radioimmunoassay.

The treatment of these two groups of patients appears to be related primarily to regaining body weight. Patients with anorexia nervosa also need psychiatric therapy.

Hypothalamic failure due to lesions of the hypothalamus

These disorders may manifest themselves as either primary or secondary amenorrhea. Lesions of the hypothalamus associated with amenorrhea include craniopharyngioma, tuberculous granuloma, and the sequelae of meningoencephalitis. These patients have a low estradiol level and will not have uterine bleeding after progesterone administration. The random serum FSH and LH levels in these patients are either very low or in the low-normal range. In this latter group, the low-normal levels of LH and FSH are insufficient to stimulate the ovarian follicles to synthesize estradiol.

Amenorrhea secondary to hyperandrogenic chronic anovulation (polycystic ovarian syndrome)

Women with hyperandrogenic chronic anovulation (HCA; commonly referred to as polycystic ovarian syndrome; PCO) most likely have a neurotransmitter-hypothalamic disorder that may result in the histologic (polycystic) changes seen in the ovary. Most patients with HCA present with oligomenorrhea but some have secondary or even primary amenorrhea. These patients are usually euestrogenic with the defect being mainly one of failure to ovulate. These patients most often but not always have some degree of clinical signs of hyperandrogenism (e.g., hirsutism). For a complete discussion of this condition see Chapter 96.

Pituitary causes

Patients with amenorrhea due to a pituitary etiology may have nonneoplastic lesions or tumors.

Nonneoplastic lesions

This group includes patients with a destructive process of the pituitary, such as seen in Sheehan and Simmond syndrome. The pituitary cells are damaged by anoxia, thrombosis, or hemorrhage. These patients have low serum levels of LH, FSH, and estradiol and therefore will not bleed following intramuscular progesterone.

Pituitary tumors

Amenorrhea may be the first sign of a pituitary tumor (nonprolactin-secreting adenoma). Patients with amenorrhea who have pituitary tumors usually have low serum estradiol and therefore do not have uterine bleeding following administration of intramuscular progesterone. A random serum level of FSH and LH may be either low or normal. However, repeated sampling of these hormones at 10- to 15-min intervals for 4 h will reveal less than a normal amount of these hormones being secreted. Clinically, repeated sampling is not practicable and therefore a "normal" value should be considered as low.

Ovarian causes of amenorrhea

There are two different ovarian causes of amenorrhea which result in ovarian failure. They are premature ovarian failure, and loss of ovarian function secondary to castration, infection, hemorrhage, or compromised blood supply.

Premature ovarian failure

This diagnosis is made when ovarian failure occurs at any age between the onset of menarche and age 40. Because the ovaries of these patients do not secrete sufficient amounts of estradiol to maintain the negative feedback on the hypothalamus, the gonadotropins are found to be elevated into the postmenopausal range. Although gonadotropin levels do fluctuate, the levels are consistently elevated and therefore a single serum FSH determination is adequate to make the diagnosis. These patients will not have uterine bleeding following intramuscular progesterone. With rare exceptions, ovulation cannot be induced in these patients with drug therapy.

Loss of ovarian function secondary to castration, intraovarian infection, or interference of blood supply

Loss of ovarian function following surgical castration is self-explanatory. On rare occasions, patients with severe bilateral tuboovarian abscesses have responded well to antibiotic therapy and do not require surgical treatment. In some, the infection completely destroys the ovarian tissue, which results in ovarian failure. After ovarian cystectomy, the ovarian blood supply sometimes is compromised, resulting in cystic degeneration. Usually this process is unilateral and therefore does not manifest itself with amenorrhea. However, it may occur bilaterally or in the only remaining ovary, resulting in loss of ovarian function. These patients are sterile and need estrogen replacement.

Diagnosis evaluation

The initial work-up of patients with secondary amenorrhea includes history and physical examination, complete blood count, and urinalysis. If the patient has any signs and symptoms of hyperthyroidism, a serum T3 and thyroxine by radioimmunoassay should be obtained. Neither dilatation and curettage nor laparoscopy is indicated for patients with secondary amenorrhea.

Withdrawal uterine bleeding, following an injection of progesterone in oil, has made it possible to divide patients with amenorrhea into two major categories (Table 92.1). In individuals with uterine bleeding, a single serum LH value of over 25 m IU/ml is indicative of hyperandrogenic chronic anovulation (HCA, PCO; Table 92.1). Patients who have LH values below 25 m IU/ml have hypothalamic dysfunction (euestrogenic amenorrhea). In these patients, serum prolactin should be ordered even in the absence of galactorrhea; if it is elevated, a computed tomography (CT) or magnetic resonance imaging (MRI) scan of the sella turcica should be performed to rule out pituitary tumors. A thyrotropin-releasing hormone (TRH) stimulation test prior to ordering a CT scan or MRI may be indicated. If the prolactin response is normal, uterine withdrawal bleeding with medroxyprogesterone (10 mg for 10 days) or 100 mg progesterone intramuscularly should be induced at least every 3 months if the patient does not desire pregnancy. If pregnancy is desired, treatment should be with clomiphene citrate. If the patient fails to ovulate on clomiphene, she should be treated with human menopausal gonadotropin (hMG) or GnRH. If pregnancy is not desired, a barrier method of contraception is recommended, as spontaneous recovery and ovulation can occur. It is unnecessary to perform a CT or MRI of the sella turcica for patients in this group unless they have galactorrhea in addition to the amenorrhea or have an elevated serum prolactin.

A single serum FSH (but not LH) in patients who do not have uterine bleeding (hypoestrogenic amenorrhea) can identify two distinct populations, one with a low or normal FSH and the other an elevated value (Table 92.1). The former group represents these patients with hypothalamic–pituitary failure, and the latter group represents patients who have ovarian failure.

All patients with hypothalamic–pituitary failure (hypoestrogenic) without a history of drugs, exercise, or weight loss should have further evaluation to demonstrate the presence or absence of a pituitary tumor, including a serum prolactin followed by a CT scan or MRI of the sella turcica. In addition, patients with a possible history of Sheehan disease should have an insulin-induced hypoglycemia test in order to determine the pituitary growth hormone, prolactin, and adrenocorticotropic hormone reserve. If cortisol fails to rise 10 μg% above baseline, 10 mg of hydrocortisone should be given twice daily as a maintenance dose. Because these patients have low levels of estradiol, they rarely respond to clomiphene citrate and therapy with hMG or GnRH should be initiated if pregnancy is desired.

Patients with ovarian failure are easily diagnosed because they invariably fail to respond to progesterone challenge and have elevated FSH values. These patients will not respond to any form of ovulatory drug therapy. However, they could become pregnant by using a fertilized donor egg. Because they do not have adequate endogenous levels of estrogens, estrogen replacement therapy should be used to prevent osteoporosis. The recommended regimen is 0.625 mg of conjugated estrogen given days 1 through 25 of each month. Provera 5.0 mg daily, given days 14 through 25, should be used in order to avoid an unopposed estrogen effect on the endometrium.

SUGGESTED READING

AIMAN J, SMENTEK C. Premature ovarian failure. *Obstet Gynecol* 1985;66:9.

ALPER MM, GARTNER PR. Premature ovarian failure: its relationship to autoimmune disease. *Obstet Gynecol* 1985;66:27.

ASHERMAN JG. Traumatic intrauterine adhesions and their effects on fertility. *Int J Fertil* 1957;2:49.

BERGA SL, MORTOLA JF, GIRTON L, et al. Neuroendocrine aberrations in women with functional hypothalamic amenorrhea. *J Clin Endocrinol Metab* 1989;68:301.

CHIAUZZI V, CIGORRAGA S, ESCOBAR ME, et al. Inhibition of FSH-receptor binding by circulating immunoglobulins. *J Clin Endocrinol Metab* 1982;54:1221.

CROWLEY WF, FILICORI M, SPRATT KI, et al. The physiology of gonadotropin-releasing hormone (GnRH) secretion in men and women. *Recent Prog Horm Res* 1985;4:473.

DIZEREGA GS, KLETZKY OA, MISHELL DR Jr. Diagnosis of patients with Sheehan's syndrome using a sequential pituitary stimulation test. *Am J Obstet Gynecol* 1978; 132:348.

KHOURY SA, REAME NE, KELCH RP, MARSHAL JC. Diurnal patterns of pulsatile luteinizing hormone secretion in hypothalamic amenorrhea: reproducibility and responses to opiate blockade and an α2-adrenergic agonist. *J Clin Endocrinol Metab* 1987;64:755.

KLETZKY OA, DAVAJAN V, NAKAMURA RM, et al. Classification of secondary amenorrhea based on distinct hormonal patterns. *J Clin Endocrinol Metab* 1975; 41:660.

KLETZKY OA, DAVAJAN V, NAKAMURA RM, et al. Clinical categorization of patients with secondary amenorrhea using progesterone induced uterine bleeding and measurement of serum gonadotropin levels. *Am J Obstet Gynecol* 1975;121:695.

KLETZKY OA, NAKAMURA RM, THORNEYCROFT IA, et al. The log-normal distribution of gonadotropins and ovarian steroid values in the normal menstrual cycle. *Am J Obstet Gynecol* 1975;121:688.

KLETZKY OA, MISHELL DR Jr, DAVAJAN V, et al. Pituitary stimulation test in amenorrheic patients with normal or low serum estradiol. *Acta Endocrinol* 1978; 87:456.

KLIBANSKI A, BILLER BMK, ROSENTHAL DI, et al. Effects of prolactin and estrogen deficiency in amenorrheic bone loss. *J Clin Endocrinol Metab* 1988;67:124.

LEDGER WL, THOMAS EJ, BROWNING D, et al. Suppression of gonadotrophin secretion does not reverse premature ovarian failure. *Br J Obstet Gynecol* 1989; 96:196.

LLOYD T, MYERS C, BUCHANAN JR, DEMERS LM. Collegiate women athletes with irregular menses during adolescence have decreased bone density. *Obstet Gynecol* 1988;72:639.

MIGNOT MH, SCHOEMAKER J, KLEINGELD M, et al. Premature ovarian failure: the association with autoimmunity. *Eur J Obstet Gynecol Reprod Biol* 1989;30:59.

MISHELL DR Jr, KLETZKY OA, BRENNER PF, et al. The effect of contraceptive steroids on hypothalamic–pituitary function. *Am J Obstet Gynecol* 1977;128:60.

PALA A, COGHI I, SPAMPINATO G, et al. Immunochemical and biological characteristics of a human autoantibody to human chorionic gonadotropin and luteinizing hormone. *Clin Endocrinol Metab* 1988;67:1317.

REBAR RW, ERICKSON GF, YEN SSC. Idiopathic premature ovarian failure: clinical and endocrine characteristics. *Fertil Steril* 1982;37:35.

SNOW RC, BARBIERI RL, FRISCH RE. Estrogen 2-hydroxylase oxidation and menstrual function among elite oarswomen. *J Clin Endocrinol Metab* 1989;69:369.

93

Galactorrhea and hyperprolactinemia

MICHAEL VERMESH

Galactorrhea is defined as nonpuerperal lactation noted whether spontaneously or following manual expression from one or both breasts. To detect galactorrhea, the breast examination should be performed by compressing the glands from the periphery of the breast toward the nipple concentrically. Galactorrhea fluid appears as either a milky or watery substance. The observation of microscopic fat globules in the fluid is a simple and accurate diagnostic test of galactorrhea.

The exact incidence of galactorrhea in women of the reproductive age group is unknown.

Pathophysiology

Prolactin (PRL) is the most important hormone involved in the pathophysiology of galactorrhea. It is evident that prolactin secretion is controlled mainly by the hypothalamus. The predominant action of the hypothalamus on PRL release in mammals is inhibitory, through dopamine acting as a prolactin-inhibiting factor (PIF). There is also some evidence in animals for the existence of a PRL-releasing factor (PRF) which could be related to serotonin. In humans, PRL is stimulated by sleep, stress, exercise, nipple stimulation, thyrotropin-releasing hormone (TRH), insulin-induced hypoglycemia, and phenothiazines. PRL is inhibited by L-dopa, dopamine, and certain ergot alkaloids, including bromocriptine mesylate (Parlodel). While TRH directly stimulates the pituitary to release PRL, chlorpromazine (Thorazine) inhibits PRL by depleting the hypothalamus of dopamine. In contradistinction, L-dopa influences PRL secretion by being first converted to dopamine in the hypothalamus. Bromocriptine, in addition to inhibiting PRL secretion by a direct action on the pituitary, also has a dopaminergic effect on the hypothalamus.

Symptoms and signs related to hyperprolactinemia

Galactorrhea is the most frequently observed abnormality. Menstrual irregularities that may be associated with hyperprolactinemia include luteal phase defect, oligomenorrhea, or amenorrhea. Interference with ovulation and normal corpus luteum formation may result either from direct action on the ovary or from PRL effect on gonadotropin-releasing hormone (GnRH) secretion. Hyperprolactinemia in men rarely causes galactorrhea, but may diminish libido and cause impotence.

Differential diagnosis

Hyperprolactinemia may be due to physiologic, pharmacologic, or pathologic factors.

Physiologic factors

PRL is secreted in a sleep-related circadian rhythm. It increases shortly after the onset of sleep, with a maximum release between 03:00 and 05:00 h. A mild increase in PRL level also occurs after lunch, particularly after a high-protein and high-fat meal. PRL levels are influenced by serum estradiol, and display positive correlation during the menstrual cycle and during pregnancy. During the menstrual cycle PRL levels are higher in the luteal phase than in the follicular phase. During pregnancy, high estradiol concentrations stimulate PRL release and induce hyperplasia and hypertrophy of the lactotrophs. As a result, serum PRL levels rise from <20 ng/ml in the nonpregnant state to about 200 ng/ml during the third trimester of pregnancy. PRL is considered a stress-induced hormone, in that stress and exercise may cause hyperprolactinemia.

Because of these influences it is recommended that when hyperprolactinemia is suspected, the serum sample for measuring PRL be obtained in the follicular phase of the cycle, in the late morning hours, and not preceded by breast examination or exercise.

Pharmacologic factors

Drug-induced hyperprolactinemia appears to be the most common cause of nonphysiologic galactorrhea and/or hyperprolactinemia. Drugs that have been shown to produce hyperprolactinemia include the major and minor tranquilizers, antihypertensive agents, and narcotics. High-dose estrogen oral contraceptives may also increase PRL levels. Hyperprolactinemia is uncommonly associated with ingestion of low-dose (35 μg estrogen) oral contraceptives.

Pathologic factors

The two most important factors are pituitary adenoma and hypothyroidism. Other causes include acromegaly, Cushing's disease, herpes zoster, chest trauma and surgery.

About 50% of patients with hyperprolactinemia will have radiographic changes of the sella turcica compatible with an adenoma. The term microadenoma has been used to describe pituitary tumors <10 mm in diameter. Those >10 mm in diameter are called macroadenomas. In approximately 10% of galactorrheic patients with an abnormal X-ray, the serum PRL levels have been reported to be normal. Nearly all of these patients have the empty sella syndrome. This syndrome results from herniation of the subarachnoid membrane into the sella turcica through a defective sella diaphragm. Patients with an empty sella have, in general, a more benign prognosis than patients with pituitary adenomas.

In approximately 2–4% of patients with galactorrhea, the etiology has been determined to be primary hypothyroidism. These patients have diminished thyroid function and therefore lack both negative feedback on the hypothalamus (TRH) and the pituitary (thyroid-stimulating hormone; TSH) axis and positive feedback on dopamine secretion. This failure results in the increased secretion of TSH and decreased secretion of dopamine which results in hyperprolactinemia. A small increase in TRH may be of secondary importance.

The diagnosis of primary hypothyroidism is made by measuring serum TSH by radioimmunoassay (RIA). In these patients, the value of TSH is elevated above the normal range (the upper limit of normal TSH varies in different laboratories, from 5 to 10 μU/ml). In addition to TSH, measurement of serum thyroxine by RIA and the free thyroxine index (FTI) is used in order to rule out the rare case of TSH-producing pituitary adenoma and to confirm the diagnosis of primary hypothyroidism.

Galactorrhea, menstrual patterns, and prolactin levels

Galactorrhea can be present in patients with either normal or abnormal menses. In fact, galactorrhea associated with a pituitary tumor has been reported in postmenopausal women. Therefore, the menstrual history alone cannot be used to select patients who need a complete work-up. However, the menstrual history in conjunction with a single serum PRL value has been used to identify patients with low or high risk of having a pituitary adenoma.

The high-risk group of patients were found to be those with PRL levels >200 ng/ml as well as those with amenorrhea/galactorrhea and low circulating levels of estrogen as determined by failure to have uterine bleeding following progesterone administration. Two-thirds of these patients were found to have radiographic findings indicating the presence of a pituitary adenoma.

The low-risk group of patients are those with galactorrhea, normal menses, and serum PRL levels of <20 ng/ml. It has been reported that none of the patients with these findings had abnormal hypocycloidal tomograms of the sella turcica. However, in galactorrheic patients with normal menses and PRL levels >20 ng/ml, abnormal tomograms compatible with microadenomas were found; thus, it is recommended that patients with galactorrhea and normal menses have a computed tomography (CT) or magnetic resonance imaging (MRI) scan of the pituitary only if serum PRL is elevated.

Diagnostic evaluation

The use of drugs or medications with PRL-stimulatory properties can be ruled out by the history. If possible, such agents should be discontinued and serum PRL measured 1 month later. If PRL is still elevated, the physician should proceed with the evaluation. If the medication (tranquilizer, antihypertensive agent) cannot be discontinued, a complete work-up to rule out a pituitary adenoma should be initiated.

The first step in the evaluation of patients with hyperprolactinemia is measurement of serum TSH. An elevated serum TSH level identifies patients who may have primary hypothyroidism as the etiology of their galactorrhea. The diagnosis is confirmed by measurement of the FTI. Patients with primary hypothyroidism will have elevated TSH and low FTI values. These patients should be given thyroxine replacement therapy, starting at a low daily dose of 0.05 mg for 2 weeks. Then the dose should be increased by 0.05 mg every 2 weeks, up to a maintenance dose.

If TSH is normal in a patient with elevated PRL, imaging of the pituitary gland with CT scan or MRI is necessary to rule out pituitary adenoma. MRI is superior to CT in the identification of the optic chiasm, optic nerves, cavernous sinuses, and carotid arteries and is the method of choice to detect an empty sella.

Treatment

The objectives of therapy in patients with galactorrhea and/or hyperprolactinemia include elimination of lactation, establishment of normal estrogen secretion, induction of ovulation, and treatment of PRL-secreting pituitary adenomas. The recommended forms of management are periodic observation, drug therapy, surgery, and radiation therapy.

Periodic observation is indicated in menstruating women with galactorrhea who have normal or idiopathic elevated serum PRL levels. Patients with oligomenorrhea can be treated with progestins to induce regular uterine bleeding. Microadenomas may be followed up with yearly measurements of serum PRL. Serial pituitary imaging is unnecessary after the diagnosis of a microadenoma or functional hyperprolactinemia, since long-term studies have shown that only a small percentage of women with a microadenoma who do not receive any treatment have an increase in size of the tumor. Furthermore, many women with microadenoma also develop markedly decreased and/or normal PRL levels over time, with an increased likelihood of this happening if they become pregnant.

Patients with primary hypothyroidism should be treated with thyroxine, as described earlier.

Bromocriptine mesylate has been found to be successful in lowering serum PRL to normal levels, stopping galactorrhea, and establishing normal ovulatory menstrual cycles. The recommended dose is 2.5–7.5 mg/day; however, we have treated patients with 20 and 30 mg daily without complications. The effects of this drug appear to be only temporary, since the majority of patients cease to menstruate and again develop hyperprolactinemia, and galactorrhea after discontinuing therapy. Thus, years of treatment may need to be considered when counseling patients. No definitive information is yet available as to bromocriptine's long-term effects in patients with PRL-secreting pituitary adenomas, although reports of tumor regression have been published. Initially, the drug may induce nausea, vomiting, postural hypotension, headaches, and nasal stuffiness. These effects are transient and can be minimized by administering the agent at bedtime and by avoiding large dosage increments. Vaginal administration of bromocriptine may be an alternative option for patients with persistent gastrointestinal side-effects.

Although estrogen therapy is successful in suppression of postpartum lactation by its direct effect on the breasts, it is not recommended for use in the galactorrheic patients, since estrogen is known to stimulate both the growth of the pituitary and the release of PRL.

Patients with hyperprolactinemia and low levels of serum estradiol (<40 pg/ml) are at risk for developing osteoporosis and should always be treated with bromocriptine. These patients will begin to have ovulatory cycles and, if pregnancy is not desired, a mechanical method of contraception should be recommended.

Surgery

At Los Angeles County–University of Southern California Medical Center, surgical therapy is recommended only for patients with macroadenomas or evidence of extrasellar extension of the tumor who fail to respond to bromocriptine therapy. Following surgery, bromocriptine therapy should be continued if the pituitary tumor is thought to be incompletely resected. If surgery is planned for a patient already on bromocriptine therapy, the drug should be maintained until the day of surgery to prevent a sudden regrowth of the adenoma. For patients with microadenomas, bromocriptine treatment alone has been used. These patients are being followed every 6–12 months with PRL measurements and every 2–3 years with CT scan. Only if there is enlargement of the adenoma should surgery be considered.

Pregnancy

Patients with PRL-secreting pituitary adenomas (prolactinomas) should be counseled prior to conceiving. Microadenomas usually do not enlarge significantly during pregnancy, whereas macroadenomas may grow rapidly and cause visual and other neurologic disturbances. Surgical removal of macroadenomas should, therefore, be considered if pregnancy is planned. An alternative method of treatment could be the continuation of bromocriptine during pregnancy to prevent a sudden increase in size of the adenoma. Such treatment has been used in several patients without apparent detriment to the fetus. While pregnant, these patients should have visual field examinations every 3 months. Utilizing this approach, nearly all patients have been delivered at term without complications. There is no contraindication to breast-feeding.

SUGGESTED READING

CROSIGNANI PG, MATTEI AM, SEVERINI V, CAVIONI V, MAGGIONI P, TESTA G. Long-term effects of time, medical treatment and pregnancy in 176 hyperprolactinemic women. *Eur J Obstet/Gynecol Reprod Biol* 1992;44:175.

DAVAJAN V, KLETZKY OA, MARCH CM, ROY S, MISHELL DR Jr. The significance of galactorrhea in patients with normal menses, oligomenorrhea and secondary amenorrhea. *Am J Obstet Gynecol* 1978;130:894.

KLETZKY OA, VERMESH M. Effectiveness of vaginal bromocriptine in treating women with hyperprolactinemia. *Fertil Steril* 1989;51:269.

KLETZKY OA, DAVAJAN V, MISHELL DR Jr, *et al*. A sequential pituitary stimulation test in normal subjects and in patients with amenorrhea-galactorrhea with pituitary tumors. *J Clin Endocrinol Metab* 1977;45:631.

MARCH CM, MISHELL DR Jr, KLETZKY OA, ISRAEL R, DAVAJAN V. Galactorrhea and pituitary tumors in post-pill and non-post-pill amenorrhea. *Am J Obstet Gynecol* 1979;134:45.

MARCH CM, KLETZKY OA, DAVAJAN V, *et al*. Longitudinal evaluation of patients with untreated prolactin-secreting pituitary adenomas. *Am J Obstet Gynecol* 1981; 139:835.

MARRS RP, BERTOLLI SJ, KLETZKY OA. The use of thyrotropin releasing hormone in distinguishing prolactin-secreting pituitary adenoma. *Am J Obstet Gynecol* 1980;138:620.

VERMESH M, FOSSUM GT, KLETZKY OA. Vaginal bromocriptine: pharmacology, and effect on serum prolactin in normal women. *Obstet Gynecol* 1988;72:693.

94

Androgen excess: differential diagnosis

ROGERIO A. LOBO

Androgen excess includes signs and symptoms which are both defeminizing (oligomenorrhea, amenorrhea, decreased breast tissue, decreased cervical mucus, decreased vaginal rugae) and masculinizing (hirsutism, temporal balding, deepening of the voice, clitoromegaly, increased muscle mass, increased libido, acne). Hirsutism should not be used interchangeably with virilization. Hirsutism is the excessive growth of body hair where it is not normally found. Virilism is used if frank masculinization and defeminizing signs are present. The progression of hirsutism to virilism implies a more severe form of androgen excess.

Hirsutism

Hirsutism is increased hair growth in a central body location or the appearance of hair in an area where it does not occur normally. This term has to be distinguished from hypertrichosis which is a generalized increase in body hair. Hirsutism has been graded by several techniques. Although no scoring system is completely adequate, we have adopted the modified scheme of Ferriman–Gallwey (Fig. 94.1). In this system, each of nine body sites is scored and then totaled. Whereas this method is important for documenting changes before and after therapy, there are other methods to assess changes in hair growth. Perhaps the best method is the use of photographs of affected areas before and after treatment.

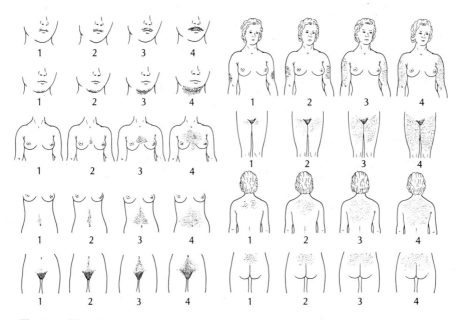

Fig. 94.1 Hirsutism scoring from 1 to 4 from nine body sites. Adapted from Ferriman and Gallwey and Lorenzo *et al.*

Physiologic changes in hair growth

It must be remembered that at three times during a woman's life (puberty, pregnancy, postmenopause) hair may appear at an accelerated rate as the result of physiologic changes in circulating sex steroids and other trophic hormones. At puberty, adrenal androgen increases before an increase in ovarian estrogen. During pregnancy, these changes remain unexplained because although total circulating testosterone levels are increased, there is a minimal change in the unbound fraction. During the postmenopausal years, the ovaries secrete virtually no estrogen; androgens continue to be produced by both the ovaries and the adrenal glands.

Androgen excess

Peripheral causes

Idiopathic hirsutism

One of the most common causes of hirsutism, if not the most frequently encountered condition, has been thought to be constitutional. As many as one-third of all women will have cosmetic complaints pertaining to excess hair growth. Women of Mediterranean ancestry are considered more likely to appear hirsute, usually with no disruption of their ovulatory menstrual pattern or evidence of virilization.

Some women with constitutional hirsutism have increased levels of one or more of several androgens (testosterone, androstenedione, dehydroepiandrosterone, dehydroepiandrosterone sulfate (DHEAS)) in their peripheral circulation. Indeed, only a minority of women will have no elevated androgen levels, particularly if several androgens are measured. Many women have an increased clearance rate of testosterone which compensates for an increased daily production rate of testosterone. Many women will have some small increase in unbound or free testosterone in the peripheral circulation. These findings suggest that these women should not be considered to have idiopathic hirsutism because they have subtle changes in androgen metabolism. How often these findings occur depends on how intensive the investigation is.

However, it has been shown that most women with idiopathic hirsutism have abnormally high androgen metabolism in peripheral tissues (such as skin), making this largely a disorder of the peripheral compartment. Under these circumstances, normally circulating androgens like testosterone are converted more efficiently to more potent androgens like dihydrotestosterone. Dihydrotestosterone is the active intracellular androgen in skin and is required for the expression of androgen effects. Thus, a high level of 5α-reductase in skin, which converts testosterone to dihydrotestosterone, explains most of the abnormality in this group. Androgen receptor levels have been found to be normal. At present, we still use the term idiopathic hirsutism but know that, regardless of any subtle increases in androgen production, skin androgen metabolism (via 5α-reductase) is increased. For practical reasons we diagnose women as having idiopathic hirsutism if they have no changes in menstrual function and if circulating androgen levels are either normal or only minimally elevated.

Ovarian causes of androgen excess

Polycystic ovary syndrome

Either idiopathic hirsutism or polycystic ovary syndrome (PCO) is the most common cause of clinical androgen excess. PCO is presented in Chapter 97.

Hyperthecosis syndrome

Women with hyperthecosis are more likely than women with PCO to have virilizing signs and symptoms and are less likely to ovulate in response to clomiphene citrate (Clomid, Serophene). Most often the history is one of long-standing, progressive hirsutism and virilization. Patients with hyperthecosis syndrome are usually older than those with PCO.

On ultrasound, enlarged ovaries are seen bilaterally without the subcortical cysts characteristic of PCO. Little cystic activity is seen within the substance of ovary and the stroma is extremely dense. The diagnosis of hyperthecosis is confirmed histologically when nests of theca cells are found in the ovarian stroma at some distance from the follicles. Because surgical wedge resections are performed rarely, the diagnosis of hyperthecosis is not often documented. Although luteinizing hormone levels are usually not high, ovarian androgen levels suppress very well with the gonadotropin-releasing hormone agonist. Adrenal androgen levels (e.g., DHEAS) are usually not elevated, in contrast to this finding in PCO.

Androgen-producing ovarian tumors

Androgen-producing ovarian tumors are rare. The largest and most common are the Sertoli–Leydig cell tumors, formerly referred to as arrhenoblastomas. These tumors occur most often in the second, third, and fourth decades of life, are usually palpable on pelvic examination and have a low-grade malignant potential.

Hilus-cell tumors occur commonly in postmenopausal women, usually are not palpable on pelvic examination and have a low-grade malignant potential. Lipoid-cell tumors also can secrete androgens. They are more common in premenopausal women and have a somewhat greater malignant potential than the others. Seventy-five percent of women with lipoid-cell tumors are virilized and 10% have Cushing's syndrome. The lipoid-cell tumor behaves endocrinologically as an adrenal androgen-producing tumor. These tumors are usually cystic. Granulosa–theca cell tumors usually secrete estrogens but infrequently have been associated with excess androgen secretion.

A general rule of thumb is to begin the investigation when testosterone levels exceed 2.5 times the upper range for testosterone, as reported by the laboratory. In addition, there must be the history of rapidity of onset and progression in defeminizing or masculinizing signs. Other ovarian tumors also may cause androgen excess by a mechanism other than secretion of androgen by the tumors cells. Any ovarian tumor has the potential of being associated with androgen secretion. Mucinous cystadenomas, Brenner tumors, cystadenocarcinomas, and Krukenberg tumors all have been associated with a functioning ovarian stroma that liberates increased amounts of androgen. The diagnosis of androgen-producing ovarian tumor should be considered whenever a woman has male levels of total serum testosterone, usually >200 ng/dl.

Adrenal causes of androgen excess

Congenital adrenal hyperplasia – adult onset

The postpubertal manifestation of hirsutism and/or virilization as the result of congenital adrenal hyperplasia (CAH) is now an established diagnostic entity. These patients may be taller than their peers early in life, but the excess sex steroids cause the distal epiphyses to close prematurely and the patients are often shorter than their peers and members of their families. These findings, while characteristic of more severe or classic cases of CAH, are less consistent in the adult (late-onset) or attenuated form. Anovulation with either oligomenorrhea or amenorrhea is a frequent finding and the diagnosis is easily confused with PCO.

Most women with adult-onset CAH have an enzyme deficiency in the cortisol pathway due to an incomplete 21-hydroxylase deficiency. This does not result in salt-wasting. A few have an incomplete 11β-hydroxylase deficiency. Both enzyme defects produce an increase in serum 17α-hydroxyprogesterone or its urinary metabolite, pregnanetriol, and inefficient cortisol production. The 11β-hydroxylase deficiency also causes an increase in 11-deoxycortisol (substance S) and clinical hypertension in some patients. Both enzyme defects may be accentuated by the administration of intravenous adrenocorticotropic hormone (ACTH) which causes a marked increase in the 17α-hydroxyprogesterone levels. Serum levels of the Δ^5 adrenal androgens, such as DHEAS, are not consistently increased. The most commonly elevated androgen is androstenedione. Administration of dexamethasone 0.5–0.75 mg/day suppresses androgen levels and relieves the clinical signs and symptoms. Spontaneous ovulation and pregnancy often occur.

A 3β-ol-dehydrogenase defect also has been diagnosed in adult women presenting with androgen excess. In this form of adult-onset CAH, patients have high levels of Δ^5 adrenal androgens such as DHEAS while androstenedione and testosterone are usually normal or low. These enzymatic disorders have been reported to occur in as many as 5–20% of the hirsute population, although the lower figure is probably more accurate.

Androgen-producing adrenal tumors

Adrenal adrenomas or carcinomas that produce androgens are rare causes of clinical androgen excess. Adrenal carcinomas are usually large enough to be detected on an intravenous pyelogram by the time they produce signs and symptoms of androgen excess. Androgen-producing adrenal adenomas may be macro- or microadenomas. The extent of symptoms bears no relation to the size of the adenomas. Patients with androgen-producing adrenal tumors have extremely high levels of adrenal androgens, with serum DHEAS levels usually over 8 µg/ml. Adrenal tumors rarely produce testosterone but may secrete increased levels of androgen.

Cushing's syndrome

Centripetal obesity, thinning of the skin, facial flushing, supraclavicular and dorsal neck fat pads, purple striae, muscle wasting, weakness, easy bruisability, ecchymoses, osteoporosis, hypertension, diabetes, alkalosis, hypokalemia, amenorrhea, and hirsutism are the clinical signs in women with Cushing's syndrome. Abnormal hair growth may have two patterns. In the first, there is increased growth of fine hairs of the face and extremities, rather than the coarse hairs. This lanugo type of hair is due to glucocorticoid excess. A true androgen-related coarse type of hirsutism also may result from excessive adrenal androgen production. Whenever signs and symptoms of Cushing's syndrome are present, this life-threatening diagnosis must be investigated.

Iatrogenic causes

Drugs

Some drugs that can cause hirsutism include phenytoin (Dilantin), diazoxide, corticosteroids, ACTH, 19-nortestosterone-derived progestins, anabolic steroids, danazol (Danocrine), and some nonprescription medications that have been found to contain androgens.

Genetic causes

Rare cases of gonadal dysgenesis in which a Y chromosome and incomplete forms of testicular feminization are present can produce clinical evidence of androgen excess and primary amenorrhea. This combination requires a karyotype examination for the detection of a Y chromosome, which in a female patient mandates surgical extirpation of the gonadal tissue because of the increased risk of neoplasia. Any woman with primary amenorrhea, gonadal failure, and clinical evidence of excess androgen should have her gonads removed for the same reasons.

Rare causes

Extremely rare causes of androgen excess include acromegaly and porphyria. These diagnoses usually have been confirmed prior to the investigation of androgen excess. Interestingly, there is an epidemiologic association between hirsutism and diethylstilbestrol exposure *in utero*.

Virilization in pregnancy

Virilization in pregnancy is a rare phenomenon. The endogenous source of the excess androgen is thought to be the ovaries in virtually all cases. The most common cause of virilization in pregnancy is the luteoma of pregnancy which usually regresses spontaneously postpartum. Conservative management is recommended. Other causes include ovarian androgen-producing tumors, ovarian tumors associated with a functional stroma, and hyperreactio luteinalis. Half of female infants born to mothers with virilization in pregnancy have ambiguous external genitalia and this is most likely to occur with functional tumors and luteomas.

SUGGESTED READING

FERRIMAN D, GALLWEY JD. Clinical assessment of body hair growth in women. *J Clin Endocrinol Metab* 1961;21:1440.

HATCH R, ROSENFIELD RL. KIM MH, TREDWAY D. Hirsutism: implications, etiology, and management. *Am J Obstet Gynecol* 1981;140:815.

HORTON R, HAWKS R, LOBO R. 3α,17β-Androstanediol glucuronide in plasma: a marker of androgen action in idiopathic hirsutism. *J Clin Invest* 1982;69:1203.

KIRSCHNER MA, ZUCKER IR, JESPERSEN D. Idiopathic hirsutism – an ovarian abnormality. *N Engl J Med* 1976;294:637.

LOBO RA. Hirsutism. In: Sciarra JJ, Speroff L, Simpson JL, eds. *Gynecology and Obstetrics*, vol 5: *Endocrinology, Infertility, Genetics*. Philadelphia: J.B. Lippincott, 1987:1.

LOBO RA. Androgen excess. In: Mishell DR Jr, Davajan V, Lobo RA, eds. *Infertility, Contraception and Reproductive Endocrinology*. 3rd edn. Cambridge, MA: Blackwell Scientific Publications, 1991:422.

LOBO RA, GOEBELSMANN U. Adult manifestation of congenital adrenal hyperplasia due to incomplete 21-hydroxylase deficiency mimicking polycystic ovarian disease. *Am J Obstet Gynecol* 1980;138:720.

LOBO RA, PAUL WL, GOEBELSMANN U. Serum levels of DHEAS in gynecologic endocrinopathy and infertility. *Obstet Gynecol* 1981;57:607.

SERAFINI P, ABLAN F, LOBO RA. 5α-Reductase activity in the genital skin of hirsute women. *J Clin Endocrinol Metab* 1985;60:349.

95

Androgen excess: evaluation

ROGERIO A. LOBO

History

In evaluating a woman with the signs and symptoms of androgen excess, a careful history is mandatory to narrow down the differential diagnosis. Iatrogenic causes and medical illnesses such as porphyria or acromegaly may be excluded easily. Rapidly progressive hirsutism and virilization would suggest a neoplastic cause such as an androgen-producing ovarian tumor. In addition, it is important to determine if hair has been removed by shaving or other means, at what age the symptoms were first noticed, and if any menstrual irregularities are present.

Physical examination

On physical examination, the presence of virilism (increased muscle mass, decreased breast size, clitoromegaly) and signs suggestive of Cushing's syndrome (central obesity, striae, bruisability) should be noted. Although it is rare for patients with Cushing's syndrome to present primarily with androgen excess, it may be ruled out by an overnight dexamethasone (DEX) suppression test or 24-h urinary free cortisol measurements. DEX (1 mg) is ingested at 23:00 h. If the patient's cortisol is suppressed to <5 µg/ml at 08:00 h the next morning, the diagnosis of Cushing's syndrome is effectively ruled out. The 24-h urinary free cortisol level is usually <100 µg/day and in Cushing's syndrome is >250 µg/day.

Weight loss, a unilateral adnexal mass, or bilaterally enlarged ovaries may be helpful in making the diagnosis of ovarian neoplasm or polycystic ovary syndrome (PCO). If the patient is shorter than her peers and has significant androgen excess and/or hypertension, the diagnosis of adult-onset congenital adrenal hyperplasia (CAH) may be considered.

Diagnostic approach

Adrenal and ovarian androgen levels

The diagnostic approach is based on whether ovarian or adrenal androgens are elevated. Adrenal androgen secretion is assessed best by measuring serum dehydroepiandrosterone sulfate (DHEAS). More than 90% of DHEAS is derived from the adrenals and its measurement is more useful and sensitive than measurements of urinary 17-ketosteroids. When clinically available, measurements of 11β-hydroxyandrosterone, another adrenal androgen, may also be assessed as this steroid has also been shown to be useful.

Serum testosterone is the best indicator of ovarian androgen production because about two-thirds of serum testosterone in women is derived from the ovaries and it rarely is produced directly by the adrenals. Measurement of free, or unbound testosterone (defined in Chapter 96) allows a more sensitive estimation of testosterone production, as sex hormone-binding globulin often is decreased in androgen excess. However, it is not essential to measure unbound or free testosterone levels in most patients. A new marker for disorders of the peripheral compartment is 3α-diol androstanediol glucuronide (3α-diol G). Serum 3α-diol G is elevated in most patients with hirsutism, and if testosterone or DHEAS is normal, suggests a peripheral disorder. Serum 3α-diol G is highly correlated with skin 5α-reductase activity. Recent work has shown that androsterone glucuronide is also a useful marker of peripheral androgen effects. Androsterone is the major 5α-reduced product of androstenedione.

The only other test to be considered is the measurement of 17α-hydroxyprogesterone (17-OHP). This test should be performed to rule out CAH if the patient is shorter than her peers, has significant hirsutism or virilization, hypertension, a strong family history of hirsutism, or circulating androgen levels above those usually encountered in hirsute patients. Adrenocorticotropic hormone (ACTH) testing is used to distinguish patients who have CAH from others, such as patients with PCO, who have elevated 17-OHP levels due to ovarian hypersecretion. In PCO, 17-OHP rarely exceeds 5 ng/ml.

Neoplasms

If total serum testosterone is in the male range (>200 ng/dl) or 2.5 times the upper limit for the laboratory, the possible presence of an ovarian androgen-secreting neoplasm should be evaluated by vaginal ultrasound. If DHEAS is above 8 μg/ml, an adrenal androgen-secreting neoplasm should be suspected. We recommend a computed tomography (CT) or magnetic resonance imaging scan to identify an adrenal neoplasm. Rarely, an adrenal testosterone-producing neoplasm will be present. In this instance, DHEAS levels are under 8 μg/ml and testosterone is in the tumor range. If testosterone is moderately elevated and the ovaries are normal on scan, an adrenal CT scan should be ordered. Selective venous catheterization studies should only be done for patients with "normal" ovaries and adrenals on scan and who have persistently elevated testosterone levels. A more recent and valuable technique for scanning ovaries and adrenals involves a radioactive injection of iodomethyl-norcholesterol (NP-59). Areas of active steroidogenesis are readily detected.

Functional diagnosis: PCO and CAH

If ovarian or adrenal neoplasms are ruled out by the combination of clinical and laboratory assessment, the remaining diagnosis falls into a functional class. Adrenal and/or ovarian androgen excess can occur in PCO as well as in some women who have been thought to have idiopathic hirsutism. Therefore, further evaluation of these patients depends on whether there is increased adrenal androgen production (reflected by DHEAS) and/or ovarian androgen production (reflected by testosterone or unbound testosterone). The specific diagnosis of PCO will not be discussed here. However, in a patient who is suspected of having adult-onset CAH, measurement of 17-OHP is very helpful. If this level is >8 ng/ml, the diagnosis is almost certain. If it is elevated >3 ng/ml, but <8 ng/ml, a diagnosis of CAH cannot be made without ACTH stimulation. Many women with PCO or adrenal androgen excess may have slight elevations of 17-OHP. However, these levels rarely exceed 5–6 ng/ml.

ACTH testing is carried out by giving 1 mg DEX at 23:00 h, as is done to rule out Cushing's syndrome. At 08:00 h the next day, 0.25 mg ACTH (Cosyntropin) is given intravenously as a bolus. Because adrenal function has been suppressed by DEX, the 08:00 h level of 17-OHP will be low, usually <3 ng/ml. If the 60-min level is elevated, usually >20 ng/ml, the diagnosis of CAH can be made. Women with PCO who have elevated basal levels of 17-OHP will not have an exaggerated response to ACTH. It has been shown that pretreatment with DEX is not necessary. New *et al.* have provided a normogram for the diagnosis of 21-hydroxylase deficiency based upon basal and ACTH-stimulated levels of 17-OHP.

With regard to the specific functional diagnosis, if total or unbound testosterone is elevated but below the male range, the diagnosis of ovarian androgen excess can be made. If DHEAS is between 2.8 and 8 μg/ml, adrenal androgen excess is diagnosed. We have used a level above 5 μg/ml to diagnose a moderate to severe form of adrenal androgen excess and patients with DHEAS levels from 2.8 to 5 μg/ml have the diagnosis of mild adrenal androgen excess. Women who have elevated unbound testosterone levels in combination with elevations in DHEAS have a mixed form of androgen excess. In our studies, the mixed group is the most common group; the ovarian androgen excess group is second (elevated unbound testosterone, normal DHEAS); and adrenal androgen excess is the least common abnormality (elevated DHEAS, normal total or unbound testosterone).

Idiopathic hirsutism

Hirsutism in association with near normal levels of unbound testosterone and DHEAS may be termed idiopathic. This term may be used in a practical way to categorize patients. However, careful study of these women indicates that most do have subtle androgen abnormalities, specifically increased androgen action in their peripheral tissues (skin and hair follicles). Serum 3α-diol G will be elevated in virtually all patients with ovarian or adrenal androgen excess but may be elevated in only 80% of patients with an idiopathic disorder. Its measurement may be useful in demonstrating peripheral involvement, but there is limited information at present to recommend its measurement for monitoring therapy.

SUGGESTED READING

ABRAHAM G. Ovarian and adrenal contributions to peripheral androgens during the menstrual cycle. *J Clin Endocrinol Metab* 1979;39:340.

ABRAHAM GE, CHAKMAKJIAN ZH, BUSTER JE, MARSHALL JR. Ovarian and adrenal contributions to peripheral androgens in hirsute women. *Obstet Gynecol* 1975;46:169.

KIRSCHNER MA, ZUCKER IR, JESPERSEN D. Idiopathic hirsutism – an ovarian abnormality. *N Engl J Med* 1976;294:637.

LIDDLE GW. Tests of pituitary adrenal suppressibility in the diagnosis of Cushing's syndrome. *J Clin Endocrinol Metab* 1960;20:1539.

LOBO RA. Hirsutism. In: Sciarra JJ, Speroff L, Simpson JL, eds. *Gynecology and Obstetrics*, vol 5: *Endocrinology, Infertility, Genetics*. Philadelphia: J.B. Lippincott, 1987:1.

LOBO RA. Androgen excess. In: Mishell DR Jr, Davajan V, Lobo RA, eds. *Infertility, Contraception and Reproductive Endocrinology*. 3rd edn. Cambridge, MA: Blackwell Scientific Publications, 1991:422.

LOBO RA, GOEBELSMANN U. Adult manifestation of congenital adrenal hyperplasia due to incomplete 21-hydroxylase deficiency mimicking polycystic ovarian disease. *Am J Obstet Gynecol* 1980;138:720.

LOBO RA, GOEBELSMANN U. Evidence for reduced 3β-ol hydroxylase dehydrogenase activity in some hirsute women thought to have polycystic ovary syndrome. *J Clin Endocrinol Metab* 1981;53:394.

LOBO RA, PAUL WL, GOEBELSMANN U. Dehydroepiandrosterone sulfate as an indicator of adrenal androgen function. *Obstet Gynecol* 1981;57:69.

LOBO RA, PAUL WL, GOEBELSMANN U. Serum levels of DHEAS in gynecologic endocrinopathy and infertility. *Obstet Gynecol* 1981;57:607.

NEW MI, LORENZEN F, LERNER AJ, *et al*. Genotyping steroid 21-hydroxylase deficiency: hormonal reference data. *J Clin Endocrinol Metab* 1983;57:320.

96

Management of hirsutism

ROGERIO A. LOBO

Physiologic hirsutism at the time of puberty, pregnancy, or the postmenopausal years requires no treatment. It is frequently difficult to discover iatrogenic causes of androgen excess, but once detected, treatment is simply removal of the offending agent. The treatment of androgen excess associated with Cushing's syndrome, acromegaly, or porphyria is directed at the primary disease. Genetic causes of excesss androgen, often in association with ambiguous genitalia, and tumors that produce androgens are managed by surgical intervention. Patients with virilization of a short duration have a better prognosis when the source of the androgen is removed than do patients with long-standing virilization. Hirsutism secondary to a tumor may respond dramatically when the tumor is removed.

Source of androgen

Stimulation and suppression of ovarian and adrenal androgens have been suggested to determine the source of the excess androgen as ovarian, adrenal, or both. We do not feel that this testing adds important information or distinguishes completely between androgens secreted by the two sets of glands. Serum dehydroepiandrosterone sulfate (DHEAS) is used to reflect adrenal androgen excess and serum testosterone is used to reflect primarily ovarian androgen excess.

Testosterone is a potent androgen in the peripheral circulation. Approximately 90% of circulating testosterone is bound to a high-affinity protein referred to as testosterone–estradiol-binding globulin, or sex hormone-binding globulin (SHBG). Testosterone bound to SHBG is biologically and physiologically inactive. The remaining 10% of the testosterone in the circulation is not bound to SHBG. Of this 10%, 9% is bound to albumin and the remaining 1% is free, not bound to any protein. The portion of testosterone in the circulation bound to the low-affinity protein albumin (weakly bound) is available to the androgen receptors and is therefore biologically active and considered unbound. As the majority of women with androgen excess have a decreased level of SHBG, serum unbound testosterone often is elevated and gives more information than the measurement of total serum testosterone.

Other assays for free testosterone include only dialyzably free testosterone (non-SHBG, nonalbumin-bound). Unbound or free testosterone may be used to access more critically the production of androgen but is not a test that needs to be ordered in most clinical situations. Although measurement of total testosterone is sufficient for clinical diagnostic purposes in most instances, patients with an idiopathic disorder may benefit from this more discriminating assay of unbound or free testosterone. We currently base the treatment of hirsutism on basal determinations of serum DHEAS, serum testosterone, and/or unbound testosterone. Selectively, we measure serum 3α-androstanediol glucuronide (3α-diol G) and 17α-hydroxyprogesterone. It is not necessary to measure androstenedione under most circumstances.

Medical management

Hirsutism may be treated with corticosteroids, combination oral contraceptives (OCs), combinations of corticosteroids and OCs, gonadotropin-releasing hormone (GnRH) agonists and receptor-blocking agents. Receptor-blocking agents include cyproterone acetate (Androcur – not available in the USA), cimetidine (Tagamet), cyproheptadine (Periactin), spironolactone (Aldactone), and flutamide (Eulexin). Several antiandrogens, such as cyproterone acetate and spironolactone, also inhibit 5α-reductase activity, which is the most important metabolic step in determining the biologic effects of androgens. New agents which specifically inhibit 5α-reductase (finasteride, Proscar) may be useful in the future.

Corticosteroids

Corticosteroids may be useful if serum DHEAS is evaluated above 5 µg/ml and/or for the diagnosis of congenital adrenal hyperplasia (CAH). We have used dexamethasone (DEX), although other corticosteroids, such as prednisone, also may be used. DEX inhibits adrenocorticotropic hormone secretion from the pituitary, and in addition, may exert a direct inhibitory effect on steroidogenesis. We use low doses (0.25–0.5 mg) and reevaluate treatment at 3-month intervals. The dose may be lowered in order to keep the 08:00 h cortisol level in a detectable range (approximately 2 µg/dl). In patients who have CAH, 0.75 mg is often necessary for treatment, although many women may be maintained adequately on 0.5 mg daily.

Oral contraceptives

To select the proper OC, it is necessary to understand the effects of sex hormones on SHBG. Estrogens increase SHBG, resulting in a rise in total testosterone but a decrease in the biologically active unbound fraction of testosterone in the peripheral circulation. Androgens, or something associated with elevated androgen levels, decrease SHBG, resulting in an increase in the biologically active unbound testosterone in the peripheral circulation. The progestin in OCs decreases luteinizing hormone-dependent production of ovarian testosterone and androstenedione. When OCs are used for the management of hirsutism, levonorgestrel, which has androgenic properties of its own and decreases SHBG, should be avoided. A combination OC that contains norethindrone or ethynodiol diacetate and ethinylestradiol 35 µg has a very favorable estrogen : gestogen ratio for the treatment of hirsutism and can be administered cyclically. The newer selective progestins (norgestimate, desogestrel, gestodene) in OCs have the advantage of having a greater progestin : androgen potency ratio compared to current formulations and offer a theoretic advantage.

Gonadotropin-releasing hormone agonists

These agents have been found to be particularly useful for treating more severe forms of ovarian hyperandrogenism or for women who have not responded to other treatments. Down-regulation of the ovary (e.g., Depo Lupron 3.75 mg im every 4 weeks) has been found to be highly effective. The only concern, apart from that of expense, is that long-term treatment leads to vasomotor symptoms and bone loss. However, the addition of estrogen or OCs to this regimen is of additional benefit and has been useful in our experience, allowing therapy to be extended to 1 year or more.

Receptor-blocking agents

Receptor-blocking agents are effective antiandrogens. Cyproterone acetate is a progestin derivative that has been used effectively together with estrogen for the treatment of hirsutism as well as for contraception but it is unavailable in the USA. In this country, cimetidine, cyproheptadine, and spironolactone have been used effectively to treat hirsutism. More is known about spironolactone than about the other two drugs and recent studies have suggested that the former two agents are not particularly effective. In addition to its effect on decreasing steroidogenesis (primarily ovarian), spironolactone increases the clearance of testosterone, blocks the androgen receptor, and inhibits skin 5α-reductase activity. Doses of 50–200 mg/day, given in two divided doses, have been used and found to be effective for most patients. There is a dose–response effect and doses of 100–200 mg/day are usually necessary. Apart from a transient diuresis, side-effects are few. Specifically, hyperkalemia does not occur in patients with normal renal function. However, many patients will complain of some irregular bleeding. This complaint is managed by the addition of an OC.

Treatment regimens

We have used a therapeutic approach based on abnormalities in serum total testosterone, unbound testosterone, and DHEAS. If only serum total testosterone or unbound testosterone is elevated, OCs are used. This is also the case even if DHEAS is elevated mildly (<5 μg/ml). However, if the elevation in serum total testosterone or unbound testosterone is associated with DHEAS levels >5 μg/ml, DEX 0.25–0.37 mg is added to the OC regimen. If DHEAS is elevated moderately (5 μg/ml or more) without significant increase in serum total testosterone or unbound testosterone, DEX is used alone. It is unusual for women to have marked elevations in DHEAS (e.g., 6–8 μg/ml) without any elevations in unbound testosterone. Therefore, most patients with higher levels of DHEAS receive DEX and OCs in combination. Women who have significant complaints of hirsutism and testosterone levels above 100 ng/dl and those who have failed treatment with OCs and other regimens are candidates for the GnRH agonist.

Women with hirsutism and no increases in serum total testosterone, unbound testosterone, or DHEAS are given spironolactone 100–200 mg/day. The existence of a peripheral disorder may be confirmed by finding elevated levels of serum 3α-diol G, but it is not necessary to measure this metabolite in most clinical instances. This dose of spironolactone has been used effectively and without side-effects. Effectiveness usually is noted within 3 months. This therapy also is used if hirsutism has not improved after 6 months of conventional therapy, as discussed above.

Our recent studies have suggested that, despite normalization of elevated androgen levels with DEX, clinical improvement is not marked unless an antiandrogen is added. Therefore, we rarely use DEX alone for the complaint of hirsutism and add spironolactone in most cases.

Monitoring

Patients being followed on therapy should have a repeat measurement of serum DHEAS and testosterone at least once about 3 months after starting therapy. The earliest clinical changes should occur by 3 months, which represents the duration of the hair cycle on the face. It is important to stress that the rate of hair growth will be affected and new hair should not appear. However, the existing hair does not fall out during therapy. Scoring systems to monitor hair changes and/or photographs are extremely valuable.

Surgery

Wedge resection of the ovaries has been recommended previously for the treatment of hirsutism due to polycystic ovary syndrome (PCO). Because ovaries that have been invaded surgically are prone to adhesions and there is no evidence of a long-term reduction in circulating androgens by this procedure, it is not recommended for the management of hirsutism. While some wedge procedures may be justified in some cases of PCO where conventional induction of ovulation has failed, it is not effective for the treatment of hirsutism. Wedge resection has been reported to be beneficial for hirsutism in only 16% of patients.

Oophorectomy may be considered in women with markedly elevated levels of serum testosterone and normal DHEAS levels. Many will have long histories of hirsutism and virilization and often the histologic diagnosis is hyperthecosis. A test for the effectiveness of oophorectomy is usually a prerequisite and involves the use of the GnRH agonist. The closer these women are in age to the time of spontaneous menopause, the more reasonable it would be to perform surgical extirpation of the ovaries.

Efficacy of treatment

Patients may not notice a decrease in hair growth due to hormonal therapy for 6–12 months. Hormonal therapy primarily inhibits the growth of new hair follicles. Temporary methods of removing or concealing excess hair include tweezing, clipping, shaving, waxing, bleaching, and depilatories. Tweezing should be avoided, as this may result in more hair growth by the surrounding follicles. Electrolysis is the only method of permanent hair removal. This procedure is limited, as only 100 hair follicles can be removed at a session and the process can result in hyperpigmentation and folliculitis. This treatment is recommended only after hormonal levels are normalized and new hair growth has been arrested.

Women with hirsutism have to be treated for many months. However, approximately 1 year after the cessation of hair growth and the normalization of hormone levels, we have attempted to discontinue therapy and reevaluate the patient. The problem often recurs, but in some women 1 year of treatment has had a long-lasting effect.

SUGGESTED READING

BOISSELLE A, TREMBLAY RR. New therapeutic approach to the hirsute patient. *Fertil Steril* 1979;32:276.

CARMINA E, LOBO RA. Peripheral androgen blockade versus glandular androgen suppression in the treatment of hirsutism. *Obstet Gynecol* 1991;78:849.

CARMINA E, JANNI A, LOBO R. Physiologic hormonal replacement enhances the effect of the GnRH-agonist in the treatment of hirsutism. *J Clin Endocrinol Metab* (submitted).

CASEY JH. Chronic treatment regimens for hirsutism in women: effect on blood production rates of testosterone and on hair growth. *Clin Endocrinol* 1975;4:313.

CUMMING DC, YANG JC, REBAR RW, YEN SSC. Treatment of hirsutism with spironolactone. *JAMA* 1982;247:1295.

GIVENS JR, ANDERSEN RN, WISER WL, UMSTOT ES, FISH SA. The effectiveness of two oral contraceptives in suppressing plasma androstenedione, testosterone, LH, and FSH, and in stimulating plasma testosterone-binding capacity in hirsute women. *Am J Obstet Gynecol* 1976;124:333.

JUDD HL, MCPHERSON RA, RAKOFF JS, YEN SSC. Correlation of the effects of dexamethasone administration on urinary 17-ketosteroid and serum androgen levels in patients with hirsutism. *Am J Obstet Gynecol* 1977;128:408.

LOBO RA. Hirsutism. In: Sciarra JJ, Speroff L, Simpson JL, eds. *Gynecology and Obstetrics*, vol 5: *Endocrinology, Infertility, Genetics*. Philadelphia: JB Lippincott, 1987:1.

LOBO RA. Androgen excess. In: Mishell DR Jr, Davajan V, Lobo RA, eds. *Infertility, Contraception and Reproductive Endocrinology*. 3rd edn. Cambridge, MA: Blackwell Scientific Publications, 1991:422.

LOBO RA, PAUL WL, GOEBELSMANN U. Serum levels of DHEAS in gynecologic endocrinopathy and infertility. *Obstet Gynecol* 1981;57:607.

LOBO RA, SHOUPE D, SERAFINI P, BRINTON D, HORTON R. The effects of two doses of spironolactone on serum androgens and anagen hair in hirsute women. *Fertil Steril* 1985;43:200.

WILD RA, UMSTOT ES, ANDERSEN RN, GIVENS JR. Adrenal function in hirsutism. II. Effect of an oral contraceptive. *J Clin Endocrinol Metab* 1982;54:676.

97

Therapy of polycystic ovary syndrome

ROGERIO A. LOBO

Polycystic ovary syndrome (PCO), previously referred to as Stein–Leventhal syndrome, is an extremely heterogeneous clinical disorder. It is characterized by the presence of menstrual irregularities such as amenorrhea, oligomenorrhea and dysfunctional (anovulatory) uterine bleeding, infertility, and hirsutism. Because the major features are those of perimenarchal onset of hyperandrogenism and chronic anovulation, whether or not the ovaries are enlarged or polycystic, we have renamed this the syndrome of hyperandrogenic chronic anovulation (HCA). Therapy depends on the patient's chief complaint. By and large, it can be stated that amenorrhea and oligomenorrhea are treated with intermittent administration of a progestin, infertility is treated with clomiphene citrate (Clomid, Serophene), and hirsutism is treated according to the abnormality in androgen secretion (Chapter 96).

Etiology

HCA or PCO is associated with prolonged periods of anovulation and extraovarian estrogen production, largely by peripheral conversion of androstenedione to estrone and elevated levels of unbound estradiol. This derangement leads to persistent acyclic estrogen overproduction associated with a lack of progesterone, which normally would be produced by the corpus luteum. Persistent acyclic estrogen overproduction in conjunction with the absence of luteal-phase progesterone causes prolonged estrogenic stimulation of the endometrium and may lead to cystic hyperplasia, atypical hyperplasia, or even endometrial carcinoma.

The untreated patient risks the development of endometrial carcinoma earlier than women with regular menstrual cycles. All therapeutic modalities for PCO must eliminate the persistent acyclic estrogen overproduction or counteract its consistent mitogenic effect on the endometrium by producing an appropriate progestogenic effect on the endometrium; this is accomplished by administering an appropriate progestogen dose for a sufficient length of time.

The true pathophysiology of PCO is unsettled because it is a heterogeneous syndrome and not all patients exhibit the same constellation of symptoms and signs. Nevertheless, a fairly characteristic biochemical abnormality is that of inappropriate gonadotropin secretion which is evidenced by elevated levels of serum luteinizing hormone (LH) and ratios of LH to follicle-stimulating hormone (FSH) often in excess of 3:1. These and other findings suggest the involvement of the hypothalamic–pituitary axis.

However, not all patients will exhibit the gonadotropin disturbances. Some are of normal weight and others may not exhibit even the skin manifestations of hyperandrogenism (acne, hirsutism). Although polycystic changes in the ovary frequently are encountered, this finding alone does not make the diagnosis of PCO, but the absence of such characteristic ovarian findings does not exclude the diagnosis either. Both adrenal and ovarian androgen levels may be increased and hirsutism need not be present. A characteristic finding which is now thought to be involved in the pathophysiology of PCO is that of insulin resistance. This occurs in up to 75% of all patients and accentuates the ovarian androgen disturbance. Most women also have lipoprotein abnormalities with low high-density lipoprotein–cholesterol levels.

For treatment purposes, a functional diagnosis is based clinically on the appreciation of the two dominant characteristics of the syndrome, chronic anovulation and hyperandrogenemia (even in the absence of hirsutism). Treatment then is based on the specific complaint.

Management

Dysfunctional bleeding and endometrial disease

PCO patients with oligomenorrhea or amenorrhea who neither desire fertility in the immediate future nor complain about increased hair growth should receive a 10-day course of medroxyprogesterone acetate (Provera) 10 mg/day orally, given conveniently for the first or last 10 days of a calendar month. Provera is a nonandrogenic progestin and is therefore preferred over 19-norprogestins which also may be used. This regimen is repeated each month in patients with PCO who present with oligomenorrhea or amenorrhea because they are unlikely to resume regular ovulatory cycles spontaneously.

It is suggested that all PCO patients who present with a history of long-standing untreated amenorrhea, oligomenorrhea, or anovulatory bleeding should have an endometrial biopsy to rule out malignancy. Endometrial findings on vaginal ultrasound have been useful in determining the need for endometrial sampling, even without a history of abnormal bleeding.

Dysfunctional uterine bleeding will be prevented by medroxyprogesterone acetate 10 mg/day taken daily for 10 consecutive days each month. Cyclic administration, as this regimen is called, does not inhibit ovulation. Spontaneous ovulation may occur occasionally in PCO; thus, women who desire contraceptive protection should be advised to use an oral contraceptive (OC). OCs are effective in preventing unopposed estrogen effects of the endometrium and are beneficial in hyperandrogenic patients with PCO.

Anovulation

Clomiphene citrate

If the patient wishes to conceive, she should be treated with clomiphene citrate. To avoid clomiphene citrate administration in early pregnancy, it is imperative to rule out an existing pregnancy in any oligomenorrheic or amenorrheic patient by history, examination, and pregnancy test. We induce menses before therapy with an intramuscular injection of 100 or 200 mg of progesterone in oil. On the third to fifth day after the onset of bleeding, clomiphene citrate therapy, at an initial dose of 50 mg/day for 5 days, is begun. We use the individualized graduated clomiphene citrate regimen which is discussed in detail in Chapter 102.

Combined drug therapy

If clomiphene citrate fails to induce ovulation, dexamethasone in combination with clomiphene citrate may be tried, as may human menopausal gonadotropins (hMG; Pergonal). Dexamethasone is indicated in patients who fail to ovulate with clomiphene citrate alone and who have elevated levels of androgens, particularly if serum dehydroepiandrosterone sulfate (DHEAS) is elevated. DHEAS is an indicator of adrenal androgen production which is controlled by adrenocorticotropic hormone and suppressed by 0.5 mg of dexamethasone or less given daily at bedtime. Dexamethasone is given in conjunction with the same dose of clomiphene citrate given before dexamethasone was started. Dexamethasone therapy should be started 2 weeks prior to the first clomiphene citrate dose and dexamethasone is usually continued throughout consecutive treatment months until a β-human chorionic gonadotropin radioimmunoassay is positive. After the first month, the dose of dexamethasone should be decreased to 0.25 mg.

Prolactin is elevated in as many as a third of patients with PCO. If hyperprolactinemia is present, the patient should be evaluated further, depending on how high the level is. However, lowering prolactin with bromocriptine may be beneficial for inducing ovulation in patients who do not respond to clomiphene alone. In patients who do not respond to clomiphene or combination therapy, Pergonal (LH and FSH) or "pure" FSH may be used. These therapies are discussed in detail in Chapter 103. Although "pure" FSH (Metrodin) has some theoretic advantages for the induction of ovulation in PCO, to date this treatment has not been shown to be more successful than the use of Pergonal. Although cystic "PCO ovaries" are not found in all patients, those who have such findings are at increased risk for hyperstimulation with hMG or FSH treatment.

Wedge resection

Wedge resection to induce ovulation rarely is indicated because the overwhelming majority of patients will ovulate when treated with clomiphene citrate. Some who do not ovulate with clomiphene citrate alone may do so when it is given in combination with dexamethasone or when treated with hMG. Wedge resection may result in ovulation in women who fail to respond to clomiphene citrate. However, wedge resection may also cause tuboovarian adhesions and thus may decrease the chances for fertility. Therefore medical treatment is the method of choice for induction of ovulation in PCO patients.

In the last few years, a resurgence of interest has occurred in using microsurgical, laser, and laparoscopic techniques for wedge resection. The most recent methods using laparoscopic electrocautery to cause multifocal tissue destruction have been successful in that most (70–90%) clomiphene citrate-resistant patients have ovulated after the procedures and unadjusted pregnancy rates of 50% have been reported. Nevertheless, these techniques are only justified with clomiphene resistance and, in our Medical Center, in those patients who have significant hyperstimulation with hMG or FSH.

Management of hirsutism

Hirsutism results from excessive androgen production of adrenal and/or ovarian origin. Chapters 94–96 discuss this subject more fully. Ovarian androgen overproduction in PCO patients is stimulated by elevated serum LH concentrations and is compounded by a decrease in circulating sex hormone-binding globulin (SHBG). The latter results in an increase in non-SHBG-bound (e.g., androgenically active) testosterone. When combination OC steroids are given, serum LH is suppressed, ovarian androgen production is reduced, and the ethinylestradiol present in combination OCs increases circulating SHBG through its effect on the liver. Thus, combination OC steroids will decrease both the absolute amount of circulating testosterone and the relative proportion of free (e.g., androgenically active) testosterone. We prescribe combination OCs that contain 35 µg of ethinylestradiol in combination with lower doses of norethindrone or ethynodiol diacetate. This amount of ethinylestradiol suffices to induce hepatic SHBG production and the combination of norethindrone and ethinylestradiol suppresses serum LH. Currently the newer selective progestins are being used.

A new treatment for hirsutism in PCO of primarily ovarian origin may be the gonadotropin-releasing hormone agonist. These compounds down-regulate the pituitary, which results in dramatic decreases in ovarian steroid production. The addition of estrogen or OCs may be used to counteract hypoestrogenism.

Corticosteroids, such as dexamethasone, suppress adrenal androgen production. Corticosteroids are indicated only in hirsute patients with elevated serum DHEAS (>5 µg/ml). OCs are sufficient to suppress adrenal androgen levels that are elevated but below this level.

Excess body hair will not disappear even when androgen excess has been corrected. On the other hand, hair will not regrow as quickly or be as coarse as before. Thus, additional mechanical methods of hair removal are indicated.

Wedge resection is followed by an immediate decrease in serum testosterone and androstenedione levels. However, the drop in serum androgens is temporary and wedge resection is therefore not recommended to treat hirsutism.

In older women who do not desire further child-bearing and who are severely affected by androgen excess of primarily ovarian origin, oophorectomy should be considered.

SUGGESTED READING

CHANG RJ, LAUFER LR, MELDRUM DR, *et al.* Steroid secretion in polycystic ovarian disease after ovarian suppression by a long-acting gonadotropin-releasing hormone agonist. *J Clin Endocrinol Metab* 1983;56:897.

GIVENS JR, ANDERSEN RN, WISER WL, UMSTOT ES, FISH SA. The effectiveness of two oral contraceptives in suppressing plasma androstenedione, testosterone,

LH, and FSH, and in stimulating plasma testosterone-binding capacity in hirsute women. *Am J Obstet Gynecol* 1976;124:333.

GOLDZIEHER JW, AXELROD LR. Clinical and biochemical features of polycystic ovarian disease. *Fertil Steril* 1963;14:631.

GREENBLATT E, CASPER RF. Endocrine changes after laparoscopic ovarian cautery in polycystic ovarian syndrome. *Am J Obstet Gynecol* 1987;156:279.

JUDD HL, RIGG LA, ANDERSON DC, YEN SSC. The effects of ovarian wedge resection on circulating gonadotropin and ovarian steroid levels in patients with polycystic ovary syndrome. *J Clin Endocrinol Metab* 1976;43:347.

KIRSCHNER MA, JACOBS JB. Combined ovarian and adrenal vein catheterization to determine the site(s) of androgen overproduction in hirsute women. *J Clin Endocrinol Metab* 1971;33:199.

LOBO RA. The syndrome of hyperandrogenic chronic anovulation. In: Mishell DR Jr, Davajan V, Lobo RA, eds. *Infertility, Contraception and Reproductive Endocrinology.* 3rd edn. Cambridge, MA: Blackwell Scientific Publications, 1991:447.

LOBO RA. Chronic anovulation and polycystic ovary syndrome. In: Keye WR, Chang RJ, Rebar PW, Soules MR, eds. *Infertility: Evaluation and Treatment.* New York: W.B. Saunders (submitted).

LOBO RA, PAUL W, MARCH CM, GRANGER L, KLETZKY OA. Clomiphene and dexamethasone in women unresponsive to clomiphene alone. *Obstet Gynecol* 1982;60:497.

LOBO RA, GYSLER M, MARCH CM, GOEBELSMANN U, MISHELL DR Jr. Clinical and laboratory predictors of clomiphene response. *Fertil Steril* 1982;37:168.

VENTUROLI S, ORSINI LF, PARADISI R, *et al.* Human urinary follicle-stimulating hormone and human menopausal gonadotropin in induction of multiple follicle growth and ovulation. *Fertil Steril* 1986;45:30.

98

Menopause

DANIEL R. MISHELL, JR

The decline of ovarian function occurs gradually, and the cessation of menses is only one facet of the climacteric process. In practice the terms menopause and climacteric are used interchangeably. The mean age of menopause in the USA is about 51 years, with a normal distribution curve and 95% confidence limits between ages 45 and 55 years.

The age at which the menopause occurs is genetically predetermined, unlike the age of menarche, which is related to body mass. The only environmental factor affecting the age of menopause is cigarette smoking, which decreases the age of menopause by about 2 years.

After the menopause, ovarian production of estrogen ceases and circulating levels fall dramatically, with estrone levels becoming greater than estradiol levels. Extraglandular conversion of circulating androstenedione accounts for almost all estrone production. After the menopause, about 85% of androstenedione comes from adrenal secretion and about 15% from the ovaries. The conversion of androstenedione to estrone takes place mainly in the fatty tissue; therefore, obese women have higher levels of estrone and are less likely to be estrogen-deficient.

Decreasing estrogen production leads to atrophy of the vagina, which can produce the distressful symptoms of senile vaginitis or atrophic vaginitis. This type of vaginitis can cause itching, burning, discomfort, dyspareunia, and also vaginal bleeding when the epithelium thins. Senile vaginitis is best treated with estrogen replacement therapy. Local therapy can be used for the first few weeks. However, because vaginal administration of estrogen results in irregular systemic absorption, for long-term prevention of vaginal atrophy as well as osteoporosis, the patient is best treated with systemic estrogen. Estrogen deprivation may also cause the structures that support the uterus — the cardinal and uterosacral ligaments — to lose their tonicity, and uterine descensus may occur.

The trigone of the bladder and the urethra are embryologically derived from estrogen-dependent tissue, and estrogen deficiency can lead to their atrophy, producing symptoms of urinary urgency, incontinence, dysuria, and urinary frequency. Another problem that can develop with decreased circulating estrogen levels is decreased synthesis of collagen that forms the connective tissue beneath the vaginal epithelium. This change may decrease the support of the posterior urethrovesicle angle and urinary stress incontinence can develop. Loss of collagen can also lead to clinically symptomatic cystoceles and/or rectoceles. These urinary symptoms can be alleviated or prevented with estrogen replacement therapy.

The pathognomonic symptom of menopause is the hot flush or flash, which is caused by a decrease in circulating estrogen levels. The change in estrogen levels leads to alterations in the hypothalamus that are probably mediated through the central nervous system. When the change in estrogen levels is not gradual but sudden, such as occurs after premenopausal oophorectomy, the individual is more likely to develop symptomatic hot flushes.

About 75% of all women going through menopause develop hot flushes. Obese individuals are less likely to develop flushes, as they do not have as great a decrease in estrogen levels.

About one-third of women with hot flushes have sufficiently severe symptoms to require medical assistance. About one-half of the patients with flushes have at least one a day, and about 20% have more than one a day. These flushes frequently occur at night, awaken the individual, and then produce insomnia. Hot flushes do not persist in most women for more than 2–3 years, and it is uncommon for a woman to have hot flushes that last more than 5 years after menopause. The hot flush is a systemic physiologic phenomenon that takes place over a period of 3–5 min.

The most effective treatment for the hot flush is estrogen. Since so many of the hot flushes occur at night, it is advisable for the patient to ingest the estrogen tablet before bedtime. Some patients, such as those with a history of cancer of the breast or a recent (<2 years) cancer of the endometrium, should not take estrogen. The next best therapy is a progestogen. Oral medroxyprogesterone acetate (MPA) in a dosage of 20 mg/day relieves hot flushes significantly more effectively than placebo. Unfortunately, MPA does not prevent vaginal or urethral atrophy, but it will diminish hot flushes in patients who cannot take estrogen. Injections of Depo-Provera (DMPA) in a dosage of 150 mg once every 3 months relieve hot flushes very well. Other agents shown to reduce hot flushes significantly include clonidine, naloxone, and methyldopa (Aldomet), but these drugs are not usually prescribed for this purpose.

Other systemic symptoms

Symptoms such as anxiety, depression, irritability, and fatigue increase after menopause. Several studies have demonstrated that estrogen improves many of these psychologic symptoms significantly better than placebo, particularly depression, in addition to relieving the hot flush and allowing the patient to sleep better. Postmenopausal estrogen users have significantly thicker skin and a greater amount of collagen in the dermis than nonestrogen users. The systemic estrogen use can retard wrinkling and thinning of the skin postmenopausally.

Osteoporosis

Osteoporosis is defined as an asymptomatic reduction in the mass-per-unit bone volume (density) so that there is a significantly increased risk of fracture in the absence of trauma. Postmenopausal osteoporosis initially affects trabecular bone which is present in the vertebral column and distal radius. Osteoporosis develops more slowly in cortical bone, which is present in the limbs. Bone mass is increased in black, obese, and tall women and is decreased in short, frail, thin-skinned, sedentary women. Thus, women in the former group usually do not develop osteoporosis, while women in the latter group are at a greater risk for developing the disorder. In the latter group of women about 1–1.5% of bone mass is lost each year after menopause. Osteoporosis is an asymptomatic disease, and its presence usually is not detected until a fracture occurs many years later. At least 25% of the bone needs to be lost before osteoporosis is diagnosed by routine X-ray examination.

At present the methods available for establishing the early diagnosis of osteoporosis in trabecular bone, specifically bone density studies and computed tomography (CT) scans, are complicated and expensive. Although dual-photon absorptiometry and CT scans effectively measure bone density in trabecular bone, the equipment necessary to perform these procedures is expensive and needs to be located in institutions. Dual-energy X-ray absorptiometry (DEXA) is a new method of measuring bone density that has greater precision and can be completed in a shorter time than CT or dual-photon absorptiometry. The technique of single-photon absorptiometry is much easier to perform, and the equipment is portable and less expensive and can be used in an office or clinic setting. Nevertheless, this technique can only be used to measure the density of structures composed primarily of cortical bone – the bone in the axial skeleton such as the radius, femur, or os calcis. Since postmenopausal osteoporosis affects trabecular bone more rapidly than it does cortical bone, utilization of single-photon absorptiometry on bones in the limbs can fail to detect the presence of loss of trabecular bone in the thoracic spine because the density of the bone being measured may remain within the normal range. Thus neither of the photon absorptiometry techniques should be utilized for routine screening of postmenopausal women.

Lindsay *et al.* have stated that bone mass measurements are indicated only when clinical decisions will be influenced by the information gained; that is, when a woman will take estrogen only if there are objective measurements of bone loss. A careful history and physical examination will determine whether risk factors for development of osteoporosis are present. Factors known to increase the risk of osteoporosis are as follows:

1 race: white or Oriental;

2 reduced weight for height;

3 early spontaneous menopause;

4 early surgical menopause;

5 family history of osteoporosis;

6 diet; low calcium intake, low vitamin D intake, high caffeine intake, high alcohol intake, and high protein intake;

7 cigarette smoking;

8 endocrine disorders such as diabetes mellitus, hyperthyroidism, and Cushing's disease;

9 sedentary lifestyle.

In women undergoing a normal menopause, fractures begin to occur about age 60 in structures composed mainly of trabecular bone, such as the vertebral spine and distal portion of the radius. By age 60, 25% of white and Oriental women develop spinal compression fractures. Loss of bone mass in cortical bone occurs at a much slower rate, so osteoporotic fractures of the femur usually do not begin to occur until about age 70 or 75.

Patients with osteoporosis have a higher bone resorption rate than normal. With a few months of estrogen treatment, bone resorption rates return to normal. Bone formation in patients with osteoporosis is normal before and after the estrogen therapy. The best way to prevent loss of calcium from bone in postmenopausal women or castrated women is to administer exogenous estrogens.

Both prospective (cohort) and several retrospective (case control) studies have shown that estrogen therapy reduces the amount of postmenopausal bone loss as well as the incidence of fracture.

Studies in which bone density was measured have shown the minimum dosage of estrogen needed to prevent osteoporosis is 0.625 mg of conjugated equine estrogens, 0.625 mg of estrone sulfate, and 0.5 mg of micronized estradiol. In addition, estrogen administered by subdernal pellets, transdermal patch, or transdermal gel has been shown to decrease the urinary calcium:creatinine ratio. These data provide indirect evidence that these parenteral routes of administration of estrogen should also decrease the loss of bone mass.

Indirect evidence suggests that progestins by themselves also reduce the rate of bone reabsorption as they decrease the amount of urinary calcium excretion. Addition of a progestin to estrogen replacement therapy does not inhibit the beneficial effect of estrogen in reducing the rate of bone reabsorption.

Ingesting the recommended daily intake of dietary calcium (800–1000 mg/day) during the adolescent years results in greater peak adult bone mass than occurs if insufficient calcium is ingested. Thus postmenopausally, with steady loss of bone, women who when premenopausal ingested the recommended intake are less likely to have sufficient reduction in bone density to cause fractures than those ingesting insufficient calcium.

However, several investigators have shown that when postmenopausal women utilize dietary calcium supplementation without estrogen, it does not prevent postmenopausal bone loss.

Controversy exists whether calcium supplementation is advisable in postmenopausal women receiving estrogen replacement. It appears that when postmenopausal women ingest an adequate amount of calcium in their diet – more than 500 mg daily – additional calcium supplementation is of no benefit, especially if they are also receiving estrogen. Calcium supplementation is only of benefit for those women who have an inadequate daily ingestion of calcium, <500 mg. It is preferable to maintain an adequate intake of calcium by eating foods containing this mineral than by supplemental calcium sources.

Exercise in the premenopausal years increases bone density. However, weight-bearing exercise alone will not prevent postmenopausal bone loss. It has been reported that neither a program of brisk walking nor back exercise altered the rate of trabecular bone loss postmenopausally. Thus calcium alone and a moderate exercise program cannot prevent the loss of bone mass in the early postmenopausal woman, but exercise is beneficial for the woman's overall health. It is not necessary for postmenopausal women to receive vitamin D, because it has been shown that women with osteoporosis treated with various regimens with and without vitamin D had no difference in the incidence of subsequent osteoporotic fractures.

In summary, estrogen increases calcium absorption and reduces the rate of bone reabsorption. It will not stimulate new bone growth but will prevent osteoporosis if therapy is started at the time of menopause. For women at risk of developing osteoporosis, specifically nonobese white or Oriental women, estrogen replacement is the best means to prevent this debilitating and painful disease.

Metabolic effects

With any drug there is a benefit:risk ratio, but the risks of estrogen replacement therapy are minimal. Exogenous estrogen administration produces effects on serum proteins, specifically an increase in serum globulins. One of these globulins, angiotensinogen, can be converted to angiotensin and produce an increase in blood pressure, whereas other globulins may produce a hypercoagulable state and possibly thrombosis. In addition, exogenous estrogens may alter lipid levels and other metabolic processes. However, these metabolic changes are related to the dosage and type of estrogen administered, and the dose and type of estrogen given for postmenopausal hormone replacement therapy are much less potent than those used in oral contraceptives. Ethinylestradiol, 30 and 35 µg, which is the dosage of estrogen in most of the currently used oral contraceptive formulations, is the equivalent of about 2.5 mg of conjugated equine estrogens. Therefore, although the usual dosage of 0.625 mg of conjugated estrogen is 20 times greater than the minimum weight of estrogen used in oral contraceptives, it is only about one-fifth as potent in terms of effects on liver globulins and postmenopausal estrogen replacement does not increase blood pressure or the risk of developing thromboembolism. Estrogen appears to have little effect on glucose metabolism, as several recent studies have shown no decrease in glucose tolerance in patients treated with doses of estrogen equivalent to 1.25 mg of conjugated equine estrogen. Although some studies have shown a statistically increased risk of gallbladder disease in postmenopausal estrogen users, others have reported no such risk. Estrogens may accelerate the formation of cholelithiasis in susceptible individuals.

Cardiovascular effects

In contrast to the increase in blood pressure that has been reported in some women using oral contraceptives, no such increase has been observed with use of estrogen replacement therapy. It is safe to prescribe estrogen replacement for postmenopausal women with hypertension, and if blood pressure increases while they are receiving this treatment, it is unlikely that the estrogen is the cause of the blood pressure elevation.

There is no epidemiologic evidence of an increased incidence of thrombophlebitis or thromboembolism in postmenopausal estrogen users as compared with control subjects. Several epidemiologic studies have reported no increased incidence of these disorders in postmenopausal women taking estrogen, in comparison to the increased incidence found in oral contraceptive users. Furthermore, there is no evidence that postmenopausal women with a past history of thrombophlebitis have an increased incidence of thrombophlebitis with estrogen replacement therapy.

In contrast to the increased risk of myocardial infarction found in women over 35 who smoke and ingest high dosages of oral contraceptives, use of estrogen replacement has been shown to reduce the risk of myocardial infarction.

Although no randomized prospective studies have been performed to date, an abundance of epidemiologic data indicates that estrogen replacement therapy retards the development of atherosclerosis in postmenopausal women and reduces their risks of developing myocardial infarction and cerebrovascular accident (stroke). Several retrospective case-control studies have demonstrated a reduction in risk of coronary heart disease in estrogen users.

In addition, as summarized by Stampfer *et al.*, many prospective studies have also demonstrated that approximately a 50% reduction in myocardial infarction occurs in estrogen users.

Additional evidence from studies of women undergoing coronary artery angiography supports the belief that estrogen use retards the development of atherosclerosis. In a retrospective study of women undergoing coronary angiography Gruchow *et al.* reported that the degree of coronary artery occlusion did not increase after age 60 among estrogen users, while it did among nonusers.

McFarland *et al.* reported that among 345 women undergoing coronary artery catheterization for suspected myocardial infarction, estrogen users were only half as likely as nonusers to have severe coronary artery disease (more than 70% occlusion). Sullivan performed a retrospective 10-year follow-up of 2268 women who had coronary angiography. Survival rates at 10 years were significantly higher among estrogen users with both mild to moderate and severe degrees of coronary artery occlusion. Among the latter group, survival was only 60% among estrogen nonusers while it was 97% among estrogen users. After appropriate adjustment for other risk factors, estrogen was found to have a significant independent effect on survival. These data indicate that estrogen prevents worsening of existing atherosclerosis and that prior cardiovascular disease is not a contraindication to estrogen replacement.

Paganini-Hill *et al.* showed in a cohort study that postmenopausal estrogen use significantly reduced the risk of death from cerebrovascular accident (stroke) among women 75–85 years of age. Thus, estrogen use protects against the development of cerebral artery atherosclerosis as well as coronary artery atherosclerosis. Cardiovascular disease is the major cause of death among women over 50. Therefore several studies have shown that estrogen reduces the risk of overall mortality among postmenopausal women.

Probably the main mechanism whereby oral estrogen replacement retards atherosclerosis postmenopausally is prevention of the adverse alterations in endogenous circulating lipid levels that normally occur after the menopause. In longitudinal studies it has been shown that total serum cholesterol, low-density lipoprotein (LDL) cholesterol and triglycerides increased postmenopausally while high-density lipoprotein (HDL) cholesterol levels declined. Several investigators have reported that ingestion of various oral estrogen formulations postmenopausally prevents these unfavorable alterations in the lipid profile.

Numerous studies have shown that administration of oral conjugated equine estrogens as well as other oral estrogens raises triglycerides and serum HDL cholesterol and lowers LDL cholesterol with minimal changes in total cholesterol. Data regarding parenteral administration of estrogen fail to show similar consistent significant lipid changes, indicating the first pass of the oral estrogen through the liver has a major influence on lipid metabolism.

The effects of combinations of estrogens and progestins for postmenopausal women on lipid metabolism depend on the doses and the potencies of both the estrogen and the progestin used in the regimen. In most studies, the beneficial changes with estrogen alone are reduced or eliminated with the addition of a synthetic progestin.

Nevertheless, estrogen may have other actions, including a direct effect on the coronary arteries to prevent atherosclerosis. Additional studies are currently being performed to determine whether parenteral estrogen and various estrogen–progestin combinations will also prevent atherosclerosis.

Neoplastic effects

Breast

Much concern has been raised about the neoplastic risks of postmenopausal estrogen replacement therapy, particularly breast and endometrial cancer, since these areas are estrogen target tissues. The possibility exists that estrogen can stimulate a nonpalpable breast cancer and carcinoma of the breast may exist in the preclinical state for as long as 8 years before it is palpable. Therefore it is advisable to obtain a mammogram to rule out subclinical breast cancer on all patients before initiating estrogen therapy and annually thereafter.

Many epidemiologic studies have investigated the relation of exogenous estrogen and the incidence of breast cancer. In 1988 Armstrong reviewed the results of all 23 studies of estrogen use and breast cancer published before 1987. He concluded that the use of estrogen does not significantly alter the risk of breast cancer (relative risk 1.01; 95% confidence interval, 0.95–1.08).

More recent metaanalyses by Steinberg *et al.*, and Dupont and Page, and Coldite *et al.* also found no significant increase in breast cancer among all estrogen users. In the former study, however, after 15 years of estrogen use the relative risk of developing breast cancer increased significantly (relative risk 1.3; 95% confidence interval, 1.2–1.6). The increased risk occurred mainly among premenopausal estrogen users or women who received an estradiol formulation, not conjugated equine estrogen.

Thus the epidemiologic data are generally reassuring as most studies show no increased risk of development of breast cancer among post-menopausal estrogen users, with the possibility of a slightly increased risk with long-term use of a high dose estradiol formulation. At present, it is not clear what effect the addition of a progestin to estrogen replacement therapy has on the risk of breast cancer, but metaanalysis of studies to date indicate no alteration in the risk of breast cancer, positively or negatively, with the use of a progestin–estrogen combination.

Endometrium

Many epidemiologic studies have reported that there is significantly increased risk of endometrial cancer developing in postmenopausal women who are ingesting estrogen without progestins, as compared with nonestrogen users. The risk increases with increasing duration of use of estrogen as well as with increasing dosage.

The endometrial cancer that develops in estrogen users is nearly always well-differentiated and is usually cured by performing a simple hysterectomy. The risk of developing endometrial carcinoma for women receiving estrogen replacement can be markedly reduced by giving the patient progestogens. The duration of progestin therapy is more important than the dosage. The use of progestins lowers the chances of postmenopausal estrogen users' developing cancer of the endometrium, and therefore progestins should be given to postmenopausal women receiving estrogen if they have a uterus. The addition of a progestin to estrogen therapy does not appear to cause an increase of any other systemic disease and acts synergistically with estrogen to cause a slight increase in bone density. The use of synthetic progestins, however, may reverse the beneficial effect of estrogen upon serum lipids.

The epidemiologic data showing a reduction in heart attacks in estrogen users were derived from women taking estrogen without a progestin. Whether the addition of a progestin to the regimen will reverse the beneficial action of estrogen upon cardiovascular disease remains to be determined. Nevertheless, it would appear prudent to use the lowest doses of progestin that will prevent the endometrial proliferation produced by estrogen.

Treatment regimens

Estrogen therapy for postmenopausal women should be given in the lowest possible dose that relieves vasomotor symptoms, prevents vaginal–urethral epithelial atrophy, maintains the collagen content of the skin, reduces the rate of bone resorption, and prevents acceleration of atherosclerosis. Estrogen therapy given to postmenopausal women should result in physiologic and not pharmacologic circulating levels of estrogen, so that the risks of hypertension and thromboembolic disease are not increased. This dose of estrogen, termed the *physiologic replacement dose*, is 0.625 mg of conjugated equine estrogen or estrone sulfate or 1 mg of micronized estradiol. The long-term effects of transdermal estradiol have not yet been determined, but it appears that the 0.05 mg skin patch provides physiologic estrogen replacement. Higher doses of estrogen may be needed for 1 or 2 years to relieve hot flushes. Vaginal administration of estrogen may be used initially to relieve atrophic vaginitis but it is best to employ other routes for long-term use as vaginal estrogen absorption is greatly variable.

If a progestin is added to the regimen in order to protect the endometrium, it does not negate the beneficial effects of estrogen on vasomotor symptoms or on bone density. The progestin may have an adverse effect on the vaginal and urethral mucosa, and may produce undesired central nervous system symptoms and adversely affect mood and the sense of well-being. Depending on the dose and biologic activity of the specific progestin, the favorable antiatherogenic lipid profile produced by estrogen may also be altered and therefore may possibly result in a partial or complete loss of the cardiovascular protective effect of unopposed estrogen. The epidemiologic studies showing a reduction in myocardial infarction with hormonal replacement only looked at groups of women taking estrogen alone, without progestins. Finally, a hormonal regimen should be selected that produces the least amount of uterine bleeding, and the bleeding should occur at regular intervals. One of the primary reasons that postmenopausal women decide not to use estrogen, or discontinue its use, is the occurrence of uterine bleeding. For this reason, combination instead of sequential estrogen–progestin regimens are being increasingly prescribed as the former regime is usually associated with no bleeding after the first few months.

The benefit of including a progestin in the estrogen replacement regimen is protection of the endometrium. Unfortunately, this benefit is accompanied by an increase in central nervous system symptoms and changes in mood and sense of well-being.

Women who have undergone a hysterectomy are no longer at risk for endometrial cancer. Until other significant benefits of progestin therapy for menopausal women are established, an unopposed estrogen regimen, cyclic or continuous, is recommended for postmenopausal women who no longer have a uterus.

For postmenopausal women who have not had a hysterectomy, there are many treatment regimens used, in addition to the combined continuous estrogen–progestin regimens. An estrogen-only regimen may be utilized to optimize protection from cardiovascular disease, in conjunction with an annual endometrial biopsy or vaginal ultrasonography to measure the endometrial thickness.

Several investigators have shown that all women with endometrial thickness of 5 mm or less measured by ultrasound had a histologic diagnosis of atrophic endometrium. Thus, if confirmed by others, this technique may be used instead of annual biopsy to screen postmenopausal women with a uterus receiving estrogen without a progestin or those who bleed with a continuous combined estrogen–progestin regimen.

Currently in clinical practice, physicians most often include a progestin in the hormonal replacement regimen of postmenopausal women who have a uterus. Various regimens, both sequential and continuous combined, have been utilized. The hormones are usually administered in a cyclic manner, with a daily dose of estrogen given the first 25 days each month and a daily dose of progestin administered concomitantly with the last 10–14 days of the estrogen. The estrogen may also be given every day of the month in a continuous fashion and the progestin given daily for the first 10–14 days of the month with the combined regimen. The latter sequential regimen is easier for patients to remember than the former. With the continuous combined regimen, both the estrogen and the progestin are administered every day of the month or 5 out of 7 days each week. The cyclic regimens usually result in monthly withdrawal bleeding, which may lessen with continued use. The continuous regimen may result in breakthrough bleeding during the first few months, but with longer use nearly all women remain amenorrheic. Because endogenous fluctuating estrogen levels in the early menopause may contribute to uterine bleeding with the continuous combined regimen, it has been recommended that the sequential regimen be used in the first 5 years after the menopause, after which the combined regimen can be utilized to increase patient compliance.

The minimal dosage and type of progestin necessary to prevent endometrial cancer have not been determined. For postmenopausal women receiving 0.625 mg of conjugated equine estrogen, 2.5 mg of medroxyprogesterone acetate reduced nuclear and cytosol estrogen receptor levels to those found before estrogen administration. Since the side-effects of progestin therapy are dose-related, reduction in dose of progestin to the minimum that still protects the endometrium may lead to improved patient compliance. Therefore, while 10 mg of medroxyprogesterone acetate is usually presented in the sequential regimen, only 2.5 mg is needed when given continuously to prevent endometrial hyperplasia.

A routine pretreatment endometrial biopsy is unnecessary, as it is not cost-effective. Also routine annual biopsies are not necessary. If breakthrough bleeding, but not withdrawal bleeding, occurs, the lining of the uterine cavity should be sampled if ultrasonography shows the endometrial thickness to be >5 mm, or vaginal ultrasonography is not available. Annual mammography should be recommended for all women aged 50 years or older, regardless of whether they are on estrogen therapy, as the incidence of breast cancer steadily increases as a woman ages. Contraindications to estrogen therapy occur infrequently. These include a history of breast cancer and thromboembolic disease associated with oral contraceptive use or pregnancy. There are no data to support these contraindications, and the American College of Obstetrics and Gynecology issued a committee opinion in 1991 stating that clinicians may elect to prescribe estrogen replacement to women with a past history of breast cancer who wish to receive the benefits of estrogen. Alternatively, progestins or clonidine can be given to reduce hot flushes and a vaginal lubricant given to relieve the symptoms of vaginal atrophy. The Centers for Disease Control have reported that women with a positive family history of breast cancer involving either a second-degree or a first-degree relative may use estrogen replacement therapy without an increased risk of breast cancer. Women with active liver disease should avoid the oral administration of estrogen.

Estrogen is the treatment of choice for the relief of vasomotor symptoms and symptoms caused by vaginal and urethral mucosa atrophy. In addition, estrogen therapy maintains the integument, improves mood, prevents postmenopausal osteoporosis and, above all, significantly reduces the morbidity and mortality associated with cardiovascular disease. Nearly all postmenopausal women can derive a substantial benefit from the use of estrogen replacement therapy and several studies have shown that estrogen users have decreased overall mortality compared to women of a similar population who were not taking estrogen.

SUGGESTED READING

ARMSTRONG BK. Oestrogen therapy after the menopause – boon or bane? *Med J Australia* 1988;148:213–214.

BARRETT-CONNOR E, BROWN WV, TURNER J, *et al.* Heart disease risk factors and hormone use in postmenopausal women. *JAMA* 1979;242:2167.

BRINCAT M, MONIZ CJ, STUDD JWW, *et al.* Long-term effects of the menopause and sex hormones on skin thickness. *Br J Obstet Gynaecol* 1985;92:256.

CAMPBELL S, BEARD RJ, McQUEEN J, *et al.* Double blind psychometric studies on the effects of natural estrogens on post-menopausal women. In: Campbell S, ed. *Management of the Menopause and Post-menopausal Years.* Lancaster, England: MTP Press, 1976:152.

COLLINS J, DONNER A, ALLEN LH, ADAMS O. Oestrogen use and survival in endometrial cancer. *Lancet* 1980;2:961.

COOPE J. Double-blind cross-over study of estrogen replacement therapy. In: Campbell S, ed. *Management of Menopause and Post-menopausal Years.* Lancaster, England: MTP Press, 1976:167.

DAVIS MR. Screening for postmenopausal osteoporosis. *Fertil Steril* 1987;156:1.

DUPONT WD, PAGE DL. Menopausal estrogen replacement therapy and breast cancer. *Arch Intern Med* 1991;151:67.

ERLIK Y, TATARYN IV, MELDRUM DR, *et al.* Association of waking episodes with menopausal hot flushes. *JAMA* 1981;245:1741.

GIBBONS WE, MOYER DL, LOBO RA, *et al.* Biochemical and histologic effects of sequential estrogen/progestin therapy on the endometrium of postmenopausal women. *Am J Obstet Gynecol* 1986;154:456.

GRUCHOW HW, ANDERSON AJ, BARBORIAK JJ, SOBOCINSKI KA. Postmenopausal use of estrogen and occlusion of coronary arteries. *Am Heart J* 1988;115:954.

HAMMOND CB, JELOVSEK FR, LEE KL, *et al.* Effects of long-term estrogen replacement therapy. II. Neoplasia. *Am J Obstet Gynecol* 1979;133:537.

HENDERSON BE, ROSS RKL, PAGANINI-HILL A, MACK TM. Estrogen use and cardiovascular disease. *Am J Obstet Gynecol* 1986;154:1181.

HULKA BS. Effects of exogenous estrogen on postmenopausal women: the epidemiologic evidence. *Obstet Gynecol Surv* 1980;35:389.

LINDSAY R, HART DM, MACLEAN A, *et al.* Bone response termination of oestrogen treatment. *Lancet* 1978;1:1325.

LINDSAY R, HART DM, FORREST C, BAIRD C. Prevention of spinal osteoporosis in oophorectomized women. *Lancet* 1980;2:1151.

McFARLAND KF, BONIFACE ME, HORNUNG CA, *et al.* Risk factors and non-contraceptive estrogenase in women with and without coronary disease. *Am J Heart* 1989;117:1209–1214.

MASCHAK CA, LOBO RA, DOLZONO-TAKANO R, *et al.* Comparison of pharmacodynamic properties of various estrogen formulations. *Am J Obstet Gynecol* 1982;144:511.

NOTELOVITZ M, KITCHENS C, WARE M, *et al.* Combination estrogen and progestogen replacement therapy does not adversely affect coagulation. *Obstet Gynecol* 1983;62:596.

PAGANINI-HILL A, ROSS RK, GERKINS VR, *et al.* A case control study of menopausal estrogen therapy and hip fractures. *Ann Intern Med* 1981;95:28.

ROSS RK, MACK TM, PAGANINI-HILL A, *et al.* Menopausal oestrogen therapy and protection from death from ischemic heart disease. *Lancet* 1981;1:858.

STAMPFER MJ, COLDITZ GA, WILLETT WC, *et al*. Postmenopausal estrogen therapy and cardiovascular disease. *N Engl J Med* 1991;325:756–762.

STEINBERG KK, THACKER SB, SMITH J, *et al*. A meta-analysis of the effect of estrogen replacement therapy on the risk of breast cancer. *JAMA* 1991;265:2985–2990.

SULLIVAN JM, VANDER ZWAAG R, HUGHES JP, *et al*. Estrogen replacement and coronary heart disease. *Arch Intern Med* 1990;150:2557–2562.

WREN BC, ROUTLEDGE AD. The effect of type and dose of oestrogen on the blood pressure of post-menopausal women. *Maturitas* 1983;5:135.

99

Premature ovarian failure

MARK V. SAUER

Premature ovarian failure (POF), more descriptively termed hypergonadotropic hypogonadism, is defined as the cessation of ovarian function after puberty but prior to the age of 40 years. The diagnosis implies that the woman is otherwise in good health, free of genetic anomalies, and has experienced normal somatic growth. POF should be distinguished from several similar conditions associated with prenatal and postnatal gonadal failure. The most common of these include Turner's syndrome and gonadal dysgenesis. Overall, beween 1 and 5% of all women of reproductive age experience the premature cessation of ovarian function.

Etiology

Premature ovarian failure is actually an expression of several disease states about which little is definitively known. Patients are characterized by a spectrum of clinical, morphologic, and endocrinologic features. The heterogeneity of clinical presentations suggests several etiologies. Reviewing the histopathology of ovarian biopsies taken from women with POF provides insight into differing mechanisms responsible for the decline in ovarian function.

Afollicular histopathology

At the time of biopsy many women with POF are noted to have few or no primordial follicles. This occurs either as a result of an increase in the rate of follicular atresia of a normal complement of follicles, or secondary to a normal atresia rate of a reduced number of follicles. The latter condition may exist secondary to a failure in primordial germ cell migration, leading to a subnormal number of follicles residing in the ovary.

Follicular histopathology

These biopsies are characterized by numerous primordial follicles, with or without any maturation delays. Postulated pathophysiologic changes include a resistance to endogenous gonadotropin stimulation due to a deficiency or an altering of follicle-stimulating hormone (FSH) receptors. The loss of FSH receptors may be autoimmune in nature. Antiovarian antibodies also occur, often in association with polyglandular failure. Lymphocytic infiltration is commonly apparent in the gonadal biopsies of these patients.

POF is associated with karyotypic abnormalities (18% of patients), and has also been described as occurring in families. The familial occurrence of POF with vertical transmission of the trait suggests a possible autosomal dominant, sex-linked inheritance pattern. In individuals possessing a Y chromosome, a 30% risk of developing a tumor by their mid 30s warrants the extirpation of the abnormal gonad. Various X-chromosome disorders are also associated with POF. A deletion or translocation of the long arm of the X chromosome (Xq) has been shown adversely to affect ovarian function. Normal function depends upon the integrity of the "critical region" on Xq from band q13 to 26 on both X-chromosomes.

Ovarian failure is known to occur in women following chemotherapy and radiation treatment for various cancers. Fractionating the dose of radiation reduces the probability of ovarian damage. Multiple-agent chemotherapy carries the highest risk for inducing amenorrhea (50–85%), a rate similar to that seen when radiation and single-dose chemotherapy are given in combination.

Endocrine profile

When examining the concentrations of FSH, luteinizing hormone (LH), estrone, estradiol, and progesterone taken from women with POF, several patterns of expression are evident. Profiles range from the traditional postmenopausal pattern of elevated gonadotropin and low sex steroid levels, to relatively normal-appearing cyclic ovulatory patterns. Unless a woman was previously rendered surgically castrate, spontaneous resumption of ovulatory cycles may occur. These cycles may be quite normal, and 5–10% pregnancy rates are observed in patients with POF independent of treatment. Commonly ovulatory patterns of hormone expression are noted, despite elevated FSH. Many menstrual cycles are short, as a result of either an attenuated follicular or luteal phase. Anovulation is frequent. The triad of infertility, regular menses, and elevated serum FSH levels describes women with occult ovarian failure, a condition of compensated granulosa cell function, which may be an early stage of POF.

Diagnosis

POF should be considered whenever there is a history of amenorrhea in a woman under the age of 40 years, especially if associated with signs and symptoms of hypoestrogenism. A single random value of FSH >40 mIU/ml traditionally has been used to make the diagnosis. However, most women experience a transitional phase of hypergonadotropic eugonadism before a hypogonadal state is reached. During this time a serum FSH obtained on day 3 of the menstrual cycle is elevated (20–40 mIU/ml). In uncertain cases, it may be helpful to obtain weekly measurements of FSH in order to characterize patients more definitively. Estradiol measurements are usually below 30 pg/ml. However, in transitional patients estradiol levels may still be in the range seen in normal ovulating women.

Autoimmune disease is prevalent in women with ovarian failure (10–40%). Therefore, it is necessary to test other organ systems for associated disease. This includes concentrations of serum calcium and phosphorus (parathyroid), thyroxine, thyroid-stimulating hormone, and antithyroid antibodies (thyroid); morning cortisol (adrenal) levels, fasting glucose (pancreas), complete blood count (parietal cells, stomach) and platelets. Hypothyroidism due to autoimmune thyroiditis is the most common endocrine disturbance occurring in association with POF. Sophisticated assays for antiovarian antibodies or antibodies to FSH receptor are difficult to obtain. However, studies have cited antibodies against gonadotropins, stromal and thecal cell antigens, and ovarian gonadotropin receptors. Other autoimmune disorders typified by the collagen vascular diseases may be coexistent. Tests such as antinuclear antibody and rheumatoid factor are helpful in identifying these patients.

Although commonly practiced in the past, ovarian biopsy is not warranted in these women. The biopsy is not always diagnostic and can be misleading, which is not surprising since only 0.5% of the total ovarian mass is represented in a single biopsy sample. Estradiol levels >50 pg/ml indicate the presence of active granulosa cells and viable follicles. However, failure to document elevations in serum estradiol, similar to the absence of follicles on ovarian biopsy, does not preclude the existence of remaining oocytes.

Treatment

Autopsy data from women who were castrated under the age of 40 demonstrate an increased incidence of coronary atherosclerosis in those surviving at least 14 years beyond the surgery. These individuals also risk accelerated bone loss, no different from that experienced by older women following natural menopause. Both of these phenomena can be slowed or reversed by administering hormone replacement therapy (estrogen/progestogen). The replacement regimens are similar to that normally prescribed to older patients. Younger women occasionally need more estrogen to alleviate symptoms. Oral contraceptive pills may be prescribed, providing a higher dose of estrogen while protecting against a rare spontaneous pregnancy. Estrogen replacement therapy is warranted in all women found to have hypergonadotropic amenorrhea, even if amenorrhea is intermittent, in order to avoid osteoporosis. Reduced spinal bone density is present at the time of diagnosis in up to 60% of women treated for POF.

There exists no proven effective method of inducing ovulation in patients with POF, as assessed by a prospective controlled study. Empiric therapies have been used frequently, despite a lack of proven benefit. These treatments include attempts at increasing ovarian stimulation using high doses of exogenous gonadotropins as well as suppression of gonadotropins by administering high-dose estrogen or gonadotropin-releasing hormone analog. Corticosteroid suppression has also been used to counteract the presumed autoimmune cause of POF. However, patients have not benefited from any of these methods, and generally experience a pregnancy rate similar to that known to occur spontaneously in women with hypergonadotropic hypogonadism.

Infertility secondary to ovarian failure is best addressed through the *in vitro* fertilization of oocytes donated by fertile women. Using donated oocytes and sex steroid hormone replacement, women with POF experience pregnancy rates following embryo transfer that approximate 35–40%. For couples willing to accept a third-party gamete, oocyte donation and assisted reproductive techniques offer the best opportunity for pregnancy.

SUGGESTED READING

AIMAN J, SMENTEK C. Premature ovarian failure. *Obstet Gynecol* 1985;66:9–14.

ALPER MM, JOLLY EE, GARNER PR. Pregnancies after premature ovarian failure. *Obstet Gynecol* 1986; 67:59S–62S.

CAMERON IT, O'SHEA FC, ROLLAND JM, HUGHES EG, DEKRETSER DM, HEALY DL. Occult ovarian failure: a syndrome of infertility, regular menses, and elevated follicle-stimulating hormone concentrations. *J Clin Endocrinol Metab*

1988;67:1190–1194.

KREINER D, DROESCH K, NAVOT D, SCOTT R, ROSENWAKS Z. Spontaneous and pharmacologically induced remissions in patients with premature ovarian failure. *Obstet Gynecol* 1988;72:926–928.

MEYER WR, LAVY G, DeCHERNEY AH, VISINTIN I, ECONOMY K, LUBORSKY JL. Evidence of gonadal and gonadotropin antibodies in women with a suboptimal ovarian response to exogenous gonadotrophin. *Obstet Gynecol* 1990;75:1795–1799.

NELSON LM, KIMZEY LM, WHITE BJ, MERRIAM GR. Gonadotropin suppression for the treatment of karyotypically normal spontaneous premature ovarian failure: a controlled trial. *Fertil Steril* 1992;57:50–55.

RABINOWE SL, RAVNIKAR VA, DIB SA, GEORGE KL, DLUHY RG. Premature menopause: monoclonal antibody defined T lymphocyte abnormalities and antiovarian antibodies. *Fertil Steril* 1989;51:450–454.

REBAR RW, CONNOLLY HV. Clinical features of young women with hyper-gonadotropic amenorrhea. *Fertil Steril* 1990;53:804–810.

REBAR RW, ERICKSON GF, YEN SSC. Idiopathic premature ovarian failure: clinical and endocrine characteristics. *Fertil Steril* 1982;37:35–41.

SAUER MV, PAULSON RJ. Human oocyte and preembryo donation: an evolving method for the treatment of infertility. *Am J Obstet Gynecol* 1990;163:1421–1424.

SURREY ES, CEDARS MI. The effect of gonadotropin suppression on the induction of ovulation in premature ovarian failure patients. *Fertil Steril* 1989;52:36–41.

100

Infertility

DANIEL R. MISHELL, JR

Infertility can be defined in general as the inability of a couple to conceive after 1 year of sexual intercourse without contraception. Infertility can also be defined specifically as a reduced capacity to conceive compared with the mean capacity of the general population. Infertility is a very common problem. It is estimated that in 1991 one in 12 couples of reproductive age in the USA or 2.4 million women suffered from infertility. About 30% of infertile couples in the USA seek therapy and 15% of these undergo some form of artificial reproductive technology. In 1990 the estimated health-care expenses for infertility were 1.3 billion dollars.

To understand what is meant by infertility, it is important to understand the concept of fecundability. Fecundability is defined as the rate of conception occurring in a population in a given time period, usually 1 month. The monthly conception rate of normal fertile couples is about 20%. Because the couples who are less fertile are those who are not pregnant after the first month of trying to conceive, the monthly fecundability rate steadily decreases in subsequent months. After 3 months of trying to conceive, about 50% of normal couples have conceived. After 6 months about 75% have conceived, and after 12 months, about 90% have conceived. Those couples who have not conceived at the end of the first year of attempting can be divided into two groups: the first group of couples are unable to conceive without therapy and they should be considered sterile. Examples include males with aspermia and females who have complete tubal occlusion. The second group includes those with low fecundability who are hypofertile and most likely will be able to conceive without any therapy in a prolonged time period. These couples include those with oligospermia or mild endometriosis, as well as those with idiopathic or unexplained infertility. Between 1 and 2 years it is estimated that without therapy about 66% of the latter group will conceive, between 2 and 3 years, about 50% of the remainder will conceive, between 3 and 4 years, about 40%, and between 4 and 5 years about 33% of these hypofertile couples will conceive without therapy. Thus conception rates of hypofertile couples without therapy are inversely related to the *duration* of infertility of the couple.

According to three surveys in the USA, the percentage of married women who are infertile is about 8% in the age group 20–29. This percentage then steadily increases to 15% in the ages 30–34, to 22% from ages 35 to 39 and to 29% between ages 40 and 44. These epidemiologic data have been confirmed by studies with women of different ages whose husbands were aspermic and conceived with donor semen. These studies found that the pregnancy rates were constant among these women up to age 31 but then steadily declined so that by age 35 only about half as many women became pregnant with a given number of inseminations compared to those under age 31, and by age 40 only about one-third of women inseminated became pregnant in the same number of insemination cycles. Therefore after 31 years of age, with increasing age the percentage of women with low fecundability steadily increases because fertilized ova from women over the age of 31 are less likely to result in a viable pregnancy than fertilized ova from younger women. Thus two factors influence fecundability rates: the duration of time during which the couple has been attempting to conceive, and the age of the female member of the couple.

Cigarette smoking is an environmental factor that contributes to infertility. Compared to women who do not smoke, or have smoked in the past, women who smoke more than 20 cigarettes a day have about a 20% less chance of conceiving in a given time period than nonsmokers matched for age.

At the time of the initial consultation the clinician should take a complete history and perform a physical examination. In addition, the normal reproductive process, the results of normal fecundability in humans, the optimal time of coitus, and the diagnostic evaluation to be performed should be discussed with the infertile couple. While reviewing the diagnostic evaluation, the clinician should disscuss not only the type of tests but also the sequence, the timing in the menstrual cycle, and the time after the initial consultation when they are to be performed as well as the discomfort and costs of the various diagnostic procedures.

It has been found by performing a single episode of artificial insemination in one cycle of women with aspermic husbands that the optimal incidence of conception occurred when the insemination was performed on the day prior to the rise in basal body temperature. Basal body temperature rises because of an increase in progesterone which occurs after ovulation has taken place. It is therefore considered optimal to perform insemination or have normal sexual intercourse on the day *prior* to the rise in basal temperature. Sperm retain their viability and fertilizing capacity for a longer time period than the ovum is capable of being fertilized after ovulation occurs. Therefore it is best to have the sperm in the oviduct awaiting the release of the egg and its transport into the tubal ampulla. The optimal time when sperm should be deposited into the oviduct is the day prior to ovulation. The hormone which has a dramatic rise 1 day *prior* to ovulation and therefore is the best predictor of ovulation is luteinizing hormone (LH). Therefore measurement of LH by urinary LH detection tests is the best way to determine the optimal time to have intercourse or insemination. Tests which measure LH in a random daily urine specimen are usually more convenient for planning natural or artificial insemination than the tests that determine the amount of LH in the first morning urine specimen, as ovulation most commonly occurs on the day following the detection of LH in a random specimen, while it occurs on the day when LH is detected in the first morning specimen, which contains urine formed during the previous night.

At the initial consultation for infertility two key terms are important to use in counseling couples. These terms are *time* and *timing*. It usually takes several cycles for normal couples to conceive and only half will have conceived after three cycles of optimal attempts to conceive.

Documented causes of infertility include anovulation, abnormalities of the sperm and/or semen, pelvic factors causing tubal obstruction, and problems with the cervical mucus and sperm interaction. Treatment of these abnormalities has been shown to improve the rates of pregnancy. Other perceived causes of infertility such as mild endometriosis and luteal deficiency have not been proven to have a causal relation with infertility as their specific treatment has not been shown to yield higher pregnancy rates than occur without treatment.

It is estimated that in about 10% of infertile couples the woman does not ovulate. About one-quarter to one-third of infertile couples have some type of abnormality in the semen analysis and in 30–40% there is severe pelvic disease such as salpingitis or endometriosis that disrupts normal tubal function. An additional 10–15% of couples have some abnormality in the sperm–cervical mucus interaction. The remaining 10–15% have unexplained causes for their infertility or, to be more precise, are hypofertile. The primary infertility diagnostic evaluation should be done sequentially from the least invasive and least costly test to the more invasive procedures to help diagnose these four etiologies of infertility.

The first five steps of the primary infertility evaluation are as follows.

1 The first step is to document ovulation by having the patient take a basal body temperature, obtain a serum specimen for progesterone on day 21 of the cycle, and obtain a serum follicle-stimulating hormone (FSH) measurement on day 3 of the cycle. A sustained basal body temperature rise of >10 days and a mid luteal phase serum progesterone level of 10 ng/ml or higher are good indirect indices of ovulation as well as adequate corpus luteum function. It has been shown when progesterone is measured daily in cycles of women who have conceived that serum progesterone levels of 10 ng/ml or higher occur on 1 day or more in the luteal phase. A basal serum follicular phase FSH is very important as it has been shown that during the 5 years before the menopause, before the clinical signs of ovarian failure, serum FSH begins to rise. When the FSH level is >25 m IU/ml, nearly all the eggs released by the ovary are incapable of being fertilized normally and developing into a normal pregnancy. Even with *in vitro* fertilization procedures, if the woman's FSH is >25 m IU/ml, pregnancies do not occur. Since about 1% of women develop ovarian failure prior to the age of 40, the finding of a persistently elevated serum FSH in the follicular phase during several cycles indicates that this woman is unable to conceive unless donor oocytes are utilized.

2 The second step in the primary infertility evaluation is the semen analysis obtained after 2 days of abstinence and examined within 1–2 h of ejaculation. The recommended normal values for the semen analysis are a volume >2 ml, and a pH between 7.2 and 7.8. Sperm density should be >20 million/ml and the total sperm count should be >40 million with a sperm motility of 50% or more and a vital stain indicating >50% live sperm. More than 50% of the sperm should have normal morphology and there should be <10 million white cells per ml of semen.

3 The third step is a postcoital test performed just prior to ovulation, which should reveal five or more actively motile sperm in the cervical mucus withdrawn from the level of the internal os. The couple should abstain from intercourse for 2 days before the test and the test should be performed at the proper time of the menstrual cycle – the day before ovulation when the mucus is thin and watery.

4 The fourth step is a hysterosalpingogram. This is best performed with water-based dye. In addition to demonstrating tubal patency, the hysterosalpingogram can indicate that there are no abnormalities in the uterine cavities and therefore excludes the need for hysteroscopy. This test can also diagnose the presence of salpingitis isthmica nodosa, can evaluate the characteristics of the tubal mucosa and, if a hydrosalpinx is present, offer prognosis of fertility after tubal reconstruction surgery.

5 The fifth step in the infertility work-up is the diagnostic laparoscopy which should be scheduled in the follicular phase of the cycle. A concurrent dilatation and curettage, as well as hysteroscopy, should not be performed as adhesions can develop after a diagnostic curettage. It is not cost-effective to perform a hysteroscopy if the hysterogram shows the endometrial cavity to be normal as the hysterosopic examination of the cavity will also be normal.

The second five steps in the infertility evaluation are: (1) to obtain a blood sample for measurement of thyroid-stimulating hormone (TSH) and prolactin; (2) perform an endometrial biopsy in the luteal phase of one cycle; (3) to perform immunologic testing for antisperm antibodies in the female and the male; (4) to perform microbiologic cultures of the cervix and/or the endometrium; and (5) to perform a hamster egg sperm penetration test. To determine if any treatment for infertility is superior to no treatment, the results of therapy need to be analyzed by life-table analysis and compared with nontreated controls or, if these are unavailable, to historical controls. Furthermore, therapy should only be offered if proven to hasten the time to conception compared to no treatment. Treatment should increase the fecundability rate. Studies have shown that, without therapy, pregnancy rates range from 30 to 50% at the end of 1 year in untreated couples in whom the first five steps in the infertility investigation revealed no abnormalities. Furthermore, two studies show that without therapy, pregnancy rates of these couples at the end of 2 years approach 70%. There is no evidence that treatment of certain perceived etiologies of infertility yield better results than those which occur without therapy. Perceived etiologies of infertility without a proven causal relation include endometriosis without tubal adhesions, luteal insufficiency, the presence of antisperm antibodies, and hyperprolactinemia in women who ovulate. Therefore, since treatment of these etiologies is not proven to be superior to no treatment, diagnosis of these conditions and their treatment is unnecessary.

Causes of infertility diagnosed by abnormalities found with the first five steps in the infertility evaluation have shown that treatment is superior to no treatment. These causes include anovulation (its therapy is discussed in Chapters 102 and 103), therapy consists of ovulatory-inducing agents—including clomiphene citrate, human menopausal gonadotropin (hMG), FSH, pulsatile gonadotropin-releasing hormone (GnRH), dexamethasone—or partial ovarian destruction. Induction of ovulation in anovulatory women with one of these agents improves pregnancy rates compared with placebo. Treatment of oligozoospermia with washed intrauterine insemination of semen treatment by swim-up or Percoll gradient with or without superovulation also increases pregnancy rates compared to natural intercourse (Chapter 105). Treatment of an abnormal postcoital test with intrauterine insemination with or without superovulation also has been shown to give superior results than with no treatment (Chapter 104).

Treatment of tubal disease should be divided into treatment of distal and proximal tubal disease (Chapters 108, 109, and 110). Mild distal tubal disease is best treated with laparoscopic surgery, while severe distal tubal disease is best treated by *in vitro* fertilization and embryo transfer. Proximal tubal disease, if mild, can be treated with transcervical techniques and, if severe, with *in vitro* fertilization and embryo transfer. Mild to moderate endometriosis without tubal or ovarian adhesions has not been shown to be a cause of infertility. Optimal therapy is not to suppress ovulation with danazol, GnRH agonists, and high doses of progestins, but rather to induce multiple ovulation with clomiphene citrate or hMG together with intrauterine insemination. Moderate or severe endometriosis can be treated by pelviscopic surgery or by laparotomy or by *in vitro* fertilization and embryo transfer (Chapter 112). All other causes of infertility and unexplained infertility should be treated by superovulation and intrauterine insemination for at least three to six cycles. If pregnancy fails to occur, then treatment with *in vitro* fertilization or some other form of assisted reproductive techniques can be utilized. Studies have shown that patients with no abnormalities in the first five steps of a diagnostic infertility evaluation, called unexplained infertility, have superior pregnancy rates when treated with clomiphene citrate alone or clomiphene citrate plus intrauterine insemination compared to placebo or observation. In a study by Dodson *et al.*, patients with unexplained infertility were randomized to treatment with clomiphene citrate plus intrauterine insemination or observation. The fecundability rate with the treatment regimen was about 0.1, while with observation it was 0.03. A review of six studies in which unexplained infertility was treated with superovulation with hMG plus intrauterine insemination showed that the combined fecundability rate was 0.23. Chaffkin *et al.* reported that treatment with a combination of hMG and intrauterine insemination yielded higher fecundability rates than treatment with either hMG or intrauterine insemination alone. Crosiginani and Walters, in a multicenter study, showed that superovulation with either intrauterine insemination or intraperitoneal insemination produced fecundability rates between 0.2 and 0.3, which were comparable to those of gamete intrafallopian transfer or *in vitro* fertilization and higher than superovulation without intrauterine insemination.

In conclusion, regarding the diagnosis and treatment of infertility, first one should perform the basic five steps to determine treatable causes of infertility. Then one should sequentially treat any abnormal finding. If the basic five-step investigation is normal, the couple is hypofertile, not infertile. Therefore, to hasten the time to conception compared to withholding therapy, superovulation plus intrauterine insemination should be offered. After six treatment cycles, if pregnancy has not occurred some kind of assisted reproductive technology should be offered.

SUGGESTED READING

BARNEA ER, HOLFORD TR, MCINNES DRA. Long-term prognosis of infertile couples with normal basic investigations: a life-table analysis. *Obstet Gynecol* 1985;66:24.

BAYER SR, SEIBEL MM, SAFFAN DS, *et al.* Efficacy of danazol treatment for minimal endometriosis infertile women: a prospective randomized study. *J Reprod Med* 1988;33:179.

BYRD W, GUZICK DS, ACKERMAN GE, *et al.* Treatment of refractory infertility by transcervical intrauterine insemination of washed spermatozoa. *Fertil Steril* 1987;48:921.

CHAFFKIN LM, NULSEN JC, LUCIANO AA, METZGER DA. A comparative analysis of the cycle fecundity rates associated with combined human menopausal gonadotropin (HMG) and intrauterine insemination (IUI) versus either MHG or IUI alone. *Fertil Steril* 1991;55:252–257.

COLLINS JA, WRIXON W, JANES LB, *et al.* Treatment-independent pregnancy among infertile couples. *N Engl J Med* 1983;309:1201.

COLLINS JA, MILNER RA, ROWE TC. The effect of treatment on pregnancy among couples with unexplained infertility. *Int J Fertil* 1991;36:140–152.

CROSIGNANI PG, WALTERS DE, SOLIANI A. The ESHRE multicentre trial on the treatment of unexplained infertility: a preliminary report. *Human Reprod* 1991;6: 953–958.

CRUZ RI, KEMMANN E, BRANDEIUS VT, *et al.* A prospective study of intrauterine insemination of processed sperm from men with oligoasthenospermia in super-ovulated women. *Fertil Steril* 1986;46:673–677.

DEATON JL, NAKAJIMA ST, GIBSON M, *et al.* A randomized, controlled trial of hormonal responses and conception rates. *Gynecol Endocrinol* 1990;4:75–83.

DIMARZO SJ, KENNEDY JF, YOUNG PE, *et al.* Effect of controlled ovarian hyper-simulation on pregnancy rates after intrauterine insemination. *Am J Obstet Gynecol* 1992;166:1607–1613.

DODSON WC, WHITESIDES DB, HUGHES CKL, *et al.* Superovulation with intra-uterine insemination in the treatment of infertility: a possible alternative to gamete intrafallopian transfer and *in vitro* fertilization. *Fertil Steril* 1987;48:441.

EVANS JE, WELLS C, GREGORY L, WALKER S, *et al.* A comparison of intrauterine insemination, intraperitoneal insemination, and natural intercourse in super-ovulated women. *Fertil Steril* 1991;56:1183.

FEDELE L, PARAZAZINI F, RADICI E, *et al.* Buserelin acetate versus expectant management in the treatment of infertility associated with minimal or mild endometriosis: a randomized clinical trial. *Am J Obstet Gynecol* 1992;166:1345–1350.

FISCH P, COLLINS JA, CASPER RF, *et al.* Unexplained infertility: evaluation of treat-ment with clomiphene citrate and human chorionic gonadotropin. *Fertil Steril* 1987;51:441.

GLAZENER CMA, KELLY NJ, HULL MGR. Prolactin measurement in the investi-gation of infertility in women with a normal menstrual cycle. *Br J Obstet Gynaecol* 1987;94:535.

HARRISON RF, DELOUVOIS J, BLADES M, *et al.* Doxycycline treatment and human infertility. *Lancet* 1975;1:605.

HENDERSHOT GE, MOSHER WD, PRATT WF. Infertility and age: an unresolved issue, *Fam Plann Perspect* 1982;14:287.

HO PC, SO W-K, CHAN Y-F, YEUNG WS-PB. Intrauterine insemination after ovarian stimulation as a treatment for subfertility because of subnormal semen: a prospective randomized controlled trial. *Fertil Steril* 1992;58:995.

HOGERZEIL HV, SPIEKERMAN CM, DEVRIES JWA, DE SCHEPPER G. A randomized trial between GIFT and ovarian stimulation for the treatment of unexplained infertility and failed artificial insemination by donor. *Hum Reprod* 1992;4:1235–1239.

HORBAY GLA, COWELL CA, CASPER RF. Multiple follicular recruitment and intrauterine insemination outcomes compared by age and diagnosis. *Hum Reprod* 1991;6:947.

HULL MGR, SAVAGE PE, BROMHAM DR. Prognostic value of the postcoital test: prospective study based on time-specific conception rates. *Br J Obstet Gynaecol* 1982;89:299.

HULL MGR, GLAZENER CMA, KELLY NJ, *et al*. Population study of causes, treatment, and outcome of inferility. *Br Med J* 1985;291:1693.

HULL MGR, EDDOWES HA, FAHY U, *et al*. Expectations of assisted conception for infertility. *Br Med J* 1992;304:1465–1469.

KARAMARDIAN LM, GRIMES DA. Luteal phase deficiency: effect of treatment on pregnancy rates. *Am J Obstet Gynecol* 1992;167:1391–1398.

KIRBY CA, FLAHERTY SP, GODFREY BM, *et al.*. A prospective trial of intrauterine insemination of motile spermatozoa versus timed intercourse. *Fertil Steril* 1991;56:102.

LALICH RA, MARUT EK, PRINS GS, SCOMMEGNA A. Life table analysis of intrauterine insemination pregnancy rates. *Am J Obstet Gynecol* 1988;158:980–984.

LENTON EA, SOBOWALE OS, COOKE ID. Prolactin concentrations in ovulatory but infertile women: treatment with bromocriptine. *Br Med J* 1977;2:1179.

LERIDON H, SPIRA A. Problems in measuring the effectiveness of infertility therapy. *Fertil Steril* 1984;41:580.

LI TC, DOCKERY P, ROGERS AW, COOKE ID. How precise is histologic dating of endometrium using the standard dating criteria? *Fertil Steril* 1989;51:759–763.

MARTINEZ AR, VERMEIDEN JPW, BERNARDUS RE, *et al*. Intrauterine insemination does and clomiphene citrate does not improve fecundity in couples with infertility due to male or idiopathic factors: a prospective, randomized, controlled study. *Fertil Steril* 1990;53:847–853.

MENKEN J, TRUSSELL IJ, LARSEN U. Age and infertility. *Science* 1986;23:1389.

PEARLSTONE AC, PANG SC, FOURNET N, BUYALOS RP, GAMBONE J. Ovulation induction in women age 40 and older: the important of basal follicle-stimulating hormone level and chronological age. *Fertil Steril* 1992;58:674.

QUAGLIARELLO J, ARNY M. Intracervical versus intrauterine insemination: correlation of outcome with antecedent postcoital testing. *Fertil Steril* 1986;46:870–875.

ROUSSEAU S, LORD J, LEPAGE Y, VAN CAMPENHOUT J. The expectancy of pregnancy for "normal" infertile couples. *Fertil Steril* 1983;40:768.

SCHWARTZ D, MAYAUX MJ. Female fecundity as a function of age: results of artificial insemination in 2193 nulliparous women with azoospermic husbands. *N Engl J Med* 1982;306:404.

SERHAL PF, KATZ M, LITTLE V, WORONOWSKI H. Unexplained infertility – the value of Pergonal superovulation combined with intrauterine insemination. *Fertil Steril* 1988;49:602.

SHOUPE D, MISHELL DR JR, LACARRA M, *et al*. Correlation of endometrial maturation with four methods of estimating day of ovulation. *Obstet Gynecol* 1988;73:88.

SILVERBERG KM, BURNS WN, JOHNSON JV, SCHENKEN BS, OLIVE DL. A prospective, randomized trial comparing two different intrauterine insemination regimens in controlled ovarian hyperstimulation cycles. *Fertil Steril* 1991;57:357.

SMARR SC, HAMMOND MG. Effect of therapy on infertile couples with antisperm antibodies. *Am J Obstet Gynecol* 1988;158:969.

TEMPLETON AA, PENNEY GC. The incidence, characteristics, and prognosis of patients whose infertility is unexplained. *Fertil Steril* 1982;37:175.

VAN NOORD-ZAADSTRA BM, LOOMAN CWN, ALSBACH H, *et al*. Delaying childbearing: effect of age on fecundity and outcome of pregnancy. *Br Med J* 1991; 302:1361–1365.

WILCOX A, WESTHOFF C, VESSEY M, *et al*. Effects of age, cigarette smoking, and other factors on fertility: findings in a large prospective study. *Br Med J* 1985; 290:1697.

101

Ovulation:
prediction and detection

CHARLES M. MARCH

During ovulatory menstrual cycles, a complex series of endocrinologic, biophysical, and structural events occur that can be monitored by clinical, chemical, and physical means. Clinical analyses include basal body temperature (BBT) determinations and measurements of changes in the quality, quantity, and ionic concentration of cervical mucus and in the alterations in the proportions of superficial and parabasal cells in the vaginal epithelium. Chemical monitoring includes measurement of luteinizing hormone (LH), follicle-stimulating hormone (FSH), estradiol (E_2), and progesterone or their metabolites in serum and/or urine as well as the histologic changes in the endometrium. Steroids have been measured in saliva also. Physical monitoring involves ovarian ultrasound to assess the number of follicles and their growth. A second physical determination is that of the electrical resistance in saliva or vaginal secretions. Separately or in concert, these techniques have been used to detect ovulation, to monitor ovulation induction, and to predict ovulation in order to time coitus or inseminations. With some modifications, these techniques also could improve the effectiveness of natural family planning.

The resurgence of interest in home diagnostic tests is due to the development of monoclonal antibody technology. These tests are based upon antigen–antibody reactions. A variety of substances that are foreign to a host can act as antigens. Antigens may be bacteria, viruses, or certain molecules (e.g., proteins and polysaccharides) that can evoke the production of antibodies by the immune system of the host. The antibody created after exposure to a certain antigen has a structure that interdigitates with a portion of that antigen's surface like the pieces of a puzzle.

The antibody binds with the antigen forming the antigen–antibody complex. If that binding is very tight, the complex serves to inactivate the antigen and to protect the host.

For purposes of hormonal testing, an antibody which can bind specifically and tightly to one certain hormone (the antigen) can detect very small amounts of the hormone. Until recently, most antibodies have been produced by immunizing animals against a hormone and using their serum as the source of the antibody. These antibody preparations are not always useful as diagnostic agents because a mixture of antibodies usually is produced by many different B lymphocytes responsible for antibody production.

Although a mixture of antibodies often can be separated into individual, more specific components, cell lines capable of producing a single type of antibody have been developed. The cells derived from the multiplication of one hybridoma cell all produce the same antibody, called a monoclonal antibody, in an unending and invariable supply. Because one antigen can trigger the formation of many different antibodies, many different monoclonal antibodies can be produced against one individual antigen. Each monoclonal antibody then can be evaluated for its specificity and affinity for that antigen, and the best antibody can be selected and used to detect accurately the desired hormone in blood or urine.

Monoclonal antibody technology has been available for detecting both human chorionic gonadotropin (hCG) and LH. Both were used initially by physicians or laboratories, and subsequently, they have been available as over-the-counter products.

One of these tests, OvuKIT, is used to measure the preovulatory LH surge in urine. This test is a semiquantitative, two-site, enzyme-linked immunospecific assay. An α-subunit specific antibody is fixed to a plastic dipstick. The LH in the urine specimen binds to that antibody and subsequently to a β-subunit specific antibody that has been linked to alkaline phosphatase. The enzyme is now bound to the dipstick and can react with the substrate solution, which causes the stick to turn blue. The result is semiquantitative because the intensity of the color of the dipstick may be compared to a control which contains 35 mIU/ml of LH. This test takes approximately 1 h to complete. There is no cross-reaction with thyroid-stimulating hormone (TSH) or FSH, but hCG does cause a false-positive test. Multiple over-the-counter drugs, as well as many prescription items, do not interfere with the tests, nor do albumin, bilirubin, glucose, hemoglobin, and other compounds.

With OvuKIT an LH surge is defined as a color change that equals or exceeds the color intensity generated in the 35 mIU/ml LH standard (the "surge guide"). Testing of the midday (10:00 h to 20:00 h) specimen is most likely to detect the LH surge. Testing is begun on a specific day of the menstrual cycle according to the usual menstrual interval. In principle, this should be about 4 days before the expected date of the LH surge. The sticks provide a permanent record and can be compared with one another. For those women with variable cycles, an instruction booklet that accompanies the tests provides guidance for the user. If more questions arise, a toll-free number may be called for assistance.

OvuQuick is a modified version of OvuKIT and requires only 4 min to complete each test. A reference spot (analogous to the "surge guide") is on each test pad. Multiple other tests with various modifications are available from other manufacturers.

This method of predicting the LH levels in a semiquantitative fashion has been shown to correlate very well with quantitative measurements of LH. The rise in urinary LH levels indicative of the LH surge lags behind the rise in serum levels by approximately 12 h. The key to over-the-counter tests is their reliability in the hands of unskilled users. These concerns have been addressed satisfactorily by the manufacturers.

The semiquantitative method of determining the LH surge allows the patient and physician to predict when that probable ovulation will occur within a 12–24-h period. The occasional LH surge that is not followed by ovulation and instances of the luteinized unruptured follicle syndrome will not be detected. The purpose of these tests is to predict ovulation so that coitus can be timed or inseminations planned. Because the tests predict ovulation shortly before it occurs, they cannot be used as a method of contraception.

The thermogenic shift, especially if it is an abrupt one and preceded by a nadir, measures a response to the production of progesterone by the corpus luteum. A slight but significant increase in progesterone production usually precedes the LH peak, but this early rise is usually insufficient to cause a BBT shift. Although in most women BBTs can be interpreted correctly, the system has a number of inherent problems: the day of ovulation may vary from one cycle to another; the day of the shift may precede or follow the day of follicle rupture (as evidenced by real-time ultrasound) by more than 2 days; basal temperatures may be altered by very many factors; and, of greatest importance, the change can be judged only retrospectively. Because most BBT shifts occur after ovulation, this technique can be used only for purposes of confirmation. The same drawback applies to luteal-phase progesterone levels and endometrial biopsies.

Follicular maturation is associated with increased production of E_2 from the granulosa cells. The exponential rise in the serum E_2 concentration leads to an E_2 peak that induces the LH peak and precedes it by 12 h. Serum tests for E_2 and LH can be used to monitor oocyte maturation and to predict ovulation. However, these are expensive and inconvenient because multiple visits to a physician or laboratory are needed. Usually results are not available for 8–24 h.

The preovulatory E_2 rise causes the cervical os to open widely with a simultaneous increase in cervical mucus production and a change in the character of the mucus. Mid-cycle mucus is clear, acellular, and has a high water concentration and a high spinnbarkeit. Usually mucus of this good quality is present only during the preovulatory period, and its increased production lags behind the marked rise in serum E_2 levels by 2 days. The changes in cervical mucus, together with those in basal temperature, form the basis of the symptothermal method of natural family planning. However, in some instances there is mucus of good quality well before ovulation, and in other women, cervical mucus production remains inadequate despite a normal E_2 peak.

The CUE Fertility Monitor was developed as an objective method of assessing changes in cervical mucus quantity and ionic content as reflected in the vaginal electrical resistance (VER). A second sensor is available to assess the salivary electrical resistance (SER). Albrecht *et al.* correlated changes in VER and SER with BBT recordings and serum LH levels during 17 ovulatory menstrual cycles. These investigations demonstrated that the mean BBT nadir occurred 3 days before the LH peak. Thus, the lowest point could be used to time coitus or an insemination. The SER values showed a double peak, the first of which occurred 4–6 days before the LH peak. This interval is sufficiently long to suggest that this technique may be useful in natural family planning. Similar results occurred whenever the CUE Monitor was used during clomiphene-induced ovulations, but these results must be confirmed by other investigators.

The preovulatory E_2 rise also causes an increase in the number of superficial cells present in the vaginal epithelium and a proportionate decline in the number of parabasal cells. Because these changes lag behind those in serum by 3 or 4 days, the cornification index or karyopyknotic index is not sufficiently sensitive to predict impending ovulation. Moreover, alterations in vaginal flora can prevent the normal epithelial responses.

Multiple studies have demonstrated an excellent correlation between E_2 levels and ovarian follicular development in spontaneous and in clomiphene- and gonadotropin-stimulated cycles. Some studies show an improved pregnancy rate when ultrasound monitoring is added to serum E_2 monitoring of gonadotropin therapy.

The application of ultrasound to reproductive endocrinology and infertility is among the most exciting uses. Because of improved technology and resolution, real-time sector scanners have been used for all of these studies. A vaginal transducer provides better images and is more comfortable than transabdominal transducers, which employ a full-bladder

technique. Real-time ultrasound can be used to monitor follicular maturation and rupture and is the only technique available to determine in
which ovary the dominant follicle is developing and to verify that ovulation has occurred.

In the ideal 28-day cycle, ovarian imaging is begun on day 10 of the
cycle and continued daily. If the patient's average cycle length is shorter
or longer, the day of the first scan is adjusted appropriately. Each ovary
should be scanned in transverse and longitudinal planes. Whenever one
or more follicles emerges and reaches 12–14 mm in diameter, an oblique
measurement also should be obtained. Evaluation of follicular growth and
development may be limited to measurement of the largest diameter of
the largest follicle or extended to calculation of follicular volume. The
volume of a follicle is determined by the formula $4/3\pi r^3$ (r = radius) if the
three diameters do not differ by >1 mm, or $4/3\pi A^2B$, where A is the long
radius and B is the short radius. If three separate diameters can be
measured, the volume would be $4/3\pi r_1 \times r_2 \times r_3$. Although assessment
of only the largest diameter of the largest follicle usually will suffice,
follicular volume is a more accurate parameter of oocyte maturity and
may be mandatory in patients with an overdistended bladder or pelvic
adhesions which may cause follicular compression (i.e., artificial elonga-
tion of the long diameter). The accuracy of these daterminations has been
confirmed by laparoscopy and follicular aspiration.

One criterion for follicular maturation includes progressive enlargement of the dominant follicle(s) in all diameters. In spontaneous ovulatory cycles, if only the largest diameter is considered, the change is from
a mean of 10 mm 5 days prior to ovulation to a mean of 21 mm on the day
of ovulation. Estimates of largest mean follicular diameter have ranged
from 14 to 28 mm. As occurs with serum E_2 levels, the rate of change is
exponential during this time period.

Ovulation may be presumed to have occurred if the events described
in the preceding paragraph are followed by: (1) disappearance of the
follicle; (2) the replacement of the dominant follicle by an irregular cystic
structure that gradually decreases in size; (3) "filling in" of the follicle
with ultrasonic echoes with or without an increase in size; or (4) collapse
of the follicle followed by the emergence of a corpus luteum cyst, which
may exceed 40 mm in diameter. Each of these changes may be accompanied by the presence of a small amount of fluid in the cul-de-sac,
indicating follicular rupture.

An excellent correlation between oocyte maturation and follicular
growth, as assessed by ultrasound, with circulating E_2 levels has been
demonstrated in both spontaneous and stimulated cycles. During clomi-
phene-stimulated cycles, the development of multiple follicles has been
noted, and commonly more than one of these will be a dominant follicle.

The dominant follicle associated with clomiphene administration tends to be 3–5 mm larger than that associated with spontaneous ovarian activity.

In contrast, the dominant follicles that emerge following gonadotropin stimulation are usually smaller than those which reach maturity during natural cycles. The response to gonadotropins varies, depending upon the patient's pretreatment E_2 level. Although in all patients multiple follicles begin to develop, only those with oligomenorrhea and those amenorrheic patients who have progesterone-induced withdrawal bleeding commonly have multiple dominant follicles. There are three or more dominant follicles in approximately 10% of treatment cycles of these women and in two-thirds of the treatment cycles there are two or more dominant follicles. In contrast, among estrogen-deficient women, only one-third of the cycles is associated with the development of two or more dominant follicles.

Vermesh *et al.* studied 14 spontaneous and 17 clomiphene citrate-induced ovulatory menstrual cycles by means of OvuSTICK, First Response, real-time ovarian ultrasound, frequent serum E_2 LH determinations, and BBT recording. Ovulation, as judged by ultrasound, occurred on the day after the serum LH peak in all cycles. The urinary LH surge, as assessed by First Response, occurred on the day of ovulation in 54% of cycles and 1 day before ovulation in another 30% of cycles. OvuSTICK predicted ovulation on the day of the surge in 88% of cycles studied. The BBT nadir occurred on the day of ovulation only 10% of the time, and in another 20% of cycles the nadir preceded ovulation by 1 day.

It appears that the BBT, ultrasound, and at-home tests for the LH surge are the best techniques to predict and confirm occurrence of the day of ovulation. Selection of technique depends upon the type of information sought and must be balanced against cost and convenience.

SUGGESTED READING

ALBRECHT BH, FERNANDO RS, REGAS J, *et al.* A new method for predicting and confirming ovulation. *Fertil Steril* 1985;44:200.

CABAU A, BESSIS R. Monitoring of ovulation induction with human menopausal gonadotropin and human chorionic gonadotropin by ultrasound. *Fertil Steril* 1981;36:178.

DE ALLENDE ILC. Endocrinological implications of colpocytology. *Obstet Gynecol Surv* 1958;13:753.

DE CRESPIGNY LC, O'HERLIHY C, ROBINSON HP. Ultrasonic observation of the mechanism of human ovulation. *Am J Obstet Gynecol* 1981;139:636.

FERNANDO RS. Prediction of ovulation with the use of oral and vaginal electrical measurements during treatment with clomiphene citrate. *Fertil Steril* 1987;47:409.

HACKELOER BJ, NITSCHKE-DABELSTEIN S. Ovarian imaging by ultrasound: an attempt to define a reference plane. *J Clin Ultrasound* 1980;8:497.

HACKELOER BJ, FLEMING R, ROBINSON HP, *et al*. Correlation of ultrasonic and endocrinologic assessment of human follicular development. *Am J Obstet Gynecol* 1979;135:122.

HOULT IJ, DE CRESPIGNY LC, O'HERLIHY C, *et al*. Ultrasound control of clomiphene/human chorionic gonadotropin stimulated cycles for oocyte recovery in *in vitro* fertilization. *Fertil Steril* 1981;36:316.

JENSEN MR, KAPLAN BJ, MARRS RP, *et al*. Maturation value as an indicator of the serum estrogen concentration during treatment with gonadotropins. *Acta Cytol* 1981;25:251.

MARRS RP, VARGYAS JM, MARCH CM. Correlation of ultrasonic and endocrinologic measurements in human gonadotropin therapy. *Am J Obstet Gynecol* 1983;145:417.

O'HERLIHY C, DE CRESPIGNY LC, LOPATA A, *et al*. Preovulatory follicular size: a comparison of ultrasound and laparoscopic measurements. *Fertil Steril* 1980; 34:24.

O'HERLIHY C, DE CRESPIGNY LJC, ROBINSON HP. Monitoring ovarian follicular development with real-time ultrasound. *Br J Obstet Gynaecol* 1980;87:613.

O'HERLIHY C, EVANS JH, BROWN JB, *et al*. Use of ultrasound in monitoring ovulation induction with human pituitary gonadotropins. *Obstet Gynecol* 1982; 60:577.

QUEENAN JT, O'BRIEN GD, BAINS LM, *et al*. Ultrasound scanning of ovaries to detect ovulation in women. *Fertil Steril* 1980;34:99.

SHOUPE D, MISHELL DR Jr, LACARRA M. Correlation of endometrial maturation with four methods of estimating the day of ovulation. *Obstet Gynecol* 1989;73:88.

SMITH KH, PICKER RH, SINOSICH M, *et al*. Assessment of ovulation by ultrasound and estradiol levels during spontaneous and induced cycles. *Fertil Steril* 1980; 33:387.

VERMESH M, KLETZKY OA, DAVAJAN V, *et al*. Monitoring techniques to predict and detect ovulation. *Fertil Steril* 1987;47:259.

102

Induction of ovulation with clomiphene citrate

CHARLES M. MARCH

Induction of ovulation with clomiphene citrate (Clomid, Serophene) should be restricted to those patients with oligomenorrhea or with primary or secondary amenorrhea who do not have ovarian failure and who wish to conceive. The administration of clomiphene citrate to an anovulatory patient who does not desire pregnancy is not warranted. Such therapy is often given to learn information regarding the dynamics of the hypothalamic–pituitary–ovarian defect responsible for the anovulation, but the results do not give prognostic information regarding the patient's ability to respond to the drug at a later date when she wishes to conceive. In addition, the small risk of side-effects and complications during clomiphene therapy is inappropriate in someone not interested in conception.

Clomiphene should be employed as therapy in patients who have either anovulation or oligoovulation. The latter group should be treated with clomiphene because it will induce ovulation more often, that is, on a monthly basis. Of even greater importance is that ovulation will occur at a relatively predictable time; therefore, the chance of conception will increase because intercourse or insemination could be timed accurately. Clomiphene citrate is the pharmacologic agent of choice for ovulation induction in most anovulatory patients. Clomiphene is safer and more effective than the administration of glucocorticoids or gonadotropins for ovulation and is cheaper and easier to use than gonadotropins.

This agent is an antiestrogen and a weak estrogen. It acts by competing with endogenous estradiol for estrogen-binding sites in the hypothalamus and displaces estradiol from these binding sites. Therefore, it blocks the static negative feedback of estradiol upon the hypothalamus, permitting an increased release of gonadotropin-releasing hormone (GnRH) which stimulates the pituitary to increase follicle-stimulating hormone (FSH) and luteinizing hormone (LH) production and release. During successful clomiphene therapy, the frequency and amplitude of GnRH pulses are increased. In turn, the gonadotropins cause oocyte recruitment and maturation with an increasing production of estradiol. The estradiol initially produces a negative feedback upon the hypothalamus and pituitary to reduce gonadotropin secretion. Then, as the endogenous estradiol level increases exponentially, it provides a positive feedback to give the LH/FSH surge which reproduces that occurring in a spontaneous ovulatory cycle.

Prior to beginning treatment, the patient should be investigated to rule out the presence of ovarian failure, associated endocrinopathies such as a pituitary tumor or thyroid or adrenal disorders, and any contraindications to pregnancy. Coincident with the first course of therapy, a semen analysis should be obtained to rule out azoospermia or severe oligospermia. Clomiphene is administered beginning between day 3 and 5 following a spontaneous or induced menstrual period. Treatment is initiated with a daily dose of 50 mg for a 5-day period. If ovulation occurs, it will usually do so within 5–10 days, with a mean of 7 days, following the last clomiphene tablet. Ovulation should be documented in each cycle of treatment. This is best done by the use of a basal body temperature (BBT) record. If a classic thermogenic shift occurs, ovulation may be presumed. Ovulation may also be presumed if the serum progesterone level is >3 ng/ml 2 weeks after the last clomiphene tablet. If the level of progesterone is determined at the time of peak production, the level is usually higher than 15 ng/ml. An endometrial biopsy may also be used to document that ovulation has occurred and that the endometrial response is appropriate. For ease, convenience and expense, a BBT is the method of choice and should be employed if satisfactory results are obtained. In addition, the BBT provides information about the timing of ovulation so that the frequency of coitus may be increased during this period. If menstrual bleeding does not occur within 4 weeks after the last clomiphene tablet and the cycle was ovulatory, a pelvic examination should be performed as well as a pregnancy test.

In each treatment cycle the patient should be evaluated in the luteal phase or following a spontaneous menstrual period. If normal menses occurred, if the cycle was ovulatory, and if the pelvic examination does not reveal ovarian enlargement, the patient should be retreated with the same dose of clomiphene beginning on the same start day used previously. If the cycle was anovulatory, whether or not bleeding has occurred, the dose of clomiphene should be increased. If there is no bleeding, give 100 mg progesterone in oil or oral medroxyprogesterone acetate 10 mg/day for 5 days to induce withdrawal bleeding. After spontaneous or induced bleeding, treatment should begin with 100 mg/day for a 5-day period. If this course of therapy is ovulatory, the same dose should be continued, and monthly examinations should be performed preceding each successive course of therapy. These examinations serve to exclude the presence of pregnancy as well as to exclude the presence of ovarian enlargement which would delay further therapy until the functional cyst(s) had regressed. If ovulation does not occur at the 100-mg dosage, the dose should be increased, in 50 mg/day increments, up to five tablets – 250 mg/day – for 5 days. If this dose is not successful in inducing ovulation, a maximal dose of 250 mg of clomiphene daily for 5 days followed 5–10 days later by 5000 IU of human chorionic gonadotropin (hCG) intramuscularly in a single dose to simulate the LH surge should be given. The ideal day for hCG administration should be determined by following oocyte maturation. This is best determined by observing follicular development using real-time ultrasound of the ovaries. A marked increase in cervical mucus production (the use of the semiquantitative cervical score is very helpful) may be used to improve timing. Recent research has demonstrated that occasional patients will respond to even higher daily doses of clomiphene or to 250 mg given for 8 days. However, if ovulation does not occur in these patients, they should be considered for therapy with bromocriptine (if they have hyperprolactinemia), human menopausal gonadotropins (Pergonal), or human menopausal FSH (Metrodin). The regimen outlined includes treatment above the 100 mg/day dosage, which is the maximum recommended in the physician's product brochure. However, approximately 25% of patients who ovulate and conceive with clomiphene citrate will do so only when these higher doses have been employed. In addition, treatment should be extended beyond the recommended three ovulatory cycles. Studies at many medical centers have proven the safety and efficacy of exceeding the manufacturer's recommendation. Once an ovulatory dose is reached, treatment should be continued on a regular basis until: (1) conception occurs; (2) other infertility factors are discovered which would preclude pregnancy; (3) serious side-effects occur; or (4) the couple wishes to discontinue therapy. However, because only 5% of all couples who conceive do so after six cycles of therapy, the empiric use of other modalities should be considered at that time.

Of all patients who conceive during therapy, three-quarters will do so within the first three ovulatory cycles. For this reason, in those whose history and physical findings do not suggest that other infertility factors are present, extensive infertility studies should be delayed until after ovulation is induced three times. Following these three ovulatory cycles, a fractional postcoital test should be performed to verify the presence of normal sperm transport. An endometrial biopsy should be obtained to ascertain if the endometrial response is normal. If this study is normal, the next step would be the investigation of the uterine and tubal factors by means of hysterosalpingography. The final infertility study would be the investigation of the pelvic factor by laparoscopy.

At the initial interview with the couple, prior to induction of ovulation, the physician should explain that, by utilizing this regimen, over 90% of patients who have oligomenorrhea may be expected to ovulate. The overall incidence of pregnancy is approximately 50%. However, if those patients with other infertility factors have been eliminated, more than 85% of those who ovulate when treated with clomiphene will conceive.

Hammond *et al.* reported that, in women who ovulate with clomiphene and in whom other infertility factors are not demonstrated, conception rates are similar to those of a normal fertile population who discontinue using a diaphragm for contraception. By life-table analysis these investigators demonstrated that the fecundability rate of these patients was 22%, compared to 25% in those who discontinued a barrier method of contraception.

There is no increased risk of congenital anomalies during clomiphene treatment, nor is there an increased risk of spontaneous abortion. However, early studies showed that when clomiphene was administered inadvertently during the first 6 weeks of pregnancy, the incidence of birth defects was 5.1%. Although this frequency is not significantly higher than the 2.4% observed in patients to whom the drug was given prior to conception, this increase is of concern – the drug may be teratogenic if given during the time of embryogenesis. Therefore, it is important that clomiphene be administered only when a patient has had *normal* withdrawal bleeding and pregnancy has been ruled out.

During therapy the risk of forming a functional ovarian cyst is between 5 and 10%. If a cyst forms it will regress spontaneously in less than 1 month, provided that clomiphene is withheld during that time. Cysts may occur at any dose and during any course of therapy. The risk of a multiple gestation – almost always twins – is also between 5 and 10%.

More than 90% of oligomenorrheic patients will ovulate. If the woman has secondary amenorrhea and she has evidence of endogenous estrogen production, as shown by the presence of withdrawal bleeding following the administration of progesterone in oil, she is advised that her chance of ovulating is approximately 70%. The estrogen-deficient amenorrheic woman, that is, the one who does not have uterine bleeding following progesterone administration and who has a normal or low level of gonadotropins, rarely has an ovulatory response to clomiphene citrate. She should be treated with human menopausal gonadotropins.

Some hyperandrogenic anovulatory women who do not respond to this treatment regimen will be found to have elevated serum levels of the adrenal androgen dehydroepiandrosterone sulfate (DHEAS). If the DHEAS level exceeds 2.8 μg/ml, treatment with dexamethasone 0.5 mg at bedtime should be started. After 2 weeks, menses should be induced and, while continuing the dexamethasone, clomiphene is given on days 5–9 of the cycle using a daily dose of 250 mg. With this combined regimen, a few more anovulatory patients may be made to respond.

SUGGESTED READING

GYSLER M, MARCH CM, MISHELL DR, *et al*. A decade's experience with an individualized clomiphene treatment regimen including its effects on the post-coital test. *Fertil Steril* 1982;37:161–167.

HAMMOND MG, HALME JK, TALBERT LM. Factors affecting the pregnancy rate in clomiphene citrate induction of ovulation. *Obstet Gynecol* 1983;67:196–202.

KERIN JF, LIU JH, PHILLIPOU G, *et al*. Evidence for a hypothalamic site of action of clomiphene citrate in women. *J Clin Endocrinol Metab* 1985;61:265–268.

LOBO RA, GYSLER M, MARCH CM, *et al*. Clinical and laboratory predictors of clomiphene response. *Fertil Steril* 1982;37:168–174.

LOBO RA, PAUL W, MARCH CM, *et al*. Clomiphene and dexamethasone in women unresponsive to clomiphene alone. *Obstet Gynecol* 1982;60:497–501.

MARCH CM, ISRAEL R, MISHELL DR Jr. Pregnancy following twenty-nine cycles of clomiphene citrate therapy: a case report. *Am J Obstet Gynecol* 1976;124:209–210.

MARCH CM, DAVAJAN V, MISHELL DR Jr. Ovulation induction in amenorrheic women. *Obstet Gynecol* 1979;53:8–11.

103

Induction of ovulation with gonadotropins and gonadotropin-releasing hormone

CHARLES M. MARCH

The use of gonadotropins for ovulation induction had been limited by insufficient knowledge regarding the indications, treatment protocols, results, and side-effects of therapy as well as the limited availability of rapid estrogen assays and ultrasound studies on a daily basis. Although most of these problems have been overcome and the indications for treatment have been liberalized, high drug and treatment costs continue to limit widespread use of these agents. The main determinant of oocyte maturation is follicle-stimulating hormone (FSH) and the effects of various urinary and pituitary sources of gonadotropins, which have varying luteinizing hormone (LH) to FSH ratios, are similar.

Human menopausal gonadotropin (hMG, Pergonal) is a purified gonadotropin preparation extracted from the urine of postmenopausal women. Each ampule contains equal amounts of FSH and LH (either 75 or 150 IU). hMG has been used for ovulation induction, for the treatment of luteal-phase defects and for the timing of ovulation in conjunction with artificial insemination, as well as for causing superovulation in women undergoing intrauterine insemination. Gonadotropins are also prescribed in order to mature multiple oocytes in women undergoing *in vitro* fertilization or gamete intrafallopian transfer. The latter two indications will be discussed in Chapter 115.

Human menopausal FSH (hFSH, urofollotropin, Metrodin) is also a purified urinary product and is produced by removing the LH from the combined FSH/LH urinary extract. Each ampule contains 75 IU of FSH and negligible amounts of LH. Metrodin is used for ovulation induction in women with polycystic ovarian syndrome (PCO) and for ovarian hyperstimulation during assisted reproductive technology therapy. Some studies have shown that the spontaneous abortion rate is high in anovulatory women treated with hMG and that Metrodin therapy may be superior.

The hypothalamic decapeptide, gonadotropin-releasing hormone (GnRH, Lutrepulse, Factrel) is also successful in the treatment of anovulatory infertility. The effects of GnRH on the release of LH and FSH were first reported in 1969; the first pregnancy was reported 2 years later. The intravenous or subcutaneous administration of this decapeptide leads to a prompt release of both LH and FSH. The absolute amount of LH released exceeds that of FSH. A dose–response relationship has been demonstrated, and maximal stimulation occurs after treatment with 400–500 μg. Regardless of the route of administration, the medication is administered by means of a small portable pump which injects a fixed amount of medication at 60–90-min intervals. The pulsatile administration of GnRH should remain at a level amount in order to mimic the permissive effect of endogenous GnRH in maintaining normal positive- and negative-feedback relations between the pituitary and ovaries. Some authors have suggested that because the pituitary–ovarian axis remains intact, the frequency of multiple gestations and other signs of hyperstimulation should approximate that following spontaneous ovulation. Although preliminary results have not confirmed these speculations, the multiple-birth rate may be lower than that following clomiphene or gonadotropin therapy.

Intravenous administration is less costly because lower doses are employed. The response to intravenous GnRH is more predictable. However, the subcutaneous route is easier for most patients because a patent peripheral vein need not be maintained and it does not result in phlebitis or vascular thrombosis. These two routes of administration are compared in Table 103.1.

The dose is dependent primarily on the route of administration. Most patients will respond to doses of 75 μg/kg iv or 300 μg/kg sc. The pulse interval should be 60–120 min. Monitoring by serum estradiol (E_2) determinations and/or ultrasound scans of the ovaries is helpful in reducing the frequency of hyperstimulation. If GnRH is discontinued after ovulation, hCG (human chorionic gonadotropin 1000–2500 IU) should be given every 3–4 days to maintain the corpus luteum. An alternative to the use of a pump is intermittent intravenous administration via a heparin lock. Most reports of GnRH therapy have indicated that ovulation may be induced in 75% of cycles and up to one-fourth of patients will conceive within a few treatment cycles. GnRH may be utilized only in patients with a hypothalamic disorder. Those patients with pituitary failure must be treated with gonadotropins. Although the rates of ovulation and of pregnancy may be lower with GnRH than with hMG, comparative studies

Table 103.1 Comparison of intravenous and subcutaneous therapy with gonadotropin-releasing hormone

	Intravenous	Subcutaneous
Dose (ng/kg)	75	300
Interval (min)	60–90	90
Cost	Less	More
Absorption	Predictable/immediate	Variable/delayed
LH/FSH response	Normal	?Variable
Convenience	Less	More
Complications	Phlebitis, thrombosis	Hematoma, local reaction

LH, Luteinizing hormone; FSH, follicle-stimulating hormone.

have not been performed. Early studies have suggested that the rates of ovarian hyperstimulation and of multiple gestations are lower after treatment with GnRH than with hMG. At present, the need for pumps, the variable responses which occur after subcutaneous administration, and the protracted course of treatment have limited the general application of GnRH and gonadotropins are prescribed more commonly for patients with anovulatory infertility.

Candidates for ovulation induction with gonadotropins or GnRH must have ovarian follicles. This criterion will include those patients with oligomenorrhea or with amenorrhea who have uterine bleeding following the administration of progesterone in oil. These patients have normal circulating estrogen levels and, therefore, have functioning follicles. Women with either primary or secondary amenorrhea who do not have uterine bleeding after progesterone are estrogen-deficient. These patients should have a serum FSH level determined. If the FSH concentration is elevated, a diagnosis of ovarian failure should be made. With rare exceptions, these women are sterile and should not be considered for treatment with ovulatory drugs.

The estrogen-deficient amenorrheic woman who has normal or low serum levels of FSH should be completely investigated to rule out the presence of a hypothalamic or pituitary tumor. If the investigation is negative, the patient should be considered for ovulation induction with one of these agents. Candidates for therapy are anovulatory women who do not ovulate when treated with clomiphene citrate followed by hCG, administered according to the regimen outlined in Chapter 102. These patients should be considered clomiphene failures. This term should be utilized for patients who fail to ovulate when treated with clomiphene, and for those who ovulate repeatedly but fail to conceive. Although the use of gonadotropins or GnRH in the latter group of patients is empiric, only 5% of patients who conceive with clomiphene therapy do so after the sixth ovulatory cycle. Because clomiphene has a long half-life, it tends to accumulate in the endometrium after months of therapy and its antiestrogenic effect may hinder endometrial proliferation despite adequate estrogen production. A second category of candidates is those anovulatory women with hyperprolactinemia who fail to respond to bromocriptine. An additional number of patients who should be treated with gonadotropins or GnRH will be those who develop serious side-effects during clomiphene or bromocriptine therapy.

Pretreatment studies should include a semen analysis to verify that the male does not have severe oligospermia, azoospermia, or another gross abnormality. The uterine and tubal factors should be investigated by obtaining a hysterosalpingogram (or hysteroscopy) and by performing laparoscopy with hydrochromopertubation. These pretreatment procedures will serve to insure that multiple causes of infertility are not present. Although multifactorial infertility is not a contraindication to therapy with gonadotropins or GnRH, the chance of a full-term gestation is reduced in such patients and the couple should be afforded a realistic prognosis before undertaking therapy.

Extensive counseling of the couple prior to therapy is mandatory. They should have a stable relationship. Therapy with gonadotropins is inconvenient and stressful for both partners, each of whom must provide support for the other. They should be advised that the chance of conceiving in any one course of therapy is approximately 20%, a rate which is similar to the conception rate in spontaneous ovulatory cycles. Of all patients who conceive during therapy, the average number of treatment courses needed to achieve a pregnancy is three. Overall, 70% of all patients treated with hMG will conceive but among women with polycystic ovarian disease, the percentage is lower. These data, together with a thorough explanation of the risks and sequelae of multiple gestations and of hyperstimulation, will insure that the couple are well informed prior to therapy.

Women with PCO are usually very sensitive to hMG. The rationale for prescribing Metrodin is based upon the belief that the high endogenous LH levels are sufficient to induce ovarian steroidogenesis and that any additional LH may contribute to excess androgen production with subsequent follicular atresia leading to lower rates of pregnancy and/or an increased risk of abortion. Other experts believe that the extra LH may promote ovarian hyperstimulation. Comparative studies are needed to substantiate these claims. However, the drug has been shown to be effective for inducing ovulation in women with PCO.

Treatment with gonadotropins involves the attempt to mimic as closely as possible the follicular development which occurs in a spontaneous cycle. An index of this development is the rising level of E_2 in serum. Therefore, treatment should only be undertaken in locations where estrogen levels may be obtained rapidly on a daily basis. Individuality in response is the hallmark of gonadotropin therapy. The amount of medication required to induce adequate follicular development, as well as the duration of therapy, varies greatly not only from one patient to another, but also from one course of treatment to another in the same patient. However, as a general rule, progesterone-negative amenorrheic patients require significantly more medication than do those who are progesterone-positive, that is, those who do have withdrawal bleeding. For this reason, treatment must be tailored individually to each patient in each cycle of therapy.

Two different treatment regimens are used for the administration of hMG: hMG only and sequential clomiphene–hMG. In both instances hCG is added to cause ovum release. Patients who have oligomenorrhea and those who have amenorrhea with withdrawal uterine bleeding following progesterone in oil should receive pretreatment with clomiphene citrate (200 mg daily) for 5 days to induce partial follicular development. On day 6 of this regimen, hMG is administered. In this group of patients the duration of treatment and the dose of hMG required will be reduced by one-half compared to treatment with hMG only. The hypogonadotropic, estrogen-deficient amenorrheic woman will not benefit from clomiphene pretreatment but should receive two treatment courses of sequential estrogen–progestin prior to beginning hMG/hCG. Conjugated estrogen, 1.25 mg, is administered daily for 25 days and medroxyprogesterone acetate, 10 mg/day, is added on days 20 through 25. This regimen will prime the endometrium and endocervix so that they may respond to the endogenous E_2 which will be secreted during gonadotropin therapy. Following the end of the second withdrawal bleeding, hMG is begun.

On the first day of gonadotropin administration, patients in both groups are seen in the morning, a serum sample is obtained for E_2 measurement, and a real-time ultrasound examination of the ovaries using an endovaginal transducer is performed to assess the number and size of ovarian follicles. A pelvic examination is performed to calculate the cervical score (quantity of cervical mucus, extent of ferning, spinnbarkeit, and size of external os) as well as to palpate the ovaries to rule out the presence of enlargement or tenderness. hMG or hFSH is administered in the evening. Treatment is usually initiated with a daily dose of two ampules (150 IU) and this dose is continued daily. The serum E_2 level, examination, and ultrasound are repeated after 3 or 4 days of treatment. If the E_2 concentration remains unchanged, the dose of hMG is increased by a factor of 0.5 and continued again at this new level for another 3 or 4 days. This stepwise increase every 3 or 4 days by a factor of 0.5 is continued until the dose is found which will cause a doubling of the serum E_2 level above baseline concentration serum E_2 levels. At this point, this "ideal dose" is maintained. When the serum E_2 level doubles and provided ultrasound permits adequate visualization of both ovaries, E_2 determinations may be eliminated and further treatment guided solely by the changes in the number and size of follicles.

Whenever a follicle reaches 14 mm, scans should be performed daily. When a single (or at most three) dominant follicle reaches 17 mm in mean diameter, ovulation is induced with hCG. The correlation between total follicular volume and serum E_2 levels is excellent but the advantages of ultrasound monitoring are the immediate results, the assurance that there are not too many (more than three) mature follicles, and verification that at least one follicle has matured (i.e., has reached a preovulatory size). Because of the many uses of ultrasound, this monitoring technique has made gonadotropin treatment available more widely than previously. Clinical methods of estimating response to gonadotropins such as cervical score or vaginal cytology are not sufficiently sensitive to be the sole guides to dosage and duration of treatment.

As an adequate degree of follicular development is achieved, the rapidly rising estrogen levels will stimulate cervical mucus production. When there is an increase in the amount of cervical mucus, as well as an increase in spinnbarkeit and ferning, a fractional postcoital test is performed. In this way, the adequacy of sperm transport is verified. If sperm transport is abnormal, an intrauterine insemination with washed sperm is performed 24–36 h following the injection of hCG. When optimal levels of estrogen are reached, and provided the ovaries are not tender or enlarged, 5000 IU of hCG is given 24 h after the last injection of gonado-tropins. The couple are instructed to have intercourse daily including the last day of hMG therapy, as well as 12 and 36 h after the hCG injection. Seven days following the first injection of hCG, 3000 IU of hCG is given to maintain the corpus luteum. The supplemental hCG is withheld if the ovaries are enlarged or tender. On the day of the second injection of hCG, a serum sample may be obtained for measurement of progesterone concentration.

By utilizing this protocol, we have been able to achieve ovulation in 99% of our courses of therapy. This high rate surpasses other published reports and reflects careful patient selection as well as a strict adherence to the protocol. Only 8% of our pregnancies have been multiple gesta-tions and only one has been of a number greater than triplets. Minimal ovarian enlargement (5–10 cm), which resolved spontaneously, occurred in 8% of our treatment cycles. We also attribute these excellent results to a strict adherence to our protocol.

Other regimens, including combinations with GnRH or with dexamethasone, have been utilized, occasionally with success. However more data are needed before an ultimate role for such protocols will be known with certainty.

In the absence of a carefully planned protocol and strict adherence to it, and in the absence of careful monitoring techniques, treatment with gonadotropins or GnRH may lead to complications. However, with an appropriate protocol and monitoring techniques, almost all patients treated may expect to ovulate safety. Pregnancy rates of 70% with a very low rate of multiple gestations and other complications may be expected. Although the rate of spontaneous abortion is increased somewhat, no increase in the incidence of congenital anomalies has been reported.

SUGGESTED READING

BERG FD, HINRICHSEN MJ. Cumulative pregnancy rates in patients treated by pulsatile administration of GnRH. In: Genazzani AR, ed. *The Brain and Female Reproductive Function*. New Jersey: Parthenon, 1987.

EVRON S, NAVOT D, LAUFER N, et al. Induction of ovulation with combined human menopausal gonadotropins and dexamethasone in women with polycystic ovarian disease. *Fertil Steril* 1983;40:183.

HOMBERG R, ESHEL A, ARMAR NA, et al. One hundred pregnancies after treatment with pulsatile luteinizing hormone releasing hormone to induce ovulation. *Br Med J* 1989;298:809.

KNOBIL E. The neuroendocrine control of the menstrual cycle. *Recent Prog Horm Res* 1980;36:53.

MCFAUL PB, TRAUB AI, THOMPSON W. Treatment of clomiphene citrate-resistant polycystic ovarian syndrome with pure follicle-stimulating hormone or human menopausal gonadotropin. *Fertil Steril* 1990;53:792.

MARCH CM. Improved pregnancy rate with monitoring of gonadotropin therapy by three modalities. *Am J Obstet Gynecol* 1987;156:1473.

MARCH CM, TREDWAY DR, MISHELL DR, Jr. Effect of clomiphene citrate upon amount and duration of human menopausal gonadotropin therapy. *Am J Obstet Gynecol* 1976;125:699–704.

MARCH CM, DAVAJAN V, MISHELL DR, Jr. Ovulation induction in amenorrheic women. *Obstet Gynecol* 1979;53:8–11.

MARRS RP, MARCH CM, MISHELL DR, Jr. A comparison of clinical and laboratory methods in monitoring human menopausal gonadotropin therapy. *Fertil Steril* 1980;34:542–547.

MARRS RP, VARGYAS JM, MARCH CM. Correlation of ultrasonic and endocrinologic measurements in human menopausal gonadotropin therapy. *Am J Obstet Gynecol* 1983;145:417.

REGAN L, OWEN EJ, JACOBS HS. Hypersecretion of luteinizing hormone, infertility, and miscarriage. *Lancet* 1990;336:1141–1144.

104

Postcoital testing: the cervical factor as a cause of infertility

VAL DAVAJAN

The incidence of infertility secondary to abnormal mid-cycle cervical mucus–spermatozoa interaction is estimated to be about 10%. Microscopic examination of preovulatory postcoital cervical mucus specimens obtained from these patients reveals few or no sperm, or only immobilized sperm. These findings are believed to be incompatible with normal reproductive processes. In the evaluation of infertility, the postcoital test (PCT) is the only *in vivo* test that brings together both partners in a testing system. In 1982, a report using life-table analysis demonstrated a significant difference in cumulative conception rates between infertile couples with normal PCT and couples with abnormal PCT.

Technique

Before the cervical mucus is aspirated, the portio vaginalis is cleansed using a dry cotton swab. Then the cervical mucus is aspirated with a large syringe attached to a polyethylene suction catheter. The catheters may be sizes 5–14 French, depending on the diameter of the external os. The tubing is grasped 2.5 cm from the distal end with an atraumatic clamp. The aspiration must be initiated just as the tip of the catheter is inserted into the external os. A constant negative pressure is maintained with the syringe as the catheter is advanced to the internal os level (2.5 cm). The aspiration then should be terminated and the clamp closed completely. The catheter is withdrawn gently, and the trailing mucus is cut away with scissors to prevent the sample from being pulled out of the catheter. The catheter segment containing the mucus then is cut into three segments.

Table 104.1 Normal postcoital test

Days of abstinence	Usual pattern
Days of examination	−3, −2, −1 Before ↑ BBT and 1 day after ↑ BBT
Hours from coitus to examination	2–2.5
Sperm/high power field (×400; internal os level)	≥5
Spinnbarkeit	≥6 cm

BBT, Basal body temperature.

The segment from the tip of the catheter contains mucus from the internal os level, and the segment closest to the clamp represents mucus from the level of the external os. A smear of the posterior vaginal fornix should always be obtained to make sure that spermatozoa were deposited in the vaginal vault.

The PCT should be performed within 2–3 h of coitus, as it has been reported that the number of sperm present in the cervical canal is at a maximum 2–2.5 h after coitus. The examination should be scheduled 1–3 days prior to the expected rise in basal body temperature (BBT) and 1 day after the rise as determined by reviewing previous temperature graphs. A mini-BBT taken from the end of menses until the temperature rises and remains elevated for 3 days should be performed in every cycle in which a PCT is performed. If the PCT is abnormal, it should be repeated every 2 days until there is a temperature rise; this will insure that the PCT is performed during the time of maximal estrogen stimulation, which is 1–3 days before the rise in BBT. Before each PCT, the couple should observe their usual period of abstinence so that the test will provide an accurate evaluation of what has occurred in the past.

A normal test will have at least five motile sperm per high-power field at the internal os level. The spinnbarkeit measured in the same mucus sample should be no less than 6 cm (Table 104.1).

Abnormal PCT with anatomic defects

The etiology of various causes of abnormal PCT is outlined in Table 104.2.

Cervical stenosis

Conization of the cervix is still the most common etiology of cervical stenosis. The diagnosis is made when attempts to pass a size 5 French catheter or wire probe into the endocervical canal encounter resistance.

Table 104.2 Categorization of causes of abnormal postcoital test (PCT)

Anatomic defects
Cervical stenosis

Abnormal cervical mucus
Poor quality
Low quantity

Abnormal PCT with normal cervical mucus
Faulty coital technique
Vaginal factor or weak sperm factor
Oligospermia and/or low motility
Low semen volume
Immobilized sperm in endocervical canal
Large semen volume
Highly viscous semen

Neither estrogen therapy nor attempts to recanalize the endocervix with dilators, cryosurgery, or laser have been successful. Small laminaria have been employed in our clinic and an occasional pregnancy has been achieved. Intrauterine insemination, using washed sperm obtained from the patient's husband, is being used extensively at present to deal with this problem.

Abnormal PCT secondary to abnormal cervical mucus

Poor quality of mucus

There are patients who secrete abnormally thick, cellular cervical mucus at mid-cycle. These patients should be treated with intrauterine washed-sperm insemination. However, if the technique is not available, a daily dose of 0.1 mg diethylstilbestrol (DES) can be given on days 5–15 of a 28-day menstrual cycle. This may improve the quality of mucus. In some of these patients, this improvement results in a normal PCT. If there is no improvement, the DES dose would be increased to 0.2 mg/day. With improvement, the appropriate dose should be given for no less than 1 year. In all patients undergoing treatment for any type of cervical problem, the treatment should result in an improved PCT. Therefore, all treatment efforts should be evaluated by performing a repeat PCT during a treatment cycle. If improvement still is not noted, the abnormal mucus should be removed by aspiration. If clear mucus is found trailing behind the thick mucus, the thick mucus should be cut away from the clear mucus and the clear mucus allowed to remain in the canal. Following this "unplugging," the patient either may have artificial insemination or be instructed to return home to have intercourse. The treatment of choice is intrauterine insemination.

Low quantity of mucus

Some women secrete only minimal amounts of mucus at mid-cycle. If the wash insemination technique is unavailable, in some of these patients DES therapy (0.1 mg/day on days 5–15 of a 28-day cycle) increases mucus secretion. If there is an increase in mucus production with DES, the PCT should be repeated at mid-cycle; if the test is normal, the therapy should be continued for at least 1 year. In unresponsive patients, the dose of DES should be increased to 0.2 mg/day. If no mucus is produced at this level, conjugated estrogens 1.25–5 mg/day should be prescribed. If this fails, the patient should be referred to a clinic where mid-cycle intrauterine inseminations can be performed.

Abnormal PCT with normal cervical mucus

Faulty coital technique

In some infertile patients, no spermatozoa can be seen in the cervical mucus following intercourse. If a smear taken from the posterior vaginal fornix contains no sperm when the husband is known to have sperm, this indicates that a faulty coital technique is highly likely. If the patient is extremely obese, the fault may be the husband's failure to penetrate into the vagina during attempted coitus. In such patients, careful review of coital technique is all that is necessary to correct the abnormality. Artificial intrauterine insemination using the husband's semen can be performed if the couple cannot correct a faulty technique.

Vaginal factor, or weak sperm factor

If the semen analysis is normal and no sperm are seen in the cervical mucus but are found in the vagina, it is important to rule out a hostile vaginal factor or weak sperm factor. If washed-sperm insemination is unavailable, cervical cup insemination followed by a PCT in 1 h should be performed. A specially designed cup (Milez Products, Chicago) is placed on the cervix, and semen then is introduced through the stem and exposed to the cervix for 1 h. The cup is removed, the portio vaginalis is cleansed, and an *in vivo* PCT is performed. If motile sperm are seen at the internal os level, the procedure can be instituted as therapy in the ensuing cycles. The exact etiology of the vaginal factor or weak sperm factor has not yet been established.

Oligospermia

Oligospermia is defined as a sperm concentration of <20 million/ml. If an abnormal PCT is a result of oligospermia, intrauterine wash insemination should be performed. If this is unavailable, cervical cup therapy as outlined should be attempted. If an improvement is noted on the postcup PCT, cup insemination should be used as therapy for at least four cycles. The best days for performing insemination now are being determined by the use of the BBT, urinary luteinizing hormone kits, and serial ultrasonography.

Low semen volume

In a certain number of couples with an abnormal PCT, lack of sperm penetration into the cervical canal may be due to an abnormally low volume of semen (<2 ml). If semen specimens are found to be consistently <2 ml and the low volume is not due to faulty collection, intrauterine wash or cervical cup insemination should be tried as therapy.

Immobilized sperm in the endocervical canal

Not infrequently, an abnormal PCT is due to immobilization of sperm. In such cases, immunologic test (immunobead) can be done, although in most of these patients there is no correlation between these positive immunologic tests and immobilization of sperm in the cervical canal. Immobilization of sperm in the cervical mucus may be due to some as yet undetermined factors or to locally secreted antibodies. Presence of *Ureaplasma urealyticum* or *Chlamydia* organisms in either the semen or the cervical mucus may play a role in this finding. If bacterial cultures are negative, intrauterine insemination should be attempted. If bacteria are present, appropriate antimicrobial therapy should be given.

Large volume of semen

If a PCT is abnormal and the only finding is a large volume of semen (>8 ml), either washed-sperm intrauterine insemination or a split-ejaculate specimen should be collected and cup insemination performed using the first 2 ml of ejaculate.

Highly viscous semen (incomplete liquefaction)

In some patients with an abnormal PCT, the only finding is failure of the semen to liquefy completely. The etiology is not completely known, but it may be due to an enzyme deficiency or abnormality. With the sperm-washing techniques now being used, almost all semen specimens can be liquefied adequately for intrauterine insemination. If total liquefaction is not achieved by the usual washing techniques, then the swim-up technique should be tried.

In vitro methods

In vitro methods of evaluating sperm–cervical mucus interaction are not as useful as the *in vivo* test. The most popular methods are the Miller–Kurzrok slide test, the capillary tube method of Kremer, and the bovine cervical mucus–human sperm penetration tests.

Preparing spermatozoa for intrauterine insemination

Washed-sperm technique

A semen specimen is collected by masturbation into a sterile jar. The specimen is transferred to a tapered centrifuge tube and washed with tissue culture medium. We prefer to use buffered "human tubal fluid" medium (HTF). The semen sample is mixed with HTF at 1:2 volume on a vortex mixer at a reading of 4. The mixture is centrifuged for 5 min at 300 g. The supernatant is discarded and sperm concentrate mixed with 3 ml of HTF solution and centrifuged for 3 min at 300 g. The supernatant is discarded again, and 0.25–0.3 ml of HTF is added to the sperm concentrate. The mixture is drawn up in a sterile 1-ml syringe, and a 5.4 Sheppard insemination catheter is used to perform the intrauterine insemination at the top of the fundus. The cervix is wiped clean with a dry swab and no sterilizing solution is used.

Percoll technique

This technique is used to separate the sperm with greatest motility and highest quality from the remainder of sperm, white blood cells, and debris. Separation is done using a one-step discontinuous gradient technique.

Swim-up technique

This technique is used for separating motile sperm from immobilized sperm, white and red blood cells, and seminal plasma debris. An aliquot of 0.5 ml of sperm is layered beneath 2 ml of HTF solution in a 12 × 75 mm culture tube. After 1 h, using a pipette, the upper 1-ml layer is aspirated carefully and discarded. After another hour, the upper 1 ml is aspirated and washed twice in HTF solution. The separated spermatozoa then are used to perform intrauterine insemination.

SUGGESTED READING

BERGER T, MARRS RP, MOYER DL. Comparison of techniques for selection of motile spermatozoa. *Fertil Steril* 1985;43:268.

DAVAJAN V. Postcoital testing: the cervical factor and a cause of infertility. In: Mishell DR Jr, Davajan V, Lobo RA, eds. *Infertility, Contraception, and Reproductive Endocrinology*, 3rd edn. Cambridge, MA: Blackwell Scientific Publications, 1991:599–611.

DAVAJAN V, KUNITAKE GM. Fractional *in vivo* and *in vitro* examination of postcoital cervical mucus in the human. *Fertil Steril* 1969;20:197.

DAVAJAN V, KHARMA K, NAKAMURA RM. Spermatozoa transport in cervical mucus. *Obstet Gynecol Surv* 1970;25:1.

DAVAJAN V, NAKAMURA RM, MISHELL DR Jr. A simplified technique for evaluation of the biophysical properties of cervical mucus. *Am J Obstet Gynecol* 1971; 109:1042.

HULL MGR, GLAZENER CMA, KELLY NJ, et al. Population study of causes, treatment and outcome of infertility. *Br Med J* 1985;291:1693.

KREMER J. A simple sperm penetration test. *Int J Fertil* 1965;10:201.

KUNITAKE GM, DAVAJAN V. A new method of evaluating infertility due to cervical mucus–spermatozoa incompatibility. *Fertil Steril* 1970;21:706.

MILLER EG Jr, KURZROK R. Biochemical studies of human semen. *Am J Obstet Gynecol* 1932;24:19.

SCOTT JZ, NAKAMURA RM, MUTCH J, et al. The cervical factor in infertility: diagnosis and treatment. *Fertil Steril* 1977;28:1289.

TREDWAY DR, SETTLAGE DS, NAKAMURA RM, et al. The significance of timing for the postcoital evaluation of cervical mucus. *Am J Obstet Gynecol* 1975;121:387.

105

Male factor in infertility

GERALD S. BERNSTEIN

The clinician who evaluates or treats the female member of an infertile couple must also have some knowledge of male reproductive physiology and the interaction between male and female factors required to achieve pregnancy. About one-third of cases of infertility are due to an abnormality of the male; in other instances combined male and female factors may be present.

To achieve pregnancy, the male must produce an adequate number of spermatozoa with normal function and deliver the sperm into the vagina. The sperm then must be able to enter the cervix and ascend into the upper female genital tract and fertilize an ovum. This requires a competent endocrine system and an intact male reproductive tract as well as the normal psychoneurovascular mechanisms required to produce erection and ejaculation. Evaluation of male fertility requires consideration of these factors.

The general work-up of the infertile couple includes two tests of male function: the semen analysis and the postcoital test (PCT). These provide information about semen quality and the interaction between spermatozoa and cervical mucus, respectively.

Evaluation of semen

Semen analyses should be done in a laboratory staffed by personnel experienced in this procedure. The ejaculate should be collected by masturbation into a wide-mouth container after 2–5 days of sexual abstinence. Special nonlatex condoms are available which, unlike contraceptive condoms, have no toxic effect on sperm motility. Sexual stimulation provided by coitus or other female assistance may produce a better semen sample than solo masturbation.

The semen should be observed within 2 h of collection, preferably within 1 h, because after 2 h sperm motility may decline. If the semen is collected at home, the specimen should be protected against cold temperatures during transport to the laboratory. The sample can be kept at body temperature by having the patient place the container in the waistband of his trousers.

If the male has frequent emissions, semen also should be obtained at this normal ejaculatory frequency without a prescribed period of abstinence. The patient may have normal semen after several days of rest, but a decreased sperm count under normal conditions of sexual activity. Several semen samples should be evaluated, as semen quality can vary over a period of time. If the analysis is abnormal, at least three specimens collected at monthly intervals should be evaluated.

Table 105.1 shows the "normal" values for semen quality. These values, however, do not define the limits of fertility. Pregnancies may occur regularly with sperm counts of <5 million/ml and with even lower values.

An important aspect of semen quality in relation to fertility is the number of morphologically normal sperm with good motility and the ability to fertilize ova. Nonmotile sperm and sperm with poor motility ordinarily do not penetrate and migrate through cervical mucus. Some morphologically abnormal sperm are excluded from the cervix because their heads are too large to fit into the channels formed by the linear macromolecules within the cervical mucus. Sperm with very small or round rather than oval heads are able to enter the cervical mucus but have no fertilizing ability because their heads have no acrosome, a structure that enables sperm to penetrate and fertilize ova.

Table 105.1 Recommended standards for semen analysis (modified from Aitken *et al.*)

Parameter	Recommended normal value
Volume	2.0 ml or more
pH	7.2–7.8
Sperm density	$\geq 20 \times 10^6$/ml
Total sperm count	$\geq 40 \times 10^6$/ml
Sperm motility	$\geq 50\%$ with progressive motility
Vital staining	$\geq 50\%$ live (exclude dye)
Sperm morphology	$\geq 50\%$ normal
White cell count	$<10^6$/ml

Functional properties of spermatozoa

The functional properties of spermatozoa are motility, the ability to penetrate cervical mucus and to ascend into the upper female genital tract, and the capacity to fertilize ova.

Motility is assessed in the semen analysis. Conventionally, an observer estimates the percent motile sperm and quality of motility. Equipment is now available for automated quantitative analysis of sperm motility by computer-assisted motion analysis, which occasionally may reveal subtle defects in movement that impair the penetration of cervical mucus and fertilizing capacity. The PCT evaluates the interaction between spermatozoa and cervical mucus. More detailed studies of sperm–mucus interaction can be done as necessary by *in vitro* test systems.

In vitro fertilization with human ova is the best laboratory measurement of fertilizing capacity, but this is impractical as a routine laboratory test. The zona-free hamster-egg penetration test can be used as an alternate evaluation.

Causes of semen abnormalities

A number of factors can cause semen to be abnormal, including the following:

1 anatomic factors, including varicocele and cryptorchidism;

2 endocrine factors;

3 genetic factors, such as Klinefelter's syndrome and other manifestations of the 47,XXY karyotype, 46,XX males, and various autosomal translocations;

4 inflammatory disease, such as prostatitis (sometimes asymptomatic) and epididymitis;

5 autoimmune phenomena, leading to the formation of autoantibodies against spermatozoa;

6 ejaculatory dysfunction, including retrograde ejaculation, which may occur in some diabetics or following bladder neck surgery, and ejaculatory failure, occurring after sympathectomy, use of ganglionic-blocking drugs, or spinal cord injury;

7 psychologic factors, such as impotence and premature ejaculation;

8 faulty coital technique;

9 exogenous factors, including drugs, radiation, chemicals, and alcohol;

10 neoplasma, such as pituitary tumors and testicular neoplasms;

11 factors of unknown etiology, including absence of germinal epithelium in the testes (Sertoli-cell-only syndrome), abnormalities of spermatogenesis (maturation arrest and hypospermatogenesis), and disorganization of the germinal epithelium.

The following relationships between specific causes and abnormalities have been noted.

1 A low sperm count may be caused by an endocrine disorder, varicocele, prostatitis, other genital infections, or exogenous agents. Sometimes the diagnostic evaluation is normal except for idiopathic histologic changes in the germinal epithelium.

2 Absence of sperm in the ejaculate may result from sex chromosome disorders, Sertoli-cell-only cell syndrome, testicular failure, endocrinopathy, or inflammatory or congenital obstruction of the male genital tract.

3 Orgasm without production of ejaculate may be due to retrograde ejaculation or ejaculatory failure.

4 Low semen volume may be due to partial retrograde ejaculation, obstruction of the ejaculatory ducts, or malfunction of the prostate or seminal vesicles.

5 Poor sperm motility may be caused by autoantibodies, infection, varicocele, or structural abnormalities of the spermatozoa (immotile cilia syndrome, Young's syndrome). The presence of white blood cells or erythrocytes in the semen suggests infection.

6 Autoagglutination of the sperm may result from either infection or autoantibodies.

7 Abnormal sperm morphology may be caused by a number of factors, including varicocele, stress, infection, and exogenous factors.

Evaluating the male with abnormal semen

Men with abnormal semen should be evaluated to determine the cause of the abnormality and to ascertain if the problem can be treated. In addition, since abnormal semen may reflect a serious underlying medical disease, the work-up should include steps to rule out such possibilities. Some examples of these conditions are pituitary tumors and malignant testicular neoplasms.

The work-up should be done by a physician competent in andrology. This may be a urologist, internist, or a gynecologist with a special interest in male reproductive disorders. The evaluation may include endocrine, microbiologic, immunologic, genetic, and other studies, depending on the results of the semen analysis, history, and physical examination. The andrology consultant and gynecologist should work in close cooperation.

Treatment

There are specific treatments for some types of male infertility, including varicocele, infection, some endocrine deficiencies, retrograde ejaculation, reversible effects of drugs or toxins, and ductal obstructions amenable to surgery. Some disorders (maturation arrest, hypospermatogenesis) are potentially correctable but owing to the limited knowledge about the control of spermatogenesis only empiric measures can be used at present. Clomiphene citrate and other hormonal interventions are unsatisfactory when there is not a specific indication for endocrine therapy.

Since the medical treatment of the infertile male is often obscure or unsatisfactory, there is an increasing tendency to use assisted reproductive technology in an effort to maximize the potential of the male partner's semen. The technology ranges from intrauterine insemination with processed sperm to more sophisticated procedures such as gamete and zygote intrafallopian transfer, and *in vitro* fertilization with embryo transfer. In general, assisted reproductive technology for male-factor problems has not been as successful as when these procedures are done for female factors.

A recent advance in the use of assisted reproductive technology has been in the management of a congenital anomaly in which the vas deferens is absent and there is no egress for spermatozoa from the epididymides. This condition was formerly treated by creating an artificial spermatocele using a plastic device and recovering sperm by aspirating this device transcutaneously. This technique was usually unsuccessful, but some pregnancies have been achieved by using sperm recovered surgically from the epididymides to achieve fertilization *in vitro*, followed by embryo transfer into the endometrial cavity.

The gynecologist should continue evaluating the female partner, while the male is being evaluated even when the semen is subnormal. Because pregnancy can occur with very low sperm counts, correction of a female factor, such as a subtle disturbance of ovulation or luteal-phase defect, may improve the couple's fertility despite the poor semen quality.

Artificial insemination with donor semen or adoption are options when the male has uncorrectable azoospermia or severe oligozoospermia, and these alternatives should be discussed with the couple. The threat of acquired immune deficiency syndrome and other sexually transmitted diseases has caused most clinicians to use frozen semen for donor insemination. Donors are tested for antibodies against the human immunodeficiency virus when semen is banked, and the specimens are quarantined for 6 months until the donor retests negative.

Whether the husband's or a donor's semen is used, artificial insemination should be done near the time of ovulation, as determined by monitoring urinary luteinizing hormone in conjunction with visualization of follicular growth by ultrasound to maximize the chance of successful fertilization.

Future developments

Current research in andrology should improve our ability to diagnose and treat disorders that are presently not treatable or that may not be detected with current technology. Some areas of interest are the regulation of spermatogenesis, the regulation of motility and fertilizing capacity, and identification of substances in the environment and workplace that may adversely affect semen quality and male fertility. Although progress has been slow in terms of diagnosis and therapy, such research will lead ultimately to better management of the infertile male.

SUGGESTED READING

AITKEN RJ, COMHAIRE FH, ELIASSON R, et al. *WHO Laboratory Manual for the Examination of Human Semen and Semen–Cervical Mucus Interaction.* Cambridge: Cambridge University Press, 1987.

BELSEY MA, ELIASSON R, GALLEGOS AJ, et al. (eds). *Laboratory Manual for the Examination of Human Semen and Semen–Cervical Mucus Interaction.* Singapore: Press Concern, 1980.

BERNSTEIN GS. Male factor in infertility. In: Mishell DR Jr, Davajan V, eds. *Infertility, Contraception and Reproductive Endocrinology.* Oradell, NJ: Medical Economics Books, 1986:423.

BERTHELSEN JF, SKAKKERBACK NE. Distribution of carcinoma-*in-situ* in testes from infertile men. In: Skakkeback NE, Berthelsen JG, Grigor KM, et al., eds. *Early Detection of Testicular Cancer.* Copenhagen: Scriptor, 1981:172.

BLASCO L. Clinical tests of sperm fertilizing ability. In: Wallach EE, Kempers RD, eds. *Modern Trends in Infertility and Conception Control,* vol 3. Chicago, IL: Year Book Medical Publishers, 1985:435.

ELIASSON R. Parameters of male fertility. In: Hafez ESE, Evans TN, eds. *Human Reproduction.* New York: Harper & Row, 1973:39.

JEQUIER A, CRICK J. *Semen Analysis: A Practical Guide.* Oxford: Blackwell Scientific Publications, 1986.

KERIN JFP, KIRBY C, PEEK J, et al. Improved conception rate after intrauterine insemination of washed spermatozoa from men with poor quality semen. *Lancet* 1984;1:533.

KNUTH VA, NIESCHLAG E. Comparison of computerized semen analysis with the conventional procedure in 322 patients. *Fertil Steril* 1988;49:881.

LIPSCHULTZ LI, HOWARDS SS (eds). *Infertility in the Male.* New York: Churchill Livingstone, 1983.

MACLEOD J, WANG Y. Male fertility potential in terms of semen quality: a review of the past. A study of the present. In: Wallach EE, Kempers RD, eds. *Modern Trends in Infertility and Conception Control,* vol 2. Baltimore, MD: Williams & Wilkins, 1982:361.

MASCOLA L, GUINAN ME. Screening to reduce transmission of sexually transmitted diseases in semen used for artificial insemination. *N Engl J Med* 1986;314:1354.

NACHTIGALL RD, FAURE N, GLASS RH. Artificial insemination of husband's sperm. In: Wallach EE, Kempers RD, eds. *Modern Trends in Infertility and Con-*

ception Control, vol 2. Baltimore, MD: Williams & Wilkins, 1982:404.

PETERSON EP, MOGHISSI KS, PAULSEN A, *et al.* New guidelines for the use of semen for donor insemination. *Fertil Steril* 1986 (Suppl. 2);46:95S.

SANTEN RJ, SWERDLOFF RS (eds). *Male Reproductive Dysfunction. Diagnosis and Management of Hypogonadism, Infertility, and Impotence.* New York: Marcel Dekker, 1986.

SILBER SJ, BALMACEDA J, BORRERO C, *et al.* Pregnancy with sperm aspiration from the proximal head of the epididymis: a new treatment for congenital absence of the vas deferens. *Fertil Steril* 1988;50:525.

SOKOL RZ, PETERSEN G, STEINER BS, *et al.* A controlled comparison of the efficacy of clomiphene citrate in male infertility. *Fertil Steril* 1988;49:865.

STEINBERGER E, RODRIGUEZ-RIGAU LJ, SMITH KD. The interaction between the fertility potential of the two members of an infertile couple. In: Frajese G, Hafez ESE, Conti C, *et al.*, eds. *Oligozoospermia: Recent Progress in Andrology.* New York: Raven Press, 1981.

STEWART DJ, TYLER JPP, CUNNINGHAM AL, *et al.* Transmission of human T-cell lymphotropic virus type III (HTLV III) by artificial insemination by donor. *Lancet* 1985;2:581.

YANAGIMACHI R, YANAGIMACHI H, ROGERS BT. The use of zona-free animal ova as a test system for the assessment of the fertilizing capacity of human spermatozoa. *Biol Reprod* 1976;15:471.

106

Intrauterine adhesions

CHARLES M. MARCH

Although intrauterine adhesions (IUAs) were described initially by Fritsch in 1894, this condition received widespread attention only after the reports by Asherman of the syndrome which bears his name. Unfortunately, most physicians do not consider the condition to be a common one, despite many reports to the contrary (Table 106.1).

There are three common antecedent factors for the development of IUAs. The most common is curettage of the pregnant or recently pregnant uterus. Almost 40% of the patients with IUAs who have been referred to this medical center have had an elective abortion of pregnancy. Patients may also develop synechiae following curettage after a spontaneous abortion. Women who have had a missed abortion are at greatest risk among all patients in the abortion category. In one study, the frequency of IUAs was 6.4% among those who had undergone curettage because of an incomplete abortion, but 30.9% if the diagnosis was a missed abortion.

Another common etiology for the subsequent development of IUAs is the presence of endometritis. Tuberculous endometritis may be the sole cause of IUAs. However, the presence of other types of bacterial infection increases the risk for the development of adhesive disease in patients who have had a curettage or other uterine surgery. Despite the opinion of Rabau and David that infection is present in all cases of traumatic amenorrhea, few of the more than 300 patients we have treated had any clinical evidence of infection. All of these few women had undergone cesarean section.

A final antecedent factor is previous uterine surgery. Adhesions have

Table 106.1 Frequency of intrauterine adhesions in various conditions

Condition	Percentage
Amenorrhea	1.7
Infertility	4.0
Incomplete abortion	6.4
Elective abortion	13.0
Postpartum hemorrhage	3.7
	23.4
Missed abortion	30.9
Recurrent abortion	39.0

been noted following cesarean sections, hysterotomies, myomectomies, metroplasties, and diagnostic curettages. The "routine" dilatation and curettage (D&C) performed at the time of laparoscopy for the infertile woman serves no purpose and may be harmful. Thus, it should be abandoned.

The common denominator for the development of uterine adhesions in all of these conditions is trauma to the basalis of the endometrium. Additive factors in the patient who has been pregnant are tetanic uterine contractions which maintain the uterine walls in close apposition and the low levels of estradiol which are present immediately following pregnancy. Because the levels of estradiol are low, the stimulus for endometrial regeneration is markedly reduced. Nursing will maintain hypoestrogenism for a longer period and increase the risk of IUA development following a postpartum curettage. The uterus is most vulnerable between the second and fourth weeks after delivery. Perhaps estrogen therapy and placement of a splint will reduce the frequency of IUA formation after a curettage during this time period.

Following curettage, white blood cells infiltrate the endometrial surface and are replaced by fibroblasts. Adhesions are thin, vascular strands initially. As they mature, the adhesions became thicker and more fibrous. The final product is an avascular, fibrous bridge of variable width and length which maintains the uterine walls in apposition. In some patients, endometrial trauma is followed by amenorrhea but not adhesions. Patients with this problem (endometrial sclerosis) have had extensive endometrial necrosis. The histology reveals only rare isolated islands of basal cells clinging to the myometrium. Because the cavity is normal, the diagnosis cannot be made by hysterosalpingography (HSG); only hysteroscopy can prove the diagnosis.

The key to establishing the diagnosis is a high index of suspicion. All women who have menstrual complaints and/or infertility and who have a history of prior endometrial trauma should be investigated for the presence of IUAs. Five techniques have been utilized to establish the diagnosis. Amenorrhea with evidence of luteal-phase activity such as a biphasic basal body temperature or an elevated level of progesterone in serum is evidence of end-organ failure. However, the same symptoms may occur in patients with cervical stenosis even in the absence of cyclic abdominal pain. Failure to have uterine bleeding following combined or sequential estrogen–progestin treatment is also evidence of endometrial insufficiency. If this test is utilized, sequential estrogen–progestin therapy is preferable to the use of oral contraceptives because the latter may cause hypomenorrhea or amenorrhea. However, because IUAs may exist in patients with normal menses, neither regimen may be used to rule out the presence of intrauterine synechiae. Difficulty in sounding the endometrial cavity or the impression of an irregular or small cavity also suggests the presence of adhesions. HSG under fluoroscopic control is the study utilized most often to establish the presence of adhesions. The finding of lacunar-shaped defects placed irregularly throughout the cavity is strongly supportive of the impression of IUAs. Unfortunately, false-positive studies occur and neither the extent nor the exact location of the adhesions may be determined with certainty. However, patients with normal HSGs do not have adhesions. The definitive diagnostic study is hysteroscopy. Under direct vision the extent, location, and density of the adhesions may be determined with accuracy and the disease may be classified (Table 106.2).

Patients with intrauterine adhesions may complain of amenorrhea or hypomenorrhea, infertility, or recurrent abortion. Others conceive and deliver without difficulty but have problems with removal of the placenta. Despite even extensive adhesions a woman may have painless, spontaneous menses of normal flow and duration. The relation between recurrent abortion and adhesions is difficult to assess. Women with recurrent abortion frequently have the diagnosis of IUAs established.

Table 106.2 Hysteroscopic classification: Asherman's syndrome (modified from March *et al.*)

Classification	Description
Severe	$>\frac{3}{4}$ of uterine cavity involved; agglutination of walls and thick bands; ostial areas and upper cavity occluded
Moderate	$\frac{1}{4}$–$\frac{3}{4}$ of uterine cavity involved; walls not agglutinated – adhesions only; ostial areas and upper fundus partially occluded
Minimal	$<\frac{1}{4}$ of uterine cavity involved; filmy adhesions; ostial areas and upper fundus minimally involved or clear

However, this diagnosis might have been made only after multiple curettages had been performed and the adhesions therefore may be the sequelae to treatment for each loss rather than the cause of recurrent abortion. Moreover, these adhesions may have developed only after the last curettage.

The therapy of IUAs is directed toward accomplishing four goals: (1) the restoration of normal uterine architecture; (2) the prevention of readherence; (3) the stimulation of endometrial regeneration; and (4) verification that the uterus is normal before conception is attempted. Under hysteroscopic visualization the surgeon may lyse all the adhesions and not traumatize normal endometrium. A panoramic hysteroscope is used and the cavity is distended with Hyskon. This medium is not miscible with blood and permits the surgeon to have a clear view of the cavity even after extensive surgery has been performed. Miniature scissors are used for incising the adhesions. Scissors produce less trauma than either a laser or electrosurgical knife and are the preferred method of lysing adhesions. Under hysteroscopic guidance, only scar tissue is incised and adjacent normal endometrium is not traumatized. This tissue becomes a source for endometrial regrowth over the freshly dissected surfaces. Each adhesive band is identified and divided. Restoration of uterine architecture to normal can be achieved even in those with complete uterine obliteration. Women who have very extensive disease should undergo simultaneous laparoscopy in order to reduce the risk of uterine perforation.

If the intensity of the light source for the laparoscope is reduced markedly, the laparoscopist will detect dissection into the myometrium sooner because the light of the hysteroscope will begin to shine through the uterine serosa at a single point. In contrast, after the cavity's configuration has been restored, the uterus will have a uniform glow. Following adhesiolysis as large a loop intrauterine device (IUD) as possible is placed in the cavity and retained for 2 months. Postoperative use of an IUD may reduce the chances that the raw, dissected surfaces will readhere. Copper-bearing IUDs and the Progestasert IUD may have too small a surface area to prevent adhesion reformation and those which contain copper may induce an excessive inflammatory reaction. Therefore their use is not advised. If a loop IUD is not available, an 8 French Foley catheter with a 3-ml balloon can be used. The balloon is inflated, the catheter remains for 1 week, and a broad-spectrum antibiotic is prescribed during that time period. Special Silastic uterine splints are also available to maintain separation of the uterine walls.

Conjugated equine estrogens, 5 mg/day, are given to all patients for 60 days, and medroxyprogesterone acetate, 10 mg, is added during the last 5 days of estrogen therapy. This high-dose steroid regimen stimulates the endometrium maximally to promote reepithelialization of the previously scarred surfaces. The adequacy of therapy should be assessed accurately by repeat hysteroscopy or by HSG following withdrawal bleeding. If the HSG is normal, complete resolution may be presumed. An abnormal HSG, however, does not definitively indicate persistent adhesions and hysteroscopy should be repeated. The importance of a postoperative study to verify normalcy of the cavity prior to permitting conception cannot be overemphasized. Severe obstetric complications have been reported in patients who conceived prior to having postoperative studies performed to document complete resolution of the adhesions. It is likely that these women had persistent disease causing the subsequent obstetric problems.

After one hysteroscopic treatment, 90% of our patients have had a normal follow-up hysteroscopy or HSG. Although most of the others have needed only a second procedure to restore normal uterine architecture, a few women have needed three to six operations. Ninety-eight percent of those who had amenorrhea or hypomenorrhea now have normal menses. The pregnancy results are excellent and surpass other types of therapy. Seventy-five percent of our patients who wished to conceive and who had no other known infertility factors have done so and >85% of the pregnancies have been successful. Two patients have had placenta previa and two required manual removal of the placenta. One patient had retained placental fragments which were detected when a curettage was performed to stop hemorrhage 3 weeks after delivery. Her follow-up HSG had been abnormal but she conceived before another hysteroscopic procedure was performed. These results are superior to those achieved by outdated treatment modalities such as blind disruption of adhesions by a sound or a curette.

The hysteroscopic approach to IUAs offers complete management: diagnosis, treatment, and follow-up. For each step the hysteroscopic approach surpasses any and all alternatives.

SUGGESTED READING

ASCH RH, ZUO WL, GARCIA M, RAMZY I, LAUFE L, ROJAS FP. Intrauterine release of oestriol in castrated rhesus monkeys induces local but not periperal oestrogenic effects: a possible approach for the treatment and prevention of Asherman's syndrome. *Hum Reprod* 1991;6:1373–1378.

ADONI A, PALTI Z, MILWIDSKY A, *et al*. The incidence of intrauterine adhesions following spontaneous abortion. *Int J Fertil* 1982;27:117.

AMERICAN FERTILITY SOCIETY. The American Fertility Society classification of adnexal adhesions, distal tubal occlusion, tubal occlusion secondary to tubal ligation, tubal pregnancies, Mullerian anomalies and intrauterine adhesions. *Fertil Steril* 1988;49:944.

CARP HJA, BEN-SHLOMO I, MASHIACH S. What is the minimal uterine cavity needed for a normal pregnancy? An extreme case of Asherman syndrome. *Fertil Steril* 1992;58:419–421.

DEATON JL, MAIER D, ANDREOLI J Jr. Spontaneous uterine rupture during pregnancy after treatment of Asherman's syndrome. *Am J Obstet Gynecol* 1989;160: 1053–1054.

FRIEDLER S, MARGALIOTH EJ, KAFKA I, YAFFE H. Incidence of post-abortion intrauterine adhesions evaluated by hysteroscopy – a prospective study. *Hum Reprod* 1993;8:442–444.

JEWELEWICZ R, KHALAF S, NEUWIRTH RS, VANDE WIELE RL. Obstetric complications after treatment of intrauterine synechiae (Asherman's syndrome). *Obstet Gynecol* 1976;47:701.

JONES WE. Traumatic intrauterine adhesions. A report of 8 cases with emphasis on therapy. *Am J Obstet Gynecol* 1964;89:304–313.

MARCH CM, ISRAEL R. Intrauterine adhesions secondary to elective abortion. *Obstet Gynecol* 1976;48:422.

MARCH CM, ISRAEL R. Gestational outcome following hysteroscopic lysis of adhesions. *Fertil Steril* 1981;36:455.

MARCH CM, ISRAEL R, MARCH AD. The hysteroscopic management of intrauterine adhesions. *Am J Obstet Gynecol* 1978;130:653.

RABAU E, DAVID A. Intrauterine adhesions: etiology, prevention and treatment. *Obstet Gynecol* 1963;22:626.

VALLE RF, SCIARRA JJ. Intrauterine adhesions: hysteroscopic diagnosis, classification, treatment, and reproductive outcome. *Am J Obstet Gynecol* 1988;158:1459–1470.

107

Management of uterovaginal anomalies

DONNA SHOUPE

Anomalies of the uterus and vagina are associated with countless and varied clinical findings. They are caused from either a genetic error or by exposure to a teratogen during embryonic development. An improved understanding of the characteristics of each distinct entity, along with availability of advanced imaging techniques and less invasive surgical procedures, has ushered in a new era in the management of uterovaginal anomalies.

Incidence

The incidence of congenital defects of the female reproductive tract is not known since an estimated 75% of these defects remain asymptomatic and undiagnosed. In a recent study, however, 679 women with normal reproductive histories underwent a hysterosalpingogram. In this "normal" population, 22 (3.4%) had congenital anomalies which included septate uteri (90%), bicornuate uterus (5%), and didelphus uterus (5%). Prior to this study, the incidence was estimated around 0.5%.

The clinician should be alerted to the possibility of a uterine anomaly in the clinical settings listed in Table 107.1.

Associated problems: urinary tract abnormalities

The close embryologic development between the urinary and reproductive systems often means that abnormal development in one will affect

Table 107.1 Conditions associated with uterovaginal anomalies

Obstetric
High presenting part
Abnormal presentation
Retained placenta
Premature birth
Dystocia
Stillbirth

Gynecologic
Recurrent first-trimester loss
Second-trimester loss
History of incompetent cervix
Broad uterus or fundal notch noted on exam
Presence of vaginal or cervical anomalies
Two separate cornua on bimanual exam
Ectopic pregnancy

Ultrasound
Two-lobed contour of uterus with asymmetric shape of fundus
Off-center amniotic sac

the other system. The incidence of combined anomalies varies, but the diagnosis of unilateral absence or underdevelopment in one system is a strong signal to investigate the other. Up to 75% of patients with unicornuate uteri have unilateral renal agenesis. Likewise, 20% of patients with unilateral renal agenesis will have major reproductive tract anomalies. Vaginal anomalies are also associated with urinary tract changes.

Every woman with uterine anomalies or vaginal septum should have either an intravenous pyelogram or ultrasound scanning of the abdominal cavity.

Associated problems: endometriosis

Retrograde menstruation appears to play a significant role in the development of endometriosis. The presence of patent tubes, functioning endometrium, and an outflow obstruction is associated with a high incidence (up to 77%) of endometriosis.

There are increases in the muscular skeletal system anomalies and increased collagen vascular diseases in these patients. Other reports show associated problems in the digestive tract, chiefly imperforate anus, cardiovascular system, eyes, and ears.

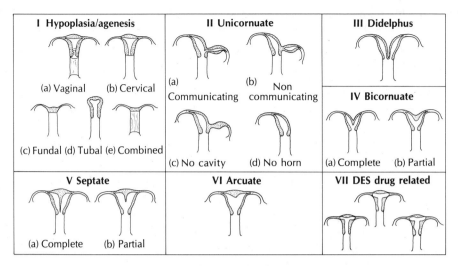

Fig. 107.1 Classification system of Müllerian anomalies developed by the American Fertility Society. DES, Diethylstilbestrol.

Classification system

The American Fertility Society developed a classification system for Müllerian system anomalies associated with fetal wastage. In this system, each group represents a structural change that has similar clinical problems, treatment, and prognosis. This classification system (Fig. 107.1) consists of seven major uterine anatomic types as well as the associated vaginal changes. The first three vaginal conditions described below are not Müllerian anomalies and not included in this classification system, but are included here as uterovaginal anomalies.

Labial fusion

Labial fusion is most often a result of exogenous androgen exposure. The most common etiology is congenital adrenal hyperplasia which is associated with clitoral enlargement and labial fusion and is most often due to a 21-hydroxylase deficiency. An elevated blood level of 17-hydroxyprogesterone necessitates cortisol replacement therapy. This condition is often diagnosed at birth or in early infancy.

Labial fusion may also result from defects in the anterior abdominal wall or from a local infectious process.

If there is a small opening in the labia fusion plane, a vaginogram prior to surgical separation informs the surgeon regarding the depth of fusion present, the dimensions of the upper vagina, and may confirm the presence of a cervix.

Imperforate hymen

Imperforate hymen is most often diagnosed at puberty when either primary amenorrhea occurs, or when hematocolpos or hematometrium causes pain or urinary retention. Occasionally, a mucocolpos or hydrocolpos causes pain and is diagnosed during infancy or childhood. The diagnosis is made by inspection of a bulging membrane at the introitus. Treatment consists of a cruciate incision in the hymen. A thick hymen may need a triangular section removed and placement of hemostatic sutures.

Transverse vaginal septum

If the area between the junction of the Müllerian tubercle and sinovaginal bulb is not properly canalized, a transverse vaginal septum may occur. This may be complete or partial and lie in the upper third or lower two-thirds of the vagina. Septa located in the upper third of the vagina are usually the thickest and most difficult to correct surgically. Transverse vaginal septa are extremely rare, occurring in only 1:75000 women.

With complete septa, hematocolpos or hematometrium may become symptomatic, similar to the imperforate hymen above. With an incomplete septum, cyclic cramping, and bleeding, a foul-smelling vaginal discharge, dystocia, or sexual problems may be the presenting complaint.

Generally, the septa are thin and <1 cm thick. If an opening is present, manual dilatation may be possible or a simple incision with suturing of the edges of the septum to the vagina on either side. If a vaginogram reveals a thick septum, either an anastomosis between the lower and upper vagina, or a split-thickness skin graft, similar to the McIndoe procedure, mentioned below, may be necessary.

Class I: hypoplasia/agenesis

Vaginal agenesis

Vaginal agenesis associated with absence of the uterus is called Rokitansky–Kuster–Hauser syndrome. Usually small masses of smooth muscular tissue, resembling a rudimentary uterus, tubes, and ovaries, remain. Occasionally, the smooth muscular tissue retains an epithelial lining and problems associated with occult menstruation occur. While complete vaginal agenesis is usual, about 25% of patients will at least have a short vaginal pouch.

The work-up includes documentation of the absence of a uterus. Magnetic resonance imaging (MRI) has been advocated for demonstrating ovaries, Müllerian and vaginal rudiments, and renal agenesis. From 25 to 40% have renal abnormalities and additionally, in one report 12% of patients had skeletal changes, including congenital fusion or absence of vertebrae.

Treatment is usually directed at the creation of a functional (>12 cm) vagina. The first choice is progressive vaginal dilators which generally take several months in well-motivated patients. A bicycle seat can be used to maintain dilator pressure for 15–20-min sessions for a total of 2 h/day. Surgical correction is usually the McIndoe procedure which utilizes a stent over which a split-thickness skin graft is sewed and placed in a dissected space between the rectum and the bladder. The success rate is 80%. The Williams procedure utilizes labial skin which is used to create a vaginal pouch. A normal vaginal axis is reported to develop eventually.

Palpation of a partially descended testis, presence of scant pubic hair, or failure to identify ovaries is an indication for karyotype testing. Androgen insensitivity syndrome (testicular feminization syndrome) has a 46,XY karyotype. A high incidence of seminomas is reported and therefore the testes need to be removed after puberty.

Cervical agenesis

Congenital absence of the cervix with functioning endometrial tissue is extremely rare. Primary amenorrhea and cyclic abdominal pain is the usual presentation. Creation of a functional cervix is difficult due to lack of cervical mucus production. Infection, stenosis, and reoperation are common. Endometriosis, presumably from retrograde flow, is an additional problem. Advanced reproductive technologies may offer some hope for these patients.

Fundal agenesis

Congenital absence of the fundal portion of the uterus with normal tubes and ovaries is extremely rare. A MRI scan may accurately identify remnants and normal structures. Surgery is rarely indicated unless endometrial tissue is present.

Tubal agenesis

The diagnosis of congenital tubal anomalies is generally made after problems of infertility. Microscopic tubal unification may be possible in cases of segmental tubal agenesis.

Combined

Treatment of combined vaginal and fundal hypoplasia is directed at creating a functional vagina, as described above.

Class II: unicornuate

Communicating rudimentary horn

Many of these anomalies are asymptomatic, although incidences between 10 and 70% of fetal loss in unicornuate uteri are reported. Cervical incompetence may account for much of the increased risk of fetal loss. Congenital alterations of uterine vascularization may compromise utero-placental blood flow, and may account for early pregnancy loss and greater risk for intrauterine growth retardation.

Recurrent first-trimester loss or a single second-trimester loss is an indication for a hysterosalpingogram. Placement of a cervical cerclage should be considered after reproductive loss. Removal of a communicating horn is necessary if it is associated with retrograde flow, an ectopic pregnancy, cyclic pain, or mass formation.

Noncommunicating rudimentary horn

In 90% of rudimentary horns, there is no communication to the uterine cavity. The presence of any endometrial tissue in a noncommunicating horn may lead to the problems listed above and is generally an indication for removal of the horn. A pregnancy in a noncommunicating horn is thought to be due to transperitoneal migration of the ova and/or sperm. Rarely a live birth occurs.

No cavity

These patients are generally asymptomatic but when a unicornuate uterus is associated with increased pregnancy losses, the patients can be managed as for communicating unicornuate uterus (see above).

No horn

Early pregnancy loss can be managed the same as for communicating unicornuate uterus (see above), often with placement of a cervical cerclage. A 30–50% incidence of unilateral renal malformation can be anticipated.

Class III: didelphus

Complete duplication of the uterus, vagina, and cervix often does not become symptomatic until a patient notices that a tampon does not obstruct menstrual bleeding. In some cases, the diagnosis is made at the time of the first pelvic exam. Didelphic uteri are usually not associated with reproductive wastage, unless associated with an incompetent cervix, but are reported to increase the risk of premature labor. A mean length of gestation of around 35 weeks is reported with a 27% incidence of breech presentation. There is also the chance that pregnancies exist in both uteri or remain in one uterus after removal of the other pregnancy for whatever medical reason.

The diagnosis is made by inspection of a double cervix and vagina and palpation of a double uterus. A metroplasty is rarely indicated or beneficial.

Class IV: bicornuate

There is generally no conception difficulty in the case of bicornuate uterus, but dystocia, premature birth, and retained placenta are common. Most studies reporting increased fetal wastage rates include septate uteri.

The diagnosis can sometimes be made on bimanual examination with detection of two completely separate cornua. Since this could also represent an exceptionally wide uterus possibly with a septum, a hysterosalpingogram or further investigation is necessary.

It is suggested that along with the defect in fusion, there is inadequate formation and functioning of the cervix. Placement of a cervical cerclage should be the primary consideration in cases of repetitive fetal loss as increased rates of incompetent cervix, as high as 38%, are reported in women with bicornuate uteri. The value of a Strassman unification procedure is questionable but the procedure has been advocated by some authors for reproductive failure.

Class V: septate

The most outstanding feature of the septate uterus is the high incidence of first-trimester fetal wastage, which is thought to be related to inadequate blood supply in the septum, resulting in placental site malnourishment. Most data suggest that the more complete the septum, the higher the frequency of fetal loss. However, there are some studies suggesting that the more complete the septum, the better the blood supply and the better the chance for a full-term pregnancy. Abnormal fetal presentation is associated with septate uteri, especially breech presentation, and also incomplete expulsion of the placenta leading to postpartum hemorrhage.

If a hysterosalpingogram cannot distinguish a septate from a bicornuate uterus then direct visualization, usually through laparoscopy, may be necessary for diagnosis. Treatment by hysteroscopic resection with laparoscopic monitoring is the treatment of choice in cases of repetitive pregnancy losses. If unsuccessful, a Tompkins operation is recommended.

Class VI: arcuate

Because the arcuate uterus is externally unified, it could be classified as a form of a partial septate uterus. However, because it behaves benignly, it is classified separately. The arcuate uterus may simply be a variant of normal.

Class VII: diethylstilbestrol drug-related

The changes associated with diethylstilbestrol exposure *in utero* include anomalies in all parts of the genital tract. At least 50% of these women have vaginal adenosis, and 20–50% have structural abnormalities of the cervix. A hypoplastic or T-shaped uterus is characteristic. Reproductive performance is reduced in these women as they have increased risk of spontaneous abortion, ectopic pregnancies, perinatal mortality, and premature labor.

Overall, patients with diethylstilbestrol exposure have a good chance for at least one viable pregnancy. After demonstration of a reproductive problem, a hysterosalpingogram is indicated. This population is at increased risk of incompetent cervix and a cervical cerclage may be indicated.

Summary

The fallopian tubes, uterus, and upper four-fifths of the vagina are created by fusion of the Müllerian ducts occurs during the 10th to 17th weeks of pregnancy. A disturbance of duct migration may create problems both anatomically and functionally. The most common site of anomalies is the vagina; these anomalies are frequently accompanied by changes in the urinary tract. Cervical and uterine abnormalities are equally common.

Most congenital uterine anomalies can be accurately defined with imaging techniques, including hysterosalpingogram, ultrasound, and MRI. It is of utmost importance that, prior to any intervention, comprehensive examinations be done to establish with certainty which complaints are due to uterovaginal pathology. Each case must then be assessed on its own merits and treated appropriately (Table 107.2). A cerclage is a simple and effective treatment and avoids major surgery.

Table 107.2 Treatments available for various classifications of Müllerian anomalies

Class	Treatments available
IA	Vaginal anastomosis, McIndoe procedure
IB	Surgery unwarranted in most cases
IC	No surgery available
ID	Early tubal unification in cases of segmental tubal agenesis
IE	Dilator therapy or artificial vagina
II	Cervical cerclage
III	Cervical cerclage, value of metroplasty unclear
IV	Cervical cerclage, value of metroplasty unclear
V	Hysteroscopic resection, Tompkins metroplasty
VI	No treatment needed
VII	Cervical cerclage

Advanced pelviscopy, microsurgical techniques, and advanced reproductive technologies may offer additional possibilities for successful reproductive outcome.

SUGGESTED READING

AMERICAN FERTILITY SOCIETY. The American Fertility Society classifications of adnexal adhesion, distal tubal occlusion, tubal occlusion secondary to tubal ligation, tubal pregnancies, Mullerian anomalies and intrauterine adhesions. *Fertil Steril* 1988;49:944.

ANDREWS MC, JONES HW Jr. Impaired reproductive performance of the unicornuate uterus: intrauterine growth retardation, infertility and recurrent abortion in five cases. *Am J Obstet Gynecol* 1982;144:173.

BIEDEL CW, PAGON RA, ZAPATA JO. Mullerian anomalies and renal agenesis: autosomal dominant urogenital adysplasia. *J Pediatr* 1984;104:861.

BUTTRAM VC, BIGGONS WE. Mullerian anomalies: a proposed classification (an analysis of 144 cases). *Fertil Steril* 1979;32:40.

DeCHERNEY AH, RUSSELL JB, BRAEBE RA, POLAN ML. Resectoscopic management of mullerian fusion defects. *Fertil Steril* 1986;45:726.

FEDELE L, DORTA M, BRIOSCHI D, GUIDIDI NM, CANDIANI GB. Magnetic resonance imaging in Mayer–Rokitansky–Kuster–Hauser syndrome. *Obstet Gynecol* 1990;76:593.

GOLAN A, LANGER R, BUKOVSKY I, CASPI E. Congenital anomalies of the mullerian system. *Fertil Steril* 1989;51:747.

GREEN LK, HARRIS RE. Uterine anomalies. *Obstet Gynecol* 1976;47:427.

HEINONEN PK, PYSTYNEN PP. Primary infertility and uterine anomalies. *Fertil Steril* 1983;40:311.

HEINONEN PK, SAARIKOSKI S, PYSTYNEN P. Reproductive performance of women with uterine anomalies. *Acta Obstet Gynecol Scand* 1982;61:157.

OLIVE D, HENDERSON DY. Endometriosis and mullerian anomalies. *Obstet Gynecol*

1987;69:412.

ROCK JA. Surgery for anomalies of the Mullerian ducts. In: Thompson JD, Rock JA, eds. *TeLinde's Operative Gynecology*. 7th edn. Philadelphia: JB Lippincott, 1992:603–660.

SIMON C, MARTINEZ L, PARDO F, TORTAJADA M, PELLICER A. Mullerian defects in women with normal reproductive outcome. *Fertil Steril* 1992;56:1192.

108

Tubal factor in infertility

ROBERT ISRAEL

Fallopian tube abnormalities, adhesive pelvic disease, and endometriosis, along with the male factor, account for the majority of infertility. In most clinics, the pelvic factor is the etiology in 30–40% of infertility cases. With indigent populations, tubal disease and pelvic adhesions may account for an even higher percentage of infertility. Although the diagnosis of tubal or pelvic disease is relatively straightforward, surgical correction of tubal obstructions does not yield satisfying results.

Diagnostic techniques for evaluating tubal function, and the pelvis in general, have become more sophisticated. However, they still indicate only patency, obstruction, or distortion – not the degree of physiologic impairment. Reproductive function remains unmeasured.

Uterotubal insufflation (Rubin's test)

In 1920, Rubin described a nonoperative method of determining tubal patency by instilling a gas, initially oxygen, via a transvaginal–transuterine route. To eliminate the possibility of air embolism, carbon dioxide soon replaced oxygen. As with any study of tubal patency, uterotubal insufflation should be carried out in the follicular phase of the menstrual cycle, after the menses and before ovulation. Investigations of tubal patency are contraindicated in the luteal phase as they may damage or delay implantation of a fertilized ovum. Also, the thicker secretory endometrium may occlude the tubal ostia at the tubal–endometrial cavity junction and yield a false result. Other contraindications are pregnancy, uterine bleeding, pelvic infection, recent curettage, and inadequate equipment.

Interpretation of uterotubal insufflation must be tempered with a great deal of caution. Cornual spasm can mimic occlusion, and indications of tubal patency can be misleading. The test gives no assurance that both tubes are open, that one tube is open, or that partial patency exists. Obviously, pelvic adhesions cannot be diagnosed. If used as a quick office screening study, its limitations must be considered and the results must not be utilized as a definitive evaluation of the tubes and pelvis.

The therapeutic benefit of repeated insufflation, or "blowing out the tubes," in three successive cycles has not been proven by any prospective study. Following distal tubal surgery, hydrotubation or uterotubal insufflation may be utilized to help maintain patency, although its use does not improve the pregnancy rate. The most important consideration in analyzing uterotubal insufflation is the realization that it does not depict the actual condition of the fallopian tubes. Decisions as to whether the tubes are open or closed or whether conservative tubal surgery should or should not be performed must not be made on the basis of a Rubin's test. Therefore, the value of carrying out this study must be seriously questioned.

Hysterosalpingography

A more definitive study of the fallopian tubes involves transuterine dye instillation under X-ray visualization. The contraindications to hysterosalpingography (HSG) are the same as for uterotubal insufflation. The study is performed after the menses, in the follicular phase, prior to ovulation. Exactness and care are essential.

The instrumentation can be the same as for uterotubal insufflation utilizing a vacuum cannula, a Jarcho cannula, or a small Foley catheter or its equivalent. The vacuum cannula causes the least patient discomfort, but often does not remain in place well. The Jarcho cannula allows the best uterine positioning. The Foley catheter is excellent with a patulous cervix, but can obscure a portion of the uterine cavity. If a radiologist is going to perform the HSG, the gynecologist should be in attendance or, at the very least, review the X-rays. Preferably, the dye instillation should be set up and administered by the gynecologist. Image intensification fluoroscopy adds to the interpretation of the final X-rays and should be part of the procedure. However, it should be carried out by a radiologist skilled in the technique. Even if 1 min of fluoroscopy is utilized during an HSG, the patient receives a radiation dose equal to that of one conventional film, about 1 rad. In actuality, a properly performed HSG requires less than 15 s of fluoroscopy time.

Two types of contrast media are available for HSG: oil-based and water-soluble. Although the oil-based solutions may improve the pregnancy rate in some infertility etiologies, they do not outline the uterine cavity or demonstrate ampullary rugation as well as the water-soluble media. In the past, serious embolization complications were reported with oil-based contrast media, especially in the presence of distal tubal obstruction. These have not been reported using the currently available oil media. With the advent of laparoscopy, the advantage of taking a 24-h delay film after oil HSG has lost its importance. As a greater amount of water-soluble medium than oil-based medium is necessary for an HSG, uterine cramps and peritoneal irritation may be a problem. However, using a solution of extremely low viscosity, e.g., diatrizoate meglumine and iodipamide meglumine (Sinografin), and warming it, will reduce uterine cramping, thus improving patient acceptance and study accuracy. In summary, water-soluble media are preferable.

In patients with a history of pelvic inflammatory disease (PID), the HSG should be deferred until the white blood count and erythrocyte sedimentation rate have returned to normal. Antibiotic coverage (doxy-cycline 100 mg b.i.d.) before and after HSG may provide additional pro-tection. A flare-up of acute salpingitis after an HSG is a poor prognostic sign regarding the success of any subsequent reparative surgery. If even attempted, surgery should be deferred at least 6 months.

The HSG is extremely valuable in the work-up of the infertile patient. In a population with a high incidence of salpingitis, an HSG, under antibiotic coverage, should be obtained relatively early in the infertility investigation. In some pathologic conditions, an HSG may be the defini-tive study. As noted by Klein and coworkers in our clinic, the HSG is diagnostic of pelvic tuberculosis. In salpingitis isthmica nodosa, an HSG defines the extent of the process even with patent tubes. In patients with hydrosalpinges, the HSG can be predictive of surgical outcome and may steer the work-up away from reconstructive surgery and toward *in vitro* fertilization (IVF). Factors such as an abnormal ampullary mucosal pat-tern, an increased ampullary diameter (>1.5 cm), and obvious dilatation of the proximal ampulla, when combined with similarly negative laparo-scopic findings, do not offer even marginally satisfactory postoperative pregnancy rates.

The discovery of extensive tubal disease may alter, and certainly speed up, the other infertility studies. Multifactor infertility does not have a very good prognosis. An abnormal HSG will hasten the time of laparo-scopy and, possibly, as noted above, bring the investigation to an early conclusion. In addition, according to studies in our institution, unsus-pected intrauterine pathology will be demonstrated in 10% of HSGs obtained for infertility. Confirmatory hysteroscopy should be done when-ever an intrauterine defect is found on HSG.

The illuminated hysterosalpingogram should be present in the operating room at the time of surgery. Although, in some series, discrepancies between HSG and definitive laparoscopy have occurred as much as 25% of the time, HSG is still a valuable study. Its technical problems can be overcome by endoscopy. For example, occasionally a tube that seems to be blocked on HSG can be proven to be patent at laparoscopy by using a probe to occlude the other tube at the uterine cornu while continuing to instill the dye transcervically. If several months have elapsed between the HSG and surgery, advancing disease or a reaction to the HSG may explain tubal occlusion found at laparoscopy which was not present on an earlier HSG. On occasion, mechanical problems with laparoscopic chromopertubation may occur, and the illuminated HSG may provide evidence of patency.

If an HSG is obtained either as the "final" evaluation in the infertility work-up or only, as in repeated uterotubal insufflations, for its "therapeutic" benefit, its continuing value must be questioned. However, as an adjuvant to laparoscopy and infertility surgery, the HSG may be of significant benefit.

Laparoscopy

The panoramic view of the pelvis provided by the laparoscope is superb. For the infertility patient, laparoscopy has become an integral part of the entire investigation, and in many instances, therapy.

An ovulatory infertile patient with a normal postcoital test and semen analysis first undergoes HSG. If the HSG is abnormal, laparoscopy should follow in the next cycle. Although discrepancies have been reported between HSG and laparoscopy up to 25% of the time, if the HSG is entirely normal, office studies and/or therapies can be undertaken for a limited time period. If pregnancy does not occur in 3–6 months, laparoscopy must be performed. An anovulatory infertile patient should be evaluated and have ovulation therapeutically induced before an extensive infertility work-up is undertaken. Although a postcoital test should be deferred until ovulatory cycles have been achieved, an early semen analysis and HSG will rule out or rule in other significant pathology. If more than one factor exists to account for the infertility, pregnancy becomes even more difficult and the entire situation should be reviewed. But if all studies have been normal and clomiphene (Clomid, Serophine)-induced ovulatory cycles have been achieved for at least 6 months, laparoscopy should be performed to eliminate the possibility of unsuspected pelvic pathology. Even in an asymptomatic patient with unexplained infertility, laparoscopy can reveal significant disease 44–75% of the time.

In addition to its value in diagnosing unsuspected pelvic pathology, laparoscopy is an essential primary step when conservative infertility surgery is contemplated. The laparoscope can reveal a normal pelvis, thus eliminating the need for further surgery. With the laparoscope, the skilled infertility surgeon can define, categorize, and surgically treat pelvic disease and distortion. In some cases, laparoscopy can reveal such extensive pelvic destruction that reconstructive surgery is contraindicated and the patient can be advised to abandon further infertility studies and consider alternatives such as adoption and/or assisted reproductive technologies, such as IVF. In view of its importance in determining the degree of pelvic pathology and the necessity for conservative infertility surgery, laparoscopy in the infertile patient should be carried out only by a gynecologic surgeon who is prepared to make endoscopic judgments and perform the required surgery.

As with any study of tubal function, laparoscopy should be performed in the follicular phase of the menstrual cycle. A thorough examination of the pelvis must be carried out, utilizing the accessory probe to lift, move, and feel all areas of the pelvis. Since the manipulations are extensive and adhesive disease is often encountered, a double-puncture and, if laparoscopic surgery is performed, a triple-puncture technique under general endotracheal anesthesia is required. Prior pelvic surgery is usually not a deterrent to an adequate laparoscopic examination. In a study from this institution, 38 of 155 infertility patients (25%) who underwent uneventful laparoscopy had a history of previous pelvic surgery, usually a salpingectomy for an ectopic pregnancy. During laparoscopy, chromopertubation is carried out with a dilute indigo carmine solution instilled via a uterine cannula.

The decision to proceed with conservative infertility surgery is made at the time of laparoscopy. Therefore, prior to laparoscopy, all possible pelvic findings and surgical risks are explained to the patient and her husband. If pelvic pathology is confirmed, or unsuspected pathology found, the patient is prepared to undergo definitive tubal or pelvic surgery either via the same laparoscopy or by a laparotomy immediately following, utilizing the same anesthetic. Various degrees of adhesions can be lysed through the laparoscope depending on the endoscopic skills of the surgeon and the relationship of these adhesions to other organs, e.g., the bowel. In well-trained hands, the laparoscope can be considered a primary surgical tool in infertility.

The presence or absence of additional infertility factors plays a prognostic role when combined with the laparoscopic findings. When laparoscopy reveals a normal pelvis, the presence of an infertility factor that has responded to treatment is an encouraging sign. Continuing to treat that problem may result in pregnancy. On the other hand, the patient who has minimal or unilateral disease at laparoscopy has a more favorable outlook for pregnancy if the pelvic pathology is not compounded by an additional infertility factor. In view of the generally poor results achieved with conservative tubal surgery, the laparoscope must be used very critically in order to select the best candidates for reparative operations.

SUGGESTED READING

BOER-MEISEL ME, TEVELDE ER, HABBEMA JDF, KARDAUN JWPF. Predicting the pregnancy outcome in patients treated for hydrosalpinx: a prospective study. *Fertil Steril* 1986;45:23.

DECHERNEY AH. "The leader of the band is tired . . .". *Fertil Steril* 1985;44:299.

DRAKE TS, GRUNERT GM. The unsuspected pelvic factor in the infertility investigation. *Fertil Steril* 1980;34:27.

GOMEL V. An odyssey through the oviduct. *Fertil Steril* 1983;39:144.

GOMEL V. *Microsurgery in Female Infertility*. Boston: Little, Brown, 1983.

ISRAEL R, MARCH CM. Diagnostic laparoscopy: a prognostic aid in the surgical management of infertility. *Am J Obstet Gynecol* 1976;125:969.

KLEIN TA, RICHMOND JA, MISHELL DR Jr. Pelvic tuberculosis in an infertility clinic. *Obstet Gynecol* 1976;48:99.

LINDEQUIST S, JUSTESEN P, LARSEN C, RASMUSSEN F. Diagnostic quality and complications of hysterosalpingography: oil- versus water-soluble contrast media – a randomized, prospective study. *Radiology* 1991;179:69.

LOY RA, WEINSTEIN FG, SEIBEL MM. Hysterosalpingography in perspective: the predictive value of oil-soluble versus water-soluble contrast media. *Fertil Steril* 1989;51:170.

PITTAWAY DE, WINFIELD AC, MAXSON W, DANIELL J, HERBERT C, WENTZ AC. Prevention of acute pelvic inflammatory disease after hysterosalpingography: efficacy of doxycycline prophylaxis. *Am J Obstet Gynecol* 1983;147:623.

RASMUSSEN F, LINDEQUIST S, LARSEN C, JUSTESEN P. Therapeutic effect of hysterosalpingography: oil- versus water-soluble contrast media – a randomized prospective study. *Radiology* 1991;179:75.

SOULES MR, SPADONI LR. Oil versus aqueous media for hysterosalpingography: a continuing debate based on many opinions and few facts. *Fertil Steril* 1982; 38:1.

STUMPF PG, MARCH CM. Febrile morbidity following hysterosalpingography: identification of risk factors and recommendations for prophylaxis. *Fertil Steril* 1980;33:487.

109

Salpingolysis and salpingostomy

ROBERT ISRAEL

Following the laparoscopic decision to perform conservative surgery, the surgeon and the patient are faced with end-results that leave much to be desired. In most instances, subsequent pregnancy rates do not exceed 50% and include abortions and ectopics as well as term gestations. With tubal closure, surgical correction can achieve patency in the majority of cases. However, a postoperative patent tube is no guarantee that pregnancy will ensue. Prior involvement of the endosalpinx or its distortion by the surgery itself may disturb the reproductive physiology of the fallopian tube to such an extent that pregnancy will never occur.

It is difficult to compare the results of conservative infertility surgery among surgeons or even among the patients of a single surgeon. The variability of pelvic pathology makes prospective, randomized studies virtually impossible. Are pelvic adhesions present or absent? If present, to what degree and in what areas? With distal tubal disease, what degree of tubal abnormality exists? Are the tubes dilated, and, if so, to what extent? Are intraluminal adhesions present? Do fimbrial remnants remain? What is the condition of the endosalpinx? Historically, in the available retrospective studies, many of these questions were never answered. However, today, with the viable alternative of assisted reproductive technology (e.g., *in vitro* fertilization; IVF), it has become more important preoperatively to assess the tubal/pelvic status as best possible so that appropriate therapeutic directions can be taken. As discussed in Chapter 108, the hysterosalpingogram (HSG) has been used more critically to delineate the condition of the fallopian tubes. Combined with laparoscopy, the two techniques have been used diagnostically to decide whether reconstructive surgery offers any realistic chance for pregnancy success. For example, when the diameter of the hydrosalpinx, in both studies, is large, e.g., >1.5 cm, the pregnancy prospects are so poor following reconstructive surgery that IVF is a better alternative. On the other hand, when one or both tubes show a normal mucosal pattern, tubal surgery should be considered as the primary mode of treatment.

Once the proper diagnostic techniques have been utilized to make as specific an assessment of the pelvic pathology as possible and to estimate the chance of pregnancy success after corrective surgery has been performed, the only remaining decision is operative laparoscopy or operative laparotomy. As the remote chance of a pregnancy is eliminated and the pelvis in general is less vascular, either form of reparative surgery should be carried out in the follicular phase of the cycle. Operative laparoscopy offers some potential advantages over laparotomy: corrective surgery during the initial diagnostic laparoscopy, avoidance of laparotomy with its increased morbidity, and shorter hospital stays with reduced health-care costs. However, the safety and efficacy of many operative laparoscopic procedures compared to laparotomy remain to be shown. Few randomized controlled trials have been performed and those that have are of low power. Most reports are of the descriptive variety. Multicenter, collaborative trials are needed to evaluate properly these new endoscopic techniques utilizing uniform protocols and outcome measures. To hasten the process, if a laparoscopic approach appears feasible, as was the case for salpingostomy treatment of ectopic pregnancy, then general use could start with provisions for continued monitoring of outcomes and complications. Laparoscopy has made important contributions, and will continue to do so, but enthusiastic proponents cannot be allowed to outshout critical appraisals.

Four basic operative procedures are utilized in conservative tubal surgery: (1) lysis of peritubal adhesions (salpingolysis); (2) opening of the occluded distal tube (salpingostomy); (3) repairing mid-segment occlusions (end-to-end anastomosis); and (4) correction of proximal obstructions. This chapter covers the first two operations; the other two are discussed in Chapter 110.

Salpingolysis

The most successful type of tubal surgery involves the lysis of peritubal and/or pelvic adhesions and does not involve primary tubal surgery. Ovum pick-up is impeded by adhesions isolating the tubes and ovaries. The tubes may spill dye into isolated pockets of adhesions, but the fimbriated ends are open and the endosalpinx is intact. The vast majority of salpingolysis surgery can be done by the skilled laparoscopic surgeon utilizing double- or triple-puncture approaches. When properly used, ancillary laparoscopic operating instruments permit adequate exposure and a wide variety of surgical manipulations. Ultimate success depends on the extent and type of adhesions encountered, and whether they reform postoperatively. In reported series, the overall pregnancy rate varies from 40 to 70% with 70–95% of the pregnancies going to term.

If significant cul-de-sac dissection is required, a uterine suspension should be part of the operative procedure in order to prevent the tubes and ovaries from falling back into areas of recently denuded adhesions. This is particularly important if the uterus is not in an anterior position at the conclusion of the surgery. Because it utilizes the distal, weaker portions of the round ligaments in the suspension, leaving the proximal, stronger areas for support, the Gilliam uterine suspension is preferred.

Various techniques are reported to reduce adhesions postoperatively. Although valid statistical support regarding their efficacy is lacking, most of these ancillary measures are strongly (perhaps emotionally) advocated by their proponents. A broad-spectrum antibiotic, e.g., doxycycline, can be administered prophylactically and should be started preoperatively in order to have an adequate tissue level at the time of surgery. During surgery, the operative field should be kept moist to prevent tissue adherence. As tissue dryness occurs more often during laparotomy than laparoscopy, the field should be irrigated with physiologic lactated Ringer's solution which has had 5000 U of heparin added to it. Historically, in an effort to dissolve any fibrinous exudate postoperatively and delay fibroblast and collagen formation, Replogle *et al.* suggested a medical regimen employing high doses of promethazine and dexamethasone. However, published results have never shown an improvement in the subsequent pregnancy rate to justify this expensive, relatively risky treatment. A *prospective* study in 1983 by Harris and Daniell confirmed this by showing no difference in the term pregnancy rate with or without corticosteroids in a group of salpingostomy patients.

Following the promethazine–dexamethasone protocol, a variety of agents have been employed to prevent adhesion formation and re-formation after conservative infertility surgery. However, two recurring themes have emerged: the site-specific efficacy of even the most promising agents has never been dramatic, and the original favorable results have never been duplicated after widespread clinical use. For most of the 1980s, the method of choice was the intraperitoneal instillation of 100 ml of a 32% solution of dextran 70 (Hyskon) just prior to closing the abdomen. As dextran 70 remains *in situ* for at least 7 days before total absorption, it is there during maximum fibroblastic proliferation. Physiologically, dextran 70 acts to separate the surfaces of recently traumatized tissues by increasing the peritoneal colloid osmotic pressure, thereby inducing an influx of fluid into the abdominal cavity. Additionally, it covers the peritoneal surfaces with a very fine, silicon-like film, which could hinder adhesion formation. In general, the long-term results with dextran 70 showed that it was much more successful in preventing new adhesion formation in the clean pelvis than preventing adhesion reformation after lysis of adhesions.

In the 1990s, barrier methods have replaced dextran 70 as the adhesion prevention technique of choice. Materials (Interceed; Gore-Tex) are placed over traumatized tissues at the conclusion of surgery (laparoscopy or laparotomy) that act as barriers to the formation or reformation of adhesions. Interceed is a biodegradable knitted fabric composed of oxidized, regenerated cellulose that is placed over the hemostatically dry surgical site, e.g., ovaries, tubes, uterus, cul-de-sac, pelvic side walls, etc., at the conclusion of surgery, moistened with saline, and left in place. It rapidly forms a soft gelatinous mass that covers the damaged peritoneum and protects it from involvement in adhesion formation. By the time it is absorbed in 2 weeks, reepithelialization of damaged peritoneal surfaces is complete. Gore-Tex surgical membrane is a permanent, inert, microporous implant of expanded polytetrafluoroethylene that is placed to overlap the peritoneal defect, e.g., myomectomy incision, by 1.0 cm and secured in an unwrinkled state by the necessary number of 7-0 or 8-0 permanent or absorbable sutures. Second-look laparoscopy is carried out and the surgical membrane retrieved. Although both these barrier methods do well in preventing the formation and reformation of adhesions, it is unlikely that they represent the final chapter in the prevention of postoperative pelvic adhesions.

Another area that lacks certainty is early second-look laparoscopy. Its proponents claim that repeat laparoscopy within 6–8 weeks of the original surgery allows easier lysis of less rigid adhesions compared to a second look 1–2 years later. However, the few papers that compare pregnancy rates between early and late follow-up laparoscopy show no statistical difference. Advocating routine second-look laparoscopy after all conservative infertility surgery is not justified.

Salpingostomy

Opening distal tubal occlusions is the least successful type of tubal surgery. A hydrosalpinx is the end-stage of generalized tubal disease. Although the surgeon may be able to open the tube, and have it remain open, residual anatomic and physiologic damage to the rest of the tube is usually sufficient to disrupt the reproductive processes necessary to achieve an intrauterine pregnancy. The fimbria are often gone, the endosalpinx is denuded partially or totally, the tubal musculature is nonfunctional, and various degrees of tubal dilatation may be present. Additionally, distal tubal closure is often associated with pelvic adhesions varying from minimal filmy to extensive thick.

With IVF success often equal to, or better than, the pregnancy rate seen after distal salpingostomy surgery, it is very important to evaluate the tubes and pelvis as critically as possible before deciding on reparative surgery. The most important prognostic factor related to surgical success is the nature of the functional anatomy present at the time of surgery. Prospective evaluation of tubal mucosa quality, the degree of distal tubal dilatation, and the extent of associated adhesions by HSG and laparoscopy permit accurate and appropriate preoperative counseling of the patient, including a comprehensive discussion of therapeutic alternatives, e.g., IVF. While patients with mild disease should strongly consider neosalpingostomy, those with moderate disease, who have a relatively high risk for subsequent ectopic pregnancy, may wish to ponder the surgical decision more carefully. Although their tubes may be functionally adequate to perform ovum capture, they may be too compromised to allow normal embryo passage. Patients with severe tubal and pelvic disease have a very poor pregnancy prognosis after neosalpingostomy and should be encouraged to consider IVF unless practical, financial, or religious constraints make IVF unacceptable.

To compound the salpingostomy problem, some surgeons include lesser degrees of fimbrial pathology in this surgical category. Fimbrial agglutination and phimosis are two of the favorites. Teasing apart filmy strands between the fimbria or dilating the fimbriated end of the tube with small bougies do not represent salpingostomy surgery. If they can be considered indicated forms of conservative infertility surgery, they should be classified in a subcategory under salpingolysis.

Surgically, by laparoscopy or laparotomy, distal tubal occlusion is approached by opening the hydrosalpinx through its central dimple with needle electrocautery or laser. Utilizing electrodissection or laser, the distal tubal scars and fimbrial bridges are lysed. Repeat chromopertubation should be carried out after the tubes have been opened and the lumen investigated for adhesions with fine probes (laparotomy) or catheters (laparoscopy). A cuff salpingostomy is performed by turning back the mucosal edges of the fimbriated end of the tube and suturing them to the serosa overlying the ampulla. Either 6-0 or 7-0 polyglycolic or polyglactic suture should be used in creating the cuff, and no more than four to six interrupted sutures should ever be necessary. Using the laser at laparoscopy, eversion of the tube is obtained by provoking retraction of the serosa distal to the incision using a defocused beam. Utilizing lactated Ringer's with heparin for irrigation, small bleeders on the mucosal edge should be specifically identified and gently fulgurated with a hand-controlled, bipolar forceps, needle electrocautery, or laser. Although recent, large case-report studies of laparoscopic salpingostomy support its efficacy, including comparable pregnancy rates with laparotomy, and shorter operations and hospital stays, there are no prospective, randomized studies available to compare microsurgery and laparoscopy. Until these are available, laparotomy remains the procedure of choice, when primary salpingostomy surgery is indicated.

In addition to the ancillary procedures – antibiotics, adhesion prevention techniques, and uterine suspension – already discussed, postoperative hydrotubation may be carried out via a number 8 or 10 intrauterine Foley catheter or Jarcho cannula, utilizing 50 ml of dextran 40. Although dextran 70 may be preferable, it is too viscous to instill transcervically through small-bore equipment. Broad-spectrum antibiotic coverage, e.g., doxycycline 100 mg orally b.i.d., should be given 2 days before, the day of, and 2 days after hydrotubation. Routinely, hydrotubation is performed once while the patient is still hospitalized and is repeated 1 week after discharge. It is continued once per cycle in the early follicular phase for 2 months. A hysterosalpingogram can be performed in the third postoperative cycle. Although hydrotubation may improve the postoperative tubal patency rate, as shown by Rock *et al.*, there is no evidence that tubal flushing improves the pregnancy rate. However, with antibiotic coverage and meticulous performance, the benefit of hydrotubation outweighs any potential risks.

From published reports, cuff salpingostomy yields overall pregnancy rates of 10–40% with term pregnancies ranging from 5 to 50%. As noted, the ultimate results depend on the anatomic and physiologic condition of the remainder of the tube rather than the specific operative method. If tubal patency was the only necessary end-point, postoperative pregnancy rates would be much higher. After cuff salpingostomy, the percentage of patent tubes varies from 50 to 90%. Usually, the surgeon can open the pipeline, but cannot restore proper function. As suggested by Umezaki *et al.* and confirmed by Russell *et al.* salpingostomy-treated tubes may require a longer healing time, so results could improve with continued follow-up.

The increased incidence of ectopic pregnancies in postsalpingostomy tubes reinforces the concept that tubal closure is not the only problem in these cases. With an indigent population prone to pelvic inflammatory disease, postsalpingostomy tubal pregnancies occur with disturbing frequency. Although the significant amount of pelvic disease found in a clinic population may explain the high tubal-to-intrauterine gestation ratio, Swolin, despite meticulously performed surgery utilizing microdissection techniques, reported comparable findings from a Scandinavian population exhibiting less extensive pelvic pathology. If an alternate fertility approach, such as IVF, achieves a *repetitive* pregnancy rate of 25–30%, the first tubal reparative surgery it will replace is distal salpingostomy.

SUGGESTED READING

CANIS M, MAGE G, POULY JL, MANHES H, WATTIEZ A, BRUHAT MA. Laparoscopic distal tuboplasty: report of 87 cases and a 4-year experience. *Fertil Steril* 1991;56:616.

DANIELL JF, PITTAWAY DE. Short-interval second-look laparoscopy after infertility surgery. *J Reprod Med* 1983;28:281.

DeCHERNEY AH. "The leader of the band is tired. . . ." *Fertil Steril* 1985;44:299.

DIAMOND MP, LINSKY CB, CUNNINGHAM T, *et al.* Adhesion reformation: reduction by the use of Interceed (TC7) plus heparin. *J Gynecol Surg* 1991;7:1.

DiZEREGA GS, HODGEN GD. Prevention of postoperative tubal adhesions. *Am J Obstet Gynecol* 1980;136:173.

DUBUISSON JB, BOUQUET DE JOLINIERE J, AUBRIOT FX, DARAI E, FOULOT H, MANDELBROT L. Terminal tuboplasties by laparoscopy: 65 consecutive cases. *Fertil Steril* 1990;54:401.

GOMEL V. Salpingo-ovariolysis by laparoscopy in infertility. *Fertil Steril* 1983; 40:607.

GOMEL V. Operative laparoscopy: time for acceptance. *Fertil Steril* 1989;52:1.

GRIMES DA. Frontiers of operative laparoscopy: a review and critique of the evidence. *Am J Obstet Gynecol* 1992;166:1062.

HARRIS WJ, DANIELL JF. Use of corticosteroids as an adjuvant in terminal salpingostomy. *Fertil Steril* 1983;40:785.

INTERCEED (TC7) ADHESION BARRIER STUDY GROUP. Prevention of postsurgical adhesions by Interceed (TC7), an absorbable adhesion barrier: a prospective, randomized multicenter clinical study. *Fertil Steril* 1989;51:933.

MURPHY AA. Operative laparoscopy. *Fertil Steril* 1987;47:1.

OPERATIVE LAPAROSCOPY STUDY GROUP. Postoperative adhesion development after operative laparoscopy: evaluation at early second-look procedures. *Fertil Steril* 1991;55:700.

RAJ SG, HULKA JF. Second-look laparoscopy in infertility surgery: therapeutic and prognostic value. *Fertil Steril* 1982;38:325.

REPLOGLE RL, JOHNSON BA, GROSS RD. Prevention of postoperative intestinal adhesions with combined promethazine and dexamethasone therapy. *Ann Surg* 1966;163:580.

ROCK JA, SIEGLER AM, MEISEL MB, *et al.* The efficacy of postoperative hydrotubation: a randomized prospective multicenter clinical trial. *Fertil Steril* 1984; 42:373.

RUSSELL JB, DeCHERNEY AH, LAUFER N, POLAN ML, NAFTOLIN F. Neosalpingostomy: comparison of 24- and 72-month follow-up time shows increased pregnancy rates. *Fertil Steril* 1986;45:296.

SCHLAFF WD, HASSIAKOS DK, DAMEWOOD MD, ROCK JA. Neosalpingostomy for distal tubal obstruction: prognostic factors and impact of surgical technique. *Fertil Steril* 1990;54:984.

SURGICAL MEMBRANE STUDY GROUP. Prophylaxis of pelvic sidewall adhesions with Gore-Tex surgical membrane: a multicenter clinical investigation. *Fertil Steril* 1992;57:921.

TEVELDE ER, BOER-MEISEL ME, MEISNER J, SCHOEMAKER J, HABBEMA JDF. The significance of preoperative hysterosalpingography and laparoscopy for predicting the pregnancy outcome in patients with a bilateral hydrosalpinx. *Eur J Obstet Gynecol Reprod Biol* 1989;31:33.

UMEZAKI C, KATAYAMA KP, JONES HW Jr. Pregnancy rates after reconstructive surgery on the fallopian tubes. *Obstet Gynecol* 1974;43:418.

110

End-to-end anastomosis and cornual (interstitial) occlusion

MICHAEL VERMESH

The most successful primary tubal surgery is the correction of mid tubal occlusion secondary to previous tubal sterilization. The remainder of the tube, proximally and distally, is normal and the pelvis is free of adhesions. Additionally, the patient has proven her fertility and is infertile only because of tubal sterilization.

As has been stressed with any form of conservative surgery, laparoscopy should precede laparotomy to confirm the normal status of the pelvis and to decide that adequate tubal segments exist for anastomosis. If the sterilization was performed by laparoscopic fulguration, with or without tubal transection, a hysterosalpingogram should be otained prior to diagnostic laparoscopy to determine the extent of the interstitial–isthmic fill. At laparoscopy, the most proximal portions of the tubes are often difficult to visualize even when they fill with dye.

Ideally, for end-to-end reconstruction, the prior tubal sterilization should have been a small, mid tubal (Pomeroy) segmental resection. If a satisfactory end-to-end anastomosis can be performed in the isthmus, success should be extremely high. In a young woman, sterilization by segmental mid tubal resection or laparoscopic sterilization with bipolar coagulation, bands, or clips should be considered the techniques of choice with 1–2 cm of proximal isthmus left undamaged. With these procedures, if the future brings a change of mind, reanastomosis success will be high.

Unfortunately, reversal of laparoscopic tubal fulguration, especially if it was performed with unipolar equipment, may be impossible because insufficient tubal segments remain. If no proximal tube can be located, even with shaving back of the uterine cornu, or if the proximal segments are abnormal as a result of poststerilization changes, microscope-assisted anastomosis of the distal tube into the endometrial cavity is the only alternative. For such surgery, the distal tubal segments should be at least 5 cm long. Fimbriectomy sterilization represents the worst reversal odds. With removal of the distal tube, only cuff salpingostomy is available as a reversal procedure, and even this approach requires a residual tube extending into the mid-ampulla.

The technique of end-to-end anastomosis requires excision of the scarred site of the previous tubal sterilization and approximation of the distal and proximal segments. Loupe magnification, or the use of an operating microscope, especially in isthmic–isthmic or isthmic–interstitial anastomoses, has improved the subsequent pregnancy rates by 10–15% compared with surgery done without magnification. The tubal ends are pulled together with three or four interrupted 8-0 polyglycolic or polyglactic sutures placed through the muscularis, but not including the mucosa. The serosa is closed over the anastomotic site utilizing interrupted 6-0 sutures of the same material. When the operating microscope is used, nonabsorbable monofilament 9-0 or 10-0 nylon sutures have been utilized.

The pregnancy rate following microsurgical end-to-end anastomosis should be in the 60–75% range. Gomel's 80% pregnancy rate remains the highest reported. The spontaneous abortion rate is unchanged from a normal obstetric population. However, the tubal pregnancy rate following end-to-end reanastomosis increases to 5%.

Proximal occlusion

The least frequently performed, and technically most complex, reparative tubal surgery is the correction of cornual (interstitial) occlusion. The anatomic site of obstruction includes a segment, or all, of the interstitial portion of the tube. Usually the patient has a history of uterine invasion, – dilatation and curettage, pregnancy with sepsis, intrauterine device insertion – or has had a sterilization procedure (as discussed above) that was maximally destructive to the proximal tube. In many instances, the uterine invasion was not accompanied by any clinical evidence of pelvic sepsis, yet interstitial occlusion was the end-result. Additionally, salpingitis isthmica nodosa, a condition unique to the interstitial and isthmic portions of the tube, may create blockage.

Proximal tubal obstruction presents a significant diagnostic problem. Conventional hysterosalpingography may not differentiate tubocornual spasm from true mechanical obstruction. Consequently, surgical evaluation by laparoscopy with chromopertubation and/or laparoscopy with concurrent hysteroscopy and tubal catheterization may be necessary to minimize the chance of a false-positive diagnosis and to assess the distal tube. Selective salpingography, an extension of conventional hysterosalpingography, may obviate the need for diagnostic laparoscopy in selected patients. A curved catheter is advanced through a trans-cervical cannula and, under fluoroscopic guidance, wedged into the tubal ostium. In patients with cornual spasm, the hydrostatic pressure of direct injection may demonstrate tubal patency, or dislodge soft, intraluminal debris, allowing tubal fill and spill. Falloposcopy, an extension of hyster-oscopy, using a small, flexible, fiberoptic endoscope, permits direct visualization of intratubal pathology.

Treatment options for proximal tubal occlusion include transabdominal tuboplasty, transcervical tubal cannulation, and *in vitro* fertilization (IVF). In patients with endometriosis and proximal tubal occlusion, hormonal suppression with danazol or gonadotropin-releasing hormone agonists should be considered before proceeding to transabdominal or transcervical tuboplasty.

All procedures to treat proximal tubal obstruction have in common an increased risk for subsequent tubal ectopic pregnancy, which should, therefore, be diagnosed and localized early. Surgical repair of proximal tubal occlusion is recommended only in cases of isolated proximal ob-struction. Reproductive outcome after surgery for proven bipolar (proximal and distal) disease in the same tube shows the fertility rate to be poor. Furthermore, correction of multifocal tubal occlusion may predispose to an unacceptably high incidence of ectopic pregnancies.

A variety of operative techniques exist for reconstruction of the prox-imal tube. Microsurgical approaches include both cornual and posterior implantation techniques performed with the uterine cavity either closed or exposed by incision. Term pregnancy rates range from 14 to 69%. Disadvantages to implantation procedures include postimplantation pelvic pain, shortening of the fallopian tube, and dehiscence of the uterine incision in subsequent pregnancies. Microsurgical tubocornual anastomosis has been consistently more successful than conventional implantation, with pregnancy rates ranging from 50 to 80%. Thus, if the transabdominal operative approach is selected to correct proximal occlusion, microsurgical tubocornual anastomosis is the procedure of choice. Postoperatively, a hysterosalpingogram can be obtained at 3 months, and, if patency is demonstrated, pregnancy can be attempted. If a tubocornual anastomosis has been performed with the operating microscope, and the uterine defect minimized, subsequent pregnancy may be completed by vaginal delivery unless a cesarean section is in-dicated for obstetric reasons. The spontaneous abortion rate is unchanged from a normal obstetric population and the tubal pregnancy rate is similar to that found after mid tubal reanastomosis.

Patients who are poor candidates for pelvic reconstructive surgery, such as those with combined proximal and distal disease or failed tubal anastomosis, are candidates for IVF. When compared to the surgical approach, IVF is a minimally invasive procedure that can be performed without general anesthesia. Pregnancy rates are variable and depend on diagnosis, patient's age, stimulation regimen, and number of embryos transferred.

Transcervical tuboplasty is less invasive and may be more cost-effective than either microsurgical tuboplasty or IVF in a selected group of patients. A prior or concurrent laparoscopy is recommended to assess the condition of the distal tube and the presence of peritoneal factors such as adhesions or endometriosis. A flexible guidewire cannulation technique to establish tubal patency has been described. The procedure can be performed under fluoroscopy with intravenous sedation, or in association with diagnostic laparoscopy using the operating channel of a hysteroscope. The two most commonly used cannulation systems are a balloon catheter system and a coaxial catheter and guidewire system. Patients with a history of previous proximal tubal surgery, salpingitis isthmica nodosa, and/or evidence of uterine myomas at or close to the uterotubal junction, are poor candidates for therapeutic tubal cannulation. In a recent study of transcervical balloon tuboplasty, 92% of 77 patients with bilateral proximal tubal occlusion had successful recanalization of at least one tube, and 23 patients subsequently conceived. Complications included pinpoint wire perforations without clinical consequences in two cases and one case of ectopic pregnancy. Six months after the procedure, the tubal patency rate was 68%. Patients who fail to conceive 6 months after tubal cannulation should undergo hysterosalpingography. If one or both tubes remain patent and conception does not occur 12 months after cannulation, other treatment options should be explored.

Microsurgery/laser surgery

Gynecologic microsurgery includes magnification with an operating microscope or binocular lenses ($\times 3$–6); its definition encompasses ophthalmic-type instrumentation, gentle tissue handling, well-controlled hemostasis, extremely fine (7-10 through 10-0) sutures, and the ancillary techniques already described to reduce postoperative adhesion formation. Although all of these procedures have enhanced conservative reproductive surgery, magnification by itself seems to have improved the pregnancy rates in only one form of reconstructive tubal surgery.

Following end-to-end tubal reanastomosis utilizing an operating microscope or binocular lens magnification, pregnancy rates have improved by 10–20% over conventional, nonmagnified end-to-end anas-

Table 110.1 Range of reported pregnancy outcomes following surgical correction of the tubal factor in infertility

Operation	Pregnancy rate %	Spontaneous abortion %	Ectopic pregnancy %	Term gestation %
Salpingolysis	40–70	10–20	1–2	70–90
Salpingostomy	10–40	10–20	15–40	45–55
End-to-end anastomosis	60–75	10–20	5–10	60–70
Tubocornual anastomosis	50–60	10–20	5–10	60–70

tomosis. However, there is no evidence that magnification is associated with higher pregnancy rates in other forms of tubal surgery, such as salpingostomy or salpingolysis.

It is difficult to compare the results of any type of conservative infertility surgery when the operations are performed by different surgeons. Ideally, variation in surgical skills could be controlled by having the same surgeon alternately perform macro- and microsurgical repairs. However, encountering varying pelvic conditions could skew even this approach. Perhaps the ultimate contribution of microsurgical principles will be the impact on gynecologic surgery in general. With the emphasis on gentle tissue handling and well-controlled hemostasis, routine gynecologic surgery, especially when it involves preservation of the uterus and adnexa, will be carried out with more care and attention to detail, so that future reproductive potential will not be compromised.

The value of carbon dioxide laser in tubal surgery is unresolved. The major advantage of laser surgery is the hemostasis obtained when tissue is vaporized. In addition, the operative time is shorter and surgical precision enhanced. However, as yet, patency and pregnancy rates following reconstructive laser surgery have shown no improvement over those achieved with microsurgery. As respected investigators continue to publish their results with the laser, the true place of this instrument in the aramentarium of the reproductive gynecologic surgeon will become clearer.

Summary

It is difficult to analyze the reported results of conservative tubal surgery. Great variation exists between the number of operative procedures performed per series, the degree of tubal and adhesive disease encountered, the specific surgical techniques utilized, and the ancillary therapeutic measures employed. In addition, many series mention only the pregnancy rate and do not break it down into a life-table analysis which would be a truer reflection of the pregnancies over time. Although the total pregnancy rate may satisfy the surgeon, the couple considering reparative surgery is interested primarily in the expected outcome of pregnancy. Postoperatively, the only happy outcome for the infertile patient is a term gestation. A review of the literature yields the ranges of pregnancy outcomes summarized in Table 110.1 for the four surgical procedures discussed in this chapter and in Chapter 109.

SUGGESTED READING

BAGGISH MS, CHONG AP. Intraabdominal surgery with the CO_2 laser. *Reprod Med* 1983;28:269.

CONFINO E, TUR-KASPA I, DECHERNEY A, *et al*. Transcervical balloon tuboplasty: a multicenter study. *JAMA* 1990;264:2079.

DANIELL JF. The role of lasers in infertility surgery. *Fertil Steril* 1984;42:815.

DANIELL JF, HERBERT CM. Laparoscopic salpingostomy utilizing the CO_2 laser. *Fertil Steril* 1984;41:558.

DANIELL JF, DIAMOND MP, MCLAUGHLIN DS, *et al*. Clinical results of terminal salpingostomy with the use of CO_2 laser: report of the intraabdominal laser study group. *Fertil Steril* 1986;45:175.

DONNEZ J, CASANAS-ROUX F. Prognostic factors influencing the pregnancy rate after microsurgical cornual anastomosis. *Fertil Steril* 1986;46:1089.

GOMEL V. Microsurgical reversal of female sterilization: a reappraisal. *Fertil Steril* 1980;33:587.

KERIN J, KAYKHOVSKY L, SEGALOWITZ J, *et al*. Falloposcopy: a microendoscopic technique for visual exploration of the human fallopian tube from the uterotubal ostium to the fimbria using a transvaginal approach. *Fertil Steril* 1990;54: 390–400.

LAVY G, DIAMOND MP, DECHERNEY AH. Pregnancy following tubocornual anastomosis. *Fertil Steril* 1986;46:21.

LEVINSON CJ. Implantation procedures for intramural obstruction. *J Reprod Med* 1981;26:347.

MCCOMB P. The determinants of successful surgery for proximal tubal disease. *Fertil Steril* 1986;46:1002.

NOVY MT, THURMOND AS, PATTON P, UCHIDA BT, ROSCH J. Diagnosis of cornual obstruction by transcervical fallopian tube cannulation. *Fertil Steril* 1988;50:343–340.

PATTON PE, WILLIAMS TJ, COULAM CB. Results of microsurgical reconstruction in patients with combined proximal and distal tubal occlusion: double obstruction. *Fertil Steril* 1987;48:670–674.

ROCK JA, BERGQUIST CA, KIMBALL AW Jr, ZACUR HA, KING TM. Comparison of the operating microscope and loupe for microsurgical tubal anastomosis: a randomized clinical trial. *Fertil Steril* 1984;41:229.

111

Endometriosis: diagnostic evaluation

ROBERT ISRAEL

In 1921, J.A. Sampson described endometriosis as: "the presence of ectopic tissue which possesses the histological structure and function of the uterine mucosa." Although the occurrence of aberrant endometrium had been described by various individuals in the 19th century, it was not until Sampson's classic contribution that there was any appreciation of the frequency, pathology, and clinical characteristics of this enigmatic gynecologic disorder.

Incidence and distribution

Since endometriosis is dependent on the ovarian steroids for its existence and proliferation, its occurrence and clinical importance are confined generally to the reproductive years. Although Kempers *et al.* have reported active postmenopausal endometriosis *without* exogenous hormone use, the peak incidence is in the fourth decade. Marriage and child-bearing have often been deferred.

The emergence and widespread use of steroidal contraceptives over the past 20 years have not reduced the incidence of endometriosis. By reducing menstrual flow, oral contraceptives also reduce tubal reflux, so they should be the contraceptive of choice in women with treated endometriosis. Operative statistics show that endometriosis is a frequent gynecologic entity. Gross or microscopic endometriosis was noted in 14–21% of all laparotomies performed for gynecologic disease between 1950 and 1980. When laparoscopy is carried out in the infertile patient, the incidence of endometriosis varies between 4.5 and 33%, with a mean of 14%.

Although in many instances the endometriosis does not appear to be interfering with the normal reproductive process, 30–40% of patients with endometriosis have concomitant infertility. Sperm ascension, ovulation, and ovum pick-up and transport can all take place, but the presence of even minimal pelvic endometriosis creates concern in the infertility patient.

Sites

The most frequent pelvic locations for endometriosis are the ovaries, uterine ligaments (round, broad, uterosacral), pelvic peritoneum, and rectovaginal septum. Other sites include the umbilicus, laparotomy scars, hernial sacs, appendix, small intestine, rectum, sigmoid, bladder, ureters, vulva–vagina–cervix, lymph nodes, extremities, pleural cavity, and lung. The multiplicity and widespread distribution of these sites make acceptance of any *one* histogenetic theory difficult. Possibly, future histochemical and immunologic investigations will provide some definitive clues to the many unanswered questions raised by the presence of endometriosis.

Gross pathology

Like everything else connected with endometriosis, the gross pathology is characterized by variability. With mild involvement, the adnexa will be free of adhesions, and a variable number of reddish-blue (raspberry) or brown, fibrin-like implants will be present on the ovaries and/or peritoneal surfaces. With progressive disease, the older implants will have coalesced and "burnt out" leaving scarred, retracted areas that may involve peritoneal surface *only* or include peritubal and periovarian involvement and fixation. With increasing reports of nonpigmented endometriosis, laparoscopic biopsy may help to establish the diagnosis histologically in areas of white opacified peritoneum, colorless subovarian adhesions, and peritoneal pocket defects. Murphy *et al.* demonstrated microscopic foci of endometriosis in 25% of patients when biopsy specimens were taken of grossly normal peritoneum.

More significant ovarian involvement means the formation of single or multiple, unilateral or bilateral endometrial cysts (endometriomas, "chocolate" cysts). Even when quite small, the cysts show a strong tendency to perforate with escape of menstrual blood and subsequent ovarian adherence to any adjacent structure, usually the posterior surface of the broad ligament or uterus. If early perforation does not occur, larger endometriomas form with thicker walls and few surrounding adhesions. When the uterine ligaments are involved, especially the uterosacrals, endometriotic nodules form that can often be palpated on bimanual or rectovaginal examination. Endometrial islands may occur on any part of the pelvic peritoneum, involving the serosal surface of any pelvic structure. Occasionally, invasion and penetration occur in the sigmoid so that progressive submucosal scarring results in luminal constriction. Mucosal involvement with associated rectal bleeding is a late phenomenon in bowel endometriosis.

Microscopic pathology

Definitive diagnosis requires microscopic demonstration of endometrial tissue, preferably both glands and stroma. However, a wide range of patterns may occur. Some specimens reveal endometrium that histologically and functionally cannot be distinguished from normal uterine epithelium. In others, the endometrium has been completely denuded due to repeated menstrual bleeding and desquamation. Hemorrhage and pigment-laden macrophages may be the only microscopic clues. No specific pathologic diagnosis can be made definitively in one-third of clinically typical endometriosis cases.

Endometriomas, when *lacking* endometrial glands and stroma, can often be identified by a broad surrounding zone rich in large phagocytic cells laden with blood pigment (hemosiderin). These pseudoxanthoma cells have a superficial resemblance to lutein cells. When *present*, the endometrial glands usually have a proliferative or cystic hyperplastic appearance containing low-lying and inactive cells. Accompanying, and often surrounding, the endometrial reaction may be a zone of hyalinized fibrous tissue.

Malignant changes occurring in endometriomas are very rare and always of low grade histologically (adenoacanthoma). Although 10% of endometroid ovarian carcinomas are associated with ovarian endometriosis, it is unusual for malignant transformation of the endometriosis to be demonstrable. However, endometriosis has a cancer-like characteristic in the insidious, invasive way it spreads, terminating in fibrosis and scarring of any, and all, pelvic structures.

Diagnosis

The symptomatology associated with endometriosis can be as variable as anything else connected with this disease. Dysmenorrhea, dyspareunia, and dyschezia may be present as a symptom complex or individually. However, even with extensive endometriosis, pain may not be a significant clinical entity. Unless rupture occurs, ovarian endometriomas can expand painlessly. On the other hand, incapacitating dysmenorrhea and pelvic pain may be associated with minimal amounts of active peritoneal surface endometriosis. Thus, the degree of endometriotic involvement and spread bears no constant relationship to the presence or absence of subjective discomfort.

Over 50% of patients with endometriosis complain of dysmenorrhea. Usually, it is the secondary or acquired variety, although if primary dysmenorrhea is present, endometriosis can worsen it. The dysmenorrhea may be attributed to secretory changes in the endometriotic islands with subsequent miniature menstruation and bleeding in areas encapsulated by fibrous tissue or to the release of prostaglandins from aberrant endometrium. With involvement of the rectovaginal septum or uterosacral ligaments, the dysmenorrhea is often referred to the rectum or the lower sacrococcygeal area and dyspareunia is a common complaint. Dyschezia results from endometriotic bleeding in the rectosigmoid muscularis or serosa with subsequent fibrosis. Occasionally, abnormal uterine bleeding, e.g., premenstrual spotting, may occur.

Although the diagnosis may be suggested by the history, it cannot be made with any certainty on symptoms alone. Even a pelvic examination, which, at times, can be quite distinctive, *cannot* be considered pathognomonic. Tender, nodular uterosacral ligaments combined with a fixed, retroverted uterus are findings highly suggestive of endometriosis, but inflammation and cancer cannot be ruled out by bimanual examination. Standard radiography, ultrasonography, computed tomography scans, and magnetic resonance imaging have had little or no impact on improving the diagnosis of endometriosis. CA-125, the antigenic determinant of the monoclonal antibody OC-125 found on the surface of coelomic epithelium and associated with epithelial ovarian cancers, can be elevated in some patients with moderate and severe endometriosis. Although the low sensitivity of the assay rules it out as a screening test for endometriosis, in the future, other cell-surface proteins specific for endometriosis tissue may be found and detected by immunoassay techniques.

For definitive diagnosis, endoscopic visualization of the pelvis must be carried out prior to the institution of therapy. When lesions are identified and doubt still remains or nonpigmented areas of cribriform scar are seen, confirmatory transendoscopic biopsy should be performed. Laparoscopy provides a panoramic view and operative capabilities via fulguration or laser (carbon dioxide, potassium-titanyl-phosphate, or argon).

Double-puncture laparoscopy should be utilized so that a careful, complete pelvic inspection can be carried out. Additionally, one of several available instruments for uterine manipulation should be secured in the cervical canal. Preferably, it should have a central cannula for subsequent transuterine–tubal dye instillation. The procedure requires a transabdominal approach under general anesthesia; to make it worthwhile, the surgeon must be compulsively thorough in the inspection and investigation of the peritoneal cavity. The palpating probe, placed through the accessory trocar, can be used as an examining finger running over various structures, e.g., the uterosacral ligaments, to detect subperitoneal implants. Each ovary must be lifted up to visualize the undersurface adjoining the broad ligaments. The appendix and the serosa of any bowel in the pelvis should be carefully inspected for any endometriotic implants.

Until Acosta *et al.* proposed a classification in 1973, the extent of pelvic endometriosis was described by individual cases. Although it may seem a small step forward, uniformity in classification has helped categorize and analyze the success or failure of the various therapeutic modalities used in the treatment of endometriosis.

The most recent and widely accepted classification is that of the American Fertility Society*, originally published in 1979, and revised in 1985. It uses four categories — stage I (minimal); stage II (mild); stage III (moderate); and stage IV (severe) — based on the degree of involvement of the peritoneum, ovaries, and tubes. Involvement is categorized as active endometriosis and/or adhesions. Points are assigned based on dimensional spread in three categories: 1, 1–3, and 3 cm. The American Fertility Society provides copies of its classification system in the form of individual tear-off sheets. They can be used in the operating room to stage immediately the extent of the disease process noted.

SUGGESTED READING

ACOSTA AA, BUTTRAM VC Jr, BESCH PK, *et al.* A proposed classification of endometriosis. *Obstet Gynecol* 1973;42:19.

BARBIERI RL, NILOFF JM, BAST RC Jr, SCHAETZL E, KISTNER RW, KNAPP RC. Elevated serum concentrations of CA-125 in patients with advanced endometriosis. *Fertil Steril* 1986;45:630.

KEMPERS RD, DOCKERTY MB, HUNT AB, *et al.* Postmenopausal endometriosis. *Surg Gynecol Obstet* 1960;111:348.

MARTIN DC, HUBERT GD, ZWAAG RV, EL-ZEKY FA. Laparoscopic appearances of peritoneal endometriosis. *Fertil Steril* 1989;51:63.

MORCOS RN, GIBBONS WE, FINDLEY WE. Effect of peritoneal fluid on *in vitro* cleavage of 2-cell mouse embryos: possible role in infertility associated with endometriosis. *Fertil Steril* 1985;44:678.

MURPHY AA, GREEN WR, BOBBIE D, *et al.* Unsuspected endometriosis documented by scanning electron microscopy in visually normal peritoneum. *Fertil Steril* 1986;46:522.

PETERSON EP, BEHRMAN SJ. Laparoscopy of the infertile patient. *Obstet Gynecol* 1970;36:363.

*American Fertility Society, 2140 Eleventh Avenue South, Suite 200, Birmingham, AL 35205-2800.

RIDLEY JH. The histogenesis of endometriosis. *Obstet Gynecol Surv* 1968;23:1.

SAMPSON JA. Perforating hemorrhagic (chocolate) cysts of the ovary. *Arch Surg* 1921;3:245.

SCHENKEN RS (ed). *Endometriosis — Contemporary Concepts in Clinical Management.* Philadelphia: JB Lippincott, 1989.

THE FERTILITY SOCIETY. Revised American Fertility Society classification of endometriosis: 1985. *Fertil Steril* 1985;43:351–352.

112

Endometriosis: treatment

ROBERT ISRAEL

The therapeutic approach to endometriosis must be individualized according to the patient's current reproductive status and desires. There are three categories: (1) therapy of endometriosis in the infertile patient; (2) therapy of endometriosis in the symptomatic patient who wishes to preserve her reproductive function, but has no interest in immediate fertility; and (3) therapy for the symptomatic patient who has extensive endometriosis and no desire to preserve reproductive function.

Therapy for infertility

Hormonal suppression and/or conservative surgery constitute the available therapeutic modalities. The diagnosis and stage (minimal, mild, moderate, severe) are established by laparoscopy and become the basis for selection of subsequent therapy.

Minimal/mild endometriosis

This is the most unsettled therapeutic area in endometriosis. Similar pregnancy rates (50–75%) have been reported with each of the following approaches: (1) laparoscopic observation only; (2) laparoscopic fulguration; (3) laparoscopic laser; (4) danazol; and (5) gonadotropin-releasing hormone (GnRH) agonist.

Numerous studies have shown that the medical or surgical treatment of minimal and mild endometriosis produces no higher pregnancy rates than no therapy at all. It may well be that mild endometriosis is the result, not the cause, of infertility, secondary to constant menstrual cycles uninterrupted by amenorrheic episodes, such as pregnancy. Although any patient with minimal or mild endometriosis does not need active therapy of her endometriosis to improve her chances for conception, endometriosis is a gynecologic process that can progress and, therefore, when laparoscopically diagnosed it should be ablated by fulguration or laser. However, laparoscopic treatment should not be assumed to have cured the infertility and all other areas of infertility diagnoses should be explored and, when indicated, directed therapy carried out.

Laparoscopic surgery can be performed by cauterization, endocoagulation, or laser (carbon dioxide, argon, neodymium-YAG, or potassium-titanyl-phosphate) therapy. No prospective, randomized studies exist comparing these various surgical approaches, but many studies have demonstrated that laparoscopic surgery, using appropriate skills and precautions, is safe and effective. If the surgeon is adept with the endoscope, even some forms of moderate endometriosis (accessible adhesions; small endometriomas) can be treated at the time of diagnostic laparoscopy. In minimal or mild endometriosis associated with infertility, operative laparoscopy is sufficient therapy even if complete eradication does not occur. Postoperative therapy with hormonal suppression will not enhance pregnancy rates and will only delay the woman's ability to conceive.

However, with the degree of moderate disease outlined above, post-laparoscopic hormone suppression may have a place. Although few studies exist to advocate or not advocate this treatment, if the operator knows active endometriosis remains, a short, 3-month course of danazol or GnRH agonist seems appropriate. The rationale would be to attempt elimination of residual disease in the immediate postoperative period and not 1 year later after no pregnancy has occurred. Using this nonscientific approach, which of the two hormonal regimens should be selected? Again, no data exist to support the superiority of either danazol or a GnRH agonist. However, if the decision is to treat hormonally, GnRH agonists have fewer side-effects and are available in more convenient forms of administration.

In summary, where infertility coexists with minimal, mild, and some forms of moderate endometriosis, the laparoscope is used both for diagnosis and treatment. Using *only diagnostic* laparoscopy followed by full-course hormonal suppression (danazol or a GnRH agonist) offers no therapeutic advantage and should not be selected. In some cases, as discussed above, these hormones can be utilized postoperatively for a short time. Otherwise, they have no place in the management of infertility associated with minimal, mild, and operatively accessible moderate endometriosis.

Moderate to severe endometriosis

In the infertile patient with significant stage III and stage IV endometriosis, conservative surgery becomes the therapeutic choice. Eliminating large (>3 cm) endometriomas and extensive adhesions cannot be accomplished by observation or hormonal therapy. The only controversial areas surrounding conservative surgery are whether to carry it out by laparoscopy or laparotomy, the status of ancillary operative procedures, and whether preoperative or postoperative suppressive hormones should be administered. With extensive pathology attributable to endometriosis, no matter what therapeutic stance has been taken up to now, the postsurgical pregnancy outlook has been 25–45% at best.

Laparoscopy or laparotomy

In minimal, mild, and laparoscopically accessible moderate endometriosis, the use and applicability of the laparoscope have been demonstrated. As complication rates rise and inadequate resections occur with "endoscopic gymnastics," extensive laparoscopic surgical manipulations in the presence of significant moderate and severe endometriosis should be carried out only by a highly trained, skilled operator. However, even in experienced hands, endometriosis with large adnexal masses, extensive adhesions, and/or symptomatic intestinal involvement is not amenable to endoscopic surgery. Unfortunately, neither prospective, randomized studies nor comparative studies exist concerning the efficacy of laparoscopic treatment for infertility associated with endometriosis. There are no studies directly comparing laparoscopy and laparotomy as regards subsequent pregnancy success. However, initial, statistically well-designed studies using laser vaporization of endometriotic lesions and associated adhesions are promising. They present pregnancy and monthly fecundity rates that are higher in treated severe disease than those seen previously after hormonal therapy or conservative laparotomy. If future comparative studies with laparotomy bear out these results, laparoscopic conservative surgery for extensive endometriosis will have to be given serious credibility.

Ancillary operative procedures

Other surgical procedures should be, or could be, carried out in conjunction with conservative surgery for endometriosis. As cervical stenosis can encourage retrograde menstruation, the cervix should be checked, and, if necessary, dilated. Fallopian tube patency should be evaluated by transuterine dye instillation through a previously placed intrauterine cannula or catheter. Lysis of adhesions, myomectomy, and, occasionally, tuboplasty may need to be done. However, additional pelvic pathology requiring correction will lower the subsequent pregnancy rate. If secondary dysmenorrhea is part of the symptomatology, presacral neurectomy and resection of the uterosacral ligaments at their uterine insertion are indicated. Both of these procedures can be performed laparoscopically by the *skilled* endoscopist, but, again, the indications are limited and there are no comparisons, short- or long-term, to the laparotomy approach. If the uterus is not anterior and significant cul-de-sac scarring/dissection has occurred, a uterine suspension should be performed. Again, this procedure can be carried out by laparoscopy or laparotomy. Appendectomy is indicated only when the appendix is obviously involved with endometriosis. When performing any, or all, of the above procedures, one should be aware that the subsequent pregnancy rate is not improved. Therefore, these procedures should be performed only when indicated.

Adjuvant therapies – prophylactic antibiotics, glucocorticoids, high molecular weight dextran, nonsteroidal antiinflammatory agents, progestational drugs, and the latest, an absorbable fabric composed of oxidized, regenerated cellulose – have all been used to reduce adhesion formation after any form of reconstructive pelvic surgery. Although each modality has its proponents, comparative studies are lacking and long-term efficacy for any of these adjuvant therapies has never been shown. As one adhesion prevention method loses its popularity, a new one seems to pop up, thus confirming that there is no totally successful method available today.

Preoperative or postoperative hormonal suppression

Although a paucity of data exists concerning the value of preoperative and/or postoperative hormonal suppression in dealing with moderate and severe endometriosis, many surgeons believe strongly in one or both of these extrasurgical approaches. *Preoperative* treatment may decrease pelvic vascularity and inflammation, thereby reducing intraoperative blood loss and postoperative adhesions. If endometriotic implants get smaller, removing them requires less dissection, thus tissue trauma is lessened. However, there are no existing studies showing that pregnancy rates are significantly better with the use of preoperative hormones than with surgery alone. *Postoperative* hormonal treatment eliminates residal disease in situations where it was impossible or ill-advised to remove all the implants. Additionally, microscopic disease might be suppressed. Although endometriosis recurrence rates vary from 2 to 47%, there are no studies available confirming that these recurrence rates are reduced by postoperative hormones.

Only improved therapeutic results should influence the decision to use *preoperative* and/or *postoperative* hormonal therapy. Either before or after surgery, danazol is the only drug that has been investigated. *Preoperatively*, all studies agree that danazol expedites the surgical technique, but its use does not improve postoperative pregnancy rates or decrease recurrence rates. Therefore, its expense, potential side-effects, and delay of surgery must be weighed carefully against its surgical benefit. No studies exist using GnRH agonist preoperatively. *Postoperatively*, few studies exist, but one retrospective study indicates that using 2–3 months of danazol after conservative surgery for severe endometriosis significantly improves the pregnancy rate. Using one retrospective study to justify therapeutic decisions is dangerous. Unless future studies show a clear-cut advantage of postoperative hormonal suppression over conservative surgery alone, its expense, potential side-effects, and ovulation suppression during an optimal time for conception contraindicate its use.

Therapy that preserves reproductive capacity

After laparoscopic diagnosis, staging, and, if accessible, initial therapy, symptomatic endometriosis in the woman who is not interested in fertility now but wishes to retain her reproductive potential should be treated with hormonal suppression. Except for a large and/or expanding endometrioma, conservative surgery should be avoided until infertility becomes an additive problem. If operative laparoscopy is used and visible endometriosis eliminated, the patient may become symptom-free. If endometriosis and symptoms still exist after laparoscopy or recur after operative laparoscopy, hormonal suppression should be utilized.

First-choice medications, combining effectiveness with low cost, should be *continuous* oral contraceptives or *oral* medroxyprogesterone acetate. Danazol, due to its increased side-effects and higher cost, should be reserved for second-line treatment, along with the GnRH agonists. As noted earlier, GnRH agonists, due to fewer side-effects and more convenient dosage forms, would be favored over danazol. Depomedroxyprogesterone acetate may be indicated in limited clinical situations.

Although pregnancy rates following the use of *oral contraceptives* are low, this relatively inexpensive form of therapy retains a front-line place in the suppression of endometriotic symptoms and signs. Any low-dose preparation (containing 50 µg or less of ethinylestradiol) with a high progestin:estrogen ratio can be selected, e.g., Ovral or Lo-Ovral. As it creates a pseudopregnancy state, the drug should be utilized *continuously* (daily) for 9 months.

A single tablet per day is sufficient. If breakthrough bleeding occurs, the dose can be doubled or tripled. The increased dosage should be continued until the bleeding has stopped. Then the dose can be dropped in a stepwise fashion back to the original. However, if bleeding recurs, the increased dosage necessary to stop it should be continued. Breakthrough bleeding may also be controlled by the short-term addition of 20 µg ethinylestradiol to the original regimen.

Obviously, any contraindications to oral contraceptives should be ascertained prior to the start of therapy. In addition, the patient should be informed that the hormonal therapy of endometriosis is suppressive rather than curative and, after an interval of nontreatment, repeat therapy may be indicated with increasing symptomatology.

The use of *medroxyprogesterone acetate* has several proponents. A daily dose of 30 mg (10 mg three times day) to 50 mg has been advocated. Irregular bleeding can occur in 30% of patients, but supplemental estrogen or an increase in the medroxyprogesterone acetate dose can usually control the problem. Other side-effects, usually mild, include nausea, breast tenderness, fluid retention, and depression. Significant pain relief occurs during therapy, but none of the studies with this drug has addressed duration of relief after cessation of treatment or the recurrence rate.

At this time, nafarelin acetate (Synarel) and leuprolide acetate (Lupron) are the only clinically available *GnRH agonists*. Both are Food and Drug Administration-approved for gynecologic use, specifically for endometriosis (pelvic pain; reduction of lesion size). Nafarelin is administered by nasal spray in a daily dose of 400 µg, 200 µg in one nostril in the morning and 200 µg in the other nostril in the evening. The drug is available in a 0.5-oz metered spray bottle containing 10 ml (2 mg/ml) that delivers 200 µg of nafarelin per spray. Leuprolide acetate is administered in a monthly depot dose of 3.75 mg every 28 days. For both drugs, treatment should be initiated between days 2 and 4 of the menstrual cycle. Hot flashes represent the most common side-effect of GnRH agonist therapy, occurring in 85–100% of patients. Less commonly seen side-effects include irregular bleeding, vaginal dryness, depression, headaches, and dyspareunia. After a treatment course of 6 months, menses usually return within 6–10 weeks of the last dose. GnRH agonists eliminate ovarian estrogen secretion creating a medical oophorectomy without the androgenic side-effects and adverse lipoprotein changes seen with danazol. Although the GnRH agonists do accelerate bone loss during a 6-month therapeutic course, the loss of bone mineral density is not significant and returns to normal with cessation of therapy.

Now far removed from the excitement and oversell generated by the drug's introduction over 12 years ago, it seems apparent that today danazol is just another pharmacologic agent in the polypharmacy of endometriosis therapy. When danazol is used to treat symptoms, 200 mg

3 or 4 times a day is the usual dose needed to create and maintain an amenorrheic state. Like the GnRH agonists, it is started between days 2 and 4 of the menstrual cycle and continued for 6 months. As with other steroidal suppressive treatments for endometriosis, danazol does not penetrate well into ovarian endometriomas and should be used with caution (informing the patient that the cyst might rupture despite hormonal therapy) in endometriomas >1 cm. More than three-quarters of patients receiving danazol will complain of one or more side-effects, and the most significant ones result from the induced hyperandrogenic state, e.g., weight gain, muscle cramps, decreased breast size, acne, oily skin, and depression. A more worrisome risk is that danazol reduces high-density lipoprotein (HDL) levels, and this reduction continues throughout the treatment period. With cessation of treatment, HDL levels return to normal pretreatment values within 8 weeks. With the availability of GnRH agonists (fewer side-effects and more convenient administration), danazol is rapidly falling out of the endometriosis therapeutic armamentarium.

When oral preparations and the GnRH agonists have failed or are not tolerated, intramuscular depomedroxyprogesterone acetate represents a viable alternative, especially in cases of deep-seated rectovaginal, bowel, and/or pelvic side wall endometriosis. It is administered initially with 100 mg/week × four doses, then 100 mg bimonthly × two doses, then 100 mg/month × 10 doses. Side-effects include weight gain, breakthrough bleeding (25–30%), and posttherapy amenorrhea (20–25%). The patient who wishes immediate resumption of fertility upon completion of therapy should be cautioned that ovulatory medication may be necessary if amenorrhea follows treatment.

Therapy following completion of child-bearing

For the woman with moderate or severe pelvic endometriosis who has completed her family, a total abdominal hysterectomy is the therapeutic choice. *If the ovaries are involved* or other endometriotic areas remain, a bilateral salpingo-oophorectomy should be performed. Any remaining endometriosis will become fibrotic and scar without ovarian stimulation. *If the ovaries must be preserved*, e.g., in a young woman or by patient desire, and residual endometriosis is present, postoperative hormonal suppression should be used for 6–9 months, depending on the therapeutic agent selected.

After hysterectomy and bilateral salpingo-oophorectomy, estrogen replacement therapy can be used. However, as low a dose as possible should be prescribed. If residual endometriosis remains *after* removal of the uterus and ovaries, oral contraceptive therapy or depomedroxyprogesterone acetate, rather than estrogen alone, should be given for 6 months. Otherwise, the estrogen-only therapy could activate any residual disease.

SUGGESTED READING

EVERS JLH. The pregnancy rate of the no-treatment group in randomized clinical trials of endometriosis therapy. *Fertil Steril* 1989;52:906.

GANT NF. Infertility and endometriosis: comparison of pregnancy outcomes with laparotomy versus laparoscopic techniques. *Am J Obstet Gynecol* 1992;166:1072.

HULL ME, MOGHISSI KS, MAGYAR DF, HAYES MF. Comparison of different treatment modalities of endometriosis in infertile women. *Fertil Steril* 1987;47:40.

KEYE WR Jr, HANSEN LW, ASTIN M, POULSON AM Jr. Argon laser therapy of endometriosis: a review of 92 consecutive patients. *Fertil Steril* 1987;47:208.

LUCIANO AA, TURKSOY RN, CARLEO J. Evaluation of oral medroxyprogesterone acetate in the treatment of endometriosis. *Obstet Gynecol* 1988;72:323.

MELDRUM DR. Management of endometriosis with gonadotropin-releasing hormone agonists. *Fertil Steril* 1985;44:581.

MOGHISSI KS, BOYCE CR. Management of endometriosis with oral medroxy-progesterone acetate. *Obstet Gynecol* 1976;47:265.

OLIVE DL, MARTIN DC. Treatment of endometriosis-associated infertility with CO_2 laser laparoscopy: the use of one- and two-parameter exponential models. *Fertil Steril* 1987;48:18.

PORTUONDO JA, ECHANOJAUREGUI AD, HERRAN C, ALIJARTE I. Early conception in patients with untreated mild endometriosis. *Fertil Steril* 1983;39:22.

SCHENKEN RS. *Endometriosis: Contemporary Concepts in Clinical Management.* Philadelphia: JB Lippincott, 1989.

SCHENKEN RS, MALINAK CR. Conservative surgery verus expectant management for the infertile patient with mild endometriosis. *Fertil Steril* 1982;37:183.

SCHMIDT CL. Endometriosis: a reappraisal of pathogenesis and treatment. *Fertil Steril* 1985;44:157.

STEINGOLD KA, CEDARS M, LU JKH, RANDLE D, JUDD HL, MELDRUM DR. Treatment of endometriosis with a long-acting gonadotropin-releasing hormone agonist. *Obstet Gynecol* 1987;69:403.

WHEELER JM, MALINAK CR. Postoperative danazol therapy in infertility patients with severe endometriosis. *Fertil Steril* 1981;36:460.

113

Recurrent abortion

DANIEL R. MISHELL, JR

The expected probability of a woman having three consecutive spontaneous abortions is about 0.3–0.4%, but the actual incidence is reported
to range from 0.4 to 0.8%, indicating that there is a specific cause for
recurrent pregnancy loss in some women.

The abortuses of women who have three or more abortions are more
likely to be chromosomally normal (80–90%) than those of women
with a single spontaneous abortion. Women with recurrent abortions also
have a tendency to abort later in gestation, with two-thirds of such
abortions occurring beyond 12 weeks' gestation, indicating that maternal
or environmental factors are a more likely cause of repeated pregnancy
loss. Recurrent abortion is also called *habitual abortion*, but this term
implies that every pregnancy will end in an abortion. If a woman has had
no live births and three abortions, she has about a 50% chance of having
a term gestation in her next pregnancy, and if she has had one live birth,
this chance is increased to about 70%. Thus the term habitual abortion
should not be used.

Couples with recurrent abortion require careful, sympathetic management by the practitioner, because an abortion is an emotionally traumatic
experience that can result in as much grief as intrauterine fetal death in
late pregnancy or a neonatal death. With recurrent abortion this emotional trauma is magnified, and the practitioner needs to express sympathy
and understanding as counseling is performed and a diagnostic regimen
is outlined.

Because the etiology of a second-trimester loss is more likely to be
uterine in origin and thus more likely to be able to be diagnosed, a

diagnostic evaluation should be performed after a woman has had only one second-trimester spontaneous abortion. There is no need to wait for a woman to have three first-trimester abortions with their accompanying emotional trauma before beginning a diagnostic evaluation. Because one early abortion is relatively common, it is recommended that diagnostic evaluation be initiated only after a woman has two first-trimester abortions.

After a history and physical examination are performed with pertinent questions regarding cervical incompetence, a complete blood count, a serum thyroid-stimulating hormone, and a mid luteal serum progesterone measurement should be obtained. A hysterogram should be performed to rule out congenital uterine anomalies, submucous leiomyomas, and intrauterine adhesions.

Diabetes mellitus

Although uncontrolled diabetes mellitus has been associated with an increased abortion rate, Crane and Wahl found the incidence of spontaneous abortion was similar in groups of women with either gestational diabetes (12.3%) or frank diabetes (12.2%) and matched control groups (10.9 and 14.5%). In this study the diabetes was controlled with insulin. They also reported that the number of women with multiple spontaneous abortions was similar in the diabetic and control groups. Thus it appears that diabetes, when controlled by diet or insulin, is not a cause of abortion. However, diabetes without good metabolic control is associated with an increased risk of early pregnancy loss, and a direct correlation exists between the level of hemoglobin A_1 and the rate of abortion.

Thyroid disease

Although older studies indicate that hypothyroidism may be a cause of abortion, a study by Montoro *et al.* reported that no abortions occurred in 11 pregnancies of nine markedly hypothyroid women. In three recent studies of large numbers of women with recurrent abortion, only a few women in one of the studies were found to have abnormal thyroid function. There is no definitive evidence that hypothyroidism is a cause of abortion in humans.

Luteal deficiency

Several investigators have treated women with recurrent abortion and evidence of luteal deficiency with progesterone vaginal suppositories 25 mg twice daily or intramuscular progesterone 12.5 mg/day beginning 3 days after ovulation and continuing throughout the first trimester. With this treatment, term pregnancy rates have been reported to range from 80 to 90%. However, no randomized placebo studies have been reported to verify the effectiveness of progesterone in preventing abortion in women with luteal insufficiency.

There is no evidence that administration of synthetic progestins, which themselves may be luteolytic, is of benefit in reducing the incidence of abortion. There is also no benefit to be derived by initiating progesterone therapy after the expected menstrual period is missed, especially if the women develop symptoms of threatened abortion. Low progesterone levels at this time are a result, not the cause, of the abortion.

Uterine cavity synechiae

Adhesions in the uterine cavity can cause partial or complete obliteration of the endometrium leading to menstrual abnormalities and amenorrhea, as well as being a cause of abortion. The latter is thought to be the result of insufficient endometrium to support adequate fetal growth. The major cause of adhesions is curettage of the endometrial cavity in association with a pregnancy or in the early puerperium.

The recommended treatment for intrauterine adhesions is lysis of the adhesions by miniature scissors during hysteroscopy. After adhesion lysis, either an intrauterine device or small Foley catheter is usually placed in the cavity, and high-dose estrogen (conjugated equine estrogen 2.5 mg b.i.d.) is administered for 60 days. Medroxyprogesterone acetate 10 mg/day is added for the last 5–10 days, and then the foreign body is removed. March and Israel reported that the abortion rate decreased from 83 to 13% after hysterographic lysis of adhesions.

Cervical incompetence

The diagnosis of cervical incompetence is best made by a history of second-trimester pregnancy loss accompanied by spontaneous rupture of the fetal membranes without preceding uterine contractions. Cervical incompetence has been found to be associated with uterine anomalies, particularly uterus didelphus, as well as with anomalies produced by fetal diethylstilbestrol (DES) exposure.

The best treatment of cervical incompetence is placement of a concentric nonabsorbable silk or Mersilene suture at the level of the internal os (cerclage), using either the technique described by Shirodkar or McDonald. Because, as reported by Harger, these techniques yield a similar rate of success, with the rate of fetal survival increasing from about 20% before suture placement to 80% after the cerclage procedure, the McDonald procedure is preferable, since this procedure is technically easier and is associated with less morbidity than the Shirodkar technique. It is recommended that the suture be placed electively between 12 and 14 weeks of gestation after major embryogenesis has been completed and the incidence of spontaneous abortion caused by genetic abnormality has markedly lessened. An ultrasound examination should be performed before cerclage to document a normal gestation. Occasionally, if there is a markedly shortened cervix or placement of the McDonald cerclage has failed to maintain the pregnancy, a transabdominal cerclage, as described by Benson and Durfee, should be performed. If the suture is placed externally, it is usually removed at 38 weeks' gestation, and vaginal delivery allowed. However, because of cervical scarring, cesarean section is required in about 15% of pregnancies.

Acquired uterine defects

Uterine leiomyomas, especially if they are submucosal, can be associated with repetitive abortion. Although a causal relationship is difficult to establish, in a review of the literature, Buttram and Reiter reported that when myomectomy was performed for recurrent abortion in a total of 1941 women, the spontaneous abortion rate was reduced from 41 to 19%. These data indicate that, on occasion, uterine leiomyomas are a cause of abortion.

Surgical correction of bicornuate and septate uteri is possible by using one of the transfundal metroplasty techniques described by Strassman, Jones, or Tompkins or by transcervical hysteroscopic resection of the uterine septum.

March and Israel reported that it was possible to incise the septum, even those thicker than 1 cm, of all 82 women with recurrent abortion, using flexible scissors placed transcervically through the hysteroscope. After this treatment the abortion rate declined from 95 to 13%. Because these results are as good as or better than those for an abdominal metroplasty without the need to perform a laparotomy or subsequent cesarean section, hysteroscopic incision should now be the treatment of choice for the septate uterus.

The endometrial cavity of women exposed to DES *in utero* has a significantly smaller surface area than normal, which could perhaps contribute to the increased spontaneous abortion rate in women exposed to DES *in utero*. No therapy, including routine uterine cerclage, has been shown to be beneficial in lowering the abortion rate in women exposed to DES who have chromosomal abnormalities of the uterine cavity and recurrent abortion. In published surveys of couples with two or more pregnancy losses, the composite prevalence of major chromosome abnormalities in either parent is about 3%, which is 5–6 times higher than the general population. Abnormalities occurred in the female parent about twice as frequently as the male. About half of all chromosomic abnormalities were balanced reciprocal translocations, and one-fourth were Robertonian translocations. About 12% were sex chromosomal mosaicism in the female, and the rest were inversions and other sporadic abnormalities. Thus both members of couples with two or more spontaneous abortions should be karyotyped. If translocation is found in one parent, about 80% of their pregnancies will abort. If abortion does not occur in a subsequent pregnancy, fetal cytogenic studies are indicated, because there is about a 3–5% incidence of unbalanced fetal karyotype in these gestations.

Immunologic factors

The foreign antigens produced by the fetus should cause it to be rejected by the mother's immune system. Although some protection from this immunologic effect is offered by progesterone, it has been hypothesized by Rocklin *et al.* and others that a maternal blocking factor, an immunoglobulin G (IgG) antibody, coats the foreign fetal antigens and prevents the fetus from being rejected. These investigators reported that women with recurrent abortion lacked this blocking factor.

Several recent studies could not confirm as a cause of abortion the sharing of major HLAs, which may cause the maternal immune system to fail to produce blocking antibodies. Caudle *et al.* and Houwert-de Jong *et al.* found no difference in the degree of HLA sharing in couples with recurrent abortion and a control group. Smith and Cowchock likewise found no difference in the incidence of HLA-sharing between a group of couples with recurrent spontaneous abortion whose etiology for the condition was determined and another group whose etiology could not be determined. Sargent *et al.* performed a prospective study of couples with recurrent abortion before and after conception and found no difference in the incidence of HLA-sharing among the couples who subsequently had a successful pregnancy and those whose pregnancies aborted. Furthermore, they could not confirm that, after pregnancy occurred in these women, as well as in normal controls, there was an increase in production of maternal immunologic factors to fetal (paternal) HLAs.

However, Mowbray *et al.* performed a randomized treatment trial in a group of women with recurrent abortion and no detectable antibody against paternal lymphocytes. Women injected with paternal white cells had a significantly greater chance of a subsequent successful pregnancy (78%) than those injected with their own white cells (37%). However, in the study by Smith and Cowchock, after immunization of women with recurrent abortion of unknown etiology with paternal white cells, the rate of successful pregnancy was only 50%, similar to the 62% rate reported by Houwert-de Jong *et al.* in a group of women with a history of recurrent abortion who received no treatment. Furthermore, in the former study, after immunization the outcome of the pregnancy was not related to the development of blocking antibodies. Four other randomized studies of infusion of women with recurrent abortion with their husband's white cells or trophoblast revealed no difference in subsequent abortion rates compared with placebo infusion. Thus the data regarding an immunologic cause of abortion are conflicting, with the majority of the evidence failing to confirm an immunologic etiology. For this reason, at present it is not cost-effective or necessary to perform the expensive HLA typing of each member of the couple with a history of recurrent abortion. Immunization of the wife with her husband's white blood cells should be performed only under experimental protocols with informed consent, because the procedure has not been proven to be beneficial and sequelae of white blood cell transfusion can have serious adverse effects.

Lupus anticoagulant activity and antiphospholipid (anticardiolipin) antibodies

The presence of lupus anticoagulant activity, as well as elevated levels of certain antiphospholipid antibodies, particularly the anticardiolipin antibody, has been found to be associated with an increased rate of spontaneous abortion and intrauterine fetal death. These antibodies are immunoglobulins of the IgG or IgM class. Although *in vitro* these immunoglobulins have anticoagulant activity by interfering with activation of the prothrombin activator complex and thus prolonging the partial thromboplastin time, clinically the presence of these antibodies is associated with thrombosis. Although the exact mechanism for an increased incidence of thrombosis is not known, some investigators have shown that, when the antibody is present, it inhibits prostacyclin production from endothelial tissues, leading to a relative excess of thromboxane, which could enhance thrombosis. The presence of lupus anticoagulant activity is usually documented by performing an activated partial thromboplastin time (aPTT). If the test is prolonged, an equal amount of normal plasma is added to the patient's plasma and the aPTT is repeated. If it is still prolonged, the presence of lupus anticoagulant is likely and can be confirmed by correcting the aPTT with addition of phospholipid. The antiphospholipid antibodies that are associated with lupus anticoagulant activity bind several phospholipids, including cardiolipin. The majority of patients with lupus anticoagulant activity, but not all, also have anticardiolipid antibodies. The presence of the anticardiolipin antibody, as well as other antiphospholipid antibodies, can be determined by specific solid-phase or enzyme-linked immunoassays.

Deleze *et al.* reported that about 80% of women with systemic lupus erythomatosus and recurrent fetal loss had antiphospholipid antibodies, whereas they were present in only 15% of women with systemic lupus erythematosus without fetal loss. These antibodies are found also in women: (1) with other immunologic disease; (2) with subclinical auto-immune disease; and (3) with recurrent abortion, thrombosis, or throm-bocytopenia. Several groups have reported that lupus anticoagulant activity is found in about 10% of women with recurrent spontaneous abortion of undetermined etiology, although other investigators report that its prevalence in such women may reach 50%. Anticardiolipin antibody has been reported to occur in 13–40% of such individuals. Lockwood *et al.* reported that the presence of lupus anticoagulant in a normal obstetric population was only about 0.3%, and about 2% of these women had anticardiolipin antibodies. It thus appears that tests to detect the presence of both lupus anticoagulant activity and anticardiolipin antibody should be performed in individuals with recurrent abortions, since a causal relation apparently exists.

Currently there is no general agreement about therapy for individuals with recurrent abortion and the presence of lupus anticoagulant activity or anticardiolipid antibodies. Investigators have used corticosteroids, aspirin, heparin, or various combinations of these agents. Corticosteroids suppress the levels of antiphospholipid antibodies, and aspirin inhibits platelet aggregation. According to a recent review by Reece *et al.*, the most widely used therapeutic regimen is daily ingestion of 20–60 mg of prednisone with 75–80 mg of aspirin. Although the total number of patients treated with this regimen reported in the literature to date is relatively small (about 100), in their summary Reece *et al.* found that the overall live birth rate with this therapy was about 80%. Nevertheless, no prospective, randomized, double-blind, placebo-controlled trials have been reported to date to document that such therapy is responsible for increasing the live birth rate. Furthermore, serious maternal, as well as fetal, complications have been reported to occur when high-dose cortico-steroid therapy is given throughout pregnancy. In a small group of women with recurrent abortion who had antiphospholipd antibodies, a multicenter randomized trial of treatment with corticosteroids and aspirin or heparin and aspirin yielded a 75% live birth rate with both regimens. The preterm birth rate and incidence of preeclampsia were higher in the group treated with corticosteroids. No placebo group was included. Therefore these therapies, although shown to be successful in several small series, must still be regarded as investigational. Precise therapeutic regimens have not been established, but, if used, the smallest dose of corticosteroid or heparin that corrects the aPPT should be given, and the dose should be adjusted periodically throughout gestation according to aPPT levels. The initial dose of heparin is usually 10 000 U given subcutaneously every 12 h.

In conclusion, tests to detect lupus anticoagulant activity and anti-phospholipid antibodies should probably be performed, but there is no evidence in randomized studies that treatment of patients with this disorder is better than no treatment.

Therapy

If any of the diagnostic tests discussed above reveals an abnormality that can be corrected with appropriate surgical or medical therapy as described, such therapy should be initiated. If a chromosomal abnormality is found, genetic counseling should be indicated. There have been three series of large numbers of couples with recurrent abortion who have undergone a comprehensive diagnostic evaluation. Although different criteria for abnormal diagnostic tests were used by each group of investigators, no specific etiologic factor for the recurrent abortion (all tests normal) was found in 35–44% of the couples studied.

If no diagnosis can be obtained, the couple should be counseled regarding the probability of abortion in a subsequent pregnancy. After conception, measurement of human chorionic gonadotropin (hCG) levels twice weekly will allow early prognosis of the outcome of the pregnancy. In normal gestations the levels of hCG double about every 2 days, and the rate of increase in a particular patient can be compared with the expected normal rate of increase. In most individuals with an early abortion, levels of hCG will rise at a slower rate than normal, plateau, and then decline. Batzer *et al.* found that, when β-hCG doubling time in the first month of gestation was normal, it predicted a good outcome 88% of the time, and, when abnormal, predicted a poor outcome 76% of the time. If hCG levels are increasing normally, an ultrasound examination should be performed after they reach 2500 mIU/ml, at which time a gestational sac should be found. A repeat ultrasound 2 weeks later should demonstrate a normal fetal heart rate. These findings are reassuring, both to the mother and to the clinician.

Some individuals recommend that prophylactic antibiotic treatment be given to the husband and wife in the conception cycle or that progesterone supplementation be given to all women with recurrent abortion in the first trimester of pregnancy. Neither of these modalities has been demonstrated to improve the outcome of the pregnancy, but strong emotional support and counseling are important for these patients.

SUGGESTED READING

AXELSSON G, RYLANDER R. Exposure to anesthetic gases and spontaneous abortion: response bias in a postal questionnaire study. *Int J Epidemiol* 1982; 11:250.

BATZER FR, SCHLAFF S, GOLDFARB AF, *et al.* Serial β-subunit human chorionic gonadotropin doubling times as a prognosticator of pregnancy outcome in an infertile population. *Fertil Steril* 1981;35:307.

BENSON RC, DURFEE RB. Transabdominal cervicouterine cerclage during pregnancy for the treatment of cervical incompetency. *Obstet Gynecol* 1965;25:145.

BUTTRAM VC Jr, GIBBONS WE. Mullerian anomalies: a proposed classification (an analysis of 144 cases). *Fertil Steril* 1979;32:40.

BUTTRAM VC Jr, REITER RC. Uterine leiomyomata: etiology, symptomatology, and management. *Fertil Steril* 1981;36:433.

CAUDLE MR, ROTE NS, SCOTT JR, *et al.* Histocompatibility in couples with recurrent spontaneous abortion and normal fertility. *Fertil Steril* 1983;39:793.

CRANE JP, WAHL N. The role of maternal diabetes in repetitive spontaneous abortion. *Fertil Steril* 1981;36:477.

DeCHERNEY AH, RUSSELL JB, GRAEBE RA, *et al.* Resectoscopic management of mullerian fusion defects. *Fertil Steril* 1986;45:726.

DELEZE M, ALARCON-SEGOVIA D, VALDES-MACHO E, ORIA CV, PONCE DE LEON S. Relationship between antiphospholipid antibodies and recurrent fetal loss in patients with systemic lupus erythematosus and apparently healthy women. *J Rheumatol* 1989;16:768–772.

HANEY AF, HAMMOND CB, SOULES MR, *et al.* Diethylstilbestrol-induced upper genital tract abnormalities. *Fertil Steril* 1979;31:142.

HARLAP S, SHIONO PH. Alcohol, smoking, and incidence of spontaneous abortions in the first and second trimester. *Lancet* 1980;2:173–180.

HEINONEN PK, SAARIKOSKI S, PYSTYNEN P. Reproductive performance of women with uterine anomalies. *Acta Obstet Gynecol Scand* 1982;61:157.

HENSLEIGH PA, FAINSTAT T. Corpus luteum dysfunction: serum progesterone levels in diagnosis and assessment of therapy for recurrent and threatened abortion. *Fertil Steril* 1979;32:396.

HORTA JLH, FERNANDEZ JG, SOTO DE LEON B, *et al.* Direct evidence of luteal insufficiency in women with habitual abortion. *Obstet Gynecol* 1977;49:705.

HOUWERT-DE JONG MH, TERMIJTELEN A, ESKES TKAB, MANTINGH A, BRUINSE HW. The natural course of habitual abortion. *Eur J Obstet Gynecol Reprod Biol* 1989;33:221–228.

JAMES WH. On the possibility of segregation in the propensity to spontaneous abortion in the human female. *Ann Hum Genet* 1961;25:207.

KAJII T, FERRIER A, NIIKAWA N, *et al.* Anatomic and chromosomal anomalies in 639 spontaneous abortuses. *Hum Genet* 1980;55:87.

KAUFMAN RH, NOLLER K, ADAM E, *et al.* Upper genital tract abnormalities and pregnancy outcome in diethylstilbestrol-exposed progeny. *Am J Obstet Gynecol* 1984;148:973.

KLINE J, STEIN ZA, SUSSER M, *et al.* Smoking: a risk factor for spontaneous abortion. *N Engl J Med* 1977;297:793.

KLINE J, SHROUT P, STEIN ZA, *et al.* Drinking during pregnancy and spontaneous abortion. *Lancet* 1980;2:176.

LOCKWOOD CJ, ROMERO R, FEINBERG RF, CLYNE LP, COSTER B, HOBBINS JC.

The prevalence and biologic significance of lupus anticoagulant and anticardiolipin antibodies in a general obstetric population. *Am J Obstet Gynecol* 1989;161: 369–373.

MALPAS P. A study of abortion sequences. *Br J Obstet Gynaecol* 1938;45:932.

MANN EC. Habitual abortion. *Am J Obstet Gynecol* 1959;77:706.

MARCH CM, ISRAEL R. Gestational outcome following hysteroscopic lysis of adhesions. *Fertil Steril* 1981;36:455.

MARCH CM, ISRAEL R. Hysteroscopic management of recurrent abortion cause to septate uterus. *Am J Obstet Gynecol* 1987;156:834–842.

MILLS JL, SIMPSON JL, DRISCOLL SG, *et al.* Incidence of spontaneous abortion among normal women and insulin-dependent diabetic women whose pregnancies were identified within 21 days of conception. *N Engl J Med* 1988;319: 1618–1623.

MONTORO M, COLLEA JV, FRASIER D, *et al.* Successful outcome of pregnancy in women with hypothyroidism. *Ann Intern Med* 1981;94:31.

MOWBRAY JF, BIGGINS C, LIDDELL H, *et al.* Controlled trial of treatment of recurrent spontaneous abortion by immunization with paternal cells. *Lancet* 1985;1:941.

MUSICH JR Jr, BEHRMAN SJ. Obstetric outcome before and after metroplasty in women with uterine anomalies. *Obstet Gynecol* 1978;52:63.

POLAND BJ, MILLER JR, JONES DC, *et al.* Reproductive counseling in patients who have had a spontaneous abortion. *Am J Obstet Gynecol* 1977;127:685.

REECE EA, GABRIELLI S, CULLEN MT, *et al.* Recurrent adverse pregnancy outcome and antiphospholipid antibodies. *Am J Obstet Gynecol* 1990;163:162.

REGAN L, BRAUDE PR, TREMBATH PL. Influence of past reproductive performance on risk of spontaneous abortion. *Br Med J* 1989;299:541–545.

ROCK JA, JONES HW. The clinical management of the double uterus. *Fertil Steril* 1977;28:798.

ROCKLIN RE, KITZMILLER JL, CARPENTER CB, *et al.* Maternal–fetal relation: absence of an immunologic blocking factor from the serum of women with chronic abortions. *N Engl J Med* 1976;295:1209.

SARGENT IL, WILKINS T, REDMAN CWG. Maternal immune responses to the fetus in early pregnancy and recurrent miscarriage. *Lancet* 1988;2:1099–1104.

SMITH JB, COWCHOCK FS. Immunological studies in recurrent spontaneous abortion: effects of immunization of women with paternal mononuclear cells on lymphocytotoxic and mixed lymphocyte reaction blocking antibodies and correlation with sharing of HLA and pregnancy outcome. *J Reprod Immunol* 1988;14: 99–113.

STEIN Z, KLINE J, SUSSER E, *et al.* Maternal age and spontaneous abortion. In: Porter IH, Hook EB, eds. *Human Embryonic and Fetal Death.* New York: Academic Press, 1980.

STRAY-PEDERSEN B, ENG J, REIKVAM TM. Uterine T-mycoplasma colonization in reproductive failure. *Am J Obstet Gynecol* 1978;130:307.

STRAY-PEDERSEN B, STRAY-PEDERSEN S. Etiologic factors and subsequent reproductive performance in 195 couples with a prior history of habitual abortion. *Am J Obstet Gynecol* 1984;148:140.

THARAPEL AT, THARAPEL SA, BANNERMAN RM. Recurrent pregnancy losses and parental chromosome abnormalities: a review. *Br J Obstet Gynaecol* 1985;92:899–914.

VIANNA NJ. Adverse pregnancy outcomes–potential endpoints of human toxicity in the Love Canal preliminary results. In: Porter IH, Hook EB, eds. *Human Embryonic and Fetal Death*. New York: Academic Press, 1980:165–168.

WARBURTON D, FRASER FC. Spontaneous abortion risks in man: data from reproductive histories collected in a medical genetics unit. *Am J Hum Genet* 1964;16:1.

WILCOX AJ, WEINBERG CR, O'CONNOR JF, *et al*. Incidence of early loss of pregnancy. *N Engl J Med* 1988;319:189–194.

114

Luteal-phase defects

CHARLES M. MARCH

Virtually every aspect of the topic of luteal-phase defects remains controversial. The definition, incidence, pathophysiology, effects, methods of diagnosis, and modes of therapy and their efficacy all have yet to be clarified completely.

A luteal-phase defect is defined as abnormal corpus luteum function associated with insufficient progesterone production. The deficiency may be in the amount of progesterone produced per day and/or in the duration of progesterone production. Estrogen production often remains normal. Classically, there are two types of luteal-phase defects: the short luteal phase (SLP) and the inadequate luteal phase (ILP). These defects have been reported in women with infertility and in those with recurrent abortion.

The short luteal phase

Women with a SLP have short ovulatory menstrual cycles, due entirely to a reduction (<10 days) in the interval between the luteinizing hormone (LH) peak and the onset of menses. In SLP patients, the patterns of follicle-stimulating hormone (FSH) and LH secretion during the menstrual cycle are normal, but the mean FSH levels and the FSH:LH ratios are reduced. The intercycle rise in FSH is reduced significantly. The peak serum concentrations of progesterone are lower and occur earlier. If an endometrial biopsy is performed and the histology of the endometrium is correlated with the LH peak or the basal body temperature (BBT) shift, the endometrial response will be in phase.

Strott *et al.* demonstrated that this defect occurs commonly in young women and may represent insufficient maturation of the hypothalamic–pituitary–ovarian axis. It is uncertain if the SLP plays a significant role in infertility, but if this defect were severe, follicular development and corpus luteum function would be grossly abnormal and infertility would result.

Treatment should be directed toward increasing the extent of FSH stimulation very early in the menstrual cycle. Clomiphene citrate (Clomid, Serophene) should be prescribed as discussed below. If this fails to restore normal luteal function, low doses (one or two ampules/day) of human menopausal gonadotropins (hMG, Pergonal) should be given beginning on day 1 of the cycle. In milder forms of the SLP, the corpus luteum can probably be maintained by the endogenous human chorionic gonadotropin (hCG) produced by a recently implanted blastocyst, and therapy would not be indicated.

The inadequate luteal phase

In contrast to the SLP, the ILP does have a significant effect upon reproductive performance. It occurs in menstrual cycles of normal length in which inadequate amounts of progesterone are produced. The diagnosis of the ILP is most difficult; various authors have used different, arbitrary criteria that do not correlate well. Abnormal follicular-phase LH secretion has been reported in patients with histologically proven luteal-phase defects, suggesting that, like the SLP, this abnormality has a central origin.

The classical diagnosis of ILP depends upon the interpretation of a properly timed endometrial biopsy. There is little risk of interrupting a pregnancy if an endometrial biopsy is obtained in the luteal phase, provided that only a single anterior or lateral fundal sample is taken. However, if a barrier method of contraception is not used during the biopsy cycle, a rapid serum pregnancy test sensitive to 5 mIU/ml should be obtained prior to performing the biopsy. The histologic pattern of the endometrium must be correlated with the apparent day of ovulation. The date of the BBT shift, the LH surge in urine or serum, changes detected by ultrasound, or the date of hCG administration may be used to mark the beginning of the luteal phase. These techniques are more reliable than using the date of the next menstrual period's onset.

For a diagnosis of ILP, the histologic pattern should be >2 days behind the expected pattern in at least two cycles. An out-of-phase endometrium has been reported to occur in one cycle in up to 20% of women. But if two cycles are examined, the incidence falls to <3%. Thus, because occasional lags in endometrial histology are frequent in normal women and because endometrial dating is imprecise and can vary depending on interpretations of different pathologists, the defect must be documented in two or more cycles. Recently, the frequency of an out-of-phase biopsy result was reported to vary depending upon both the type of instrument used to obtain the specimen and the individual interpreting the specimen.

To establish the diagnosis, the endometrial biopsy is best obtained 12 days after the estimated day of ovulation, i.e., on day 26 of an idealized 28-day cycle. At this time, almost the entire estrogen and progesterone secretion by the ovary has been completed. Therefore, the endometrium reflects most of the steroid production of that cycle.

Single, multiple, and even daily luteal-phase progesterone assays have also been used to diagnose the ILP. If only histologic criteria are used, not all women with reduced luteal-phase progesterone production will be detected. Although total luteal-phase progesterone production is reduced in women with retarded histologic patterns, the overlap with patients with normal biopsies is too great to permit easy discrimination. Thus, some investigators have rejected the biopsy criteria and have used a single peak luteal-phase serum concentration of <10 or 15 ng/ml. Others use three pooled specimens from between postovulatory days 4 and 11, and consider a level <15 ng/ml diagnostic. It is likely that a continuum of defects is being detected by these different techniques. Because serum progesterone concentrations and endometrial histology do not always correlate, both should be obtained in the same cycle. The progesterone level is obtained 7 days after the thermogenic shift. If it is 10 ng/ml or greater, a biopsy is performed 5 days thereafter. Both are correlated with the day of the basal body temperature use and the first day of the next menses. Home urinary LH measurements or ovarian ultrasound may be substituted for the BBT record to establish the day of ovulation. If the peak serum progesterone level is low (5 ng/ml or less), treatment with clomiphene citrate should be prescribed and a biopsy performed only after the mid luteal-phase progesterone level is ≥15 ng/ml.

Atypical BBT charts showing a "stepladder" pattern or erratic shifts cannot be used to establish the diagnosis of ILP. The BBT does not reflect a specific serum progesterone concentration, and a maximal increase in BBT may occur with a serum progesterone level of only 3 ng/ml.

The incidence of the ILP is unknown. It probably occurs in only a very small percentage of infertile patients, perhaps <2%. However, ILP is more commonly associated with recurrent abortion. Now that the more sensitive β-subunit assays for hCG are available, the true incidence of occult abortions may become known. It is likely that the etiology in some cases of recurrent occult abortion involves a luteal-phase defect. The cause of reproductive failure in women with luteal-phase defects is uncertain. Progesterone deficiency may interfere with tubal transport mechanisms, uterine motility, and/or proper development of the nidation site.

Etiology

Luteal-phase defects may have their origin in the central nervous system or are secondary to hypothalamic lesions or pituitary, ovarian, or endometrial causes. Because the roles of higher cerebral centers and the hypothalamus are poorly understood at this time, only pituitary, ovarian, and endometrial causes will be considered.

Pituitary causes

Four types of pituitary lesions may lead to luteal insufficiency: (1) inadequate or asynchronous FSH/LH stimulation during the follicular phase or, more importantly, during the luteal phase of the preceding menstrual cycle; (2) asynchronous or inadequate surges of LH at mid-cycle; (3) inadequate luteal-phase LH stimulation to maintain the corpus luteum, either primary; or (4) secondary to sustained hyperprolactinemia. It has been demonstrated that elevated prolactin levels interfere with progesterone synthesis by the corpus luteum. Additionally, a number of investigators have reported that some patients with luteal-phase defects have hyperprolactinemia. Treatment with the dopamine receptor agonist bromocriptine (Parlodel) has been used with some degree of success.

Ovarian causes

There are four possible ovarian causes of luteal-phase defects: (1) chromosome abnormalities associated with reduced numbers of follicles and, therefore, inadequate steroidogenesis; (2) recruitment and development of an insufficient number of follicles during the early follicular phase of the menstrual cycle; (3) inadequate ovarian response to a normal gonadotropin stimulus; and (4) poor corpus luteum function secondary to defective or inadequate numbers of ovarian LH receptors.

Endometrial causes

An endometrial lesion can cause an apparent luteal insufficiency. Such a defect would not satisfy the definition of an inadequate corpus luteum, but the histologic pattern would be the same. With a defect in endometrial receptors, the response to normal sex hormone stimulation would be reduced and recurrent abortion or infertility would result.

Treatment

Five modalities of therapy have been recommended most often to treat the inadequate luteal phase: (1) progesterone; (2) hCG; (3) clomiphene; (4) hMG; and (5) bromocriptine. Isolated reports of treatment with FSH, gonadotropin-releasing hormone, and other progestins do not indicate improved efficiency.

Progesterone therapy may be started with one 25-mg suppository* inserted intravaginally b.i.d. beginning on the day of BBT rise and continuing until menses begin. If pregnancy occurs, therapy should continue until the 10th week of gestation. This time period extends somewhat beyond the time when placental steroidogenesis replaces that of the corpus luteum. Progesterone in oil may be used, 12.5 mg im daily, for the same duration as described for the suppositories. Oral micronized progesterone, 200 mg b.i.d., has also been utilized but no data are available to demonstrate efficacy.

Parenteral hCG 2500–5000 IU may be administered every other day beginning on the day of BBT rise, for the same duration as described for progesterone. This therapy is less successful than progesterone substitution because it cannot maintain an abnormal corpus luteum. hCG can only be used for patients whose lesions are mild and are central in origin. One successful end-point of therapy is a normal endometrium. Therefore, the adequacy of therapy can be documented by repeating the endometrial biopsy after treatment has been initiated.

Although clomiphene citrate has been recommended by some authors for management of the ILP, it has also been incriminated as causing ovulatory cycles with luteal-phase insufficiency. The latter claim has not been well substantiated.

Treatment is begun with one 50-mg tablet on day 2 of the menstrual cycle and continued for 5 days. The onset of treatment is earlier than the conventional schedule of clomiphene administration for ovulation induction. It is employed to provide an early FSH surge necessary for follicular recruitment and development. If the diagnosis was established by a low luteal-phase progesterone level, the progesterone assay should be repeated during the treatment cycle to verify correction. The daily dose of clomiphene should be maintained if normalcy has been restored. If the defect persists, the dose should be increased sequentially in 50-mg/day increments in each successive cycle until correction has been achieved.

---

*Progesterone suppositories are not commercially available and must be made by a pharmacist. Suppositories with a concentration of 25 mg each are made using this formula: progesterone powder, 25 mg per suppository, in a water-soluble base of polyethylene glycol 400, USP, 60%, and polyethylene glycol 6000, USP, 40%. A rectal suppository mold is used.

Other luteal-phase defects may respond to therapy with hMG in low doses. This therapy may be used if clomiphene treatment fails. Treatment should be begun with 1 or 2 ampules/day, starting on day 2 of the cycle. These patients should be monitored as are anovulatory patients treated with hMG/hCG. Too few data are available to know the true value of hMG in the therapy of luteal-phase defects.

Bromocriptine has been used in both hyperprolactinemic patients with ILP and those whose prolactin levels were normal. The reported results of therapy are quite varied but appear to be superior in those with hyperprolactinemia.

Treatment selection

Luteal-phase defects may occur because of hypothalamic, pituitary, ovarian, or endometrial abnormalities. A complete investigation, including serum progesterone and prolactin levels and endometrial biopsy,

Table 114.1 Selection of treatment for a patient with a luteal-phase defect (from Marsh and Shaupe)

Abnormality	Treatment	Follow-up
Low progesterone Normal prolactin Endometrium in phase	Clomiphene citrate	Progesterone
Low progesterone Normal prolactin Retarded endometrium	Clomiphene citrate	Progesterone Endometrial biopsy
Low progesterone Elevated prolactin Endometrium in phase	Bromocriptine	Prolactin Progesterone
Low progesterone Elevated prolactin Retarded endometrium	Bromocriptine	Prolactin Progesterone Endometrial biopsy
Retarded endometrium Elevated prolactin Normal progesterone	Bromocriptine	Prolactin Endometrial biopsy
Retarded endometrium Normal progesterone Normal prolactin	Progesterone	Endometrial biopsy

Low progesterone, Peak serum progesterone level <10 ng/ml; Retarded endometrium, >2 days out of phase. Follow-up peak serum progesterone levels should be ≥15 ng/ml. Combination therapy may be necessary in some patients.

is necessary before treatment can be planned. After therapy is begun, the response can be considered adequate only if all chemical or histologic abnormalities have been corrected. Table 114.1 illustrates the methods for selecting therapy and monitoring response in patients with luteal-phase defects. Patients who have a peak serum progesterone level which is <10 ng/ml should be treated initially with clomiphene citrate, regardless of endometrial histology. Patients with marked hyperprolactinemia will usually need bromocriptine; however, those patients with minimal prolactin elevations could also be treated with clomiphene. Progesterone supplementation is recommended only for those who have normal serum prolactin and progesterone levels but retarded endometrial histology. It is mandatory to document that defects are corrected at follow-up. Combination therapy is necessary for some patients. hMG should be used only for those patients whose defect was not successfully corrected by clomiphene, whether or not other drugs were also used, and those who have drug-related complications. This approach is likely to result in term pregnancy in up to 75% of patients. Because randomized placebo-controlled studies to assess the efficacy of these various modalities have not been performed, the proportion of pregnancies which occur independent of therapy is not known at the present time.

SUGGESTED READING

BORENSTEIN R, KATZ Z, LANCET M, *et al*. Bromocriptine treatment of hyperprolactinemic infertility with ovulatory dysfunction. *Int J Gynaecol Obstet* 1980; 18:195.

COOK CL, RAO CV, YUSSMAN MA. Plasma gonadotropin and sex steroid hormone levels during early, midfollicular, and midluteal phases of women with luteal phase defects. *Fertil Steril* 1983;40:45.

GOLDSTEIN D, ZUCKERMAN H, HARPAZ S, *et al*. Correlation between estradiol and progesterone in cycles with luteal phase deficiency. *Fertil Steril* 1982;37:348.

HONORE LH, CUMMING DC, FAHMY N. Significant difference in the frequency of out-of-phase endometrial biopsies depending on the use of the Novak curette or the flexible polypropylene endometrial biopsy cannula ("Pipelle"). *Gynecol Obstet Invest* 1988;26:338.

HUANG K-E. The primary treatment of luteal phase inadequacy: progesterone versus clomiphene citrate. *Am J Obstet Gynecol* 1986;155:824.

JONES GS. The luteal phase defect. *Fertil Steril* 1976;27:351.

JONES GS, AKSEL S, WENTZ AC. Serum progesterone values in the luteal phase defects. Effect of chorionic gonadotropin. *Obstet Gynecol* 1974;44:26.

KARAMARDIAN LM, GRIMES DA. Luteal phase deficiency: effect of treatment on pregnancy rates. *Am J Obstet Gynecol* 1992;167:1391.

KELLER DW, WIEST WG, ASKIN FB, *et al*. Pseudocorpus luteum insufficiency: a local defect of progesterone action on endometrial stroma. *J Clin Endocrinol Metab* 1979;48:127.

LI T-C, DOCKERY P, ROGERS AW, *et al*. How precise is histologic dating of endometrium using the standard dating criteria? *Fertil Steril* 1989;51:759.

MARSH CM, SHOUPE D. Luteal-phase defects. In: Mishell DR Jr, Davajan V, Lobo RA, eds. *Infertility, Contraception and Reproductive Endocrinology.* 3rd edn. Cambridge, MA: Blackwell Scientific Publications, 1991:805.

MCNATTY KP, SAWYERS RS, MCNEILLY AS. A possible role for prolactin in control of steroid secretion by the human Graafian follicles. *Nature* 1974;250:653.

MCNEELY M, SOULES M. The diagnosis of luteal phase deficiency: a critical review. *Fertil Steril* 1988;50:1.

NOYES RW, HERTIG AT, ROCK J. Dating the endometrial biopsy. *Fertil Steril* 1950;1:3.

SHANGOLD M, BERKELEY A, GRAY J. Both midluteal serum progesterone levels and late luteal endometrial histology should be assessed in infertile women. *Fertil Steril* 1983;40:627.

SHOUPE D, MISHELL DR Jr, LACARRA M. Correlation of endometrial maturation with four methods of estimating the day of ovulation. *Obstet Gynecol* 1989;73:88.

SOULES MR, STEINER RA, CLIFTON DR, et al. Abnormal pattern of pulsatile luteinizing hormone in women with luteal phase deficiency. *Obstet Gynecol* 1984;63:626.

STROTT CA, CARGILLE CM, ROSS GT, et al. The short luteal phase. *J Clin Endocrinol Metab* 1970;30:246.

WENTZ AC, HERBERT CM III, MAXSON WS, et al. Cycle of conception endometrial biopsy. *Fertil Steril* 1986;46:196.

115

Human *in vitro* fertilization and related assisted reproductive techniques

RICHARD J. PAULSON

Introduction

Extracorporeal fertilization of human oocytes was first reported by the British team of Steptoe and Edwards, who were also the first to achieve a successful birth following human *in vitro* fertilization (IVF) on July 25, 1978. In the relatively few years since then, thousands of pregnancies have been achieved worldwide by IVF and its modifications, now generally combined under the term assisted reproductive techniques or ARTs.

Patient selection

In its most basic sense, IVF replaces and performs the function of the fallopian tube. Initially offered to patients with tubal disease which could not be corrected surgically, with time, IVF was made available to patients with other infertility diagnoses, including endometriosis, male factor, and unexplained infertility. Patients with normal fallopian tubes have the option of IVF as well as any of the other ARTs.

The follicular phase: superovulation

Increasing the number of follicles prior to aspiration increases the likelihood of successful follicle aspiration, oocyte fertilization, and, ultimately, likelihood of pregnancy in the aspiration cycle. For this reason, controlled ovarian hyperstimulation is generally used in order to increase the number of oocytes and embryos available for transfer.

Controlled ovarian hyperstimulation is achieved by increasing circulating follicle-stimulating hormone (FSH) levels by administering either clomiphene citrate or human menopausal gonadotropin (hMG). Cycles are monitored with daily transvaginal ultrasound measurement of the size of the developing follicles and serum estradiol determinations. The dose of medication is then modified according to the patient's response. Ovulation is triggered with human chorionic gonadotropin (hCG) when follicle maturity criteria are attained. The timing of hCG administration is important since, if it is given too soon, immature oocytes may be obtained; if given too late, the oocytes may be lost to spontaneous ovulation.

To enhance cycle control and maximize oocyte yield, agonistic analogs of gonadotropin-releasing hormone (GnRH) agonists have recently come into use for pituitary down-regulation prior to the initiation of and during the course of gonadotropin therapy. While treatment cycle length has increased, as has the need for larger numbers of ampules of hMG, the prevention of spontaneous release of luteinizing hormone (LH) prior to hCG administration has resulted in decreased cycle cancellation rates and increased pregnancy rates per initicated cycle.

Unstimulated IVF

Most recently, the University of Southern California (USC) IVF program has focused on the viability of performing IVF in unstimulated cycles. Whereas the first birth after IVF occurred in a natural cycle, these cycles were subsequently abandoned because of the increased efficiency of oocyte retrieval and higher pregnancy rates of stimulated cycles. However, stimulated cycles are not without their costs; in addition to the financial cost of the ovarian stimulatory drugs, the cycles are lengthened, especially if the GnRH analogs are used for pretreatment down-regulation; the ovaries are hyperstimulated, frequently necessitating increased intercycle intervals; and endometrial receptivity seems to be decreased. Additionally, some patients who are otherwise normally ovulatory do not respond to hyperstimulation, while others may experience the complications of ovarian hyperstimulation syndrome. In order to achieve good pregnancy rates with stimulated cycles, multiple embryos must be replaced, which in some instances leads to multiple implantations, causing obstetric complications and/or the need for selective fetal reduction. For all of these reasons, the unstimulated cycle presents an attractive alternative.

The USC unstimulated IVF protocol consists of serial monitoring of a spontaneous ovulatory cycle, with hCG administration in the mid-cycle designed to deliver a predictable LH-like stimulus to the follicle and to time follicle aspiration accurately, yet allow its scheduling for a convenient time of day. After hCG administration, the cycles are conducted in a manner identical to that of stimulated cycles.

Follicle aspiration

Oocyte recovery is scheduled for 34–36 h after hCG administration. Follicle aspirations are generally performed on an outpatient basis without the need for an operating-room environment.

Laparoscopy was historically the first method of follicle aspiration and still has the advantage of giving the surgeon a limited visual inspection of the pelvis. It therefore continues to be used for IVF by some centers when there is a concurrent reason for visualization of the pelvis. It is also needed for ARTs during which the distal end of the fallopian tube is catheterized. However, since they have different goals, the concurrent performance of any ART with diagnostic laparoscopy necessarily compromises one or the other procedure. Therefore, we do not recommend that the first diagnostic laparoscopy for infertility evaluation be scheduled concurrently with an ART cycle. However, a second-look laparoscopy when only a limited inspection of the pelvis is required may be acceptable at the time of an ART.

Oocytes are separated from the follicular fluid in the laboratory under a dissecting microscope. The size of the oocytes (approximately 70–100 µm diameter) allows their visualization and mechanical transport with a pipette to a wash dish and subsequently a holding test tube containing culture medium. When all of the oocytes have been identified and isolated, they are transferred to the incubator where they are kept until insemination approximately 6 h later.

Sperm preparation

Semen is generally obtained following a 48-h sexual abstinence on the day of follicle aspiration. If oligospermia or other indications of a male infertility factor are present, the couple is cautioned about the possibility of lack of fertilization and is offered the option of using a donor sperm specimen as back-up. An additional semen specimen is obtained from the husband 24 h before the procedure and stored overnight at 4°C in test yolk buffer. A second specimen is obtained on the day of follicle aspiration. In this manner, two specimens are available for fertilization. Additionally recent studies have suggested that storage of sperm in test yolk buffer may enhance fertilization of human oocytes *in vitro*.

Spermatozoa have to be separated from the seminal plasma in order to be suitable for use in IVF. The sperm specimen is mixed with culture medium in a 1:2 ratio and centrifuged at 300 g for 10 min. The supernatant is discarded and the pellet resuspended in fresh culture medium. A second centrifugation step is followed by an incubation in which the spermatozoa contained in the pellet are allowed to swim up into approximately 1–2 ml of fresh culture medium.

A total of 200 000 motile sperm is added to each oocyte in 1 ml of culture medium approximately 6 h after oocyte collection. The gametes are then replaced in the incubator overnight. Fertilization is confirmed by visualization with a dissecting microscope of two pronuclei (2PN) in the fertilized zygote 16–20 h later. If no fertilization is noted at the end of 24 h of coincubation of oocytes with both prepared specimens, a third specimen from the husband or the prepared back-up donor specimen may be used in an effort to achieve fertilization.

Embryo transfer

Following fertilization, embryos are maintained in culture for an additional 24 h. Normally developing embryos are at least at the two-cell stage at this point, with some embryos having four or more blastomeres.

The embryos are placed 0.5 cm from the top of the uterine fundus in a small volume (10–25 μl) of transfer medium. The patient is kept recumbent in mild Trendelenburg position for 3 h to allow the transfer fluid to absorb. Alternately, the embryos may be replaced in the fallopian tubes, as with zygote intrafallopian transfer (ZIFT) and tubal embryo transfer (TET).

The luteal phase

As most failures of IVF occur after embryo transfer, it has been suggested that altered endometrial receptivity plays a major role in embryo implantation. The most convincing data supporting this contention come from oocyte donation. When embryos resulting from IVF are transferred to unstimulated recipients, the procedure results in markedly improved implantation rates. In an effort to improve endometrial receptivity in standard IVF cycles, progesterone is administered either intramuscularly, in a dose of 25 mg daily, or by vaginal suppositories, 50 mg twice daily.

Other ARTs

After it became apparent that IVF could be successfully applied to unexplained infertility as well as other conditions in which the fallopian tubes were open, other investigators attempted to modify the original IVF concept in an effort either to simplify the process and/or to increase its success in this group of patients.

The ARTs all utilize similar ovarian stimulation regimens, oocyte retrieval techniques, and methods of sperm preparation. They vary in two aspects: the first variable affects whether fertilization takes place in the laboratory or within the fallopian tube (i.e., whether embryos or gametes are replaced in he body of the female partner), and the second variable is where the gametes or embryos are physically placed (endometrial cavity, fallopian tubes, peritoneal cavity).

Two ARTs use gamete replacement and allow fertilization to take place within the body. As a result, oocyte collection and replacement are generally performed in the same setting. Their principal advantage is that a second visit for the embryo transfer is not necessary. Since fertilization cannot be verified by direct visualization, they are generally not recommended for male factor, except when donor sperm is used.

GIFT

The gamete intrafallopian transfer (GIFT) procedure uses IVF methodology for follicle stimulation and oocyte retrieval. Thereafter, oocytes and spermatozoa are replaced directly in the fallopian tube, generally by laparoscopy. Pregnancy is dependent upon fallopian tube function for early embryonic development and embryo transfer to the uterus. Ovulation, oocyte pick-up by the fallopian tube, and gamete intermixing are assisted by this ART. In the early years of IVF, follicle aspirations were performed almost exclusively with laparoscopic visualization. Thus, the option of placing the gametes in the fallopian tubes rather than requiring the patient to return for the embryo transfer represented a significant simplification of IVF. The markedly shortened time of the gametes in the laboratory environment (several minutes rather than 48 h) also meant that less could go wrong. With today's ultrasound-guided aspirations which require neither general anesthesia nor an operating-room environment, and improved laboratory techniques, the putative advantages of GIFT must be weighed against the additional cost incurred as a result of the added laparoscopy. Some centers are now investigating the possibility of gamete replacement in the fallopian tubes by the transcervical route. While success has been limited, this new modification may make GIFT a more viable alternative to the less invasive IVF-embryo transfer.

POST

Peritoneal ovum–sperm transfer (POST) is a further simplification of GIFT. Oocytes are recovered by the transvaginal route and are then mixed with sperm and injected into the pouch of Douglas by culdocentesis. Pregnancy is thus dependent upon fallopian tube function not only for transport to the uterus but also for oocyte pick-up. Only ovulation and mixing with sperm are assisted by this ART. Its success implies that in some infertile individuals, a relatively small defect in the function of the reproductive system can be the cause of long-standing idiopathic infertility. A controlled comparison with superovulation/intrauterine insemination would help delineate the additional impact on fertility of gamete intermixing to the effect achieved by superovulation alone.

The remaining ARTs are more like IVF in that they utilize fertilization of the oocytes *in vitro*. However, the resultant embryos are replaced in the fallopian tubes rather than in the uterine cavity.

ZIFT or PROST

ZIFT or pronuclear-stage tubal transfer (identical procedures given different acronyms by different centers) utilizes standard IVF technology for all phases up to the first 24 h after oocyte retrieval. By this point of embryonic life, fertilization is apparent by the visible presence of the male and female pronuclei within the zygote. The embryo is replaced at this stage of development into the fallopian tube. Pregnancy is dependent upon further embryo development and embryo transfer to the uterus. Proponents of these techniques acknowledge the advantage of the verification of fertilization *in vitro*, and point to the more "natural" quality of early embryonic development taking place within the tube rather than in the uterine cavity, as occurs with standard IVF. Most centers offering ZIFT replace the embryos by laparoscopy, although success with transcervical cannulation has been reported and is undergoing further clinical trials.

TET

TET is differentiated from ZIFT in that embryos are replaced after cleavage has taken place, 48 or 72 h after follicle aspiration. Similar arguments as for ZIFT are used by proponents to advocate the additional laparoscopy or minilaparotomy which is used for the delivery of the embryos into the female reproductive tract rather than transcervical transfer into the uterine cavity.

It is difficult to compare the relative efficiencies of the various ARTs. Different centers experience different success rates with different procedures due to a wide range of factors and variables. To date, only two randomized prospective trials have been undertaken to compare different ARTs in the same institution. Leeton *et al.* compared IVF and GIFT among patients with male factor and idiopathic infertility. No difference in pregnancy rates was found, though the study was rather small, thus limiting the power of the negative conclusion. Balmaceda *et al.* compared embryo implantation rates among recipients in an oocyte donation program who were randomly assigned to embryo transfer by either the transcervical or transabdominal intrafallopian route. No difference in implantation rates was found and, though the number of patients was not large, the combination of high pregnancy rates in both groups and an examination of per embryo implantation rates (rather than pregnancy rates) gave the study good power.

As a result of these negative studies, the philosophy of the USC IVF program has been a bias toward the least costly and least traumatic ART option. In the vast majority of cases, this means "traditional" IVF with transvaginal follicle aspiration and nonsurgical embryo transfer. GIFT and TET are reserved for IVF failures and for patients with a mechanical block to transcervical embryo transfer.

Outcome and pregnancy success following IVF

Pregnancy rates reported for IVF are highly variable, due in part to selection bias, small sample sizes, and a lack of standardization of criteria for reporting outcome. In 1986, the Society for Assisted Reproduction Technology, formed under the sponsorship of the American Fertility Society, established a national IVF registry, which collects and reports data from its member clinics. According to this survey, in the USA in 1989, a total of 15 392/oocyte retrievals for IVF resulted in 13 523 embryo transfers and 2811 clinical pregnancies (18% per retrieval). There were 655 (23%) spontaneous abortions and 154 (5%) ectopic pregnancies, leading to 2104 deliveries (14%/oocyte retrieval). At USC during 1989, 84 retrievals resulted in 78 embryo transfers, 23 clinical pregnancies (27%), and 14 deliveries (17%). The effects of age and male factor are readily evident, as 55 of these cycles were in women under the age of 40 without male factor infertility, resulting in 20 clinical pregnancies (36%) and 12 deliveries (22%). The unstimulated IVF protocol is limited to women under age 40 and without male factor. To date (1988–1990), 78 follicle aspirations have resulted in 11 clinical (14%) and nine ongoing (12%) pregnancies, or approximately one-half the rate of stimulated cycles.

Thus, on a per-cycle basis, IVF is not very efficient. However, using life-table analysis, the per-cycle pregnancy rate has been shown to be relatively constant for a least six stimulated cycles and our own data indicate the same trend for at least three unstimulated cycles. Therefore, IVF may be attempted on a repetitive basis and a considerably higher cumulative success rate achieved.

The other ARTs are also included in the registry report. GIFT pregnancy rates have consistently averaged higher than IVF, with 3652 procedures in 1989 resulting in 1112 (30%) clinical pregnancies and 848 (23%) deliveries. ZIFT, PROST, and TET data have been combined and in 1989, 908 oocyte retrievals were reported to result in 696 transfers and 190 (21%) clinical pregnancies. There were 151 (17% per retrieval) deliveries, a value similar to that of IVF.

Oocyte donation

Since IVF allows oocytes and sperm to be combined in the laboratory, oocyte donation is conceptually a simple extension of the IVF process. Intended primarily for women with ovarian failure, the technique can be applied to any woman with endometrium capable of responding to gonadal steroids. Pregnancy without ovaries was first shown to be possible in monkeys in 1983, and the first human pregnancy was reported in 1984. A variety of successful steroid regimens used to effect artificial cycles has been reported. Donated oocytes are fertilized *in vitro* with the recipient's husband's sperm and embryo replacement is scheduled for the appropriate day of the (artificial) luteal phase. When a pregnancy is established, steroid supplementation must be maintained until the 7th week of gestation, although supplementation has generally been given for several additional weeks. Pregnancies with this technique have been reported in patients with premature ovarian failure, surgical castration, and gonadal dysgenesis.

A remarkable feature of oocyte donation is its apparent high degree of success. The recipient endometrium is stimulated by an artificial steroid regimen designed to mimic a natural cycle and proven by biopsy to have normal secretory characteristics in a prior cycle. It is not exposed to the high steroid levels associated with ovarian hyperstimulation, and appears to be more receptive to implantation. In our experience, the frequency of embryo implantation in women so treated is observed to be threefold higher than in a matched group of ovulatory hyperstimulated women treated by IVF. This increased implantation rate has resulted in live birth rates of nearly 50% per embryo transfer in the donor oocyte program at USC. Additionally, the uterus of women over the age of 40 appears to retain its ability to respond to exogenous steroids and to be receptive to donated embryos. At the present time, oocyte donation appears to be the most successful method of achieving pregnancy in older patients.

Embryo and oocyte cryopreservation

Advanced stimulation regimens and retrieval techniques now result in large numbers of oocytes being retrieved from a single procedure of follicle aspiration. Since only a limited number of embryos can be transferred in any given cycle, there exists a need for long-term storage. Embryo cryopreservation was first achieved in the mouse and has been widely utilized in the animal husbandry industry. The first successful human pregnancy following cryopreservation was reported in 1983. Today, most programs utilize cryopreservation for embryos that are not transferred. The registry survey reported 2124 frozen embryo transfer cycles in 1989, with 234 (11%) clinical pregnancies and 172 (8%) deliveries.

Because of the delicate nature of the meiotic spindle present in the unfertilized mature oocyte, and because of an unfavorable surface-to-volume ratio, oocyte cryopreservation is a much less efficient process. The first human pregnancy following oocyte cryopreservation was reported in 1986. The experience with this technique is limited and it has not reached widespread use.

Future considerations

In general, the ultimate success of IVF can be increased in two ways. One way is to increase the per-cycle pregnancy rate. This can be achieved by optimizing methods of oocyte stimulation and embryo culture and by enhancing endometrial receptivity to help increase the implantation rate. The second way in which overall success can be increased is to simplify the procedure, so that individual patients may undergo a greater number of procedures for the same cost and/or inconvenience. A more meaningful way to measure pregnancy success rates in the future will be to report pregnancy rates per patient-cost and per patient-year, rather than the current practice of reporting success per cycle.

SUGGESTED READING

ANDERSON GB. Embryo transfer in domestic animals. *Adv Vet Sci Comp Med* 1983;27:129.

ASCH RH, ELLSWORTH LR, BALMACEDA JP, WONG PC. Pregnancy after translaparoscopic gamete intrafallopian transfer. *Lancet* 1984;2:1034.

BALMACEDA JP, ROTSZTEIN DA, ORD T, JUNK S, ASCH RH. Embryo implantation rates in oocyte donation: a prospective comparison of tubal versus uterine transfers. Abstract presented at the annual meeting, Society for Gynecologic Investigation, 1991.

BATEMAN BG, NUNLEY WC Jr, KITCHIN JD. Surgical management of distal tubal obstruction – are we making progress? *Fertil Steril* 1987;48:523.

BEN RAFAEL Z, MASHIACH S, DOR J, RUDAK E, GOLDMAN B. Treatment-independent pregnancy after *in vitro* fertilization and embryo transfer trial. *Fertil Steril* 1986;45:564.

CHEN C. Pregnancy after human oocyte cryopreservation. *Lancet* 1986;1:884.

CHILLIK CF, ACOSTA AA, GARCIA JE, *et al*. The role of *in vitro* fertilization in infertile patients with endometriosis. *Fertil Steril* 1985;44:56.

COHEN J, EDWARDS R, FEHILLY C, *et al*. *In vitro* fertilization: a treatment for male infertility. *Fertil Steril* 1985;43:422.

COULAM CB, PETERS AJ, GENTRY M, GENTRY W, CRITSER ES, CRITSER JK. Pregnancy rates after peritoneal ovum-sperm transfer. *Obstet Gynecol* 1991;164:1447.

DE ZIEGLER D, CEDARS MI, RANDLE D, LU JKH, JUDD HL, MELDRUM DR. Suppression of the ovary using a gonadotropin releasing-hormone agonist prior to stimulation for oocyte retrieval. *Fertil Steril* 1987;48:807.

EDWARDS RG, STEPTOE PC, PURDY JM. Establishing full-term human pregnancies using cleaving embryos grown *in vitro*. *Br J Obstet Gynecol* 1980;87:737.

GUZIK DS, WILKES C, JONES HW Jr. Cumulative pregnancy rates for *in vitro* fertilization. *Fertil Steril* 1986;46:663.

HAMORI M, STUCKENSEN JA, RUMPF D, *et al*. Zygote intrafallopian transfer (ZIFT): evaluation of 42 cases. *Fertil Steril* 1988;50:519.

HODGEN GD. Surrogate embryo transfer combined with estrogen-progesterone therapy in monkeys: implantation, gestation, and delivery without ovaries. *JAMA* 1983;250:2167.

In vitro fertilization/embryo transfer (IVF-ET) in the United States: 1989 results from the National IVF-ET registry. *Fertil Steril* 1991;55:14.

KATAYAMA KP, STEHLIK E, ROESLER M, JEYENDRAN RS, HOLMGREN WJ, ZANEVELD LJD. Treatment of human spermatozoa with an egg yolk medium can enhance the outcome of *in vitro* fertilization. *Fertil Steril* 1989;52:1077.

KOVACS GT, ROGERS P, LEETON JF, TROUNSON AO, WOOD C, BAKER HW. *In vitro* fertilization and embryo transfer: prospects of pregnancy by life-table analysis. *Med J Aust* 1986;144:682.

LEETON J, ROGERS P, CARO C, *et al*. A controlled study between the use of gamete intrafallopian transfer (GIFT) and *in vitro* fertilization and embryo transfer in the management of idiopathic and male infertility. *Fertil Steril* 1987; 48:605.

LUTJEN P, TROUNSON A, LEETON J, FINDLAY J, WOOD C, RENOU P. The establishment and maintenance of pregnancy using *in vitro* fertilization and embryo donation in a patient with primary ovarian failure. *Nature* 1984;307:174.

LUTJEN PJ, FINDLAY JK, TROUNSON AO, LEETON JF, CHAN LK. Effect on plasma gonadotropins of cyclic steroid replacement in women with premature ovarian failure. *J Clin Endocrinol Metab* 1986;62:419.

MATSON PL, YOVICK JL. The treatment of infertility associated with endometriosis by *in vitro* fertilization. *Fertil Steril* 1986;46:432.

NAVOT D, LAUFER N, KOPOLOVIC J, *et al*. Artificially induced endometrial cycles and establishment of pregnancies in the absence of ovaries. *N Engl J Med* 1986; 314:806.

PATTON PE, WILLIAMS TJ, COULAM CB. Results of microsurgical reconstruction in patients with combined proximal and distal tubal occlusion: double obstruction. *Fertil Steril* 1987;48:670.

PAULSON RJ, MARRS RP. Ovulation stimulation and monitoring for *in vitro* fertilization. *Curr Prob Obstet Gynecol Infertil* 1986;IX:497.

PAULSON RJ, SAUER MV, LOBO RA. *In vitro* fertilization in unstimulated cycles: a new application. *Fertil Steril* 1989;51:1059.

PAULSON RJ, SAUER MV, LOBO RA. Embryo implantation following human *in vitro* fertilization. importance of endometrial receptivity. *Fertil Steril* 1990;53: 870–874.

PAULSON RJ, SAUER MV, LOBO RA. Factors affecting embryo implantation following human *in vitro* fertilization. *Am J Obstet Gynecol* 1990;163:2020.

PAULSON RJ, SAUER MV, FRANCIS MM, MACASO TM, LOBO RA. IVF in unstimulated cycles: a clinical trial utilizing human chorionic gonadotropin to time follicle aspiration. *Obstet Gynecol* 1990;76:788–791.

PAULSON RJ, SAUER MV, FRANCIS MM, MACASO TM, LOBO RA. Use of test-yolk buffer (TYB) to enhance fertilization during human *in vitro* fertilization (IVF) in cases of suspected male infertility. *Fertil Steril* 1992;58:551.

RANOUX C, FOULOT H, DUBUISSON JB, *et al*. Returning to spontaneous cycles in *in vitro* fertilization. *J in vitro Fertil Embryo Transfer* 1988;5:304.

ROH SI, AWADALLA SG, FRIEDMAN CI, *et al*. *In vitro* fertilization and embryo transfer: treatment-dependent versus -independent pregnancies. *Fertil Steril* 1987;48:982.

RUTHERFORD AJ, SUBAK-SHARPE RJ, DAWSON KJ, MARGARA RA, FRANKS S, WINSTON RML. Improvement of *in vitro* fertilization after treatment with buserelin, an agonist of luteinising hormone releasing hormone. *Br Med J* 1988;296:1765.

SAUER MV, PAULSON RJ. Human oocyte and pre-embryo donation: an evolving method for the treatment of female infertility. *Am J Obstet Gynecol* 1990;163:1421.

SAUER MV, MACASO TM, HERNANDEZ MF, LOBO RA, PAULSON RJ. Establishment of a nonanonymous donor oocyte program: preliminary experience at the University of Southern California. *Fertil Steril* 1989;52:433.

SAUER MV, LOBO RA, PAULSON RJ. Successful twin gestation following donor embryo transfer to a patient with XY gonadal dysgenesis. *Am J Obstet Gynecol* 1989;161:380.

SAUER MV, PAULSON RJ, LOBO RA. A preliminary report on oocyte donation extending reproductive potential to women over forty. *N Engl J Med* 1990;323:1157.

SAUER MV, PAULSON RJ, MACASO TM, FRANCIS MM, LOBO RA. Oocyte and pre-embryo donation to women with ovarian failure: an extended clinical trial. *Fertil Steril* 1991;55:39.

SAUER MV, STEIN AL, PAULSON RJ, MOYER DL. Endometrial responses to various hormone replacement regimens in ovarian failure patients preparing for embryo donation. *Int J Obstet Gynecol* 1991;35:61.

STEPTOE PC, EDWARDS RG. Reimplantation of a human embryo with subsequent tubal pregnancy. *Lancet* 1976;1:880.

STEPTOE PC, EDWARDS RG. Birth after the reimplantation of a human embryo. *Lancet* 1978;2:336.

TROUNSON AO, MOHR L. Human pregnancy following cryopreservation, thawing and transfer of an eight-cell embryo. *Nature* 1983;305:707.

WHITTINGHAM DG, LEIBO SP, MAZUR P. Survival of mouse embryos frozen to −196°C and −269°C. *Science* 1972;178:411.

YOVICH JL, BLACKLEDGE DG, RICHARDSON PA, *et al*. Pregnancies following pronuclear stage tubal transfer. *Fertil Steril* 1987;48:851.

116

Diagnosis of early pregnancy

SUBIR ROY, FRANK Z. STANCZYK & RICHARD J. PAULSON

Introduction

The diagnosis of pregnancy can be aided by an understanding of the role of human chorionic gonadotropin (hCG) and serum progesterone in early gestation and their measurements. Ultrasound is another important aid. This chapter will discuss each of these aids in the diagnosis of early pregnancy.

The evaluation of pregnancy tests requires an understanding of the normal production of hCG in pregnancy. With this as background, it then becomes possible to choose the most appropriate test based on the interval between the onset of the last menstrual period and the time of the test. Sensitivity, specificity, accuracy, requirements for special equipment, speed, availability, and cost are some factors to consider in choosing the most suitable pregnancy test for a given clinical situation.

Production of hCG in pregnancy

β-hCG has been detected in the serum of pregnant women as early as 8–11 days after the luteinizing hormone (LH) peak, or 7–9 days after ovulation. The trophoblast production of hCG has been estimated to double within 1.4–1.6 days up to the 35th day from the onset of the last menstrual period (LMP) and within 2.0–2.7 days from day 35 to 42, reaching a serum concentration of approximately 100 mIU/ml about 2 days after the expected menses would have begun. The hCG peaks at 8–10 weeks from the LMP at 10 000–80 000 mIU/ml and then drops and remains at approximately 10 000 mIU/ml for the remainder of pregnancy.

The hCG values stated above are based on a 28-day cycle. As is well known, the follicular phase of the menstrual cycle may be variable. When the follicular phase is prolonged, ovulation is delayed, and the levels of hCG are lower than expected during approximately the first 25 days of pregnancy as compared to a patient with a pregnancy based on a 28-day cycle. A pregnancy test with a sensitivity selected to detect a certain level of β-hCG, therefore, might give false-negative results because of the delayed ovulation.

Reliability criteria of pregnancy tests

Sensitivity

The sensitivity of the various pregnancy tests depends to a large extent on the reference standard chosen. Because highly purified hCG has not been prepared in sufficient amounts, its supply has been limited. In 1964, the Second International Standard (second IS) for hCG for bioassay, a relatively impure standard obtained from the urine of women in the first trimester of pregnancy, was employed. It was estimated that this standard contained only 20% pure intact hCG. In an effort to improve the reference material, in 1974, the World Health Organization established the First International Reference Preparation (first IRP) of hCG for immunoassay, which is estimated to contain 95% pure intact hCG, and recommended that this standard be used to calibrate commercial hCG kits.

Although the first IRP is more purified than the previous standard, comparable results using both standards cannot be obtained. The clinically important consequence of this difference in standards is that hCG tests calibrated against different standards cannot be compared in terms of their sensitivity. Indeed, there may be a potential variation in the values measured for hCG of 1.5–5:1 (first IRP:second IS). Thus, without knowledge of which standard was employed, a clinician may assume incorrectly that a test was more sensitive (calibrated against the second IS) than another (calibrated against the first IRP). For example, a test utilizing the second IS may measure hCG as 25 mIU/ml, while the same sample may be reported as 50 mIU/ml when the first IRP is used. At present, a third preparation of hCG (third international standard) is being used in some hCG kits because the second IS has been exhausted. This standard is the same as the second IS.

Agglutination technology for the measurement of hCG (hemagglutination or latex agglutination), which was the first attempt at development of a rapid pregnancy test, has for all practical purposes been superseded by modern immunoassay methods. Initially, a considerable amount of experience was generated by radioimmunoassay procedures utilizing iodine 125 (^{125}I) with polyclonal antibodies to hCG or β-hCG. In order to develop a more specific assay for hCG or β-hCG, monoclonal antibodies were developed. These monoclonal antibodies have been utilized to detect hCG or β-hCG by radioimmunoassay (RIA) or immunoradiometric assay (IRMA). These tests (either RIA or IRMA), when employed quantitatively, have sensitivities as low as 1–1.5 mIU/ml and can be utilized for monitoring gestational trophoblastic disease. However, when used in a semiquantitative manner, as is possible by using β-hCG kits with preset sensitivities of 15–50 mIU/ml, they can be used as pregnancy tests.

Because the ^{125}I-based hCG or β-hCG tests require costly equipment and radioactive disposal, immunoassays utilizing nonradioactive markers or tags were soon developed. These tags may use fluorescein in the fluoroimmunoassay (FIA), luminol in the chemiluminescent assay (CIA), and an alkaline phosphatase conjugate in the enzyme immunoassay (EIA). Quantification of these nonradioactive tags requires special equipment: fluorometer for the FIA, luminometer for the CIA, and spectrophotometer for the EIA. Office and home hCG tests use the enzyme-linked immunosorbent assay (ELISA) technology, which permits quantification visually or by use of a spectrophotometer. These tests employ immunoabsorbent assays using one or more monoclonal antibodies to intact or different regions of hCG or β-hCG. They have sensitivities of around 50 mIU/ml (first IRP standard). Among the most commonly used ELISA tests in offices are the Icon II and the TestPack. Home pregnancy tests, using ELISA technology, include Clearblue Easy with a sensitivity of 100 mIU/ml standardized against the third IS; e.p.t. Stick Test, with a sensitivity of 50 mIU/ml standardized against the first IRP; Fact Plus, with a sensitivity of 250 mIU/ml; Daisy 2, with a sensitivity of 250 mIU/ml, and Advance, with a sensitivity of 250 mIU/ml, are each standardized against the third IS.

The Icon II has an internal standard, a membrane dot separate from the unknown dot, set at 50 mIU/ml for urine specimens and at 25 mIU/ml for serum (not plasma) specimens, which turn blue when the reagents have been added correctly, regardless of whether the specimen contains hCG or not and against which the degree of blue coloration for the unknown dot can be compared. The Icon II has the capability of detecting levels of hCG <50 mIU/ml (around 20–25 mIU/ml for urine or serum specimens, depending on the reader's ability to detect faint blue changes during the test interval); does not require centrifugation or filtration prior to assay; reportedly does not cross-react with extraneous materials; and it takes only 4–5 min to perform the six-step test procedure.

The TestPack, designed to detect hCG in urine, does not have a specific internal standard as an integral part of the test, but it does have a built-in filter that should not be removed. It shows a positive sign (+) if levels of hCG are >50 mIU/ml. Occasionally, specimens containing <50 mIU/ml also can test as positive. A negative sign (−) indicates the absence of detectable hCG. This six-step test also reportedly does not cross-react with extraneous materials and also can be performed in about 4–5 min.

The two ELISA tests just described are similar in terms of accuracy and ease of use. If the reagents for the RIA of β-hCG being performed within a facility are the same as for one of the ELISA tests, that ELISA test should be used to provide internal consistency.

Specificity

Generally speaking, serum tests are more specific than urine tests for the detection of hCG. Substances such as proteins, blood, some drugs, metabolites of drugs such as phenothiazines and methadone, soaps, and detergents may interfere with some of the older urine pregnancy tests, such as the latex pregnancy tests where agglutination gives false-positive results. Because of the interference, these tests required prior centrifugation or filtration of the urine specimen. The monoclonal antibodies used in the ELISA tests appear to be specific to the hCG molecule or β-hCG chain and hence do not cross-react with this extraneous material.

Although it is well established that false-negative results usually occur with tests that are not sufficiently sensitive, bacterial contamination, heat, extreme pH shifts, metabolic inactivation in the body, and dilute urine also can lead to negative tests. A concentrated first-voided specimen of morning urine nearly approximates the serum concentration of hCG and should be used for testing whenever possible.

Accuracy

The accuracy of a urine test for pregnancy can be checked by comparing its result with β-hCG levels in a serum sample drawn at the same time. However, this procedure has not been performed for every available test. Therefore, the accuracy of some tests (as a function of number of days from the onset of last period) is unknown.

The practice of some manufacturers of adding known amounts of hCG to negative sera (male or nonpregnant female serum) to create artificial concentrations of hCG, which then are tested and found to detect hCG at concentrations lower than the internal standard, may not reflect the ability of these tests to detect similar concentrations of naturally occurring hCG in urine.

With the advent of the ELISA tests, an alkaline phosphatase or horseradish peroxidase colorimetric reaction is produced. The visual acuity of the person performing the test may be the limiting factor (at the lowest detectable limits of the assay), especially as it requires the detection of a faint blue or red reaction. Tests with positive or negative controls provide an internal standard for easier comparison of end-points.

Characteristics of representative tests

Serum tests for the diagnosis of pregnancy include the RIA for hCG or the more specific β-subunit of hCG. The RIA tests, until recently, were research tools not ordinarily used as pregnancy tests. Now clinical laboratories are able to use β-hCG kits with sensitivity levels varying from 1 to 30 mIU/ml, which require less than an hour of laboratory time to perform, although customarily they are available only once daily. Radioactive iodine-labeled hCG and a γ-counter are required.

The ELISA tests typically use one of the antibodies as a coat on a membrane that captures and immobilizes the hCG molecule, if it is present in the urine or serum specimen to be tested and an aliquot of the specimen is placed on the membrane. The second antibody is linked chemically to an enzyme, and this combination binds to another site of the immobilized hCG molecule, "sandwiching" the hCG molecule between the antibody bound to the membrane and enzyme-linked antibody. Following a washing step that removes unbound enzyme-linked antibodies, a color developer is added that turns blue or red (depending on the enzyme used in the system) and denotes the presence of hCG. The intensity of the color reaction is proportional to the amount of enzyme present on the membrane and is correspondingly proportional to the amount of hCG that is present in the urine or serum specimen.

Because the sensitivity of the semiquantitative RIA β-hCG kit and ELISA pregnancy tests are so nearly equal and the latter can be performed in a few minutes in any office or laboratory rather than in a research laboratory, it is becoming customary to perform these latter assays in lieu of the serum RIA tests in most but not all circumstances (see below).

Requirements for special equipment

Equipment

The semiquantitative RIA for hCG or β-hCG is a laboratory (not office) test requiring capabilities for handling and disposing radioactive materials and a γ-counter. Furthermore, many pregnancy tests recommend that the urine specimen be centrifuged or filtered (with specific filter paper) prior to the performance of the test.

Speed

The semiquantitative RIA for β-hCG kit tests require about an hour of laboratory time, but in practice they are available from most commercial laboratories only once or, at most, twice daily. In contrast, the ELISA tests can be used by office or laboratory personnel who can be trained easily; these tests require only about 5 min to perform.

Availability

All the ELISA tests are available as kits and can be used in the office, home or laboratory. The β-hCG RIA kit tests are commercially available through almost all diagnostic laboratories.

Cost

The cost of the ELISA tests to the patient will depend upon bulk purchase price and the amount that the office or laboratory adds to acquisition price; however, the usual purchase price is about $2 per test. Laboratories charge $15–20 for the semiquantitative RIA for β-hCG.

Clinical uses of hCG measurements

Relationship between hCG levels and ultrasound

Generally, abnormal gestations are associated with abnormal (low) levels of hCG secretion. The half-life of hCG in serum is about 36 h (range 12–50 h). The value of hCG may drop on average one order of magnitude per week. This fact may be helpful in monitoring the normal regression of hCG (e.g., following a spontaneous miscarriage or molar gestation evacuation). Recently, transvaginal ultrasound performed with a 5-MHz probe suggests that a gestational sac should be evident with hCG at 1400 mIU/ml, a fetal pole should be evident at 5100 mIU/ml, and fetal heart motion detected at 17 200 mIU/ml. A note of caution: a 4-mm sac looks similar to 4 mm of fluid. A false-positive sac may represent late follicular-phase endometrium, pseudosac associated with an ectopic gestation, or a venous lake in myometrium. If the circulating hCG is >5000 mIU/ml and the transvaginal ultrasound finds nothing in the uterus, an ectopic gestation should be suspected.

Ectopics

Ectopic pregnancies have an abnormal rise of hCG; however, a normal pattern of increase of hCG does not rule out an ectopic. An abnormal pattern of increase of hCG in an asymptomatic patient should be documented by two abnormal values 1 week apart. If the patient is symptomatic, and the value of hCG is above 6500 mIU/ml, then transvaginal ultrasound should be performed. Transvaginal ultrasound should be able to locate an intrauterine pregnancy when such levels of hCG are in the circulation. Laparoscopy is indicated if the patient is symptomatic, the hCG is rising, and there is no intrauterine pressure by ultrasound, or if the hCG plateaus and there are no chorionic villi on endometrial curettage, or the patient is symptomatic or has a pelvic mass (>6 cm).

Threatened abortion

A single value of hCG ⩾10 000 mIU/ml is associated with a good prognosis. Vaginal probe ultrasound may be a useful adjunct by demonstrating cardiac motion.

Missed abortion

This condition is associated with very low levels of hCG and a disproportion between gestational age and fundal height (low size for dates). Ultrasound can be used to confirm the diagnosis by demonstrating no cardiac motion.

Multiple gestations

Twins are frequently, but not always, reported to have higher levels of hCG than singletons based upon the number of days from the onset of the LMP. Some reports have shown no higher levels of hCG with triplets or even sextuplets as compared to twin pregnancies.

Progesterone

During early pregnancy only the corpus luteum produces significant amounts of progesterone. This source predominates during the first 9 weeks of pregnancy, but thereafter is surpassed by the placenta. During the first few weeks of pregnancy, maternal plasma progesterone levels are in the range of 10–35 ng/ml. In case of disruption of the corpus luteum prior to 9 weeks of gestation, supplemental progesterone should be administered (50 mg im daily or 100 mg suppositories b.i.d., vaginally). Serum progesterone can be measured by RIA (ng/ml) or its principal urinary metabolite, pregnanediol glucuronide by ELISA colorimetric dipstick (with sensitivity to 3 μg/ml). Although varying with hydration, 1 μg/ml of pregnanediol glucuronide in urine corresponds approximately to 1 ng/ml of progesterone in serum.

Clinical uses of progesterone measurements

Abnormal gestation (ectopics or abortions)

Abnormal gestation is associated with abnormal progesterone secretion. Since progesterone is a steroid, it has a short half-life (in minutes), especially as compared to hCG, a protein, whose half-life is in hours. Therefore, progesterone levels may drop while hCG levels are still high. Dipstick pregnanediol glucuronide assays may be employed to aid in the diagnosis of abnormal gestations.

Conclusions

Until the ELISA tests for detecting hCG became available, it was necessary to use the more sophisticated and time-consuming laboratory RIA tests for early detection of pregnancy. Now the ELISA tests are clearly the pregnancy tests to be used for most circumstances. Not all available pregnancy tests have been mentioned, but some of the more common ones have been used as examples of the basic types or to demonstrate common features. The need for quantitative hCG assays to monitor gestational trophoblastic disease, where the greatest level of sensitivity to detect hCG is required (i.e., $<1\,\mathrm{mIU/ml}$), clearly indicates that the ELISA or RIA kit pregnancy tests are inadequate because of their sensitivity. The trophoblast can be producing hCG in amounts not detectable by these tests. Dipstick pregnanediol glucuronide tests may aid, especially with the use of vaginal probe ultrasound, in the diagnosis of abnormal gestations, including ectopic pregnancies.

SUGGESTED READING

BARNES RB, ROY S, YEE B, *et al.* Sensitivity of urinary pregnancy tests in surgically proven ectopic pregnancies. *J Reprod Med* 1985;30:827.

BRAUNSTEIN GD, RASOR J, ADLER D, *et al.* Serum human chorionic gonadotropin levels throughout normal pregnancy. *Am J Obstet Gynecol* 1976;126:678.

CATT KJ, DUFAU ML, VAITUKAITIS JL. Appearance of hCG in pregnancy plasma following the initiation of implantation of the blastocyst. *J Clin Endocrinol Metab* 1975;40:537.

FOSSUM GT, DAVAJAN V, KLETZKY OA. Early detection of pregnancy with transvaginal ultrasound. *Fertil Steril* 1988;49:788.

FREDERICK JL, CHENETTE PE, PAULSON RJ, STANCZYK FZ, SAUR MV. Random urinary pregnanediol glucuronide measurements in pregnancy: lack of utility for evaluation of first-trimester vaginal bleeding. *Hum Reprod* 1990;5:468.

JOHANSSON EDB. Plasma levels of progesterone in pregnancy measured by a rapid competitive protein binding technique. *Acta Endocrinol (Kbh)* 1969;61:607.

KADAR N, DEVORE G, ROMERO VR. Discriminatory hCG zone: its use in the sonographic evaluation for ectopic pregnancy. *Obstet Gynecol* 1981;58:156.

KADAR N, CALDWELL BV, ROMERO R. A method of screening for ectopic pregnancy and its indications. *Obstet Gynecol* 1981;58:162.

LENTON EA, NEL LM, SULAIMAN R. Plasma concentrations of human chorionic gonadotropin from the time of implantation until the second week of pregnancy. *Fertil Steril* 1982;37:773.

MARRS RP, KLETZKY OA, HOWARD WF, MISHELL DR Jr. Disappearance of human chorionic gonadotropin and resumption of ovulation following abortion. *Am J Obstet Gynecol* 1979;135:731.

MISHELL DR Jr, WIDE L, GEMZELL CA. Immunologic determination of human chorionic gonadotropin in serum. *J Clin Endocrinol* 1963;23:125.

NYGREN K-G, JOHANSSON EDB, WIDE L. Evaluation of the prognosis of threatened abortion from the peripheral plasma levels of progesterone, estradiol, and human chorionic gonadotropin. *Am J Obstet Gynecol* 1973;116:916.

SAUER MV, VERMESH M, ANDERSON RE, VIJOD AG, STANZCYK FZ, LOBO RA. Rapid measurement of urinary pregnanediol glucuronide to diagnose ectopic pregnancy. *Am J Obstet Gynecol* 1988;159:1531.

SAUER MV, PAULSON RJ, FREDERICK CJ, STANCZYK FZ. Effect of hydration of random levels of urinary pregnanediol glucuronide. *Gynecol Endocrinol* 1990; 4:145.

WEHMANN RE, NISULA BC. Metabolic and renal clearance rates of purified human chorionic gonadotropin. *J Clin Invest* 1981;68:184.

PART 7

Family Planning

117

Oral contraceptives: indications, contraindications, formulations, and monitoring

DANIEL R. MISHELL, JR

Oral contraceptives (OCs), the copper T 380A intrauterine device, depot medroxyprogesterone acetate, and Norplant implant are the most effective methods of reversible contraception currently available for use by women in the USA. OCs can be prescribed for the majority of women in the reproductive age group because they are young and healthy; however, there are certain absolute contraindications for their use. These include a present and past history of vascular disease, including thromboembolism, thrombophlebitis, atherosclerosis, stroke, and systemic vascular disease, such as lupus erythematosus or hemoglobin sickle cell (SS) disease. In addition, uncontrolled hypertension, diabetes mellitus with vascular disease, as well as women over 35 who smoke, are contraindications to OCs because use of high-dose OCs in women with these disorders was reported to increase the risk for stroke or myocardial infarction. One of the contraindications for OC use listed by the US Food and Drug Administration (FDA) is cancer of the breast or endometrium, although no data indicate that OCs are harmful in women with these diseases. In addition, patients who are pregnant should not ingest OCs because of the theoretic masculinizing effect of the gestagens on the external genitalia of the female fetus.

Concerns that ingestion of OCs during pregnancy produces other congenital abnormalities such as limb reduction defects and heart defects have not proven to be valid.

Patients with functional heart disease should not use OCs, since the fluid retention produced by these agents could produce congestive heart failure. However, there is no evidence that asymptomatic mitral valve prolapse is a contraindication. Patients with active liver disease should not use OCs, since steroids are metabolized in this organ. However, patients who have had liver disease (e.g., viral hepatitis) in the past but whose liver function tests have returned to normal can receive these agents.

Relative contraindications to OC use include heavy cigarette smoking under the age of 35, migraine headaches, undiagnosed amenorrhea, and depression. Migraine headaches can be made worse by OC use. Some patients who suffered a stroke while taking high dose OCs have reported an increased incidence of headaches of the migraine type, fainting, loss of vision or speech, or paresthesias before development of the cerebrovascular accident. If any of these symptoms develop in OC users, the patient should stop ingesting these agents until the diagnosis for this symptom is established. OCs are effective therapy for polycystic ovarian syndrome and can also be used to treat premature ovarian failure. There is no evidence that OCs should not be given to women with hypothalamic amenorrhea.

Anyone who develops galactorrhea while taking OCs should discontinue these agents, and after 2 weeks, a serum prolactin level should be measured. If the prolactin level is elevated, further diagnostic evaluation is indicated. OC use has not been shown to affect adversely the natural history of patients with prolactin-secreting microadenomas. Therefore the presence of these small benign tumors is not a contraindication to OC use.

Patients with a history of gestational diabetes can also take low-dose OC formulations because these agents do not affect glucose tolerance or accelerate the development of diabetes mellitus. Insulin-dependent diabetes without vascular disease, although previously a relative contraindication to OC use, is no longer considered to be so. Use of low-dose OCs in women with insulin dependence does not accelerate the disease process and these women are at high risk for pregnancy complications.

Initiating OC therapy in adolescents

In deciding whether the pubertal, sexually active girl should use OCs for contraception, the clinician should be more concerned about compliance than possible physiologic harm. Provided the postmenarcheal girl has demonstrated maturity of the hypothalamic–pituitary–ovarian axis by having at least three regular, presumably ovulatory, cycles, it is safe to prescribe OCs without being concerned about causing permanent damage to the reproductive process. OCs can also be prescribed for women with oligomenorrhea, especially those with polycystic ovarian syndrome and dysfunctional bleeding due to anovulation. OCs will inhibit the manifestation of hyperandrogenism and produce regular uterine bleeding without excessive blood loss. One need not be concerned about accelerating epiphyseal closure in postmenarcheal females. Their endogenous estrogens have already initiated the process a few years before menarche, and the contraceptive steroids will not hasten it.

Following pregnancy

Ovulation occurs sooner after a spontaneous or induced abortion, usually between 2 and 4 weeks, than after a term delivery, when ovulation is usually delayed beyond 6 weeks but may occur as early as 4 weeks in a woman who is not breast-feeding.

Thus after spontaneous or induced abortion of a fetus of less than 12 weeks' gestation, OCs should be started immediately to prevent conception following the first ovulation. For patients who deliver after 28 weeks and are not nursing, the combination pills should be initiated 2–3 weeks after delivery. If the termination of pregnancy occurs between 12 and 28 weeks, contraceptive steroids should be started 1 week later. The reason for the delay in the latter instances is that the normally increased risk of thromboembolism occurring postpartum may be further enhanced by the hypercoagulable state associated with contraceptive steroid ingestion. Because the first ovulation is delayed for at least 4 weeks after a term delivery, there is no need to expose the patient to this increased risk. If a woman takes bromocriptine to inhibit milk production she may ovulate as soon as 3 weeks postpartum and should initiate OCs 2 weeks postpartum.

It is probably best for women who are nursing not to use combination OCs, as their use, even with the low-estrogen-dose formulations, has been shown to diminish the amount of milk produced, as estrogen inhibits prolactin's action on the breast. Women who are breast-feeding every 4 h, including at nighttime, will not ovulate until at least 10 weeks after delivery and thus do not need contraception before that time. Once any supplemental feeding is introduced after 4 weeks postpartum, ovulation can resume promptly. Since only a small percentage of fully breast-feeding women will ovulate within 6 months postpartum, as long as they continue full nursing and remain amenorrheic, either a barrier method or a progestin-only OC can be used. The latter does not diminish the amount of breast milk and is effective in this group of women. However, a small portion of these synthetic steroids have been detected in breast milk. The long-term effects (if any) of these progestins on the infant are not known, but none has been detected to date.

All women

At the initial visit, after a history and physical examination have determined that there are no medical contraindications for OCs, the patient should be informed about the benefits and risks. For medicolegal reasons it is best to use either a written informed consent signed by the patient or note on the patient's medical record that the benefits and risks have been explained to her and she has been told to read the patient package insert.

Type of formulation

In determining which formulation to use, it is best to prescribe initially a formulation with less than 50 μg ethinylestradiol, since these agents are associated with less cardiovascular risk, as well as fewer estrogenic side-effects. It would also appear reasonable to use formulations with the lowest dosage of a particular progestin because less progestogenic metabolic and clinical adverse effects would be associated with their use. The development of multiphasic formulations has allowed the total dose of progestin to be reduced compared with some monophasic formulations without increasing the incidence of breakthrough bleeding. However, several monophasic formulations have a lower total dose of progestin per cycle than the multiphasic formulations.

The FDA has stated that the product prescribed should be one that contains the least amount of estrogen and progestin that is compatible with a low failure rate and the needs of the individual patient. Because few randomized studies have been performed comparing the different marketed formulations, until large-scale comparative studies are performed, the clinician must decide which formulation to use based on which formulations have the least adverse effects among patients in his or her practice. If estrogenic or progestogenic side-effects occur with one formulation, a different agent with less estrogenic or progestogenic activity can be given.

The contraceptive formulations containing progestins without estrogen have a lower incidence of adverse metabolic effects than the combination formulations. Because the factors that predispose to thromboembolism are caused by the estrogen component, the incidence of thromboembolism in women ingesting these compounds is probably not increased. Furthermore, blood pressure is not affected, nausea and breast tenderness are eliminated, and milk production and quality are unchanged. Despite these advantages, these agents have the disadvantages of a high frequency of intermenstrual and other abnormal bleeding patterns, including amenorrhea, and a lower rate of effectiveness. The use failure rate of these preparations is higher than with the combined formulations, and a relatively high percentage of the pregnancies that do occur are ectopic. Because nursing mothers have reduced fertility and are amenorrheic, the major disadvantages of these preparations are minimized for these patients. Furthermore, because milk production and quality are unaffected, in contrast to the changes produced by combination OCs, the formulations with only a progestin may be offered to these women while they are nursing. However, a small portion of these synthetic steroids have been detected in breast milk. The long-term effects (if any) of these progestins on the infant are not known, but none has been detected to date. A long-term follow-up study of breast-fed children, in which mothers ingested 50 µg of estrogen in combined OCs while they were lactating, revealed no difference in weight gain or height increase up to 8 years of age when compared with breast-fed children whose mothers did not ingest OCs. Also, the occurrence of disease or intellectual or psychologic behavior was no different between the two groups.

Follow-up

If the patient has no contraindications to OC use, no routine laboratory tests are needed. However, cervical cytology should be obtained or repeated annually, as in all women of reproductive age. At the end of 3 months, the patient should be seen again. At this time a nondirected history should be obtained and the blood pressure measured. After this visit the patient should be seen annually, at which time a nondirected history should again be taken, blood pressure and body weight measured, and a physical examination (including breast, abdominal, and pelvic examination with cervical cytology) performed. It is important to perform annual cervical cytologic examinations on OC users, since they are a relatively high-risk group for development of cervical neoplasia. The routine use of other laboratory tests is not indicated unless the patient has a family history of diabetes or vascular disease, because the incidence of positive results is extremely low. However, if the patient has a family history of vascular disease, such as myocardial infarction occurring in family members under the age of 50, it would be advisable to obtain a lipid panel before OC use is started, since hypertriglyceridemia may be present and OC use will further raise triglycerides.

Since the low-dose formulations do not alter the lipid profile, except for triglycerides, it is not necessary to measure lipids, other than the routine cholesterol screening every 5 years in women without cardiovascular risk factors, even if they are over age 35. If the patient has a family history of diabetes or evidence of diabetes during pregnancy, a 2-h postprandial blood glucose test should be performed before OCs are started and, if elevated, a glucose tolerance test performed. If the patient has a past history of liver disease, a liver panel should be obtained to make certain that liver function is normal before OCs are started.

Drug interactions

Although synthetic sex steroids can retard the biotransformation of certain drugs (e.g., phenazone and meperidine) as a result of substrate competition, such interference is not important clinically. OC use has not been shown to inhibit the action of other drugs. However, some drugs can clinically interfere with the action of OCs by inducing liver enzymes that convert the steroids to more polar and less biologically active metabolites. Certain drugs have been shown to accelerate the biotransformation of steroids in the human. These include barbiturates, sulfonamides, cyclophosphamide, and rifampicin. Back *et al.* have reported a relatively high incidence of OC failure in women ingesting rifampicin, and these two agents should not be given concurrently. The clinical data concerning OC failure in users of other antibiotics (e.g., penicillin, ampicillin, and sulfonamides) and antieleptic drugs (e.g., phenytoin and barbiturates) are less clear. A few anecdotal studies have appeared in the literature, but there is no reliable evidence for a clinical inhibitory effect of these drugs, such as occurs with rifampicin. Women with epilepsy requiring medication possibly should be treated with formulations containing 50 µg estrogen, since a higher incidence of abnormal bleeding has been reported in these women with the use of lower-dose estrogen formulations.

Noncontraceptive health benefits

In addition to being the most effective method of contraception, OCs provide many other health benefits. Some occur because the combination OCs contain a potent, orally active progestin as well as an orally active estrogen and there is no time when the estrogenic target tissues are stimulated by estrogens without a progestin (unopposed estrogen).

Both natural progesterone and the synthetic progestins inhibit the proliferative effect of estrogen, the so-called antiestrogenic effect. Estrogens increase the synthesis of both estrogen and progesterone receptors, while progesterone decreases their synthesis. Thus one mechanism whereby progesterone exerts its antiestrogenic effects is by decreasing the synthesis of estrogen receptors. Relatively little progestin is needed to do this, and the amount present in OCs is sufficient. Another way progesterone produces its antiestrogenic action is by stimulating the activity of the enzyme estradiol 17β-dehydrogenase, within the endometrial cell. This enzyme converts the more potent estradiol to the less potent estrone, reducing estrogenic action within the cell.

Benefits from antiestrogenic action of progestins

As a result of the antiestrogenic action of the progestins in OCs the height of the endometrium is less than in an ovulatory cycle, and there is less proliferation of the glandular epithelium. These changes produce several substantial benefits for the OC user. One is a reduction in the amount of blood loss at the time of endometrial shedding. In an ovulatory cycle the mean blood loss during menstruation is about 35 ml, compared with 20 ml for women ingesting OCs. This decreased blood loss makes the development of iron-deficiency anemia less likely. OC users are about half as likely to develop iron-deficiency anemia as controls.

Because the OCs produce regular withdrawal bleeding, OC users are significantly less likely to develop menorrhagia, irregular menstruation, or intermenstrual bleeding. Because these disorders are frequently treated by curettage and/or hysterectomy, OC users require these procedures less frequently.

Because progestins inhibit the proliferative effect of estrogens on the endometrium, women who use OCs have been found to be significantly less likely to develop adenocarcinoma of the endometrium even after their use is discontinued.

Estrogen exerts a proliferative effect on breast tissue, which also contains estrogen receptors. Progestins probably inhibit the synthesis of estrogen receptors in this organ as well, exerting an antiestrogenic action on the breast. Several studies have shown that OCs reduce the incidence of benign breast disease, and two prospective studies have indicated that this reduction is directly related to the amount of progestin in the compounds.

Current users of OCs have an 85% reduction in the incidence of fibroadenomas and 50% reductions in chronic cystic disease and non-biopsied breast lumps, as compared with controls using intrauterine devices or diaphragms. The risk of developing these three diseases decreases with increased duration of OC use and persists for about 1 year following discontinuation of OCs, after which no reduction in risk was observed.

Benefits from inhibition of ovulation

Other noncontraceptive medical benefits of OCs result from their main action — inhibition of ovulation. Some disorders, such as dysmenorrhea and premenstrual tension, occur much more frequently in ovulatory than anovulatory cycles. In fact, inhibition of ovulation by exogenous steroids has been used as therapy for severe dysmenorrhea for decades. OC users have 63% less dysmenorrhea and 29% less premenstrual tension than controls.

Another serious adverse effect of ovulatory menstrual cycles is the development of functional ovarian cysts — specifically, follicular and luteal cysts — that frequently require laparotomy because of enlargement, rupture, or hemorrhage. When ovulation is inhibited, functional cysts do not usually develop. In a survey performed by the Boston Collaborative Drug Surveillance Program, less than 2% of women with a discharge diagnosis of functional ovarian cysts were taking OCs, in contrast to 20% of controls. However, 20% of women with nonfunctional cysts were taking OCs, an incidence similar to that observed in the controls. Although authors of one small case series postulated that the formation of functional ovarian cysts may be increased in users of multiphasic OCs, the rate of hospitalization for ovarian cysts in the USA has remained unchanged following the widespread use of multiphasic formulations.

Another disorder linked to incessant ovulation is ovarian cancer. The development of ovarian cancer is significantly reduced in OC users with a duration-dependent decrease in risk. The reduction in risk persists after OC use is discontinued.

Other benefits

Several studies have shown that the risk of developing rheumatoid arthritis in OC users was only about half that in controls. Another benefit is protection against salpingitis, often referred to as pelvic inflammatory disease (PID). The relative risk of developing PID among OC users in most studies is about 0.5. It has been estimated that 15–20% of women with cervical gonorrhea will develop PID. In a Swedish study all cases of suspected PID were confirmed by laparoscopic visualization 1 day after hospital admission. Of women who used contraception other than the intrauterine device and OCs, 15% developed PID; only about half as many – 8.8% – of those who used OCs developed PID. The results of this study indicated that OCs reduce the clinical development of PID in women infected with gonorrhea.

Although the incidence of cervical infection with *Chlamydia trachomatis* is increased in OC users compared with controls, the incidence of chlamydial PID in OC users was only half that in control subjects. This protection may be related to the decreased duration of menstrual flow, which permits a smaller number of organisms to ascend to the upper genital tract and allows the body's defenses to eliminate them more easily. One sequela of PID is ectopic pregnancy, an entity that has tripled in incidence in the past 15 years. OCs reduce the risk of ectopic pregnancy by more than 90% in current users and may reduce the incidence in former users by decreasing their chance of developing PID.

Because of these many noncontraceptive benefits, as well as the fact that there is no evidence that the low-dose OCs are associated with an increased incidence of serious cardiovascular disease, particularly myocardial infarction, stroke, and fatal pulmonary embolism in nonsmoking women, an FDA advisory committee recommended that OCs can be used by nonsmoking women without vascular disease beyond the age of 40. Accordingly, in 1991, the class labeling for OCs was changed to read: "Therefore, the committee recommended that the benefits of oral contraceptive use by healthy nonsmoking women over 40 may outweigh the possible risks. Of course, older women as all women who take oral contraceptives should take the lowest possible dose formulation that is effective."

OCs can be prescribed until the woman becomes postmenopausal, as determined by an elevated follicle-stimulating hormone level (>30 mIU/ ml) on a serum sample obtained on the day before starting the next cycle of contraceptives. At this time treatment should be switched to estrogen–progestin hormone replacement because of the lower potency of the latter steroids upon liver globulin synthesis compared to OCs.

SUGGESTED READING

BACK DJ, BRECKENRIDGE AM, CRAWFORD FE, *et al.* The effects of rifampin on the pharmacokinetics of ethinylestradiol in women. *Contraception* 1980;21:135.

BERAL V, NANNAFORD PC, KAY C. Oral contraceptive use and malignancies of the genital tract. *Lancet* 1988;2:1331.

BRACKEN MB, VITA K. Frequency of non-hormonal contraception around conception and association with congenital malformations in offspring. *Am J Epidemiol* 1983;117:281.

CANCER AND STEROID HORMONE STUDY OF THE CENTERS FOR DISEASE CONTROL AND THE NATIONAL INSTITUTE OF CHILD HEALTH AND HUMAN DEVELOPMENT. The reduction in risk of ovarian cancer associated with oral-contraceptive use. *N Engl J Med* 1987;316:650.

CENTERS FOR DISEASE CONTROL. Combination oral contraceptive use and risk of endometrial cancer. *JAMA* 1987;257:796.

CROFT P, HANNAFORD PC. Risk factors for acute myocardial infarction in women: evidence from the Royal College of General Practitioners' oral contraception study. *Br Med J* 1989;298:165.

DIAMOND MP, GREENE JW, THOMPSON JM, *et al.* Interaction of anticonvulsants and oral contraceptives in epileptic adolescents. *Contraception* 1985;31:623.

HAZES JMW, DIJKMANS BAC, VANDENBROUCKE JP, *et al.* Reduction of the risk of rheumatoid arthritis among women who take oral contraceptives. *Arthritis Rheum* 1990;33:173.

KENNEDY KI, RIVERA R, MCNEILLY AS. Consensus statement on the use of breastfeeding as a family planning method. *Contraception* 1989;39:477.

KJOS SL, SHOUPE D, DOUHAM S, *et al.* Effect of low-dose oral contraceptives on carbohydrate and lipid metabolism in women with recurrent gestational diabetes: results of a controlled randomized prospective study. *Am J Obstet Gynecol* 1990;163:1822.

KOETSAWANG S. The effects of contraceptive methods on the quality and quantity of breast milk. *Int J Gynaecol Obstet* (Suppl) 1987;25:115.

MEADE TW. Oral contraceptives, clotting factors, and thrombosis. *Am J Obstet*

Gynecol 1982;142:758.

MEADE TW, GREENBERG G, THOMPSON SG. Progestogens and cardiovascular reactions associated with oral contraceptives and a comparison of the safety of 50- and 30-μg oestrogen preparations. *Br Med J* 1980;280:1157.

MISHELL DR Jr. Noncontraceptive health benefits of oral steroidal contraceptives. *Am J Obstet Gynecol* 1982;142:809.

NILSSON S, MELLBIN T, HOFVANDER Y, *et al.* Long-term follow-up of children breast-fed by mothers using oral contraceptives. *Contraception* 1986;34:443.

ORY HW. The noncontraceptive health benefits from oral contraceptive use. *Fam Plann Perspect* 1982;14:182.

PITUITARY ADENOMA STUDY GROUP. Pituitary adenomas and oral contraceptives: a multi-center case-control study. *Fertil Steril* 1983;39:753.

RYDEN G, FAHRAEUS L, MOLIN L, *et al.* Do contraceptives influence the incidence of acute pelvic inflammatory disease in women with gonorrhoea? *Contraception* 1979;20:149.

SENNAYAKE P, KRAMER DG. Contraception and the etiology of pelvic inflammatory disease: new perspective. *Am J Obstet Gynecol* 1980;138:852.

VESSEY M, METCALFE A, WELLS C, *et al.* Ovarian neoplasma, functional ovarian cysts, and oral contraceptives. *Br Med J* 1987;294:1518.

WILD RA, DEMERS LM, APPLEBAUM-BOWDEN D, LENKER R. Hirsutism: metabolic effects of two commonly used oral contraceptives and spironolactone. *Contraception* 1991;44:113.

WILSON JG, BRENT RL. Are female sex hormones teratogenic? *Am J Obstet Gynecol* 1981;141:567.

WOLNER-HANSSEN P, SVENSSON L, MARDH P-A, *et al.* Laparoscopic findings and contraceptive use in women with signs and symptoms suggestive of acute salpingitis. *Obstet Gynecol* 1985;66:233.

WORLD HEALTH ORGANIZATION TASK FORCE ON ORAL CONTRACEPTIVES. Effects of hormonal contraceptives on milk volume and infant growth. *Contraception* 1984;30:505.

118

Noncontraceptive effects of oral contraceptives: neoplastic, reproductive, and metabolic

DANIEL R. MISHELL, JR

Introduction

Oral contraceptives (OCs) have been marketed since 1960 and millions of women have used these products during the past 33 years. Much information has accumulated regarding the various actions of these steroids in addition to their primary effect of inhibition of ovulation. These effects can be arbitrarily divided into three categories: (1) neoplastic; (2) reproductive; and (3) metabolic.

Neoplastic effects

Numerous epidemiologic studies have been performed studying the relation of use of OCs with the most common genital neoplasms, breast, cervix, endometrium, and ovary, as well as several extragenital tumors, namely, hepatic, pituitary, and malignant melanoma. Because as yet few elderly women used OCs during their early reproductive years, the studies thus far published usually restrict the analysis to women under age 60.

Breast cancer

No study has reported a significant increase or decrease in the risk of developing breast cancer among the entire population of OC users. The combined risk estimate of the 16 case-control studies and four cohort studies summarized by Peterson and Wingo in 1992 was 1.0. In Schlesselman's review of 17 different studies in which the risk of developing breast cancer in women under 60 years of age was compared with the duration of OC use, no overall dose–response was found to exist and long-term use did not increase the risk of developing breast cancer.

The issue of latency, time since first use of OCs, and risk of breast cancer has also been studied. In groups of women using OCs for more than 10 years there was found to be no change in risk of breast cancer with increasing duration of time since first use. Thus, there is no evidence supporting a long-term latent effect. Several studies have presented data regarding the risk of developing breast cancer under age 45 by duration of OC use prior to age 25. The combined data fail to show a dose–response, indicating that early age of first OC use is not by itself a risk factor for development of breast cancer. The preponderance of data in studies estimating risk of breast cancer in women under 60 years of age by duration of OC use prior to first term pregnancy also failed to show an increased risk or a dose–response. However, analysis of the studies which estimated the relative risk of developing breast cancer in women under 45 years of age suggested that there was a trend of increasing risk with increasing duration of overall use, as well as increasing duration of use prior to first term pregnancy, with the increased risk in both groups becoming most evident after 8 years of use.

Three large studies have suggested that prolonged use of high-estrogen-dose OCs might increase the risk of developing breast cancer, but only when initially diagnosed at an early age.

Because of the concern raised by these studies, Wingo *et al.* reanalyzed the extensive data obtained by the Cancer and Steroid Hormone study organized by the Centers for Disease Control (Table 118.1). These investigators found that women who used OCs had a slightly increased risk of developing breast cancer between the ages of 20 and 34 compared to non-OC users. OC use did not alter the risk of developing breast cancer between the ages of 35 and 44, and was associated with a slightly decreased risk of developing breast cancer between the ages of 45 and 54. Because breast cancer is more common between ages 45 and 54 than under 45, OC use could be associated with an increase of about 10 cases of breast cancer per 100 000 women under age 45 but a decrease of 18 cases per 100 000 women in the 45–54-year age group.

These data are consistent with the belief that long-term use of high-dose OCs could have promoted the age at which breast cancer was diagnosed clinically among susceptible women. This promotional effect was transient, not persistent, and thus had no appreciable effect on the aggregate lifetime risk of developing breast cancer under age 60 in the population, despite the widespread use of OCs.

Because formulations with low-dose estrogen have been used by most

Table 118.1 Hypothetical annual age-specific breast cancer incidence rates in the USA in women aged 20–54 in 1982 (from Wingo *et al.*)

Age (years)	History of OC use	OC use (%)	RR (95% CI)	Annual incidence per 100 000 women	Rate difference per 100 000 women
20–34	Never	24.0	Referent	8.5	
	Ever	76.0	1.4 (1.0–2.1)	11.9	3.4
	All women	100.0		11.1	
35–44	Never	28.6	Referent	74.8	
	Ever	71.4	1.1 (0.9–1.3)	82.2	7.4
	All women	100.0		80.1	
45–54	Never	53.1	Referent	177.5	
	Ever	46.9	0.9 (0.8–1.0)	159.8	−17.7
	All women	100.0		169.2	

OC, Oral contraceptive; RR, relative risk; CI, confidence interval.

women ingesting OCs only since 1983, the effect of these agents, if any, on early development of breast cancer can be determined only several years from now. However, the data reviewed thus far by the Food and Drug Administration resulted in a statement that no change in OC use or prescribing practice was warranted.

In addition, there have been several studies of OC use and breast cancer risk in women at increased risk of developing the disease, those with a family history of breast cancer, as well as those with existing benign breast disease. The results of these studies indicate that OC use by each of these high-risk groups is not associated with any increased risk of developing breast cancer. In summary, epidemiologic data available to date indicate neither an increased nor decreased overall risk of breast cancer in OC users with any type of formulation or with long-term use of these formulations.

Cervical cancer

The epidemiologic data obtained thus far indicate that long-term use of OCs is associated with an increased risk of preinvasive cervical neoplasia as well as both epidermoid and adenocarcinoma of the cervix, when compared with matched control groups. Confounding factors, such as the woman's age at first sexual intercourse, the number of sexual partners, exposure to human papillomavirus (possibly greater among users of OCs), cytologic screening (more frequent among OC users), and the use of barrier contraceptives or spermicides (primarily by women in the control group) as well as cigarette smoking (an independent risk factor for this disease) could have influenced these results. Most of these studies made statistical corrections for these confounding factors, and in many of them the control group did not use barrier methods of contraception.

As shown in Schlesselman's review, the overall pattern of epidemiologic results suggests an approximate doubling of risk of development of carcinoma-*in-situ* with use of OCs for more than 1 year, with three studies showing increasing risk with increasing duration of use. The data for invasive cervical cancer suggest no increased risk with <5 years of OC use, but a gradually increasing risk after 5 years' use, which results in a twofold increase with 10 years of use. Data from the Royal College of General Practitioners cohort study by Beral *et al.* support the results of these case-control studies, since there was a steadily increasing risk of both preinvasive and invasive cancer of the cervix with increasing duration of OC use. Thus, although it is uncertain whether OCs themselves increase the risk of cervical cancer, act as a cocarcinogen, or have no effect, users of OCs as a group are at high risk for cervical neoplasia and require at least annual screening of cervical cytology, especially if they have used OCs for more than 5 years.

Endometrial cancer

OCs contain progestins as well as an estrogen and the progestins inhibit the synthesis of estrogen receptors in the endometrium and thus inhibit the growth-promoting mitotic action of estrogen upon endometrial tissue. At least 11 studies have been published on the relation between OCs and endometrial cancer, and nine of these studies have indicated that the use of these agents has a protective effect against endometrial cancer, the third most common cancer among US women. Women who use OCs for at least a year have an age-adjusted relative risk of 0.5 of developing endometrial cancer between ages 40 and 55 as compared with nonusers. This protective effect is related to duration of use, increasing from a 20% reduction in risk with 1 year of use to a 40% reduction with 2 years of use to a 60% reduction with 4 years of use. This protective effect appears within 10 years of initial use and persists for at least 15 years after stopping use of OCs, at least until age 60. The greatest protective effect is in nulliparous women (relative risk 0.2) or women of low parity, who have the greatest risk of acquiring this disease.

Ovarian cancer

The incidence of developing ovarian cancer is directly related to the number of times a woman ovulates in her lifetime. Thus, inhibition of ovulation by both pregnancy and OCs reduces the risk of ovarian cancer. At least 30 published reports relate the use of OCs with subsequent development of ovarian cancer and each of these shows a reduction in risk, specifically of the most common type – epithelial ovarian cancers. OCs reduce the risk of the four main histologic types of epithelial ovarian cancer: (1) serous; (2) mucinous; (3) endometrioid; and (4) clear cell. The relative risk of ovarian cancer is 0.6 for women who use OCs for 3 or more years, and as little as 6 months of use provides protection. The magnitude of the decrease in risk is directly related to the duration of use, increasing from a 50% reduction with 4 years' use to a 60–80% reduction with 7 or more years' use. The protective effect begins within 10 years of first use and continues for at least 15 years after the use of OCs ends, at least until age 60. As with endometrial cancer, the protective effect occurs only in women of low parity (four children or less), who are at greatest risk for this type of cancer.

Liver adenoma and cancer

The development of a benign hepatocellular adenoma is a rare occurrence in long-term users of OCs. The increased risk of this tumor was associated with prolonged use of high-dose formulations, particularly those containing mestranol. Although two British studies reported an increased risk of liver cancer among users of OCs, the number of patients was small and the results could have been influenced by confounding factors. Data from a large multicenter epidemiologic study coordinated by the World Health Organization found no increased risk of liver cancer associated with OC users in countries with a high prevalence rate of this neoplasm. This study found no change in risk with increasing duration of use or time since first or last use. The rate of death from this disease has remained unchanged in the USA over the past 25 years, a period when millions of women have used these agents.

Pituitary adenoma

OCs mask the predominant symptoms produced by prolactinoma, amenorrhea, and galactorrhea. When OC use is discontinued these symptoms occur, suggesting a causal relation. However, data from three studies indicate that the incidence of pituitary adenoma among users of OCs is not higher than that among matched controls.

Malignant melanoma

Several epidemiologic studies have been undertaken to assess the relation of OC use and the development of malignant melanoma. The results are conflicting, since an increased risk, a decreased risk, and no effect have all been reported. In a review by Prentice and Thomas, the summary relative risk for eight case-control studies was 1.0 and for three cohort studies 1.4, an insignificant increase. Thus there is no convincing evidence that OC use increases the risk of developing malignant melanoma.

In summary, there is an increased risk of cervical neoplasia among OC users (but no correlation has been established), as well as development of a benign liver adenoma. The incidence of breast cancer, pituitary adenomas, and melanoma is the same in OC users and control groups and there is a decreased risk of two lethal cancers – endometrial cancer and ovarian cancer – with reduction in risk persisting after OC use is discontinued.

Reproductive effects

The magnitude and duration of the delay in the return of fertility are greater for women discontinuing use of OCs with 50 µg of estrogen or more than with those containing lower doses of estrogen. However, Bracken *et al.* reported that use of the low-dose formulations still resulted in a reduction in conception rates for at least the first six cycles after discontinuation. In women stopping use of OCs in order to conceive, the probability of conception is lowest in the first month after stopping their use and increases steadily thereafter. There is little, if any, effect of duration of OC use upon the length of delay of subsequent conception but the magnitude of the delay to return of conception after OC use is greater among older premenopausal women.

Thus, for 2–3 years after the discontinuation of contraceptives in order to conceive, the rate of return of fertility is lower for users of OCs than for women who have used barrier methods. Eventually the percentage of women who conceive after ceasing to use each of these contraceptive methods becomes the same. Thus, the use of OCs does not cause permanent infertility.

Because the resumption of ovulation is delayed for variable periods after OCs are stopped, it is difficult to estimate the expected date of delivery if conception takes place before spontaneous menses return. For this reason, when women stop OCs in order to conceive, it is probably best that they use barrier methods for about 1–2 months until regular cycles resume. If conception occurs before resumption of spontaneous mensus, gestational age should be estimated by serial sonography. Neither the rate of spontaneous abortion nor the incidence of chromosomal abnormalities in abortuses is increased in women who conceive in the first or subsequent months after ceasing to use OCs.

Several cohort and case-control studies of large numbers of babies born to women who stopped using OCs have been undertaken. These studies indicate that these infants have no greater chance of being born with any type of birth defect than infants born to women in the general population, even if conception occurred in the first month after the medication was discontinued. If these steroids are ingested during the first few months of pregnancy, a recent review by Bracken and Vita of all the prospective epidemiologic studies with a control group of women not using OCs reported that there was no increased risk of congenital malformations overall among the offspring of OC users. Furthermore there was no increased risk of congenital heart defects or limb reduction defects in OC users. An increased risk of these anomalies had been reported in early case-control studies of women ingesting OCs after conception. However, the results could have been influenced by recall bias. A statement warning of a possible teratogenic effect of ingestion of OCs during pregnancy has been deleted from current product labeling for OCs.

Metabolic effects

Different metabolic effects of contraceptive steroids are produced by the estrogenic component, ethinylestradiol, as well as the progestin. In general, the severity of these adverse metabolic effects is directly correlated with the dosage and potency (biologic activity) of steroid in the formulation. During the past 30 years the amount of both the estrogenic and progestogenic component of formulations has decreased markedly and has been accompanied by a lower incidence and severity of the adverse metabolic effects.

Protein

The synthetic estrogens used in OCs increase the hepatic production of several globulins, some of which are involved in the coagulation process. Another globulin, angiotensinogen, may be converted to angiotensin and increase blood pressure in some users. The circulating levels of each of these globulins correlate directly with the amount of estrogen in the OC formulation. Epidemiologic studies have shown that the incidence of both venous and arterial thrombosis is also directly related to the dose of estrogen.

Angiotensinogen levels are lower in women who ingest formulations with 30–35 µg ethinylestradiol than in those who ingest formulations with 50 µg. However, there is still a significant increase in blood pressure in women who receive the lower dosage. Thus, blood pressure should be monitored in all users of OCs. Indirect evidence suggests that the progestin component may also affect blood pressure. However, women who receive progestins without estrogen do not have an increase in blood pressure over time, indicating that the estrogen component is the major factor in causing elevated blood pressure in certain users of OCs.

Carbohydrate

When formulations with a high dose of progestin are administered, 4–16% of women (depending on their age) have an abnormal response to the glucose tolerance test. The incidence of abnormal test results is related to the dose and potency of the progestin, since estrogen does not affect carbohydrate metabolism. Some studies have shown that formulations with a low dose of progestin do not significantly alter levels of glucose, insulin, or glucagon after a glucose load in healthy women or in those with a history of gestational diabetes. However, other studies indicate that the multiphasic formulations with norgestrel, but not those with norethindrone, produce some deterioration of glucose tolerance in normal women, as well as in those with a history of gestational diabetes.

When one is prescribing these agents for women with a history of glucose intolerance, it is preferable to use formulations with a low dose of a progestin. Kjos *et al.* have shown that women with a previous history of gestational diabetes ingesting these agents have no greater risk of developing diabetes than a control group using other methods of contraception. Data from 20 years' experience with use of mainly high-dose formulations in the large Royal College of General Practitioners study revealed no increased risk of developing diabetes mellitus among current OC users (relative risk 0.80) or former OC users (relative risk 0.82), even among those women who had used OCs for 10 years or longer.

Lipids

Adverse alterations in high-density lipoprotein (HDL) cholesterol and low-density lipoprotein (LDL) cholesterol are produced by all the progestins currently used in OCs available in the USA, and the degree of change in the levels of these cholesterols is related to the amount and potency of the progestin. Because the estrogen component has an effect opposite to that of the progestin, a decrease in HDL cholesterol levels after the ingestion of various formulations containing 50 µg of estrogen has been noted only for a formulation containing norgestrel. Studies have measured lipid levels before and after the ingestion of several low-dose estrogen–progestin formulations, including the triphasic formulation containing levonorgestrel. These found no adverse alterations in the levels of HDL or LDL cholesterol or in the ratio of total cholesterol to HDL cholesterol. In two prospective randomized studies of the 3 triphasic formulations currently being marketed in the USA, it has been reported that each had similar effects which were clinically insignificant upon carbohydrate and lipid metabolism, including changes in HDL, HDL_2 and LDL cholesterol. Studies with formulations containing the three newly synthesized progestins indicate that these also produce no alteration in lipid or carbohydrate metabolism. Thus, the most recently developed low-dose OCs have no adverse effects on carbohydrate or lipid metabolism.

Other metabolic effects

The symptoms most frequently produced by the estrogenic component include nausea (a central nervous system effect), breast tenderness, and fluid retention, which usually does not exceed 1–2 kg body weight, due to decreased sodium excretion. Minor, clinically insignificant changes in circulating vitamin levels also occurred after ingestion of the higher-dosage OCs. These changes include a decrease in levels of the B-complex vitamins and ascorbic acid and increases in levels of vitamin A. Even with use of the high-steroid-dose agents, dietary vitamin supplementation was not necessary as the changes in circulating vitamin levels were small and clinically insignificant. Estrogen can also cause chloasma (pigmentation of the malar eminences), which is accentuated by sunlight and usually takes a long time to disappear after OCs are discontinued. The incidence of all these estrogenic side-effects is much lower now than occurred previously because the formulations in use today contain only one-fifth as much estrogen as the formulations used in the 1960s.

The estrogen component of OC agents also accelerates the development of the symptoms of gallbladder disease in young women but does not increase the overall incidence of cholelithiasis. In a very large, retrospective cohort study by Strom *et al.*, the risk ratio for gallbladder disease in OC users was only 1.14, which barely achieved statistical significance. Among women using formulations with less than 50 μg of estrogen, the risk ratio for gallbladder disease was 0.97.

Data from studies of postmenopausal women receiving estrogen therapy alone, as well as estrogen–progestin sequential therapy, indicate that estrogen alone improves the mood of women, whereas the addition of a progestin increases the amount of depression, irritability, tension, and fatigue. These studies also indicate that the progestin component may be the major cause of the adverse mood changes and tiredness observed in some women after ingestion of OCs. It has not been definitely established, however, whether estrogen or progestin is the major factor in producing adverse mood changes. Possibly both are involved.

The progestins, because they are structurally related to testosterone, also produce certain adverse androgenic effects, including weight gain, acne, and a symptom perceived by some women as nervousness. Some women gain a considerable amount of weight when they take OCs, and this weight gain is produced by the anabolic effect of the progestin component. Although estrogens decrease sebum production, progestins increase sebum production and can cause acne to develop or worsen. Thus patients who have acne should be given a formulation with a low progestin:estrogen ratio. The final symptom produced by the progestin component is failure of withdrawal bleeding or amenorrhea. Because the progestins decrease the synthesis of estrogen receptors in the endometrium, endometrial growth is decreased, and some women have failure of withdrawal bleeding. Although this symptom is not important medically, since bleeding serves as a signal that the woman is not pregnant, it is desirable to have some amount of periodic withdrawal bleeding during the days she is not taking these steroids.

Both steroid components can act together to produce irregular bleeding. Breakthrough bleeding (which is usually produced by insufficient estrogen, too much progestin, or a combination of both), as well as failure of withdrawal bleeding, can be alleviated by increasing the amount of estrogen in the formulation or by switching to a more estrogenic formulation. Many women taking OCs complain of an increased frequency of headaches. The exact relation, if any, between OC use and headaches has not been determined.

Cardiovascular effects

One must be concerned about the adverse changes in lipid levels produced by the progestin component of certain high-progestin-dose OC formulations. However, the cause of the increased incidence of both venous and arterial cardiovascular disease, including myocardial infarction, in users of OCs appears to be thrombosis and not atherosclerosis.

Estrogens can increase blood viscosity by raising plasma fibrinogen levels as well as hematocrit. The synthetic progestins also increase blood viscosity by raising hematocrit and decreasing erythrocyte deformability. Increased blood viscosity, produced by either of these two steroid-dose-related mechanisms, could cause an increased incidence of thrombosis. This could explain the findings in several epidemiologic studies, including the Royal College of General Practitioners study, that the incidence of both venous and arterial thrombotic events is directly related independently to both the dose of estrogen and the dose of progestin.

Neither epidemiologic studies of humans nor experimental studies with subhuman primates have observed an acceleration of atherosclerosis with the ingestion of OCs. Three large epidemiologic studies found that there is no increased risk of myocardial infarction among former users of OCs. The incidence of cardiovascular disease is also not correlated with the duration of OC use.

Studies suggest that the estrogen component of OCs may have a protective effect on coronary arteriosclerosis that would otherwise be accelerated by decreased levels of HDL cholesterol.

The epidemiologic studies that reported an increased incidence of myocardial infarction in older users of OCs were published in the late 1970s and thus used as a database women who ingested only formulations with 50 µg or more of estrogen. In these case-control and cohort studies, a significantly increased incidence of myocardial infarction was found mainly among older users who had risk factors that caused arterial narrowing, particularly smoking, as well as preexisting hypercholesterolemia, hypertension, or diabetes mellitus.

Data accumulated during the first 10 years of the Royal College of General Practitioners study, 1968–1978, in which most users ingested formulations with >50 µg of estrogen and high doses of progestin, showed that a significantly increased relative risk of death from circulatory disease occurred only among women over age 35 who also smoked. A more recent analysis of data obtained during the first 20 years of this study, 1968–1988, revealed no significant increased relative risk of acute myocardial infarction among current or former OC users who did not smoke cigarettes. Even though most of the women in this study used high-dose formulations, a significantly increased risk of myocardial infarction occurred only among both mild (<15 cigarettes a day) and heavy cigarette smokers, with the latter group having a greater relative risk. In this and other studies, cigarette smoking was an independent risk factor for myocardial infarction, but the use of OCs by cigarette smokers greatly enhanced their risk of developing a myocardial infarction, with the two factors acting synergistically.

Although epidemiologic data from studies performed in the 1970s indicated that a possible causal relation existed between ingestion of high-dose OC formulations and cerebrovascular accident (CVA, stroke), the data were conflicting. Some studies showed a significantly increased risk of thrombotic CVA, others an increased risk of hemorrhagic CVA, and others no significantly increased risk of either entity. Furthermore, as with myocardial infarction, the studies showing a significantly increased risk of CVA in OC users indicated that the increased risk was mainly limited to older women who also smoked and/or were hypertensive.

Data from the epidemiologic studies of OC use and cardiovascular disease performed in the 1960s and 1970s are not relevant to current OC use, since the dose of both steroid components in the formulations now being marketed is much less and women with cardiovascular risk factors, such as hypertension, are no longer receiving these agents. Furthermore, it is strongly recommended that OCs should not be prescribed to women over age 35 who also smoke. All the epidemiologic studies performed during the past 14 years have shown no significantly increased risk of arterial vascular events such as myocardial infarction or stroke in OC users, as well as a steadily decreasing risk of venous thrombosis.

Data accumulated during the first 10 years of the Royal College of General Practitioners study, 1968–1978, in which most users ingested formulations with more than 50 µg of estrogen and high doses of progestin, showed that a significantly increased relative risk of death from circulatory disease occurred only among women over age 35 who also smoked.

After analyzing all the published epidemiologic data, it appears that healthy nonsmokers can continue to use OCs up to menopausal age, without having an increased risk of cardiovascular disease, provided they are using formulations with less than 50 µg of estrogen and a low dose of progestin. There is no evidence of an increased risk of cardiovascular disease associated with increasing duration of use of OCs or previous use of OCs. Thus women can take OCs for an unlimited time period, no matter how old they are when they start taking them. There is no need for a rest period after a few years of OC use, as it does not serve any value.

SUGGESTED READING

BERAL V, NANNAFORD PC, KAY C. Oral contraceptive use and malignancies of the genital tract. *Lancet* 1988;2:1331.

BRACKEN MB, VITA K. Frequency of non-hormonal contraception around conception and association with congenital malformations in offspring. *Am J Epidemiol* 1983;117:281.

BRACKEN MB, HELLENBRAND KG, HOLFORD TR. Conception delay after oral contraceptive use: the effect of estrogen dose. *Fertil Steril* 1990;53:21.

BOTTINGER LE, BOMAN G, EKLUND G, et al. Oral contraceptives and thromboembolic disease: effects of lowering oestrogen content. *Lancet* 1980;1:1097.

BRINTON LA, HUGGINS GR, LEHMAN HF, et al. Long-term use of oral contraceptives and risk of invasive cervical cancer. *Int J Cancer* 1986;38:339.

CENTERS FOR DISEASE CONTROL CANCER AND STEROID HORMONE STUDY. Long-term oral contraceptive use and the risk of breast cancer. *JAMA* 1983;249:1591.

DITKOFF EC, CRARY WG, CRISTO M, LOBO RA. Estrogen improves psychological function in asymptomatic postmenopausal women. *Obstet Gynecol* 1991;78:991.

HANNAFORD PC, KAY CR (Royal College of General Practitioners). Oral contraceptives and diabetes mellitus. *Br Med J* 1989;299:1315–1316.

KJOS SL, SHOUPE D, DOUHAM S, *et al*. Effect of low-dose oral contraceptives on carbohydrate and lipid metabolism in women with recurrent gestational diabetes: results of a controlled randomized prospective study. *Am J Obstet Gynecol* 1990;163:1822.

KUNG AW, MA JT, WONG VC, *et al*. Glucose and lipid metabolism with triphasic oral contraceptives in women with history of gestational diabetes. *Contraception* 1987;35:357–369.

LAYDE PM, BERAL V, KAR CR. Further analysis of mortality in oral contraceptive users. Royal College of General Practitioners Oral Contraceptive Study. *Lancet* 1981;1:1541.

LUYCKX AS, GASPARD UJ, GRIGORESCU F, DEMEYTS P, LEFEBVRE PJ. Carbohydrate metabolism in women who used oral contraceptives containing levonorgestrel or desogestrel: a 6-month prospective study. *Fertil Steril* 1986;45:635–642.

MEADE TW. Oral contraceptives, clotting factors, and thrombosis. *Am J Obstet Gynecol* 1982;142:758.

MEADE TW, GREENBERG G, THOMPSON SG. Progestogens and cardiovascular reactions associated with oral contraceptives and a comparison of the safety of 50- and 30-µg estrogen preparations. *Br Med J* 1980;1:1157.

NOTELOVITZ M, FELDMAN EB, GILLESPY M, *et al*. Lipid and lipoprotein changes in women taking low-dose, triphasic oral contraceptives: a controlled, comparative, 12-month clinical trial. *Am J Obstet Gynecol* 1989;160:1269.

PATSCH W, BROWN SA, GOTTO AM, *et al*. The effect of triphasic oral contraceptives on plasma lipids and lipoproteins. *Am J Obstet Gynecol* 1989;161:1396.

PIKE MC, HENDERSON BE, KRAILO MD, *et al*. Breast cancer in young women and use of oral contraceptives: possible modifying effect of formulation and age at use. *Lancet* 1983;2:926.

PITUITARY ADENOMA STUDY GROUP. Pituitary adenomas and oral contraceptives: a multi-center case-control study. *Fertil Steril* 1983;39:753.

PORTER JB, HUNTER JR, DANIELSON DA, *et al*. Oral contraceptive and nonfatal vascular disease – recent experience. *Obstet Gynecol* 1982;59:299.

PORTER JB, HUNTER JR, JICK H, *et al*. Oral contraceptives and nonfatal vascular disease. *Obstet Gynecol* 1985;66:1.

PRENTICE RL, THOMAS DB. On the epidemiology of oral contraceptives and disease. *Adv Cancer Res* 1987;49:285.

RAMCHARAN S, PELLEGRIN FA, RAY RM, HSU J-P. *The Walnut Creek Contraceptive Drug Study: A Prospective Study of the Side Effects of Oral Contraceptives*, vol 3, NIH Publication no 181-584. Washington DC: US Government Printing Office, 1981.

ROSENBERG L, PALMER JR, LESKO SM, SHAPIRO S. Oral contraceptive use and the risk of myocardial infarction. *Am J Epidemiol* 1990;131:1009–1016.

SCHLESSELMAN JJ. Cancer of the breast and reproductive tract in relation to use of oral contraceptives. *Contraception* 1989;40:1.

SHERWIN BB, GELFAND MM. A prospective one-year study of estrogen and progestin in postmenopausal women: effects on clinical symptoms and lipoprotein lipids. *Obstet Gynecol* 1989;73:759–766.

SKOUBY SO, KUHL C, MOLSTED-PEDERSEN L, PETERSEN K, CHRISTENSEN MS. Triphasic oral contraception: metabolic effects in normal women and those with previous gestational diabetes. *Am J Obstet Gynecol* 1985;153:495–500.

STADEL BV, RUBIN GL, WEBSTER LA, *et al.* Oral contraceptives and breast cancer in young women. *Lancet* 1985;2:970.

STAMPFER MJ, WILLETT WC, COLDITZ GA, *et al.* A prospective study of past use of oral contraceptive agents and risk of cardiovascular diseases. *N Engl J Med* 1988;3329:1313.

STROM BL, TAMRAGOURI RN, MORSE ML, *et al.* Oral contraceptives and other factors for gallbladder disease. *Clin Pharmacol Ther* 1986;39:335–341.

THOROGOOD M, MANN J, MURPHY M, VESSY M. Is oral contraceptive use still associated with an increased risk of fatal myocardial infarction? Report of a case control study. *Br J Obstet Gynecol* 1991;98:1245–1253.

THOROGOOD M, MANN J, MURPHY M, VESSY M. Risk factors for fatal venous thromboembolism in young women: a case-control study. *Int J Epidemiol* 1992; 21:48.

THOROGOOD M, MANN J, MURPHY M, VESSY M. Fatal stroke and use of oral contraceptives: findings from a case-control study. *Am J Epidemiol* 1992;136: 35–45.

VAN DER VANGE N, KLOOSTERBOER HJ, HASPELS IAA. Effect of seven low-dose combined oral contraceptive preparations on carbohydrate metabolism. *Am J Obstet Gynecol* 1987;156:918–922.

VESSEY MP, DOLL R, PETO R. A long-term follow-up study of women using different methods of contraception – an interim report. *J Biosoc Sci* 1976;8:373.

VESSEY MP, WRIGHT NH, MCPHERSON K, *et al.* Fertility after stopping different methods of contraception. *Br Med J* 1978;1:265.

WILSON JG, BRENT RL. Are female sex hormones teratogenic? *Am J Obstet Gynecol* 1981;141:576.

WINGO PA, LEE NC, ORY HW, BERAL V, PETERSON HB, RHODES PR. Age-specific differences in the relationship between oral contraceptive use and breast cancer. *Obstet Gynecol* 1991;78:161.

WORLD HEALTH ORGANIZATION. Combined oral contraceptives and liver cancer. *Int J Cancer* 1989;43:254.

119

Norplant contraceptive system

PAUL F. BRENNER

The Norplant contraceptive system is a long-term, sustained release of progestin, estrogen-free, reversible method of family planning. Norplant consists of six capsules made of Silastic tubing which contain levonorgestrel. Each capsule is 34 mm in length and 2.4 mm in outside diameter. Each Silastic tube is filled with 36 mg of crystalline levonorgestrel and each end of the tube is sealed with a Silastic plug. The amount of steroid released per unit time is related to the surface area of the Silastic delivery system. The release rate of levonorgestrel in each six-capsule Norplant system is 80 µg/day initially, 50 µg/day at the end of the first year of use, and 30 µg/day from the second through the fifth year of use. The duration of action is related to the amount of steroid contained within the Silastic delivery system. Norplant provides a highly efficacious family planning method lasting for 5 years.

The Norplant capsules are placed subdermally in the volar surface of the upper arm. This location seems to provide an area which favors the retrieval of the capsules and yet the site is concealed, lessening the chance of any embarrassment to the acceptor. The insertion procedure does not require a great deal of manual dexterity. The site chosen for insertion is cleansed with Betadine and injected with a local anesthetic. A 3-mm stab wound in the skin is made with a scalpel and through this incision a 10–12-gauge trocar is advanced subdermally. A capsule is inserted into the trocar and directed to the tip of the trocar with a stylet. The stylet is held steady and the trocar is withdrawn back toward the incision leaving the capsule in the desired location. As the trocar is moved in a fan-like pattern, a total of six capsules containing levonorgestrel is placed. The stylet and trocar are removed and a butterfly plaster is placed over the incision. A suture is not necessary. A pressure dressing is placed and left on for 24 h.

When synthetic steroids are administered orally there is a rapid rise in the steroid concentration in the blood which peaks in 0.5–2 h and then declines to a nadir just before the ingestion of the next dose. Birth-control pills administered orally once a day must contain a sufficient dose of steroid so that the blood levels, even at the nadir, are sufficient to maintain the contraceptive efficacy of the method. Norplant offers a sustained, relatively constant release of steroid, thus resulting in much less fluctuation of blood levels throughout the day. The major mechanism of action of Norplant in the first year is the inhibition of ovulation. In succeeding years the incidence of ovulatory cycles increases in Norplant users and other mechanisms involving the cervical mucus and the endometrium maintain the high effectiveness of the method. Norplant does not suppress estrogen levels to the menopausal range. Estrogen levels fluctuate during the use of Norplant and generally are in the range usually seen in the early proliferative phase of a normal menstrual cycle.

Norplant is a highly effective contraceptive system with a pregnancy rate of 0.2 per 100 women-years for the first year of use and a cumulative pregnancy rate of 1.1 per 100 women-years for 5 consecutive years of use. This high degree of effectiveness is at least equal to if not superior to combination oral contraceptives. The women who experience amenorrhea while using Norplant have an even lower pregnancy rate than those acceptors who have menstrual bleeding. There was some concern that efficacy was inversely related to body weight and particularly women who weighed more than 70 kg had diminished efficacy while using Norplant. Implants made of dense Silastic tubing are associated with higher pregnancy rates than the implants made of soft tubing. All Norplant capsules now available to the consumer are composed of soft Silastic tubing. With these later capsules body weight is no longer a factor affecting the efficacy of the method. When the Norplant capsules are removed there is a prompt return of fertility for those wishing to conceive.

Norplant users report an increase in the number of bleeding and spotting days. While a very rare Norplant acceptor may experience very heavy uterine bleeding, as a large group women using the Norplant capsules do not experience an increase in the mean menstrual blood loss per month or a drop in their hemoglobin and hematocrit even in the first month of use. With each successive year of use the mean number of bleeding and spotting days per month decreases, as does uterine blood loss, and hemoglobin and hematocrit levels increase slightly. With continued use of the subdermal contraceptive capsules the incidence of amenorrhea increases. Still the greatest inconvenience of this method of contraception is the unpredictability of the menstrual pattern.

Norplant is a contraceptive modality that offers several advantages: it is a completely reversible, highly effective, estrogen-free method. Levonorgestrel is released at a relatively constant rate, avoiding the peaks and nadirs of oral administration of steroids. This allows for the maintenance of constant serum levels of steroid in the peripheral circulation which provide highly effective contraception even though the administered dose has been reduced. The reduced blood levels of steroid provide a progestin-only method of contraception which has a minimal impact on carbohydrate and lipid metabolism. The few changes in carbohydrate and lipid metabolism which have been reported result in values which remain within the reference range and have no practical clinical significance. Because the patient cannot discontinue Norplant on her own, but must seek medical intervention, this family-planning method has a high continuation rate.

There are some disadvantages associated with the use of Norplant, including cycle control, with an increase in the number of days of bleeding and spotting initially and amenorrhea the longer the method is maintained. Norplant use is associated with some nuisance side-effects, including headache, depression, weight gain, acne, hirsutism, and anxiety. The subdermal capsules require both a surgical insertion and a surgical removal. At times the removal procedure may be more difficult than the insertion. If the capsules are not placed subdermally at the time of insertion then retrieval may be difficult. At times the capsules are covered with a fibrous sheath which must be incised to extricate the capsules. Norplant can be an expensive contraceptive method. There is a charge for the set of six capsules, a charge for the first visit–history–physical examination–pelvic exam–Pap smear, an insertion fee, and a removal fee. For those women who use the Norplant system for 5 years and the total expense is amortized over 60 months, the expense of Norplant compares very favorably to the use of oral contraceptives for the same period of time. Some women report that the visibility of the elevation of the skin ridges overlying the Norplant capsules is embarrassing.

There are several criteria which define appropriate candidates for Norplant. Women who seek long-term birth spacing will find Norplant an important option. Women who desire not to have any more children, but who are not ready to opt for a permanent method of family planning, will also find Norplant appealing. Women who have experienced problems with other contraceptive modalities are particularly good candidates for Norplant. Women who have demonstrated poor compliance with other contraceptive modalities will find Norplant, which requires virtually no monitoring by the acceptor once the capsules are placed, a reasonable alternative. Women who have contraindications for an intrauterine device will also be well advised to consider Norplant. Women who have reason to avoid estrogen should be counseled concerning the use of Norplant. This would include women who are 6 or more weeks postpartum, continue to breast-feed, and are sexually active. Women who have a history of several pregnancy terminations are also appropriate candidates for Norplant.

At a time when there is a desperate need for highly effective, long-term contraceptive modalities, Norplant is an important addition to family-planning techniques.

SUGGESTED READING

BRACHE V, ALVAREZ-SANCHEZ F, FAUNDES A, TEJADA AS, COCHON L. Ovarian endocrine function through five years of continuous treatment with Norplant[r] subdermal contraceptive implants. *Contraception* 1990;41:169–177.

DARNEY PD, KLAISLE CM, TANNER S, ALVARADO AM. Sustained-release contraceptives. *Curr Probl Obstet Gynecol Fertil* 1990;13:87–125.

DIAZ S, CROXATTO HB, PAVEZ M, BELHADJ H, STERN J, SIVIN I. Clinical assessment of treatments for prolonged bleeding in users of Norplant[r] implants. *Contraception* 1990;42:97–109.

DIAZ J, RUBIN J, FAUNDES A, DIAZ M, BAHAMONDES L. Comparison of local signs and symptoms after the insertion of Norplant[r] implants with and without a scalpel. *Contraception* 1991;44:217–221.

HARDY E, GOODSON P. Association between contraceptive method accepted and perception of information received: a comparison of Norplant and IUD acceptors. *Contraception* 1991;43:121–128.

KLAVON SL, GRUBB GS. Insertion site complications during the first year of Norplant[r] use. *Contraception* 1990;41:27–37.

KONJE JC, OTOLORIN EO, LADIPO OA. Changes in carbohydrate metabolism during 30 months on Norplant[r]. *Contraception* 1991;44:163–172.

SINGH K, VIEGAS OAC, LOKE DFM, RATNAM SS. Effect of Norplant[r] implants on liver, lipid and carbohydrate metabolism. *Contraception* 1992;45:141–153.

SIVIN I. International experience with Norplant[r] and Norplant[r]-2 contraceptives. *Stud Fam Plann* 1988;19:81–94.

120

Depo-Provera

PAUL F. BRENNER

Introduction

Depo-Provera (Depo-medroxyprogesterone acetate, DMPA), is a long-acting reversible hormonal method of family planning which is administered as an intramuscular injection. The hormone used in this contraceptive method is medroxyprogesterone acetate, which is an acetoxyprogesterone derivative. This is a progestin-only form of contraception. Worldwide there have been more than 30 million users of DMPA since 1960. Currently it is estimated that there are 3.5 million users in more than 90 countries. DMPA has been widely studied. There are more than 1000 scientific papers published pertaining to this injectable progestin contraceptive.

DMPA is a long-acting, highly convenient family-planning method which is easy to administer. DMPA is an aqueous suspension of micro-crystals administered by an intramuscular injection every 12 weeks. The injection site should not be massaged immediately following each injection. For women who are not current contraceptive acceptors, the first injection of DMPA should be given within the first 5 days after the onset of the last regular menstrual cycle. Contraception protection in this setting begins with the initial injection and the concomitant use of a second method is not necessary in order to enhance the prevention of pregnancy. DMPA does not protect against sexually transmitted diseases (STDs). DMPA users who are at risk for STDs should be advised to use a barrier method of contraception which contains nonoxynol 9 in addition to their injectable contraceptive. Women who are currently using either oral contraceptives or an intrauterine device and wish to switch to DMPA may receive the first injection at any time in the pill or intrauterine device cycle. Oral contraceptive use should continue after the injection until all 21 active birth-control pills are ingested. Intrauterine device removal is delayed following the first DMPA injection until the onset of the next menses.

Postpartum women may receive DMPA. Nonlactating new mothers can begin DMPA within 5 days following delivery. Postpartum women desiring to breast-feed should delay the first injection of DMPA until lactation is established, which is usually 4–6 weeks postpartum. DMPA does not adversely affect the volume or the composition of the breast milk. The growth and the development of infants born to lactating women using DMPA are normal. Women who have had a therapeutic abortion may also use DMPA. The administration of the initial injection should occur immediately after the pregnancy termination procedure is completed.

Mechanism of action

The most important mechanism whereby DMPA protects against unwanted pregnancy is the inhibition of ovulation. The mid-cycle surge of gonadotropins is eliminated. Estrogen levels in the peripheral circulation of DMPA acceptors are within the range usually found in the early follicular phase of a normal menstrual cycle. Additional antifertility effects include the formation of an atrophic endometrium which is unfavorable for implantation and a thick, viscous cervical mucus which impedes sperm penetration. Fallopian tube motility may also be decreased.

Based on studies which measured gonadotropin levels in DMPA users, ovulation is suppressed for at least 14 weeks following each intramuscular injection of 150 mg DMPA. Therefore repeat injections of DMPA should be within 14 weeks to optimize efficacy and reduce the opportunity for unwanted pregnancies. In clinical practice 150 mg injectable DMPA is administered every 12 weeks. Since ovulation is very unlikely during the 13th and 14th week following the last injection, women may be reinjected during this period of time. If the woman delays follow-up for more than 14 weeks since her previous administration of DMPA, the possibility that she may be pregnant must be considered before further DMPA is offered. Following either a single dose or multiple trimonthly injections of 150 mg DMPA, the levels of medroxyprogesterone acetate in the peripheral circulation increase, and reach peak concentrations at approximately 10 days following the last injection. The serum concentrations of DMPA then gradually decline for the remainder of the 12-week dosing interval. Depending on the sensitivity of the assay, medroxyprogesterone acetate may be found in the serum more than 200 days following a single injection of 150 mg DMPA. Repeat injections of intramuscular DMPA at 12-week intervals do not result in an accumulation of drug, as determined by the assay of medroxyprogesterone acetate at frequent intervals. Mean estradiol levels in DMPA users for 1–2 years, 2–4 years, and 4–5 years were 36 ± 2.0, 38 ± 2.1 and 42 ± 1.6 pg/ml respectively. These estrogen concentrations are not significantly different and indirectly indicate the lack of the accumulation of drug or drug effect over an extended number of years.

DMPA 150 mg administered as an intramuscular injection at 3-month intervals has a pregnancy rate (failure rate) in actual clinical use of 0.4 per 100 women-years. The reported pregnancy rate with DMPA is very similar to that of the Norplant contraceptive system and lower than that of the Paragard intrauterine device (0.7), oral contraceptives (3.0), condom (12.0), diaphragm (18.0), and foam (21.0).

DMPA users experience a disruption of cycle control. Menstrual irregularities are one of the most common reasons for the discontinuation of this method of family planning. Pretherapy counseling which prepares potential DMPA acceptors for abnormal bleeding patterns and amenorrhea will reduce the termination rates of DMPA for this reason. In the first 3-month treatment interval, one-third of the newly starting DMPA users experience an increased number of days of bleeding and spotting, one-third have a normal number of days of bleeding and spotting, and one-third have an absence of menstruation. With continued use of DMPA the percent of women experiencing amenorrhea increases and the percent experiencing increased bleeding and spotting decreases.

Table 120.1 Side-effects experienced in women taking DMPA

Side-effect	Percentage
Headache	17.1
Abdominal discomfort	13.4
Nervousness	10.8
Dizziness	5.4
Decreased libido	5.4
Asthenia	3.8
Varicose vein pain	3.6
Nausea	3.4
Vaginal discharge	2.8
Breast discomfort	2.7
Peripheral edema	2.1
Backache	2.1
Dysmenorrhea	1.8
Depression	1.7
Acne	1.3
Hair loss	1.2

Because DMPA is a potent inhibitor of ovulation, clinically dysmenorrhea is significantly reduced in DMPA users. There is a positive correlation with the duration of use of DMPA and the percent of women experiencing amenorrhea. Therefore women who continued to use DMPA are less likely to be anemic. The side-effects and the percent of women reporting side-effects while receiving DMPA are given in Table 120.1. Women using DMPA may experience an average of 2 kg (approx. 5 lb) weight gain in the first year and 1.5 kg (approx. 3 lb) more by the end of the second year.

DMPA was developed in 1954 for the treatment of endometriosis and habitual abortion. In 1960 this drug was approved by the Food and Drug Administration (FDA) for use in treating these two disease entities and in 1968 it was approved by the FDA as a contraceptive. Concerns about the delay in the return to fertility when DMPA acceptors discontinue the drug, possible teratogenicity, and carcinogenesis prompted the FDA in 1972 to stay the approval of DMPA as a contraceptive. In the same year DMPA gained FDA approval for use as adjunctive endometrial cancer therapy.

DMPA users may expect to experience a delay in return of fertility when they discontinue the use of DMPA in order to conceive. Recovery of the reproductive axis and pregnancy are quite variable from patient to patient. Pregnancy may occur as early as 4 months after the last DMPA injection and as late as 31 months or longer after stopping DMPA in order to conceive. The return of fertility is unrelated to the number of DMPA injections the patient has received. The median time interval from the last injection to conception is approximately 10 months.

Information has been collected pertaining to the pregnancy outcome of 241 of 285 pregnancies which have occurred in DMPA users. The incidence of congenital anomalies, spontaneous abortion, ectopic pregnancy, premature births, stillborn infants, and multifetal gestations was not increased in women who conceived while using DMPA compared to women who conceived at a time when they were not using any method of family planning. *In utero* exposure to DMPA does not appear to be teratogenic or detrimental to pregnancy outcome.

Approval of DMPA for contraceptive use in the USA was delayed primarily due to findings that DMPA exposure in beagle dogs increased the presence of benign and malignant mammary tumors. These findings were extrapolated to suggest that DMPA use in the human female might cause breast cancer. The World Health Organization Collaborative Study was conducted in part to determine the cancer risk in DMPA acceptors. This study concluded that women using DMPA for contraception were not at increased risk for breast cancer, cervical cancer, or ovarian cancer. Furthermore there was no association between the risk of breast cancer and the duration of use of DMPA. A weak association between DMPA use and breast cancer may be present in women under 35 years of age who had first used the drug within the previous 4 years. The risk of cervical cancer was also not related to the extended use of DMPA. Use of DMPA as a female contraceptive does significantly reduce the risk of endometrial cancer. DMPA has no neoplastic effects in women, with the exception of the protection which it provides in reducing the risk of endometrial cancer.

As with any steroidal form of family planning, the metabolic impact of DMPA must be considered. Steroids administered in sufficient doses and potency are known to alter carbohydrate and lipid metabolism and the coagulation cascade. The effects of DMPA on the lipid profile have varied from one study to another. Depending on the study, total serum cholesterol has been reported to be unchanged, increased or decreased. Low-density lipoprotein cholesterol concentrations were reported as unchanged or increased during DMPA use. Most studies have concluded that high-density lipoprotein cholesterol levels decrease during DMPA use. A slight impairment of glucose tolerance occurs in DMPA acceptors. These changes in glucose metabolism, while statistically significant, are mild and most likely lack any clinical relevance. The effect of DMPA injected as a hormonal contraceptive every 3 months is almost nil on a large number of coagulation parameters. A significant reduction in antithrombin III levels after 15 months of DMPA use has been reported but virtually all other parameters remain unaffected by DMPA use. In conclusion, DMPA would appear to produce no significant changes in the coagulation cascade, a mild impairment of carbohydrate metabolism, and a decrease in serum high-density lipoprotein cholesterol levels.

One study has reported a 7% reduction in bone density in users of DMPA for the purpose of contraception compared to controls. There is a question as to whether this is an effect of DMPA due to the lowering of endogenous estrogen levels or due to flaws in the experimental design of the study.

DMPA is a contraceptive modality which is particularly suited for women who desire a long-acting, coital-independent, convenient, highly efficacious method of family planning. Women who have experienced unacceptable side-effects or contraceptive failures while using other methods of family planning or who have contraindications to the use – particularly to estrogen – of other methods of contraception may wish to consider the use of DMPA. For women with sickle cell disease DMPA is the contraceptive method of first choice. These women experience a decrease in anemia and a decrease in the crises which occur with this disease process.

There are some women who should not receive DMPA. These include women with undiagnosed abnormal vaginal bleeding, women who are pregnant or suspected of being pregnant, women with known or suspected breast cancer, women with a past history of deep vein thrombophlebitis, pulmonary embolus, or stroke, women who are allergic to DMPA, women who are unable to comply with the injection schedule, and women with active liver disease.

In conclusion, DMPA is a contraceptive method which is highly efficacious, easy to administer, highly acceptable to patients, does not contain estrogen, and minimizes patient responsibility. The only disadvantages to this form of contraception are the disruption of the normal menstrual pattern and the delay in the return of regular menses and fertility when the method is discontinued. DMPA is an important addition to the contraceptive choices of women.

SUGGESTED READING

FAHMY K, KHAIRY M, ALLAM G, GOBRAN F, ALLOUSH M. Effect of depo-medroxyprogesterone acetate on coagulation factors and serum lipids in Egyptian women. *Contraception* 1991;44:431–444.

GARZA-FLORES J, DELA CRUZ DL, VALLES DE BOURGES V, *et al*. Long-term effects of depot-medroxyprogesterone acetate on lipoprotein metabolism. *Contraception* 1991;44:61–71.

HUOVINEN K, TIKKANEN MJ, AUTIO S, *et al*. Serum lipids and lipoproteins during therapeutic amenorrhea induced by lynestrenol and depo-medroxyprogesterone acetate. *Acta Obstet Gynecol Scand* 1991;70:349–354.

LIEW DFM, NG CSA, YONG YM, RATNAM SS. Long-term effects of Depo-Provera on carbohydrate and lipid metabolism. *Contraception* 1985;31:51–64.

LOBO RA, MCCORMICK W, SINGER F, ROY S. Depo-medroxyprogesterone acetate compared with conjugated estrogens for the treatment of postmenopausal women. *Obstet Gynecol* 1984;63:1–5.

MISHELL DR Jr, KHARMA KM, THORNEYCROFT IH, NAKAMURA RM. Estrogenic activity in women receiving an injectable progestogen for contraception. *Am J Obstet Gynecol* 1972;113:372–376.

ORTIZ A, HIROI M, STANCZYK FZ, GOEBELSMANN U, MISHELL DR Jr. Serum medroxyprogesterone acetate (MPA) concentrations and ovarian function following intramuscular injection of depo-MPA. *J Clin Endocrinol Metab* 1977;44:32–38.

SCHWALLIE PC, ASSENZO JR. Contraceptive use – efficacy study utilizing medroxyprogesterone acetate administered as an intramuscular injection once every 90 days. *Fertil Steril* 1973;24:331–339.

WHO COLLABORATIVE STUDY OF NEOPLASIA AND STEROID CONTRACEPTIVES. Breast cancer and depot-medroxyprogesterone acetate: a multinational study. Lancet 1991;338:833–838.

ZACHARIAS S, AGUILERA E, ASSENZO JR, ZANARTU J. Effects of hormonal and nonhormonal contraceptives on lactation and incidence of pregnancy. *Contraception* 1986;33:203–213.

121

Postcoital contraception/interception

PAUL F. BRENNER & DANIEL R. MISHELL, JR

Some women, for a variety of reasons, are unable to anticipate the need for adequate contraception until after coitus has occurred. This may be the result of the failure of a contraceptive method, sexual assault, or, most commonly, both partners' neglect to practice contraception. Pregnancy may result from the first sexual encounter if the coital experience was unprotected or inadequately protected. The risk of pregnancy from one coital exposure at any time during the menstrual cycle, irrespective of the regularity of the patient's cycles and at any age in the reproductive years, has been estimated at 2–4%. The risk of pregnancy from one coital exposure at mid-cycle has been estimated to be 7%. Thus, there is a need for reversible pregnancy prevention that can be administered after coitus has occurred. These methods are referred to as postcoital contraception (PCC), interception, or morning-after estrogen therapy.

Diethylstilbestrol

The first hormonal formulation used for postcoital contraception was the synthetic estrogen diethylstilbestrol (DES). This agent was administered to women of child-bearing age who requested treatment within 72 h of a single unprotected or inadequately protected coital experience since the onset of the last menses. The therapeutic regimen consisted of 25 mg DES administered by mouth twice a day for 5 days. A dual mechanism of action was suggested for DES: the estrogen affects tubal physiology and hastens the transport of the ovum through the fallopian tube, at the same time making the endometrial environment unfavorable for implantation.

The DES regimen proved to be highly effective. The University of Michigan Health Service reported a series of 1410 women who received DES; of this group, complete follow-up was obtained from 1298 women. No pregnancies occurred in the 1217 women who had a single coital exposure within 72 h before receiving DES. Of this group, approximately 90% used no method of contraception, and coitus was judged to have occurred at mid-cycle in 70%. Eighty-one women had multiple coital exposures and/or sought medical advice more than 72 h after coitus, and six of this group became pregnant.

Fewer than half (45%) reported an absence of side-effects. Approximately half complained of nausea and vomiting. The incidence of all other side-effects (headaches, dizziness, diarrhea, bloating, breast discomfort, leukorrhea, mild lower abdominal cramping pain, weight gain, irritability, darkening of the breast areola, rash, increased libido, anorexia, leg cramps, and depression) was 1% or less. The timing and character of the menstrual flow following the administration of DES were not greatly altered.

The observation that maternal ingestion of DES in the first trimester of pregnancy increases the risk of vaginal adenosis and adenocarcinoma years later in the female progeny of these pregnancies, and is associated with other untoward effects on fetuses of either sex has led to the recommendation that DES should not be used as PCC when the patient does not agree to an abortion if the method fails. A comprehensive informed consent should be obtained from all women electing to use PCC.

Other estrogens

The possibility of teratogenic and other serious side-effects in babies of either sex born to women treated with DES in the first trimester of pregnancy, as well as the high incidence of gastrointestinal side-effects, provided the stimulus to investigate other agents for use as PCC. Under the same criteria as for the use of DES, ethinylestradiol 2–5 mg for 5 days and conjugated estrogen 30–50 mg daily for 5 days have been used for PCC. The results for >9000 women with mid-cycle coital exposures treated with postcoital estrogen indicate there were 29 pregnancies, for a failure rate of 0.3%. The concomitant use of an antiemetic with postcoital estrogens greatly reduces the nausea and emesis frequently reported with these formulations.

Fasoli *et al.* performed a comprehensive literature review in 1989 and summarized the results of the 21 articles published in English, Italian, and French between 1975 and 1977 on the subject of PCC. In the six studies of high-dose estrogen, 4143 women were included and most (3168) received ethinylestradiol. Pregnancy rates among the women treated with ethinylestradiol were 0.6%, with DES 0.7%, and with conjugated estrogen 1.6%. None of these rates was significantly different from the overall mean failure rate of 0.7%. None of the trials included a control group, but it has been estimated that the clinical pregnancy rate following mid-cycle coitus is approximately 7%. Thus high-dose estrogen is an effective method of PCC.

Combined therapy

Because compliance with the 5-day estrogen regimen is not optimal, a combination of norgestrel 1 mg and ethinylestradiol 100 µg, with a second identical dose repeated 12 h after the first, has been used as a PCC regimen. The initial dose must be given within 72 h after a single unprotected coital exposure.

Fasoli *et al.* summarized the results of 11 studies with this treatment regimen involving 3802 women. Failure rates varied widely, from a low of 0.2% in a Canadian study to a high of 7.4% in an Italian study. The total pregnancy rate in the 11 studies was 1.8%, which was similar to the individual failure rate in the largest studies in this review. In one large Canadian study, 30% of the subjects treated with this regimen reported having nausea without vomiting and another 20% had nausea with vomiting. These investigators included an antiemetic, 50-mg tablet of dimenhydrinate in the package and instructed the women to take it together with the second dose of contraceptive steroid if they experienced nausea following the first dose. They also reported that the time to onset of the subsequent menses was slightly shortened in the users of this regimen.

Thus, the effectiveness of this method appears to be slightly less than that of higher dosages of estrogen alone, but a lower incidence of abnormal bleeding, delayed menses, and gastrointestinal side-effects occurs with this regimen than the high-dose estrogen. Also, because of the 1-day treatment regimen, patient compliance is greater with this technique. Thus this method is more widely used than the high-dose estrogens.

Danazol

Another method of PCC, the administration of danazol, 400–600 mg in two doses separated by 12 h, has been tried by two groups of investigators. A total of 998 women were treated in these trials and the pregnancy rate of 2.0% was similar to that with the two doses of combined oral contraceptives. However, the incidence of side-effects, particularly nausea, was less with danazol and thus patient acceptability was high. If the patient has a continuing need for contraception after the cycle in which either of these techniques is used, one of the conventional methods should be prescribed.

Several authors have advocated that intrauterine insertion of a copper intrauterine device within 5–10 days of mid-cycle coitus is an effective method to prevent continuation of the pregnancy. Fasoli *et al.* summarized the results of nine published studies in four countries involving 879 women. Only one pregnancy occurred after a copper intrauterine device was inserted in these women.

Summary

PCC should be considered emergency therapy only, not a primary method of ongoing, long-term contraception. DES, ethinylestradiol alone or in combination with norgestrel, and conjugated estrogens on a short-term basis can be used safely and effectively to achieve postcoital contraception. Insertion of a copper intrauterine device and administration of high-dose estrogens are the most effective methods of PCC, but side-effects limit acceptance of the latter technique and cost and concern about introducing pathogens into the upper genital tract with intrauterine device insertion limit its widespread use. Therefore the currently preferred regimen is two doses of norgestrel 1 mg with ethinylestradiol 100 μg, 12 h apart. The closer to the time of coitus the method is initiated, the more effective it is. Therapy should be started as early as possible and no later than 72 h following coitus. If the expected menstrual period is 2 weeks late following the use of a PCC regimen, a pregnancy test should be done.

SUGGESTED READING

DIXON GW, SCHLESSELMAN JJ, ORY HW, *et al.* Ethinyl estradiol and conjugated estrogens as postcoital contraceptives. *JAMA* 1980;244:1336.

FASOLI M, PARAZZINI F, CECCHETTI G, *et al.* Post-coital contraceptions: an overview of published studies. *Contraception* 1989;39:459.

HASPELS AA. Interception: post-coital estrogens in 3016 women. *Contraception* 1976;14:375.

HERBST AL, ULFELDER H, POSKANZER DC. Adenocarcinoma of the vagina. Association of maternal stilbestrol therapy with tumor appearance in young women. *N Engl J Med* 1971;284:878.

JOHNSON JH. Contraception – the morning after. *Fam Plann Perspect* 1984;16:266.

JOHNSTON TA, HOWIE PW. Potential use of postcoital contraception to prevent unwanted pregnancy. *Br Med J* 1985;290:1040.

Rowlands S, Guillebaud J, Bounds W, *et al*. Side effects of danazol compared with an ethinylestradiol/norgestrel combination when used for postcoital contraception. *Contraception* 1983;27:39.

Van Santen MR, Haspels AA. Interception II: postcoital low-dose estrogens and norgestrel combination in 633 women. *Contraception* 1985;31:275.

Yuzpe AA, Smith RP, Rademaker AW. A multicenter clinical investigation employing ethinyl estradiol combined with dl-norgestrel as a postcoital contraceptive agent. *Fertil Steril* 1982;37:508.

122

Intrauterine devices: benefits and risks

DANIEL R. MISHELL, JR

The main benefits of intrauterine devices (IUDs) are: (1) a high level of effectiveness; (2) a lack of associated systemic metabolic effects; and (3) a single act of motivation required for long-term use. In contrast to other types of contraception, there is no need to ingest a pill daily or regularly to use a coitus-related method. These characteristics, as well as the fact that a visit to a health facility is required for discontinuing the method, account for the fact that IUDs have the highest continuation rate of all currently available reversible methods of contraception. Together with oral contraceptives, Depo-Provera, and Norplant, the IUD is one of the four most effective reversible methods of contraception available to US women.

First-year failure rates with copper-bearing IUDs have been reported to range from less than 1 to 3.7%. Pregnancy rates are related to the skill of the physician. With experience, correct high fundal insertion occurs more frequently, and there is a lower incidence of partial or complete expulsion with resultant lower pregnancy rates. Furthermore, the annual incidence of accidental pregnancy decreases steadily after the first year of IUD use. After 5 years of use of the copper-bearing copper T 380A IUD, the cumulative failure rate is only 1.4%.

The incidence of all major adverse events with IUDs, including pregnancy as well as expulsion or removal for bleeding or pain, steadily decreases with increasing age. Thus the IUD is especially suited for older parous women who wish to prevent further pregnancies.

Mechanism of action

The IUD's main mechanism of contraceptive action in the human is spermicidal, produced by a local sterile inflammatory reaction caused by the presence of the foreign body in the uterus. Small IUDs do not produce as great an inflammatory reaction as larger ones do. However, the addition of copper increases the inflammatory reaction and with increasing amounts of copper the IUD efficacy also increases. Because of the spermicidal action of IUDs very few, if any, sperm reach the oviducts, and the ovum usually does not become fertilized. The IUD does not mainly act as an abortifacient, as is commonly believed. Upon removal of both copper-bearing and noncopper-bearing IUDs, the inflammatory reaction rapidly disappears. Resumption of fertility is not delayed and it occurs at the same rate following discontinuation of use of barrier methods of contraception.

Types of IUDs

In the past 30 years, numerous models of IUDs have been designed and used clinically. The devices developed and initially used in the 1960s were made of a plastic polyethylene impregnated with barium sulfate to make them radiographic. In the 1970s smaller plastic devices covered with copper wire, such as the copper T, were developed and widely used. In the 1980s devices bearing a larger amount of copper, including sleeves on the horizontal arm, such as the copper T 380A and the copper T 220C, were developed. These devices had a longer duration of high effectiveness and thus had to be reinserted at less frequent intervals than the devices bearing a smaller amount of copper. Although many types of IUDs developed are still available for use in Europe, Canada, and elsewhere, at present only the copper T 380A and the progesterone-releasing IUD are being marketed in the USA. Although the barium-impregnated plastic loop and the copper-bearing copper 7 and copper T 200B are still approved by the Food and Drug Administration (FDA) for use in the USA, they are no longer being sold. Production and distribution of the shield device with a multifilament tail were discontinued in 1974. Because of the increased risk of infection reported with shield IUDs, if any are still in place, they should be removed. All IUDs now approved for distribution by the FDA have monofilament tails.

There is no need to change the noncopper-bearing plastic IUDs unless the patient develops increased bleeding after the IUD has been in place for more than 1 year. Calcium salts are deposited on the plastic in time, and their roughness can cause ulceration and bleeding of the endometrium. If increased bleeding develops after a noncopper-bearing plastic

IUD has been in the uterus for 1 year or more, the old IUD should be removed and a new one inserted.

Because of the constant dissolution of copper, which amounts daily to less than that ingested in the normal diet, all copper IUDs must be replaced periodically. The copper T 380A IUD is now approved for 8 years' use by the US FDA.

At the time of scheduled removal, one device can be removed and a new one inserted at the same visit.

Adding a reservoir of progesterone to the vertical arm also increases the effectiveness of the T-shaped device. The presently marketed progesterone IUD releases 65 μg of progesterone daily. This amount is sufficient to prevent pregnancy by local action in the endometrial cavity but is not enough to cause a measurable increase in peripheral serum progesterone levels. The currently approved model of the progesterone releasing IUD must be replaced annually, because the reservoir of progesterone becomes depleted after about 18 months of use.

Although it is widely believed that the optimal time for insertion of an IUD is during the menses, there are data indicating that if a woman is not pregnant, the IUD can be safely inserted on any day of the cycle. Event rates of copper IUDs inserted between 4 and 8 weeks postpartum and more than 8 weeks postpartum are similar, indicating that copper IUDs can be safely inserted at the time of the routine postpartum visit. A withdrawal technique of insertion should be used to avoid perforation.

Although one report suggested that the perforation rate may be higher if the IUD is inserted when a woman is lactating, this finding has not been confirmed in other studies. The effect of breast-feeding on performance of the copper T 380A IUD was evaluated from data obtained from a large multicenter clinical trial. Significantly less pain and fewer bleeding problems occurred at insertion in the breast-feeding group. The explusion rate, which was low, and continuation rate, which was high, were lower in the breast-feeding than the nonbreast-feeding groups 6 months after insertion.

Adverse effects

Incidence

In general, in the first year of use, IUDs have a <1% pregnancy rate, a 10% expulsion rate, and a 15% rate of removal for medical reasons, mainly bleeding and pain. The incidence of each of these events, especially expulsions, diminishes steadily in subsequent years.

Type

Uterine bleeding

Nearly all medical reasons accounting for IUD removal involve one or more types of abnormal bleeding: heavy or prolonged menses or intermenstrual bleeding.

The amount of blood lost in each menstrual cycle is also significantly greater in women wearing inert as well as copper-bearing IUDs than in nonwearers. In a normal cycle, the mean amount of menstrual blood loss is about 35 ml. After insertion of several types of copper-bearing devices, mean menstrual blood loss has been found to vary from about 50 to 60 ml. In contrast, with the progesterone-releasing IUD the amount of blood loss is actually reduced to about 25 ml per cycle.

Although mean values of hemoglobin concentration, serum iron, and total iron-binding capacity usually do not change after IUD insertion, there is usually a significant decrease in serum ferritin levels, a sensitive noninvasive indicator for measuring tissue iron stores. Low serum ferritin levels are a good predictor of the development of anemia. Therefore, it is best that both ferritin and hemoglobin be measured annually in all wearers of nonsteroid-releasing IUDs. If either parameter decreases significantly, supplemental iron should be administered to the patient.

Patients who experience excessive bleeding in the first few months after IUD insertion should be treated with reassurance and supplemental oral iron. The bleeding may diminish with time as the uterus adjusts to the presence of the foreign body. Patients with excessive bleeding that continues or develops several months or more after IUD insertion may be treated by systemic administration of one of the prostaglandin synthetase inhibitors, such as mefenamic acid, in a dosage of 500 mg 3 times daily. If bleeding continues despite this treatment, the device should be removed. After a 1-month interval, another device may be inserted if the patient still wishes to use an IUD for contraception. If the original device was nonmedicated, the new device should be a copper- or progesterone-releasing IUD, because these smaller devices are associated with less blood loss than the larger plastic devices.

Perforation

Although it is uncommon, one of the potentially serious complications associated with use of the IUD is perforation of the uterine fundus. Perforation initially occurs at insertion and can best be prevented by straightening of the uterine axis with a tenaculum and then probing of the cavity with a uterine sound before IUD insertion, which is best performed by the withdrawal technique. Sometimes only the distal portion of the IUD penetrates the uterine muscle at insertion, and then the uterine contractions over the next few months force the IUD into the peritoneal cavity. IUDs correctly inserted entirely within the endometrial cavity do not wander through the uterine muscle into the peritoneal cavity.

The incidence of perforation is generally related to the shape of the device or the amount of force used during its insertion, as well as the experience of the clinician. Perforation rates with the copper IUD have been reported to be about 1 in 3000 insertions. The clinician should always suspect that perforation has occurred if a patient states she cannot feel the appendage but did not notice the device was expelled. One should not assume that an unnoticed expulsion has occurred. Occasionally the device has rotated in the uterine cavity and the appendage has been withdrawn into the cavity. In this situation, after pelvic examination is performed, and the possibility of pregnancy excluded, the uterine cavity should be probed. If the device cannot be felt with a uterine sound or biopsy instrument, a pelvic sonogram or X-ray film should be obtained. If the device is not visualized with pelvic ultrasonography, an X-ray film of the entire abdominal cavity should be performed, since IUDs that have been pushed through the uterus may be located anywhere in the peritoneal cavity, even in the subdiaphragmatic area.

If the IUD is found to be outside the uterus, it should be electively removed, because complications such as adhesions and bowel obstruction have been reported with intraperitoneal IUDs. Both the copper IUDs and shields have been found to produce severe peritoneal reactions. Therefore, it is best to remove these devices as soon as possible after the diagnosis of perforation is made. Unless severe adhesions have developed, most intraperitoneal IUDs can be removed by means of laparoscopy, avoiding the necessity of laparotomy.

Perforation of the cervix has also been reported to occur with devices having a straight vertical arm such as the copper T or 7. The incidence of downward perforation of these devices into the cervix has been reported to range from about 1 in 600 to 1 in 1000 insertions. When follow-up examinations are performed on patients with these devices, the cervix should be carefully inspected and palpated, as frequently the perforation does not extend completely through the ectocervical epithelium. Cervical perforation is not a major problem, but devices that have perforated downward should be removed through the endocervical canal with uterine packing forceps in the clinic, because their downward displacement is associated with a reduced contraceptive effectiveness.

Complications related to pregnancy

Congenital anomalies

When pregnancy occurs with an IUD in place, implantation occurs away from the device itself, so the device is always extraamniotic. There is no evidence of an increased incidence of congenital anomalies in infants born with an IUD *in utero*. There is also no evidence to indicate that the presence of copper in the uterus exerts a deleterious effect on fetal development. Although relatively few infants have been found with a progesterone-releasing IUD in the uterus, careful examination of these infants has also revealed no increased incidence of cardiac or other anomalies.

Spontaneous abortion

In all series of pregnancies with any type of IUD *in situ*, the incidence of fetal death was not significantly increased; however, a significant increase in the incidence of spontaneous abortion has been consistently observed. If a patient conceives with an IUD in place and the IUD is not removed, the incidence of spontaneous abortion is about 55% – approximately three times greater than would occur if the patient conceives without an IUD.

If after conception the IUD is spontaneously expelled or if the appendage is visible and the IUD is removed by traction, the incidence of spontaneous abortion is significantly reduced to about 20%. Thus, if a woman conceives with an IUD *in situ* and she wishes to continue the pregnancy, the IUD should be removed if the appendage is visible in order significantly to reduce the chance of spontaneous abortion.

If the appendage is not visible, probing of the uterine cavity may increase the chance of abortion, as well as sepsis. However, several recent reports indicate that with careful ultrasonography and meticulous technique, it is possible to remove some IUDs without a visible appendage during early pregnancy and have a normal outcome of gestation.

Septic abortion

If the IUD cannot be easily removed or the appendage is not visible, evidence suggests that the risk of septic abortion may be increased if the IUD remains in place. Most of the evidence indicating an increased risk of sepsis is based on data from women who conceived with the shield-type of IUD that had a multifilament tail. Currently, there is no conclusive evidence that a patient conceiving with an IUD with a monofilament tail has an increased risk of septic abortion, except for the fact that the spontaneous abortion rate is increased, and about 2% of all abortions become septic.

Thus if a patient who conceives with an IUD *in utero* wishes to continue the pregnancy and the device cannot be removed without entering the uterine cavity, she should be informed of the possibility of an increased incidence of sepsis and, if she wishes to continue the pregnancy, of the need to report symptoms of infection promptly. If intrauterine infection does occur with an IUD in the pregnant uterus, the endometrial cavity should be evacuated after a short interval of appropriate antibiotic treatment, similar to the treatment of uterine sepsis without an IUD in place.

Ectopic pregnancy

As stated earlier, the IUD's main mechanism of contraceptive action is the production of a continuous sterile inflammatory reaction in the uterine cavity because of foreign body presence. Because more inflammatory reaction is present in the endometrial cavity than the oviducts, the IUD prevents intrauterine pregnancy more effectively than it prevents ectopic pregnancy.

Several epidemiologic studies have confirmed that if pregnancy occurs with an IUD in place, it is more likely to be ectopic than if pregnancy occurs in the absence of an IUD. Despite the increased incidence of ectopic pregnancy in women conceiving with an IUD in place, overall the IUD reduces the incidence of ectopic pregnancy, compared to women exposed to pregnancy using no method of contraception or barrier techniques.

If a patient conceives with an IUD in place, her chances of having an ectopic pregnancy range from 3 to 9%. This incidence is about 10 times greater than the reported ectopic pregnancy frequency of 0.3–0.7% of total births in similar populations.

Thus if a patient conceives with an IUD in place, there should be a high index of suspicion of ectopic pregnancy. There is a higher frequency of ectopic pregnancies with use of the progesterone-releasing IUD than the copper IUDs. Patients conceiving with any IUD should have sonography performed early in gestation. Also, the possibility of ovarian pregnancy should always be considered. Patients wearing an IUD who have a clinical diagnosis of ruptured corpus luteum may in fact have an unrecognized ovarian pregnancy. If any patient with an IUD has an elective termination of pregnancy, the evacuated tissue should be examined histologically to be certain that the gestation was intrauterine.

The effect of the IUD on increased development of ectopic pregnancy while it is in place appears to be temporary and does not persist after removal of the IUD. In two large European studies, women wishing to conceive after they had an ectopic pregnancy had a much greater chance of having a successful intrauterine pregnancy if they were using an IUD at the time of their ectopic pregnancy than those who have an ectopic pregnancy without an IUD.

Prematurity

Several studies indicate that the rate of preterm delivery is higher if an IUD remains in the uterus throughout gestation. If it is not possible to remove the IUD and the patient wishes to continue her pregnancy, she should be warned of the possible increased risk of prematurity in addition to the increased risk of spontaneous abortion. She should also be informed about an increased risk of ectopic pregnancy and possibly septic abortion and should be instructed to report the first signs of pelvic pain or fever. There is no evidence that pregnant women with an IUD *in utero* have an increased incidence of other obstetric complications. In addition, there is no evidence that prior use of an IUD results in a greater incidence of complications in subsequent pregnancies.

Pelvic infection in the nonpregnant patient

Although bacteriologic and epidemiologic studies with the loop IUD, performed in the 1960s, indicated that it did not increase the risk of salpingitis >30 days after insertion, results of retrospective studies in the 1970s indicated that there was a three- to fivefold increased risk of developing clinical salpingitis in certain women who use an IUD. These studies overestimated the risks because the diagnosis of salpingitis was based on clinical criteria (which are frequently erroneous), the controls were using a method of contraception that reduced the risk of salpingitis, and the shield-type of IUD was used by a large percentage of the IUD-wearing subjects.

Furthermore, in all of these studies there was no differentiation between episodes of salpingitis developing in the first few months after IUD insertion, which had previously been shown to be related to insertion of the IUD, and episodes developing a few months after insertion. Lee *et al.* reported results from a multicenter case-control study of the relationship of the IUD and pelvic inflammatory disease (PID). When the PID risk of IUD users (other than the shield) was correlated with duration of use, it was found that a significantly increased risk of PID for the loop and copper 7 was present only during the first 4 months after insertion. After that period there was no significantly increased risk of PID in users of IUDs other than the shield. Results of a recently published large multicenter study coordinated by the World Health Organization revealed similar findings. In this study of 22 908 women inserted with IUDs, the PID rate was highest in the first 3 weeks after insertion, but remained constant during the 8 years thereafter. Thus, the findings of these more recent studies agree with those of earlier studies, which indicate that salpingitis occurring more than a few months after insertion of an IUD is due to a sexually transmitted disease and not related to the IUD.

An IUD should not be inserted into a patient who may have been recently infected with gonococci or *Chlamydia*. Insertion of the device will transport these pathogens from the cervix into the upper genital tract. If there is clinical suspicion of infectious endocervicitis, cultures should be obtained and the IUD insertion delayed until the results reveal that no pathogenic organisms are present. It does not appear to be cost-effective to administer systemic antibiotics routinely with every IUD insertion, but the insertion procedure should be as aseptic as possible.

The populations at high risk for developing PID include those who have a prior history of PID, nulliparous women under 25 years of age, and women with multiple sexual partners. The risk of impairing future fertility because of the increased possibility of developing salpingitis in the first few months after IUD insertion must be considered when deciding on use of an IUD in a nulliparous woman, but nulliparity is not an absolute contraindication for IUD use.

Symptomatic salpingitis may be successfully treated by antibiotics without removal of the IUD until the patient becomes free of symptoms. In patients who have clinical evidence of a tuboovarian abscess or who have a shield in place, the IUD should be removed after a therapeutic serum level of appropriate parenteral antibiotics has been reached and preferably after a clinical response has been observed. An alternate method of contraception should be used in patients who develop salpingitis with an IUD in place.

Evidence suggests that IUD users may have an increased risk for colonizing actinomycosis organisms in the upper genital tract. The relationship of actinomycosis to PID is unclear, since many women without IUDs have actinomycosis in their vagina. If these organisms are identified on the routine annual cytologic smear of IUD users, their existence should be confirmed by culture, since cytologic diagnosis of actinomycosis is not very precise. If the culture confirms their presence in the cervix, appropriate antimicrobial therapy should be used to eradicate the organisms, but the IUD does not have to be removed.

Overall safety

Several long-term studies have indicated that the IUD is not associated with an increased incidence of endometrial or cervical carcinoma. The main causes of morbidity among IUD users are complications of pregnancy, uterine perforation, and hemorrhage, as well as pelvic infection. Despite the increased morbidity with IUDs, the actual incidence of these problems is very low. IUDs are not being inserted in women at risk for developing PID, and physicians are aware of the potential complications associated with IUDs in pregnancy. The IUD is a particularly useful method of contraception for women who have completed their families and do not wish permanent sterilization and have contraindications to or do not wish to use oral contraceptives, Depo-Povera, or Norplant.

SUGGESTED READING

ALVAREZ F, GUILOFF E, BRACHE V, *et al.* New insights on the mode of action of intrauterine contraceptive devices in women. *Fertil Steril* 1988;49:768.

ANDERSON ABM, HAYNES PJ, GUILLEBAUD J, *et al.* Reduction of menstrual blood loss by prostaglandin synthetase inhibitors. *Lancet* 1976;1:774.

CHI I-C, POTTS M, WILKENS LR, *et al.* Performance of the Copper T-380A intrauterine device in breastfeeding women. *Contraception* 1989;39:603.

CHOW W-H, DALING JR, WEISS NS, *et al.* IUD use and subsequent tubal ectopic pregnancy. *Am J Public Health* 1986;76:536.

FARLEY TMM, ROSENBERG MJ, ROWE PJ, *et al.* Intrauterine devices and pelvic inflammatory disease: an international perspective. *Lancet* 1992;339:785–788.

GUILLEBAUD J, BARNETT MD, GORDON YB. Plasma ferritin levels as an index of iron deficiency in women using intrauterine devices. *Br J Obstet Gynaecol* 1979; 86:51.

HEIKKILA M, NYLANDER P, LUUKKAINEN T. Body iron stores and patterns of bleeding after insertion of a levonorgestrel- or a copper-releasing intrauterine contraceptive device. *Contraception* 1982;26:465.

LEE NC, RUBIN GL. The intrauterine device and pelvic inflammatory disease revisited: new results from the women's health study. *Obstet Gynecol* 1988; 72:1.

LEE NC, RUBIN GL, ORY HW, *et al.* Type of intrauterine device and the risk of pelvic inflammatory disease. *Obstet Gynecol* 1983;62:1.

MAKINEN JI, SALMI TA, NIKKANEN VPJ, *et al.* Encouraging rates of fertility after ectopic pregnancy. *Int J Fertil* 1989;34:46.

MISHELL DR Jr, ROY S. Copper intrauterine contraceptive device event rates following insertion 4 to 8 weeks postpartum. *Am J Obstet Gynecol* 1982;143:29.

MISHELL DR Jr, BELL JH, GOOD RG, *et al.* The intrauterine device: a bacteriologic study of the endometrial cavity. *Am J Obstet Gynecol* 1966;96:119.

ORY HW. Ectopic pregnancy and intrauterine contraceptive devices: new perspectives. The Women's Health Study. *Obstet Gynecol* 1981;57:137.

PERSSON E, HOLMBERG K, DAHLGREN S, *et al. Actinomyces israelii* in genital tract of women with and without intrauterine contraceptive devices. *Acta Obstet Gynecol Scand* 1983;62:563.

PIEDRAS J, CORDOVA MS, PEREZ-TORAL MC, *et al.* Predictive value of serum ferritin in anemia development after insertion of T Cu 220 intrauterine device. *Contraception* 1983;27:289.

STUBBLEFIELD PG, FULLER AF, FOSTER SC. Ultrasound-guided intrauterine removal of intrauterine contraceptive devices in pregnancy. *Obstet Gynecol* 1988;72:961.

VESSEY MP, LAWLESS M, McPHERSON K, *et al.* Fertility after stopping use of intrauterine contraceptive device. *Br Med J* 1983;286:106.

WHITE MK, ORY HW, ROOKS JB, *et al.* Intrauterine device termination rates and the menstrual cycle day of insertion. *Obstet Gynecol* 1980;55:220.

WORLD HEALTH ORGANIZATION (WHO). The TCu220C, multiload 250 and Nova T IUDs at 3, 5, and 7 years of use. Results from three randomized multicentre trials. *Contraception* 1990;42:141.

123

Barrier methods of contraception

PAUL F. BRENNER & GERALD S. BERNSTEIN

For properly motivated couples a barrier method of family planning is a reasonable option. While use effectiveness rates with barrier methods of contraception are not as good as with oral contraceptives, Norplant, and Depo-Provera, the barrier methods do have the advantages of decreasing the risk of sexually transmitted diseases, the absence of adverse metabolic alterations, and they can be obtained over-the-counter without a prescription. In addition, barrier methods of contraception can be used concomitantly with other more effective contraceptive modalities in order to provide enhanced protection against sexually transmitted diseases. The use of barrier methods reduces the frequency of clinical infections that are transmitted by either bacteria or viruses.

Condoms

Only sterilization of either partner and oral contraceptives are selected more frequently as a family-planning method than condoms by sexually active married couples living in the USA. The use of condoms as a contraceptive modality is reported to have a first-year failure rate of 2–20%. Lower failure rates are observed by women over the age of 30 years, women who have completed their families, and women who have achieved a high socioeconomic status and level of education. Use of the condom by highly motivated couples has a failure rate of 3–6%.

Couples electing to use the condom should be instructed: (1) apply the condom before attempting vaginal penetration; (2) cover the entire length of the erect penis with the condom; (3) the condom should fit snugly over the penis; it is not necessary to leave a reservoir to catch the ejaculate; (4) use adequate lubrication to prevent tearing of the condom or vaginal irritation but do not use petroleum-based lubricants as they cause the rubber to deteriorate; (5) hold the condom against the base of the penis and withdraw the penis and condom simultaneously before the penis becomes flaccid; and (6) use the condom at every coital exposure.

A defect in the condom occurs once in approximately every 166 times a condom is used. Condom breakage increases when the condom is not correctly applied to the penis, in hot and humid climates, and possibly with increased exposure to ozone. Most failures with this method of contraception occur because the condoms were used improperly or not at all.

The advantages of using condoms as a method of contraception include participation by the male partner and availability over-the-counter without a prescription; it is a disposable method, it is inexpensive, and there is an absence of systemic effects. The disadvantages associated with the use of condoms relate to the necessity for user responsibility, the interruption of sexual foreplay, and decreased sensation for the male partner during coitus. Rarely this method may produce local irritation and, very infrequently, an allergic reaction. The use of a condom is therefore contraindicated in those instances when either partner manifests an allergic reaction to the condom or for those men who are unable to maintain an erection while using this method of birth control.

For women with multiple sexual partners, use of condoms as the only method of contraception or in combination with other methods should be encouraged. In this setting the risk of sexually transmitted disease is high and the condom is the contraceptive method that provides the greatest protection for the male as well as his partners against venereal disease, both bacterial and viral. Condoms prevent the transmission of *Neisseria gonorrhoea* and *Chlamydia trachomatis*. These organisms are frequent causes of clinical salpingitis and the sequelae of tubal damage, including chronic pelvic pain, tubal infertility, and an increased risk of ectopic pregnancy. Condoms also prevent the transmission of the herpes virus, the human immunodeficiency virus, and the human papillomavirus. It is the impedance of the transmission of the human papillomavirus in women whose sexual partners use condoms that reduces the risk of cervical neoplasia in these women.

Diaphragm

The diaphragm method of family planning usually consists of two components, the diaphragm and the spermicidal agent. While it is recommended to use the diaphragm and the spermicide together, it is uncertain whether this is any more efficacious than the use of the diaphragm alone. The diaphragm is reported to have a first-year failure rate of 2–20%. The efficacy of this method of contraception is related to the motivation of the diaphragm user and her ability to master the techniques of insertion and removal. Highly motivated women who repeatedly practice the insertion and removal of the diaphragm under the supervision of trained personnel and who return for a 1-week follow-up visit have failure rates as low as 2–7%.

When properly fitted, the diaphragm is located just behind the symphysis pubis and deep into the cul-de-sac so that the cervix is completely covered and ideally behind the center of the membrane. The largest diaphragm that fills this space without discomfort is selected. To opt for a smaller-size device will only increase the chance of failure. The arcing diaphragm is preferable for those women with a markedly ante- or retroverted uterus. The training of the women selecting this method is best accomplished using actual diaphragms rather than open rings. In this manner the woman learns the correct placement in the vagina with the membrane arched in the right direction, the amount of spermicidal jelly or cream to use, and where to place it. The spermicide is placed in the center of the membrane and along the outer edge. In addition, the woman is instructed on palpating her cervix behind the membrane. The woman should practice the insertion and removal of the diaphragm until she has mastered the technique. After each insertion the contraceptive provider should examine the woman to ascertain her ability to achieve proper placement. If the diaphragm is correctly positioned, the upper edge is behind the symphysis and the cervix is behind the membrane as determined by palpation, and the diaphragm acceptor does not experience discomfort when she stands or walks. Within the first cycle after receiving the diaphragm a woman should have a follow-up visit to evaluate her proper use of the method.

The diaphragm should be inserted into the vagina 6 h or less before intercourse and left in place for at least 8 h following coitus. An additional placement of spermicide is recommended for each coital exposure which occurs before the diaphragm is removed. The diaphragm is not repositioned or removed in order to add additional spermicide. Each time prior to insertion, the diaphragm is inspected for perforations and, if there is any doubt, the diaphragm is filled with water to test for defects. The determination of the correct size of a diaphragm for a specific woman should be repeated at each annual visit, if the woman experiences a weight change in excess of 4.5 kg (10 lb), following an abortion or a full-term pregnancy, and if the woman has symptoms of vaginal pain, bladder or uretheral discomfort, difficulty voiding, and a urinary tract infection.

A diaphragm that is too large or is left in the vagina for more than

24 h may produce vaginal pain and ulceration. Infrequently a diaphragm acceptor will experience bladder discomfort, urethral burning, and recurrent bladder infections. The increase in urinary tract infections in diaphragm users is most likely due to increased colonization of the vagina with coliform bacteria. Very rarely a woman is allergic to the spermicide and, even less frequently, to the latex diaphragm. Toxic shock syndrome has been reported in diaphragm users but it does not occur more frequently with this method of family planning than in the general population.

The diaphragm has the advantages that it is free of systemic effects and does not involve coital interference. The diaphragm is another barrier method of family planning that impedes the transmission of bacteria and viruses. Diaphragm acceptors have a reduced risk of salpingitis, tubal factor infertility, and cervical neoplasia. Highly motivated women who are correctly fitted and instructed find the diaphragm a very acceptable means of contraception.

Vaginal foam, suppositories, and creams

Vaginal spermicides usually consist of two components. The first component is a spermicidal agent and the second is a carrier substance such as foam, suppository, or cream which acts as a barrier impeding access of sperm to the cervical canal. The most commonly used spermicidal compound in the USA admixt with all three of the carriers is nonoxynol-9 (nonylphenoxy polyoxyethylene ethanol). Spermicidal agents are reported to have first-year failure rates ranging from 13 to 30%. The use of these methods may interrupt sexual foreplay and they are considered untidy. These inconveniences have the potential to decrease the motivation of couples using spermicides, leading to higher failure rates. The only adverse reaction attributed to the use of vaginal spermicides is the rare occurrence of an allergic reaction of either partner. One study suggested that the use of spermicidal agents at the time of conception increased the risk of congenital anomalies. More recent studies have convincingly refuted this association and found no increase in chromosomal aberrations in abortuses or birth defects in the newborn of women who conceived while using vaginal spermicides.

Women electing to use vaginal spermicidal agents should be instructed as follows: (1) use the agent every time you have intercourse; (2) place the agent in the vagina in as close proximity to the cervix as feasible; (3) insert the agent into the vagina as near to the time of coitus as possible and no longer than 1 h before coitus; (4) do not douche for at least 8 h following intercourse; (5) if foam is used, be sure the container is shaken well; (6) if foam is used, have a second full container available; and (7) the use of vaginal suppositories requires a delay of 10 min from the time of placement in the vagina until coitus to allow the suppository to melt.

Indications for the use of vaginal spermicides as a single contraceptive agent include women having infrequent coitus, an unplanned coital exposure when an alternative method is not available, and women who are at a time in their reproductive years when their fertility is reduced, either immediately postpartum or past the age of 40 years. Spermicidal agents can be used as an adjunctive method in the first contraceptive cycle of birth-control pills in the event the pill user has a short cycle with early ovulation and they can be administered concomitantly with oral contraceptives when there has been an omission of one or two tablets. Spermicidal agents can be used as an adjunctive method in the initial intrauterine device cycles when unnoticed expulsions are most common. Foam used concomitantly with condoms may improve the effectiveness of the method. Contraindications to the use of spermicidal agents include individuals allergic to the spermicide and couples practicing oral–genital sex, when the taste is unpleasant.

Contraceptive vaginal sponge

The Today contraceptive vaginal sponge was approved as a general method of contraception in the USA in 1983. The consumer may obtain the sponge, which is disposable, over-the-counter without the necessity of a prescription. The sponge is a dome-shaped device with a central depression in the side facing the cervix. This configuration facilitates the placement and maintenance of the device in the vagina. On the side of the sponge facing the introitus there is a polyester loop which is used to remove the sponge. The sponge is made of polyurethane foam and is impregnated with 1 g nonoxynol-9. Once the sponge is activated, approximately 125 mg of nonoxynol-9 is released over the next 24 h. The sponge is effective for a 24 h period and, unlike other spermicides, it does not have to be inserted into the vagina before each coital exposure.

The contraceptive vaginal sponge is reported to have a first-year failure rate of 10–30%. The failure rate for the sponge in clinical trials was reported to be greater than for the diaphragm. When the data were reanalyzed, correcting for previous use of barrier contraceptives, the pregnancy rates were not different for the two methods. One study concluded that the higher failure rates with the sponge compared to the diaphragm occurred only in parous women. In those women who already had a child, the failure rate in the sponge users was twice that of the diaphragm users. Other studies have failed to find a difference in failure rates in these two methods related to parity. Some sponge-users have observed that the sponge may change color when it is removed from the vagina. The change in color does not alter either the effectiveness or the safety of the method.

The contraceptive vaginal sponge comes in only one size, and therefore does not have to be fitted to the individual woman. It must be activated by being moistened with warm tap water prior to insertion. The sponge is inserted in a manner similar to that of the diaphragm. When correctly placed deep in the vaginal vault, the sponge completely covers the cervix. The sponge may be placed in the vagina up to 24h prior to intercourse. Within the 24h interval that the sponge is correctly situated intravaginally it can be used for multiple coital episodes. The sponge should not be repositioned, removed, or reactivated between coital exposures. For optimal effectivenesss the sponge should remain in the vagina at least 6h after intercourse, but the maximum time a single sponge is left in the vagina should not exceed 30h.

The sponge is well tolerated by most women who elect to use it as their family-planning method. Women who have used the diaphragm and the sponge at different times in their reproductive years find the sponge a less messy method. Some sponge acceptors experience side-effects, including difficulty removing the sponge from the vagina, displacement of the sponge so that it does not cover the cervix, expulsion of the sponge from the vagina, vaginal discomfort, vaginal itching, awareness of the sponge by the sexual partner, penile irritation, and dyspareunia. Very infrequent adverse experiences include cervical abrasion, urinary retention, and vaginal ulceration. Very rarely a sponge-user may have an allergic reaction to the spermicide and, even less frequently, a reaction to polyurethane. Toxic shock syndrome has been reported to occur in contraceptive vaginal sponge users. As long as the sponge is not used during menses or the puerperium and the time the sponge is left in the vagina does not exceed 24h, the incidence of toxic shock syndrome is not increased in women electing to use the sponge. The incidence of toxic shock syndrome is estimated to be one case for every 2 million sponges.

The advantages of the contraceptive sponge are the simplicity of the method, the absence of systemic effects, the fact that the method is not related to coitus, that it is less messy than other barrier methods, that it is available over-the-counter without a prescription, and that it is disposable.

Cervical cap

The cervical cap is a cup-shaped device that, when correctly applied, fits over the cervix. The Prentif cavity-rim cervical cap was approved for use as a method of contraception in the USA in 1988. Compared to the diaphragm, the cervical cap is technically more difficult for the family-

planning provider to learn to fit properly and for the contraceptive acceptor to learn to use correctly. The cervical cap can be left *in situ* for a longer
interval and is reported to be more comfortable than the diaghragm. The
Prentif cavity-rim cervical cap is available in four sizes. A spermicide
should always be placed inside the cap before it is applied to the cervix
and the maximum time that the cap is left on the cervix should not exceed
48 h. If continuous use of the cervical cap exceeds the 48 h interval, an
unpleasant odor, infection, and even cervical ulceration may appear.

The cervical cap is reported to have a failure rate between 7 and 18%
during the first year of use. The failure rate is similar to that of the
diaphragm. Two-thirds of the unwanted pregnancies which occur in
women using the cervical cap are the result of user-related errors and the
remaining one-third are due to method failures. As the result of concerns
that the presence of the cervical cap may adversely affect cervical cytology, women with an abnormal Pap smear should not receive the
cervical cap as their method of contraception. In addition, women with
normal cervical cytology who opt to use the cervical cap should be advised to have a repeat Pap smear 3 months after beginning the use of this
contraceptive modality.

SUGGESTED READING

CELENTANO DD, KLASSEN AC, WEISMAN CS, ROSENHEIN NB. The role of contraceptive use in cervical cancer: the Maryland cervical cancer case control study.
Am J Epidemiol 1987;126:592.

CONANT M, HARDY D, SERNATINGER J, SPICER D, LEVY JA. Condoms prevent
transmission of AIDS-associated retrovirus. *JAMA* 1986;255:1706.

EDELMAN DA, NORTH BB. Updated pregnancy rates for the Today contraceptive
sponge. *Am J Obstet Gynecol* 1987;157:1164–1165.

FAICH G, PEARSON K, FLEMMING D, SOBEL S, ANELLO C. Toxic shock syndrome
and the vaginal contraceptive sponge. *JAMA* 1986;255:216–218.

FINN SD, LATHAM RH, ROBERTS P. Association between diaphragm use and
urinary tract infection. *JAMA* 1985;254:240.

FINN SD, JOHNSON C, PINKSTAFF C, *et al.* Diaphragm use and urinary tract
infections: analysis of urodynamic and microbiological factors. *J Urol* 1986;136:
853.

HICKS DR, MARTIN LS, GRETCHELL JP, *et al.* Inactivation of HTLV III/LACV-
infected cultures of normal human lymphocytes by Nonoxynol-9 *in vitro*. *Lancet*
1985;2:1422–1423.

KLITSCH M. FDA approval ends cervical cap's marathon. *Fam Plann Perspect* 1988;
20:137–138.

LOUIK C, MITCHELL AA, WERLER MM, HANSON JW, SHAPIRO S. Maternal
exposure to spermicides in relation to certain birth defects. *N Engl J Med* 1987;
317:474–478.

POWELL MG, MEARS BJ, DEBER RB, FERGUSON D. Contraception with the cervical cap: effectiveness, safety, continuity of use, and user satisfaction. *Contraception* 1986;33:215–232.

STROBINO B, KLINE J, LAI A, *et al.* Vaginal spermicides and spontaneous abortion of known karyotype. *Am J Epidemiol* 1986;123:431.

124

Natural family-planning methods

PAUL F. BRENNER

Abstaining from sexual intercourse during the days of the menstrual cycle when ovulation is most likely to occur and therefore the period when the ovum can be fertilized is a method used by highly motivated couples to prevent pregnancy. These methods, which rely on abstinence during a woman's fertile period, are referred to as periodic abstinence or natural family-planning methods. These methods avoid the use of hormones, surgery, intrauterine, intracervical, or intravaginal devices, barriers or spermicides.

Until recently the timing of ovulation has either been expensive and impractical when based on daily hormonal laboratory assays or imprecise when based on signs and symptoms experienced by the subject. While these later methods had the advantage of being self-determined, they required a rather extensive interval of abstinence to compensate for the lack of precision of the method. There are four natural family-planning techniques: (1) the calendar rhythm method; (2) the temperature method; (3) the cervical mucus method; and (4) the symptothermal method. The pregnancy rates associated with the natural family-planning methods are relatively high when compared to hormonal contraception, intrauterine devices, Norplant, and barrier methods of contraception. The high failure rates occur when couples find that they are unable to consistently avoid coitus for the relatively long interval which is required each cycle.

The calendar rhythm method estimates the interval during which ovulation and fertilization are most likely to occur based on the length of the preceding menstrual cycles. Three physiologic principles serve as the foundation for the calendar rhythm method. First, in ovulatory menstrual cycles, ovulation occurs 12–16 days (14 ± 2) before the onset of the next menses. Second, the ovum is capable of being fertilized for 24 h or less after ovulation. Third, the sperm is able to fertilize an ovum for 72 h or less following ejaculation. After documenting the length of her menstrual cycle for several months, a woman using the calendar rhythm method determines her fertile period (interval of abstinence) by subtracting 18 days from the length of her previous shortest cycle and 11 days from the length of her previous longest cycle. As an example, if the length of a woman's menstrual cycle varied from 26 to 30 days, her fertile period, when intercourse should be avoided, would start on day 8 (26 − 18) and continue through day 19 (30 − 11). The calendar rhythm method is contraindicated for women whose menstrual cycle length is ≤25 days or varies 8 or more days from cycle to cycle. Pregnancy rates with this particular family planning method, which usually requires abstinence for almost half the menstrual cycle, are high and range from 14.4 to 47 per 100 woman-years. Use of the calendar rhythm method alone as the sole means of contraception is no longer recommended due to the high failure rate.

The temperature method utilizes changes in the basal body temperature (BBT), during an ovulatory menstrual cycle, to determine the interval of abstinence from sexual intercourse. The BBT increases 0.5–1°F following ovulation and reflects the thermogenic properties of progesterone. The woman using the temperature method is instructed to place a thermometer and a clock next to her bedside. Special thermometers are available for taking the BBT. When she awakens and before getting out of bed, the woman takes her temperature for 3 min and then records the reading on a graph. Women using the temperature method abstain from sexual intercourse for a period starting with the onset of menses and lasting until the third consecutive day of an elevation of the BBT. The temperature method alone is seldom recommended because of the long interval of abstinence which is required.

The presence and the consistency of cervical mucus change in response to the cyclic alterations in estrogen and progesterone levels throughout the ovulatory menstrual cycle. High levels of unopposed estrogen result in the formation of copious, slippery cervical mucus. As progesterone production increases from the corpus luteum, the estrogen effects on cervical mucus are blunted and the amount and consistency of the mucus regress. Women using the cervical mucus method are taught to detect the presence of cervical mucus and to distinguish the changes in the consistency of their cervical mucus. A woman using this method abstains from intercourse during menses and every other day after the cessation of menses until the first day that she notices copious, slippery cervical mucus is present. She avoids sexual intercourse every day thereafter until 4 days after the last day when the characteristic mucus is present. The last day when copious, slippery cervical mucus is present is referred to as the peak mucus day. Following three to five cycles of training, pregnancy rates for women using the cervical mucus method during the first year varied between 20 and 24%. Women using this method are required to abstain from sexual intercourse for more than one-half the days of each menstrual cycle. Most pregnancies occurred when the couples failed to abstain from sexual intercoure during all the times prescribed by the method.

The symptothermal method uses multiple parameters to define the fertile period. The onset of the fertile period is determined from calculations based on the lengths of previous menstrual cycles and the detection of changes in cervical mucus. Cervical mucus changes and the BBT are used to estimate the end of the fertile period. The advantages of the multiple-indices method over those methods which rely on a single physiologic change are that the symptothermal method is more effective and has higher continuation rates. The disadvantage is that the more complex method is more difficult to learn than a single-index method. The pregnancy rates after 1 year of use of the symptothermal method range from 11 to 20% and the continuation rate is approximately 50%.

Natural family-planning methods have not gained wide acceptance by American women of reproductive age who desire to avoid pregnancy. The prolonged number of days each menstrual cycle during which couples using natural family-planning methods must abstain from sexual intercourse is the major factor in the poor acceptance of these methods and the relatively high failure rates. These methods of periodic abstinence are desperately in need of adjunctive technology which more precisely defines and limits the fertile period so that the interval of abstinence can be reduced. One approach has been the concomitant use of a barrier method of contraception during the fertile period, along with the use of a natural family-planning method. The pregnancy rate reported when both methods are used concurrently is approximately 10% at the end of 1 year and two-thirds of the women continue to use the combination of methods.

A second approach to broaden the acceptability and improve the efficacy of natural family-planning methods is the development of simple, rapid, self-administered (home), economic, hormonal tests. The timing of hormonal events prior to ovulation – rupture of the ovarian follicle – has been better defined with the availabilty of vaginal probe ultrasonography. Ultrasound studies provide a noninvasive method of determining when follicle rupture occurs and then allow a more precise timing of changes in steroids and gonadotropins in relation to ovulation (Table 124.1). Enzyme immunoassay tests for urinary estrogens and pregnanediol glucuronide, a

Table 124.1 Hormonal events prior to ovulation

Hormonal event	Hours preceding ovulation	
	Mean	Range
Defined rise in serum estradiol	82	54–100
Defined rise in serum luteinizing hormone	32	24–56
Defined rise in urine luteinizing hormone	30	20–44
Peak rise in serum estradiol	24	17–32
Peak rise in serum luteinizing hormone	16	8–40

major metabolite of pregesterone, have been developed. A test kit for home use to assay urinary pregnanediol glucuronide (Phase-Check) has just recently become available. Enzyme-linked immunosorbent assays for gonadotropins have been developed and several test kits for home use to measure urinary luteinizing hormone (OvuStick, OvuQuick, First Response, Q-Test, Quidell) are available. Use of these home self-administered assays over approximately 12 days each cycle should reduce the interval of abstinence to 1 week each cycle.

As these hormone tests become available to the public, their impact on the acceptance of natural family-planning methods is eagerly awaited. The current home test kits are able to detect hormonal changes which occur within 48 h or less prior to ovulation. The next step is to develop hormonal test kits which will accurately predict ovulation 4 or 5 days before the actual rupture of the follicle.

SUGGESTED READING

BROWN JB, BLACKWELL LF, BILLINGS JJ, *et al.* Natural family planning. *Am J Obstet Gynecol* 1987;157:1082–1089.

MEDINA JE, CIFUENTES A, ABERNATHY JR, SPIELER JM, WADE ME. Comparative evaluation of two methods of natural family planning in Columbia. *Am J Obstet Gynecol* 1980;138:1142–1147.

ROGOW D, RINTOUL EJ, GREENWOOD S. A year's experience with a fertility awareness program: a report. *Adv Planned Parenthood.* 1980;15:27–33.

SAUER MV, VERMESH M, ANDERSON RE, VIJOD AG, STANCZYK FZ, LOBO RA. Rapid measurement of urinary pregnanediol glucuronide to diagnose ectopic pregnancy. *Am J Obstet Gynecol* 1988;159:1531–1535

VERMESH M, KLETZKY OA. Longitudinal evaluation of the luteal phase and its transition into the follicular phase. *J Clin Endocrinol Metab* 1987;65:653–658

VERMESH M, KLETZKY OA, DAVAJAN V, ISRAEL R. Monitoring techniques to predict and detect ovulation. *Fertil Steril* 1987;47:259–264.

WORLD HEALTH ORGANIZATION. A prospective multicentre trial of the ovulation method of natural family planning. II. The effectiveness phase. *Fertil Steril* 1981;36:591–598.

WORLD HEALTH ORGANIZATION. A prospective multicentre trial of the ovulation method of natural family planning. III. Characteristics of the menstrual cycle and of the fertile phase. *Fertil Steril* 1983;40:773–778.

125

Management of complications of first-trimester pregnancy termination

PAUL F. BRENNER & CHARLES A. BALLARD

Early complications

The complications of first-trimester pregnancy termination may be divided into two groups: early and late. Early complications occur at the time of evacuation of the products of conception and consist of uterine perforation, bleeding, inability to dilate the cervix, failure to obtain tissue, and underestimation of uterine size.

Uterine perforation

Uterine perforation is a potentially serious complication. Its management depends on the site of perforation, the instrument that caused the perforation, and the likelihood of injury to the bowel.

If a midline perforation occurs with a suction cannula, with the suction turned off or with a sharp curette the procedure should be terminated and the patient observed overnight. During this time, the patient's vital signs should be taken at least every 2 h and her peripheral hematocrit determined every 4 h. Signs of peritonitis or hemorrhage indicate the need for immediate laparotomy.

If a midline perforation occurs with a suction cannula, with the suction turned on and without obvious injury to the omentum or bowel, the surgeon has two options: the patient may be observed closely for peritoneal signs and/or blood loss, or the surgeon may proceed immediately to laparotomy to assess potential injury to the abdominal organs. The latter alternative is recommended.

The lateral perforation requires, at a minimum, laparoscopy to evaluate the possibility of uterine vessel damage and the development of a broad ligament hematoma. Quite frequently, a broad ligament hematoma expands rapidly and can be palpated with a pelvic examination.

Perforations occur most frequently in severely anteverted or retroverted uteri or in patients with uterine anomalies such as a bicornuate uterus. If perforation occurs with a large instrument such as a dilator, the surgeon should not proceed to suction curettage. If the membranes are intact, the procedure should be terminated, and the patient may return in 2 weeks for evacuation of the pregnancy. If the membranes are ruptured and the procedure is to be continued after perforation of the uterus with a dilator, sharp curettage may be performed with simulataneous laparoscopic visualization. A small midline perforation with a uterine sound usually is managed by continuing the procedure.

A perforation in which bowel or omental tissue is obtained requires laparatomy and repair of the damaged structures. Perforation with a suction cannula, with the suction turned on, may lead to injury of the bowel and/or omentum. The most serious perforations are lateral perforations, perforations with a suction cannula with the suction turned on, and perforations causing injury to the bowel and/or omentum.

The use of laminaria to dilate the cervix slowly, steady traction applied to the tenaculum attached to the cervix to align the cervical canal and endometrial cavity properly, performing the procedure under local anesthesia, and, most importantly, a surgeon experienced with the technique are all factors which reduce the risk of cervical and uterine injury during a pregnancy termination.

Uterine bleeding

Heavy vaginal bleeding is a rare complication of pregnancy termination. When it occurs, the pregnancy usually has progressed to the end of the first trimester or beyond. Causes such as incomplete evacuation, uterine perforation, and laceration of the uterine vessels must be considered. Carefully sound the uterine cavity to determine if a perforation has occurred. If there is no evidence of a perforation, dilate and aspirate the endometrial cavity with a larger cannula. If this does not control the bleeding, perform a sharp curettage of the uterine cavity. If the vaginal bleeding persists, the management is intravenous oxytocin (Pitocin) 20 U/l of 5% dextrose in water with or without the addition of intramuscular ergonovine (Ergotrate) 0.2 mg. If the uterine bleeding continues, one-half ampule (10 U) of vasopressin (Pitressin) mixed with 20 ml of saline can be injected into the cervix.

Inability to dilate the cervix

Inability to dilate the cervix occurs most frequently in primigravidas. This condition may be alleviated by the insertion of laminaria, Lamicel, or Dilapan and delaying the evacuation of the products of conception for at least 6–24 h.

Failure to obtain tissue

If no tissue is obtained, the surgeon should repeat the pregnancy test and obtain a pelvic ultrasound study. Occasionally, uterine fibroids or adenomyosis mimic a pregnant uterus. Other diagnostic possibilities include a complete abortion that occurred before the surgery, ectopic pregnancy, a uterine anomaly (bicornuate uterus), and uterine perforation.

Underestimation of uterine size

Under anesthesia the uterus may be found to be considerably larger than was anticipated. The diagnostic possibilities include advanced gestational age, multiple gestation, associated gynecologic pathology (leiomyomata uteri, adenomyosis), and trophoblastic disease. If the uterus is larger than a 12-week gestational size, the operator should not proceed until the precise diagnosis is obtained and adequate blood replacement is available.

If the correct diagnosis is a second-trimester pregnancy and the membranes have not been ruptured, the surgeon can elect to stop the procedure and instead terminate the pregnancy by standard second-trimester abortion methods. If the abortion has proceeded to a stage where the membranes are ruptured, the evacuation of the products of conception must be completed. Intramuscular or vaginal administration of prostaglandins can be used in this situation.

Late complications

Late complications are those occurring any time after the evacuation procedure is terminated. Late complications of first-trimester pregnancy termination consist of infection, bleeding, retained tissue, continuation of pregnancy, ectopic pregnancy, persistent amenorrhea, and postabortal pain syndrome.

Infection

Infection frequently occurs when the products of conception are evacuated incompletely from the uterus, but it may occur even without retained tissue. Fever, chills, myalgia, fatigue, uterine cramping, foul-smelling or purulent cervical discharge, and pelvic pain are symptoms suggesting a postabortal infection. Prophylactic antibiotics are frequently used to reduce the occurrence of postabortal infections. One regimen is the administration of doxycycline 100 mg twice a day for 5–7 days. This regimen can be started prior to the procedure to evacuate the uterus, or shortly after the procedure is completed. Aggressive treatment of gonorrhea and/or *Chlamydia* prior to the abortion and careful evaluation and treatment of cervicitis will also lessen the chance of a postabortal infection.

If the patient has developed a postabortal infection, appropriate antibiotic therapy should be instituted. If her temperature is <38.3°C and the physical findings indicate a diagnosis of a postabortal infection confined to the uterus only (endometritis), she may be treated as an outpatient with a 10-day course of ampicillin 0.5 g 4 times a day.

If the patient's temperature exceeds 38.3°C and/or there are findings suggestive of parametritis or peritonitis, she should be hospitalized and should receive nothing by mouth. Vital signs should be monitored at frequent intervals, and daily fluid intake and output measured. Initial laboratory evaluation includes complete blood count, total platelet count, serum fibrinogen, and prothrombin time. Supine and upright X-rays of the abdomen should be taken to determine if uterine perforation has occurred and if there is free air in the peritoneal cavity. Two units of blood should be cross-matched for transfusion. A gonorrhea culture and *Chlamydia* culture of the cervix and aerobic and anaerobic blood cultures should be obtained.

An intravenous infusion of 1000 ml of 5% dextrose with lactated Ringer's solution should be initiated. Antibiotic therapy should include aqueous penicillin G 5 million units iv over 30 min every 6 h, clindamycin (Cleocin) 300–600 mg iv over 30 min every 6–8 h, and gentamicin (Garamycin) 80 mg over 30 min every 8 h. When the patient has been afebrile for 48 h, she can be switched to oral doses of ampicillin 0.5 g 4 times a day and clindamycin 300 mg 4 times a day for a total course of 10 days of antibiotics.

Any remaining products of conception should be evacuated from the uterus by dilatation and curettage after therapeutic levels of antibiotics are attained (2 h). An ultrasound study may be of assistance in determining if any products of conception remain within the uterine cavity. The primary treatment entails removal of the focus of infection. If the patient fails to respond to antibiotic therapy and no retained tissue is found, or if she develops a pelvic abscess, the possibilities of uterine perforation and bowel injury must be considered.

Bleeding

Bleeding frequently follows an incomplete abortion, although it can occur without tissue being left behind. Bleeding less than the patient's normal menstrual flow can persist up to 6 weeks postabortion. If bleeding is more than the normal menstrual flow, retained tissue, cervical vessel injury, uterine vessel injury, or trophoblastic disease should be considered. If the bleeding exceeds normal menstrual flow, if the cervix is dilated, if the uterus is still enlarged, or if tissue is present in the cervix or vagina, a repeat curettage is advocated.

Retained tissue

Uterine bleeding, cramping pain, and/or infection frequently signal that evacuation of the uterus was incomplete and that some tissue was left in the uterus. The uterus still may be enlarged and tender to palpation. If there is retained tissue, another curettage should be performed.

Continuation of pregnancy

Rarely does the surgical procedure performed to terminate pregnancy fail (2:1000). Patients who continue to have symptoms suggestive of early pregnancy, who fail to menstruate within 6 weeks of a therapeutic abortion, and who have an enlarging uterus at their follow-up examination should be evaluated with a pelvic exam, pregnancy test, and ultrasound study to determine if the pregnancy is continuing. Careful examination of the tissue obtained at the initial attempt to evacuate the uterus in order to identify tissue of fetal origin (fetal parts or chorionic villi) will prevent the failure to recognize an unsuccessful attempt to terminate a pregnancy at the conclusion of the surgery. Continuation of pregnancy is more likely when only decidua has been obtained on the initial curettage, but it has also been known to occur even when some villi have been obtained. When a pregnancy has continued after a therapeutic abortion, uterine anomalies must be considered strongly. The surgeon always must be aware of the possibility of a blind horn when it is impossible to complete the procedure vaginally. Another consideration when a pregnancy termination procedure has failed is a multiple gestation. Continuation of pregnancy is managed by another attempt to evacuate the products of conception from the uterus. Ultrasound surveillance during the second procedure may increase the probability of success.

Ectopic pregnancy

After each abortion, the surgeon must confirm the presence of fetal tissue. Absence of tissue of fetal origin indicates that the attempted termination of pregnancy failed, that the pregnancy was aborted prior to the surgical procedure, or that the patient has an ectopic pregnancy. An ectopic pregnancy is suggested in any patient whose pathologic specimen is reported as decidua tissue only or who exhibits the Arias-Stella reaction. Finally, the rare possibility of coexisting intrauterine and ectopic pregnancies must be considered.

Persistent amenorrhea

Patients with persistent amenorrhea following a first-trimester abortion usually have a continuing pregnancy or intrauterine synechiae. These patients are best managed by repeating the pregnancy test and obtaining an ultrasound study. If there is a continuing pregnancy, another curettage should be performed, preferably under ultrasound guidance. If the uterus is normal in size and the pregnancy test is negative, intrauterine synechiae should be suspected. Inability to sound the uterine cavity, a biphasic basal body temperature graph, or one of four consecutive weekly serum progesterone determinations exceeding 3 ng/ml (indicating an ovulatory cycle) further suggests the diagnosis of intrauterine synechiae. A hysterosalpingogram or hysteroscopy is recommended to confirm the diagnosis (see Chapter 106).

Postabortion pain syndrome

Infrequently, a postabortion pain syndrome occurs in which the patient develops cramping abdominal pain several hours to several days after her abortion. In association with the pain, the uterus is large and boggy. Postabortion pain syndrome is best managed by a repeat suction curettage to remove retained blood clots. This syndrome is usually prevented by using intravenous oxytocin, which is administered at the time of the original curettage.

SUGGESTED READING

BURKMAN RT, MASON KJ, GOLD EB. Ectopic pregnancy and prior induced abortion. *Contraception* 1988;37:21–27.

GRIMES DA, SCHULZ KF, CATES WJ Jr. Prevention of uterine perforation during curettage abortion. *JAMA* 1984;251:2108–2111.

GRIMES DA, SCHULZ KF, CATES W Jr. Prophylactic antibiotics for curettage abortion. *Am J Obstet Gynecol* 1984;150:689–694.

HOGUE CJ, CATES W Jr, TIETZE C. Effects of induced abortion on subsequent reproduction. *Epidemiol Rev* 1982;4:66–94.

HOLT VL, DALING JR, VOIGT LF, *et al.* Induced abortion and the risk of subsequent ectopic pregnancy. *Am J Public Health* 1989;79:1234–1238.

KAUNITZ AM, ROVIRA EZ, GRIMES DA, SCHULZ KF. Abortions that fail. *Obstet Gynecol* 1985;66:533–537.

SCHULZ KF, GRIMES DA, CATES W Jr. Measures to prevent cervical injury during suction curettage abortion. *Lancet* 1983;1:1182–1184.

STUBBLEFIELD PG. Surgical techniques of uterine evacuation in first-and-second-trimester abortion. *Clin Obstet Gynecol* 1986;13:53–70.

RADESTAD A, CHRISTENSEN NJ. Magnesium sulphate and cervical ripening: a biomechanical double-blind, randomized comparison between a synthetic polyvinyl sponge with and without magnesium sulphate. *Contraception* 1989;39: 253–263.

WHO TASK FORCE ON PROSTAGLANDINS FOR FERTILITY REGULATION. Randomized comparison of different prostaglandin analogues and laminaria tent for preoperative cervical dilatation. *Contraception* 1986;34:237–251.

126

Female sterilization: choice of technique

ROBERT ISRAEL

Sterilization is the final step in preventing procreation. As it plays such a prominent role in fertility termination, sterilization must be an integral part of any family-planning program. Over the past two decades, voluntary sterilization has emerged from public unawareness and medically restrictive guidelines to become a widely used method throughout the world.

Of the 900 000 sterilizations performed in 1972, male operations accounted for 60% of the total. Parity was achieved in 1973, and the male:female ratio was subsequently reversed. Since 1977, over 1 million sterilizations per year have been carried out in the USA and women have undergone 60% of these procedures. In addition, according to the National Center for Health Statistics, sterilization was selected as a family-planning method by 35% of couples in 1988, compared with only 9% in 1965.

Reversibility

Along with increased acceptance of sterilization, a better understanding of the physiologic and psychologic changes connected with such surgery has developed. Although sterilization is utilized as a final, permanent contraceptive technique by individuals concluding their reproductive potential, reversible sterilization may become a family-spacing technique of the future. Male and female sterilization methods that permit reversibility are under investigation in a very preliminary fashion. However, the most effective techniques owe their success to their high degree of *nonreversibility*. A reliably reversible technique must retain the maximum pregnancy prevention associated with currently available sterilization methods. Because sterilization should be considered permanent, thorough counseling of the individual is mandatory prior to performing the procedure.

Methodology

Postpartum tubal ligation

The Pomeroy and Irving tubal ligations performed through a small subumbilical incision remain the procedures of choice in the immediate postpartum period. They can be performed on the delivery table, often utilizing the same anesthesia; they are simple and rapid with an "acceptable" failure rate – well below 1:1000 for the Irving – and they do not prolong the postpartum hospital stay. Although the modified Irving tubal sterilization (the proximal stump buried in the myometrium, the distal stump tied off but not buried in the broad ligament) requires more time than the Pomeroy, it is worth the extra effort, as only one pregnancy is documented in the literature. When the Pomeroy procedure has been performed postpartum (a mid-segment excision after placement of catgut sutures), the failure rate has been reported to be about 0.4%. Cesarean hysterectomy should not be performed unless removal of the uterus is indicated medically by multiple myomas, cancer, or irreparable uterine damage. Excessive blood loss and an increased incidence of ureteral/bladder injury preclude cesarean hysterectomy as a routine method of female sterilization.

Vaginal hysterectomy

In the past, although vaginal hysterectomy was performed for sterilization, this primary operative indication was often camouflaged by convenient secondary diagnoses often found in parous women, e.g., pelvic relaxation. Although vaginal hysterectomy is associated with greater blood loss, higher morbidity, and a longer hospital stay than tubal sterilization, these are short-term disadvantages and must be balanced against the long-term benefits seen with vaginal hysterectomy: the guarantee of absolute sterility, the ability to correct concomitant pelvic relaxation problems often found in the over-30 multipara, and the prevention of future uterine disease. Although not secondary to the tubal ligation, subsequent gynecologic disorders will occur, necessitating further pelvic surgery 25% of the time, and hysterectomy might represent 50% of these operations. It seems apparent that sterilization could be the sole indication for vaginal hysterectomy, and in the properly selected, properly prepared patient, it might be the procedure of choice. Today, however, in cases where governmental funding is the payment source for sterilization, hysterectomy is prohibited as a method of sterilization. In addition, the totality of sterilization by hysterectomy completely eliminates future child-bearing, and, in today's transient, changeable society, such finality is not a very viable option.

Classical methods of tubal ligation or standard gynecologic operations offer reliability but little innovation. Laparoscopic, transvaginal, and, in the future, transuterine methods of sterilization represent approaches that highlight current concepts in female sterilization.

Laparoscopy

Laparoscopic sterilization is a combination of two procedures – laparoscopy and tubal sterilization – both devised for different purposes, but combined in this century and improved in the past 20 years by new technologies and new enthusiasms.

Technique

There are wide variations in preoperative preparation, the majority of which are not crucial to the success of the operation. Unless there are significant medical problems (diabetes, hypertension, etc.) or excessive obesity (90 kg (200 lb) or over), or both, there is no reason why laparoscopic tubal sterilization cannot be performed as an outpatient (1-day) procedure. The operation should take place in an operating room equipped and staffed for general anesthesia – and for exploratory laparotomy, if it proves necessary. Although a cross-match is unnecessary, blood-bank accessibility is prudent.

Although laparoscopic sterilization can be carried out under local anesthesia, most laparoscopists favor a short-acting general anesthetic with endotracheal intubation and controlled ventilation. It is unnecessary to shave either the abdomen or the perineum. The bladder is catheterized, but an indwelling catheter is unnecessary. At laparoscopy, it is often helpful to be able to elevate and rotate the uterus via a vaginal "handle." Various instruments can be utilized.

The creation of a satisfactory pneumoperitoneum is the keystone to any successful laparoscopic procedure. A Veress needle should be used to insufflate the peritoneal cavity, as its spring action combines a sharp outer point for penetrating tissue planes and a retractable, blunt inner stylet for peritoneal puncture and intraabdominal safety. With the laparoscope in place, a brief overview of the pelvis should confirm the normal structures visualized in almost all sterilization procedures.

Various instruments and methods of tubal occlusion are available. Whatever tubal occlusion technique is utilized, tissue destruction should be confined to the mid-isthmus. In this way, if sterilization reversal is subsequently requested, enough proximal and distal tubal segments will remain for end-to-end anastomosis.

Bipolar fulguration, usually with transection, remains the most widely used technique. Before transection, fulguration must be complete and must include a portion of the adjacent mesosalpinx to avoid bleeding at the transection site. After transection, each cut tubal stump (especially both proximal ends) should be recoagulated briefly to prevent tubal fistulas or recanalization.

Utilizing bipolar equipment for fulguration eliminates the electrical hazards associated with unipolar coagulation in which the current must pass through the patient to the grounding plate. In bipolar conduction, the electrical current passes in and out through the forceps, thus eliminating electrical scatter within the abdominal cavity and avoiding bowel burns. The introduction of the Falope ring, whereby a Silastic band is used to occlude the tube, as well as the spring-loaded clip, provides alternatives to electrocoagulation which eliminate electrical hazards. Postoperative abdominal discomfort is experienced for 24–48 h in 20–25% of the patients undergoing occlusive ring or clip tubal sterilization. However, both these methods destroy less tube than laparoscopic fulguration and may offer better potential for reversibility.

Laparoscopic sterilization can be performed through a single-incision technique utilizing the operating laparoscope. The accessory instrument for performing the tubal sterilization is inserted in the laparoscope itself. Therefore, the forceps moves only when the laparoscope moves and cannot move separately. Pelvic manipulation, e.g., identification of tubal fimbria, is more restricted with the operating laparoscope than with an accessory instrument inserted at a second puncture site. The single-incision technique should be attempted only after the laparoscopist has become thoroughly familiar with the two-incision approach.

Pregnancy rate

When laparoscopic tubal sterilization is correctly performed, either by fulguration or fulguration and transection, the risk of subsequent pregnancy is approximately 2–4:1000. This pregnancy rate does not include luteal-phase failures, where the patient was already pregnant at the time of surgery, or surgical errors, such as coagulating the round ligament. To avoid luteal pregnancies, sterilization can be limited to the follicular phase of the menstrual cycle, accompanied by a negative blood pregnancy test on the day preceding surgery. If effective contraception precedes the sterilization request, it is unnecessary to restrict surgery to the follicular phase of the cycle, assuming a day-before blood pregnancy test is negative. Unless medically indicated, adding a dilatation and curettage to the laparoscopic sterilization is an unnecessary expense and, if a luteal pregnancy exists, the curet may well miss it. Pregnancies secondary to surgical errors can be eliminated by properly identifying the fallopian tubes.

Although fewer Silastic band sterilizations than laparoscopic fulgurations have been performed, the pregnancy rates seem comparable. However, the failure rates published in preliminary studies utilizing the spring-loaded clip have been higher. Design modifications may improve the efficacy of clip tubal sterilization.

Any pregnancies occurring after tubal sterilization must be carefully evaluated to rule out ectopic gestation. Published reports indicate that 15% of pregnancies following all types of tubal sterilization procedures will be ectopic. However, following laparoscopic fulguration, the risk that any subsequent pregnancy will be ectopic rises to 25%, with a literature range of 9–67%.

Colpotomy

Transvaginal (colpotomy) tubal ligation still has a few proponents. It can be performed between pregnancies (interval) or following a curettage for abortion in patients with a normal or 6–8-week-sized, mobile uterus without known or palpable adnexal masses. Usually, general anesthesia is used, although conduction anesthesia (spinal or epidural) can be utilized. Each tube is secured and ligated by means of a standard technique, usually the Pomeroy. Fimbriectomy should not be performed for sterilization. Although the occasional high failure rate seen after fimbriectomy sterilization may be operator-related, the technique destroys an essential area of the tube that cannot be reversed with any degree of success.

Despite its apparent simplicity, historically, higher morbidity rates have been associated with vaginal tubal sterilization than with any other surgical approach. The morbidity has been secondary to colpotomy incision site infections (about 1:10 cases) and delayed tuboovarian abscess formation (about 1:100 cases). However, the use of prophylactic antibiotics and a rapid, precise surgical approach will all but eliminate the previously reported infectious morbidity. In well-trained, adept surgical hands, colpotomy tubal sterilization can be a reasonable alternative to laparoscopic and minilaparotomy approaches.

Transuterine approach

To bring absolute safety and simplicity to female sterilization, it would be necessary to avoid penetration of the abdominal cavity. Laparoscopy has provided the gynecologist with a sophisticated endoscopic technique, but as an instrument of tubal sterilization, it should not be the final answer. The transuterine approach to the fallopian tubes may be the ultimate solution, but at the moment it represents a good idea in search of the right technique.

Hysteroscopy has permitted direct visualization of each tubal orifice. An electrode can be threaded through the operating channel of the hysteroscope and guided under visual control to each tubal ostium. Unfortunately, too many failures have occurred to consider hysteroscopic tubal fulguration a satisfactory technique of female sterilization. Even bilateral cornual occlusion 3 months postoperatively may represent only unilateral or bilateral cornual spasm, not true closure. In addition to subsequent pregnancies, including some cornual ectopics, bowel burns have been reported due to the varying degrees of myometrial thickness present at the time of ostial fulguration.

To eliminate electrocoagulation, investigators have turned their efforts toward developing a Silastic tubal plug that would be placed as liquid silicone rubber in each orifice under hysteroscopic guidance. The liquid silicone would "cure" to form a soft plug conforming to the oviductal lumen. Tubal plugs must remain in place and provide complete blockage, which may prove difficult over time because of the known contractile strength of tubal and uterine musculature. The Silastic tubal plug has been tested at several locations in the USA and Europe. Tubal plugs, like tubal clips, offer the possibility of reversible sterilization. However, absolute effectiveness of sterilization is more important than potential reversibility, and the former must be demonstrated in any new sterilization technique before the latter can even be considered.

Chemical sterilization

The ultimate goal in transuterine sterilization would be to eliminate instrumentation like hysteroscopy altogether. By means of a syringe, catheter, or a specialized delivery system, a chemosterilant that acts on the mucosa of the fallopian tube could be instilled via the uterine cavity. Two groups of chemical agents have been investigated. One consists of nonspecific tissue adhesives or sclerosing agents that produce oviductal obstruction through scar formation. Methylcyanoacrylate, the most promising of these compounds, polymerizes in the tubes and causes a local reaction leading to fibrotic occlusion over a period of 3 months, during which time the methylcyanoacrylate is degraded and eliminated from the body. Spillage into the peritoneal cavity seems to have no deleterious effects. Bilateral tubal occlusion has been achieved over 80% of the time with a single application, and over 95% of the time with two applications. Clinical trials with pregnancy prevention as an end-point are ongoing.

The other chemosterilant group consists of highly specific chemical agents capable of inducing morphologic changes in the interstitial tubal epithelium. Quinacrine has been the most tested compound in this group, and from human studies, by Zipper *et al.* utilizing three insertions of quinacrine pellets placed high in the endometrial cavity via an intrauterine device inserter, the pregnancy rate at 48 months is 3.7 ± 2.1. In several respects, quinacrine sterilization is unique among all carefully studied sterilization procedures. No ectopic pregnancies have occurred in over 200 reported pregnancies in women who have had one or more quinacrine instillations and not one serious complication has been reported in over 25 000 cases worldwide. The possibility of a nonsurgical sterilization technique with a chemical agent of very low toxicity, which can be employed by paramedical personnel without sophisticated delivery equipment, opens exciting perspectives in the area of female sterilization.

Conclusion

Female sterilization has become an accepted, integral part of family planning. Laparoscopic sterilization techniques have simplified the surgery and introduced new operative approaches to the fallopian tubes. The future is represented by transuterine sterilization that promises to avoid anesthesia, complicated instrumentation, and penetration of the peritoneal cavity. When evaluated against the comparable standard criteria for contraception (acceptability, safety, effectiveness, and cost), surgical sterilization, even as it is performed today, appears to be one of the best family-planning methods available.

SUGGESTED READING

AMERICAN COLLEGE OF OBSTETRICIANS AND GYNECOLOGISTS. Sterilization. *ACOG Tech Bull* 1988:113.

ARANDA C, DEBADIA D, MAHRAN M, FELDBLUM PJ. A comparative clinical trial of the tubal ring versus the Rocket clip for female sterilization. *Am J Obstet Gynecol* 1985;153:755.

BHATT R, WASZAK CS. Four-year follow-up of insertions of quinacrine hydrochloride pellets as a means of nonsurgical female sterilization. *Fertil Steril* 1985; 44:303.

HUGGINS GR, SONDHEIMER SJ. Complications of female sterilization: immediate and delayed. *Fertil Steril* 1984;41:337.

MOSHER WD, PRATT WF. *Contraceptive Use in the United States, 1973–88*, vol 182. (PHS) 90-1250. Washington DC: National Center for Health Statistics, 1990.

MUMFORD SD, KESSEL E. Sterilization needs in the 1990s: the case for quinacrine nonsurgical female sterilization. *Am J Obstet Gynecol* 1992;167:1203.

NEUWIRTH RS, RICHART RM, STEVENSON T, *et al.* An outpatient approach to female sterilization with methylcyanoacrylate. *Am J Obstet Gynecol* 1980;136:951.

POINDEXTER AN III, ABDUL-MALAK M, FAST JE. Laparoscopic tubal sterilization under local anesthesia. *Obstet Gynecol* 1990;75:5.

REED TP, ERB R. Hysteroscopic tubal occlusion with silicone rubber. *Obstet Gynecol* 1983;61:388.

SHUBER J. Transcervical sterilization with use of methyl 2-cyanoacrylate and a newer delivery system (the FEMCEPT device). *Am J Obstet Gynecol* 1989;160:887.

SMITH RP, MAGGI CS, NOLAN TE. Morbidity and vaginal tubal cautery: a report and review. *Obstet Gynecol* 1991;78:209.

SODERSTROM RM. Sterilization failures and their causes. *Am J Obstet Gynecol* 1985;152:395.

SODERSTROM RM, LEVY BS. Bipolar systems – do they perform? *Obstet Gynecol* 1987;69:425.

ZIPPER J, MEDEL M, GOLDSMITH A, *et al.* The clinical efficacy of the repeated transcervical instillation of guinacrine for female sterilization. *Int J Gynaecol Obstet* 1976;14:499.

127

Vasectomy

GERALD S. BERNSTEIN

Vasectomy is one of the few methods currently available for the control of male fertility. It is a popular procedure; in the USA approximately 418 500 men had vasectomies in 1984, according to the latest survey of the Association for Voluntary Surgical Contraception. The operation is simple, it can be performed as an office procedure under local anesthesia, and it does not involve invasion of the peritoneal cavity. The failure rate in the past was generally about 0.5%, or 1:200 procedures. However, use of techniques that involve separating the two ends of the severed vas by enclosing one within the sheath of the vas deferens and leaving the other free has reduced the failure rate to zero in the hands of some surgeons. Some physicians no longer excise a segment of the divided vas. Whether or not a segment is removed, the ends of the divided vas must be sealed by ligatures, electrocautery of the lumen using a fine cautery tip, or various types of clips. Surgery is considered to be successful if two successive semen samples obtained a month apart are free of sperm; the couple can feel free to have unprotected intercourse after that time.

Complications

The complications of vasectomy are usually minor and include pain, swelling, ecchymoses, and superficial wound infections. More severe complications include epididymitis, excessive bleeding with hematoma formation, and the development of a sperm granuloma at the proximal end of the vas that may cause pain in the scrotum. There have been no deaths due directly to vasectomy in the USA. In the past, some deaths have been reported in underdeveloped countries, where the facilities for sterilizing instruments have not been adequate or patients have neglected to practice adequate postoperative hygiene.

Reversal

Progress also has been made in reversing vasectomy to restore fertility. The success of the surgery depends partly on how the original surgery was performed and the degree of inflammatory reaction that followed. If a long segment of the vas was excised or if a segment was removed from the convoluted portion of the vas, near the epididymis, the reconstruction is less likely to be successful. With conventional surgical techniques, sperm are restored to the ejaculate in 80% of cases, but only about 35% of all patients who have had the reversal procedure impregnate their wives.

Better results have been obtained with microsurgical techniques, and it is possible to restore sperm to the ejaculate in >90% of cases when sperm are present in the distal vas deferens at the time of surgery. The pregnancy rate, however, varies from 40 to 70%.

There is some controversy as to why the pregnancy rate is less than the success of restoring continuity of the vas deferens, but there is inadequate information to resolve it. Follow-up data do not always include a complete evaluation of both partners to determine the factor responsible for failure to conceive.

Epididymal obstruction due to granuloma formation is one cause of failure of vasovasostomy. If sperm are not present in the vas at the time of reoperation, a careful exploration must be done to determine if a vasoepididymostomy is required rather than a vasovasostomy.

Potential risks

In the late 1950s and early 1960s, two groups of investigators reported that some men whose vas deferens had been obstructed, whether by surgery or natural causes, developed circulating antibodies against spermatozoa. A number of investigators subsequently have shown that up to 70% of vasectomized men develop circulating antibodies that can agglutinate or immobilize spermatozoa. The antibodies usually can be found in the serum within the first 3 months after the surgery. In some cases, the antibodies can no longer be detected 2 years following the operation.

Initially, this immunologic reaction was considered to be only an interesting laboratory phenomenon without any clinical significance. In 1968, however, Roberts described seven young men who developed various medical problems after they had been vasectomized. One had multiple sclerosis, three had thrombophlebitis, and three had a variety of diseases and systemic symptoms. Roberts proposed that these disorders resulted from activation of the immune system caused by the vasectomy, and he suggested that vasectomy may be more dangerous than had previously been thought.

There have been numerous animal and clinical studies in the intervening years. In laboratory investigations, rabbits that develop high titers of sperm antibodies following vasectomy also may develop autoimmune orchitis and have immune complexes deposited in their kidneys. Other rodents also may have marked immunologic reactions following vasectomy.

In 1978, it was reported that monkeys fed a high-fat, atherogenic diet and then vasectomized developed more extensive atherosclerosis than control animals that were fed the same diet but who were not vasectomized. This study was conducted because there is some evidence that immune complexes can damage the arterial intima and thereby initiate change that can lead to the development of atheromas. There may be a similar difference between vasectomized and nonvasectomized monkeys not fed an atherogenic diet.

Safety for humans

The information described above prompted a variety of clinical studies to evaluate the effect of vasectomy on general health and the occurrence of autoimmune and cardiovascular disease. These studies, which have been summarized by Petitti, have not demonstrated any major health risk as a result of vasectomy apart from the known minor complications of the surgery.

In the largest study to date, 10 590 vasectomized men were compared with the same number of controls. The vasectomized group had no increase in morbidity or mortality except for the occurrence of epididymitis/orchitis, a recognized sequel of vasectomy.

The consensus has been that there is probably no risk that vasectomy will cause significant alterations in human health. However, several recent reports have suggested that vasectomized men are at increased risk of developing cancer of the prostate. These reports have renewed the debate about possible adverse effects of vasectomy and have made critical the need for further, well-designed studies directed to the issue of vasectomy and prostate neoplasia.

SUGGESTED READING

ALEXANDER NJ, CLARKSON TB. Vasectomy increases the severity of diet-induced atherosclerosis in *Macaca fascularis*. *Science* 1978;201:538.

ANONYMOUS. Vasectomy and prostate cancer. *Lancet* 1991;337:1445.

BERNSTEIN GS, CHOPP R, COSGROVE M, *et al.* A controlled prospective study of the effects of vasectomy. In: Lepow IH, Crozier R, eds. *Vasectomy: Immunologic and Patho-physiologic Effects in Animals and Man.* New York: Academic Press, 1979:473–489.

BIGAZZI PE. Immunologic effects of vasectomy in men and experimental animals. In: Gleicher N, ed. *Reproductive Immunology.* New York: Alan R Liss, 1981:461–476.

CLARKSON TB, ALEXANDER NJ. Vasectomy: effects on the occurrence and extent of atherosclerosis in rhesus monkeys. *J Clin Invest* 1980;65:15.

DERSIMONIAN R, CLEMENS J, SPIRTAS R. Vasectomy and prostate cancer risk: methodological review of the evidence. *J Clin Epidemiol* 1993;46:163.

GIOVANNUCCI E, TOSTESAN TD, SPEIZER FE, *et al.* Retrospective cohort study of vasectomy and prostate cancer. *JAMA* 1993;269:878.

GIOVANNUCCI E, ASCHERIO A, RIMM EB, *et al.* Prospective cohort study of vasectomy and prostate cancer. *JAMA* 1993;269:873.

GOEBELSMANN U, BERNSTEIN GS, GALE JA, *et al.* Serum gonadotropin, testosterone, estradiol, and estrone levels prior to and following bilateral vasectomy. In: Lepow IH, Crozier R, eds. *Vasectomy: Immunologic and Pathophysiologic Effects in Animals and Man.* New York: Academic Press, 1979:165–181.

GUESS HA. Vasectomy and prostate cancer. *Am J Epidemiol* 1990;132:1062.

HONDA GD, BERNSTEIN L, ROSS RK, *et al.* Vasectomy, cigarette smoking, and age at first sexual intercourse as risk factors for prostate cancer in middle-aged men. *Br J Cancer* 1988;57:326.

HOWARDS SS. Surgery of the scrotum and its contents. In: Walsh PC, Gittes RF, Perlmuter AD, *et al.*, eds. *Campbell's Urology.* Philadelphia: WB Saunders, 1986: 2965–2967.

HOWARDS SS. American Urological Association response to two articles on the relationship of vasectomy and prostate cancer. *Oncology* 1991;5:78.

HOWARDS SS, PETERSON HB. Vasectomy and prostate cancer. Chance, bias, or a causal relationship? *JAMA* 1993;269:913.

MASSEY FJ, BERNSTEIN GS, O'FALLON WM, *et al.* Vasectomy and health. Results from a large cohort study. *JAMA* 1984;252:1023.

METTLIN C, NATARAJAN N, HUBEN R. Vasectomy and prostate cancer risk. *Am J Epidemiol* 1990;132:1056.

PERLMAN JA, SPIRTAS R, KELAGHAN J. Re: "Vasectomy and the risk of prostate cancer". *Am J Epidemol* 1991;134:107.

PETITTI DB. Long-term risks of vasectomy. In: Sciarra JJ, ed. *Gynecology and Obstetrics*, vol 6. Philadelphia: Harper & Row, 1986:1–14.

ROBERTS HJ. Delayed thrombophlebitis and systemic complications after vasectomy: possible role of diabetogenic hyper-insulinism. *J Am Geriatr Soc* 1968;16:267.

ROSENBERG L, PALMER JR, ZANBER AG, *et al.* Vasectomy and the risk of prostate cancer. *Am J Epidemiol* 1990;132:1051.

SCHMIDT SS. Prevention of failure in vasectomy. *J Urol* 1973;109:296.

SILBER SJ. Vasectomy and vasectomy reversal. In: Wallach EE, Kempers RD, eds. *Modern Trends in Infertility and Conception Control*, vol 1. Baltimore, MD: Williams & Wilkins, 1979:285–301.

SILBER SJ. Pregnancy after vasovasostomy. *J Androl* 1987;8:47.

SPECIAL PROGRAMME OF RESEARCH, DEVELOPMENT, AND RESEARCH TRAINING IN HUMAN REPRODUCTION. Sequelae of vasectomy. *Contraception* 1982;25:119.

128

Fetal demise

CHARLES A. BALLARD & PAUL F. BRENNER

Fetal demise is defined by the World Health Organization as the death of the fetus occurring prior to delivery, irrespective of gestational age. The classical definition of missed abortion is fetal demise in the first or second trimester without expulsion of the fetus for a minimum of 8 weeks after fetal death. It would seem more logical, however, to consider any fetal demise in the first or second trimester to be a missed abortion. The fetal death rate is the number of fetal deaths per 1000 infants born. In 1988 the fetal death rate in the USA was 7.5/1000 total births.

Diagnosis

A diagnosis of fetal demise is suggested in any patient in whom there is no fetal growth or cessation of fetal movement. The patient also may complain of loss of breast tenderness, nausea, frequency of urination, and lassitude.

After 20 weeks' gestation, the inability to hear fetal heart sounds with a DeLee stethoscope or fetoscope and, after 12 weeks' gestation, with an office Doppler device, suggests fetal death. Neither procedure is diagnostic and may yield a small rate of false-negative results. The urinary pregnancy test is unreliable because, even though the fetus may have expired, the placenta may still function, resulting in a persistently positive pregnancy test.

An X-ray can be extremely helpful, but only when fetal demise has occurred several days previously, and only after 18–20 weeks' gestation. The diagnostic radiologic signs to look for are intravascular fetal gas, overlapping of the cranial bones, or halo sign, and an abnormal increase in width of the cranial soft tissues as a result of maceration. Also, with the loss of fetal muscle tone, the fetal spine may collapse. A more rapid and the most reliable means of determining fetal demise is the use of ultrasound. A real-time sonogram may determine the presence of absence of fetal cardiac activity.

Management

Expectant waiting

Management of fetal demise consists of expectant waiting or active intervention. Previously, expectant management was the more frequent modality for management of fetal demise because of complications of active intervention. The assumption with expectant waiting was based on the rationale that 75% of patients would deliver spontaneously within 2 weeks, and all but 7% would deliver by 3 weeks.

Because 93% of patients would deliver within 3 weeks, the major complication of a consumptive coagulopathy was significant only in a small percentage of patients. The prolonged retention of a dead fetus *in utero* leads to the depletion of clotting factors V and VIII, fibrinogen, prothrombin, and platelets. Plasma fibrinogen is the most reliable predictor of disseminated intravascular coagulopathy. Furthermore, it usually did not occur before 5 weeks after the demise, and then in only approximately 25–40% of patients. As the length of time a dead fetus is retained in the uterus continues to increase, the percent of patients who develop a coagulopathy increases progressively. It is important to obtain a weekly fibrinogen level in patients who are being observed for the spontaneous onset of labor. Fortunately, if a drop in fibrinogen occurs, it is gradual. Monitoring fibrinogen levels weekly should allow the detection of a coagulopathy in the subclinical phase before it becomes clinically significant. A clinically relevant coagulopathy does not occur until fibrinogen levels fall below 100 mg/dl.

Active intervention

With modern means of pregnancy termination, active intervention becomes more attractive as therapy for patients with fetal demise. In fact, in a very small percent of patients, the emotional impact of carrying a dead fetus is overwhelming to the point of severe depression.

In patients whose gestational age at the time of fetal death was <12 weeks, active surgical intervention is the treatment of choice. The choice between sharp curettage or suction curettage is up to the individual operator. Routine preoperative laboratory tests must include a hematocrit and fibrinogen level. If either or both are below normal, type and cross-matching the patient for several units of blood are imperative.

The major problem in termination occurs when fetal death occurs after 12 weeks' gestation. Oxytocin frequently has been used for patients in the second and third trimesters. At least in the second trimester, however, the pregnant uterus resists oxytocin stimulation. Serial attempts at induction over several days often are necessary, with the concomitant risk of water intoxication and even a possibility of uterine rupture. To increase the success rate, a combination of amniotomy and continuous intravenous oxytocin has been recommended, but if the patient fails to abort, she runs an increased risk of uterine infection with prolonged ruptured membranes.

To prevent these problems, hysterotomy has been suggested to terminate the gestation in patients where fetal death occurs after 12 weeks' gestation. This operative procedure carries all the inherent risks of general anesthesia, the risk of uterine rupture in subsequent pregnancies, and the likelihood of repeat cesarean section.

An alternative approach to terminating pregnancies after 16 weeks' gestation has been the use of intraamniotic hypertonic saline or prostaglandin $F_{2\alpha}$. Intraamniotic saline probably should not be used because of its risk of causing hypofibrinogenemia, which may be accelerated in a patient with an already low fibrinogen level. Also, there frequently is not much amniotic fluid, and this increases the difficulty of obtaining a successful tap.

Suppositories containing 20 mg prostaglandin E_2 have been approved for use in patients of <29 weeks' gestation. They are administered intravaginally at 3–5-h intervals, depending on the frequency of uterine contractions. Use of these suppositories has been shown to be highly effective (>95%), with a mean time of 10–12 h from installation to delivery. In patients whose fetal death occurred at <13 weeks' gestation, the success rate has been poor; in fact, prostaglandin suppositories offer no advantage over dilatation and curettage.

Complications

Complications depend on the length of demise and the mode of termination. Patients with prolonged demise have a risk of developing hypofibrinogenemia. Intravenous oxytocin places the patient at risk of uterine rupture and hyponatremia, possibly leading to water intoxication. Dilatation and curettage increases the risk of hemorrhage and uterine perforation. Uterine instillation of either prostaglandin or saline carries the risk of infection.

The use of vaginal suppositories produces a high incidence of gastrointestinal side-effects, such as vomiting and diarrhea; patients may develop temperatures as high as 40°C and frequently may experience chills. Rarely, uterine rupture may occur, especially in patients in the third trimester and those with an abnormal fetal lie. Vaginal suppositories probably should not be used after 28 weeks' gestation in patients who have had a cesarean section or hysterotomy, or in patients with an abnormal fetal lie. These patients may be managed expectantly or delivered by cesarean section.

Etiology and evaluation of fetal demise

Determining the cause of fetal death can be a great benefit to the parents in coping with their loss and may be essential in the counseling they receive regarding future pregnancies, particularly if the cause is associated with recurrent pregnancy wastage. Maternal diseases associated with fetal demise include chronic hypertension, pregnancy-induced hypertension, uncontrolled diabetes mellitus, specific viral and bacterial infections, and Rh-isoimmunization. Placental and fetal conditions associated with fetal demise include prolapse of the umbilical cord, placenta previa, abruptio placentae, uterine rupture, and congenital malformations. With these contributing factors in mind, the prenatal, labor, and delivery records are reviewed. Special attention is directed toward maternal blood pressure recordings, blood sugar levels, time of rupture of the membranes, maternal signs and symptoms of chorioamnionitis, blood type and Rh, and serology. The appearances of the fetus, placenta, and umbilical cord are very relevant. An autopsy is the most important study which may elucidate the cause of fetal death. Karyotype determination of the fetus should be considered, especially when there is a history of recurrent fetal demise, abnormal offspring, and gross malformations of the fetus in the current pregnancy. The success of chromosomal studies is inversely related to the interval from the time of fetal death to delivery. Additional studies which may be helpful in identifying a case of fetal demise are cultures taken from the oropharynx of the fetus and the insertion site of the umbilical cord to the placenta and a skeletal survey if permission for an autopsy can not be obtained. The presence of fetal erythrocytes in the maternal circulation due to a transplacental fetus-to-mother bleed can be tested for with the Kleihauer–Betke staining of the peripheral blood smear. An association has been found between the presence of lupus anticoagulant and anticardiolipin antibodies and the occurrence of fetal death. The search for these antibodies can be added to the overall evaluation of patients who have recently experienced a fetal demise. Overall, in more than half the cases of fetal demise a specific etiology can not be found.

SUGGESTED READING

BAILEY DH, NEWMAN C, ELINAS SP, *et al.* Use of prostaglandin E₂ vaginal suppositories in intrauterine fetal death and missed abortion. *Obstet Gynecol* 1975; 45:110.

CLAMAN P, CARPENTER RJ, REITER A. Uterine rupture with the use of vaginal prostaglandin E₂ for induction of labor. *Am J Obstet Gynecol* 1984;150:889.

DUBUISSON JB, ZORN JR, FRETAULT J, *et al.* Fetal death: coagulation defects and management of 20 cases with study of the half-life of ¹²⁵I fibrinogen. *Eur J Obstet Gynaecol Reprod Biol* 1977;7:147.

LASALA AP, STRASSNER HT. Fetal death. *Clin Obstet Gynecol* 1986;29:95.

PATTERSON SP, WHITE JH, REAVES EM. A maternal death associated with prostaglandin E₂. *Obstet Gynecol* 1979;54:123.

PHELAN JP, MEGULIAR RV, MATEY D, *et al.* Dramatic pyrexic and cardiovascular response to intravaginal prostagladin E₂. *Am J Obstet Gynecol* 1978;132:28.

RUTLAND A, BALLARD CA. Vaginal prostaglandin E₂ for missed abortion and intrauterine fetal death. *Am J Obstet Gynecol* 1977;128:503.

SOUTHERN EM, GUTKNECHT GD. Management of intrauterine fetal demise and missed abortion using prostaglandin E₂ vaginal suppositories. *Obstet Gynecol* 1976;47:602.

ZLATNIK FJ. Management of fetal death. *Clin Obstet Gynecol* 1986;29:220.

Index